AOTRAUMA

Editors Michael Schütz | Carsten Perka
Senior Editor Thomas P Rüedi

Periprosthetic Fracture Management

AOTRAUMA

Editors Michael Schütz | Carsten Perka
Senior Editor Thomas P Rüedi

Periprosthetic Fracture Management

734 illustrations/images, and 54 cases

Library of Congress Cataloging-in-Publication Data is available from the publisher.

Hazards

Great care has been taken to maintain the accuracy of the information contained in this publication. However, the publisher, and/or the distributor, and/or the editors, and/or the authors cannot be held responsible for errors or any consequences arising from the use of the information contained in this publication. Contributions published under the name of individual authors are statements and opinions solely of said authors and not of the publisher, and/or the distributor, and/or the AO Group.

The products, procedures, and therapies described in this work are hazardous and are therefore only to be applied by certified and trained medical professionals in environments specially designed for such procedures. No suggested test or procedure should be carried out unless, in the user's professional judgment, its risk is justified. Whoever applies products, procedures, and therapies shown or described in this work will do this at their own risk. Because of rapid advances in the medical sciences, AO recommends that independent verification of diagnosis, therapies, drugs, dosages, and operation methods should be made before any action is taken.

Although all advertising material which may be inserted into the work is expected to conform to ethical (medical) standards, inclusion in this publication does not constitute a guarantee or endorsement by the publisher regarding quality or value of such product or of the claims made of it by its manufacturer.

Legal restrictions

Check hazards and legal restrictions on www.aofoundation.org/legal

Distribution by Georg Thieme Verlag, Rüdigerstrasse 14, DE-70469 Stuttgart and Thieme New York, 333 Seventh Avenue, US-New York, NY 10001

ISBN: 978-3-13-171511-1
e-ISBN: 978-3-13-171521-0

1 2 3 4 5 6

Editorial

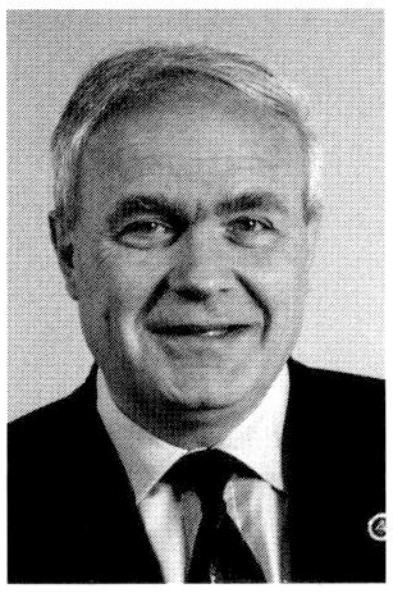

Norbert P Haas, Prof, Dr med

Berlin, May 2013

Periprosthetic fractures belong to the most complex, expensive and—for our individual patients—risky challenges in orthopedic surgery. The surgeon needs to have a profound knowledge about biomechanics and characteristics of the artificial joint, but he also needs the craftsmanship and skills of an acute care expert. As the number of periprosthetic fractures rises due to the general increase in arthroplasties and a massive demographic change in most countries, the socioeconomic impact is enormously high. Apart from this more abstract viewpoint, it is catastrophic for our elderly patients.

The term "periprosthetic fracture" contains two notions that have long been a rather uneven pair: "fracture" and "prosthesis". For many years, everyday life for—orthopedics and trauma surgeons alike—consisted either of fractures and acute trauma care; or we worked as "classic" orthopedic surgeons, busy with the implantation of various endoprostheses and caring to a lesser extent about nonelective procedures. Both divisions in our great profession were living, working, researching and treating patients in parallel universes, even if formally under one professional roof.

However, in recent years changes in our working lives have posed questions as to whether we should continue in this manner. One of the challenges, for which a closer cooperation between "state-of-the-art" trauma care and "state-of-the-art" joint replacement is crucial, is in the successful management of periprosthetic fractures. This new merger of reconstruction and replacement is underlined by the collaboration of the editors of this new book, each of them an outstanding expert in his field.

The AO family has acknowledged these challenges from very early on, continuously developing new approaches in teaching and research to optimize patient care and safety. This new book for the first time combines the latest global knowledge on periprosthetic fractures, including all relevant anatomic regions, surgical pitfalls, complex cases, and a brand new comprehensive classification on periprosthetic fractures.

Classifications have always been important cornerstones in the AO agenda as without suitable classification systems, efficient teaching and education is impossible. Thoroughly supervised by a renowned and dedicated group of authors, the AO foundation has again released a ground breaking publication with this book. Well-structured chapters and high-quality images allow a quick glance between two surgical procedures, but also deliver comprehensive scientific background information back home in front of your fireplace. We hope you will find this new book as much fun to read and as inspiring and helpful as we do in our daily routine and look forward to your comments.

Foreword

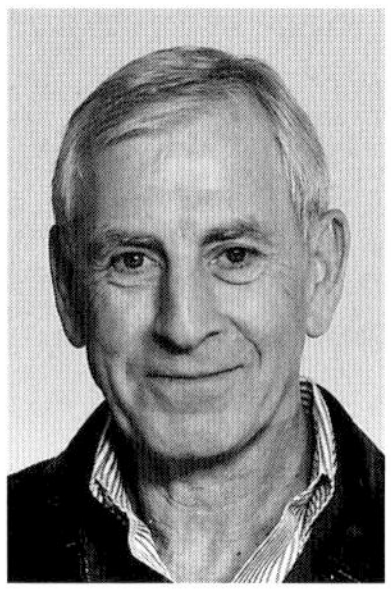

David L Helfet, MD

New York, June 2013

It gives me great pleasure to write an introduction to the "Periprosthetic Fracture Management" by Michael Schütz, MD and Carsten Perka, MD. This book on periprosthetic fractures is unique, as it represents a true collaboration between the world of Joint Arthroplasty and the world of Orthopedic Trauma. In addition, this is truly a volume that represents the collective experience from around the world. Both Dr. Perka in the Arthroplasty realm and Dr. Schütz in the AO Network have been able to put together a really unique high-profile collection of authors.

The format includes a section on Classification, based on the Vancouver experience and presented by Duncan and Haddad. The subsequent general section gives an overview of periprosthetic fractures and the management of patients with such injuries. Subsequently, the book focuses on specific periprosthetic fractures of both upper and lower extremities, their problems and management, including surgery. This includes not just the open reduction and internal fixation options, but also techniques for complex revision arthroplasty and salvage. Particularly appealing to the reader, but especially a surgeon, are the excellent and most illustrative case examples covering the whole spectrum of periprosthetic fracture types and their problems.

In conclusion, I would like to congratulate the editors and all the authors on a timely and remarkably well done volume and would recommend to all who manage these periprosthetic fractures this AO Manual as an absolute must.

Acknowledgments

The editors, Michael Schütz and Carsten Perka, wish to express their gratitude to Thomas P Rüedi, whose unwavering, constant support, ideas and encouragement resulted in this pioneering publication. As a founding member and, in the true spirit of the AO Foundation, he helped us in his calm and modest way to assemble an experienced team of authors and contributors to voluntarily contribute to the book. His wealth of experience and unique insight rendered him invaluable to the quality of this project.

The editors also wish to express their thanks to the many authors who compiled the latest knowledge on periprosthetic fractures and made this book a truly joint project of arthoplasty and trauma surgeons from around the globe. The special contribution of the comprehensive new "Unified Classification System, UCS" from Clive Duncan and Fares Haddad greatly enhanced the educational content of the publication for the surgeon community.

The AO team coordinated the overall production. Sigrid Unterberg, who meticulously planned and executed this advanced publication, deserves our very special appreciation. The publications manager, Patricia Codyre solved production obstacles as they arose, ensuring a smooth collaborative process. Jecca Reichmuth provided the superb illustrations throughout the book, while Roger Kistler delivered outstanding work on the book's layout of text, graphic design and tables. Vidula Bhoyroo, Carl Lau and Barbara Gernert supported the editorial process.

"Periprosthetic Fracture Management" is the first comprehensive book on this topic with the aim to enrich current knowledge, contribute to understanding the complex detail and surgical techniques that produce best clinical results for our patients.

Contributors

Editors

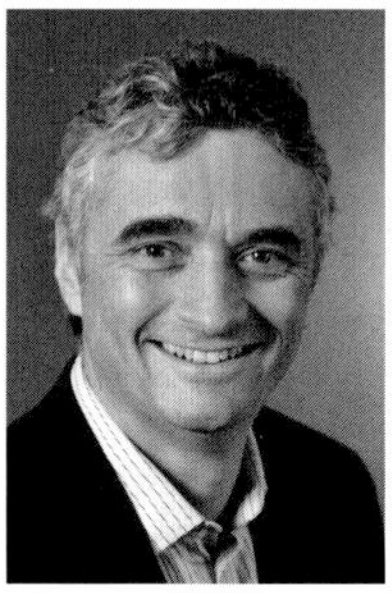

Michael Schütz, MD, FRACS, FAOrthA
Director of Trauma
E50 Hospital
Metro South Health Service District
Professor and Chair in Trauma
Institute of Health & Biomedical Innovation
Queensland University of Technology
199 Ipswich Road
Woolloongabba, Brisbane, QLD 4102
Australia

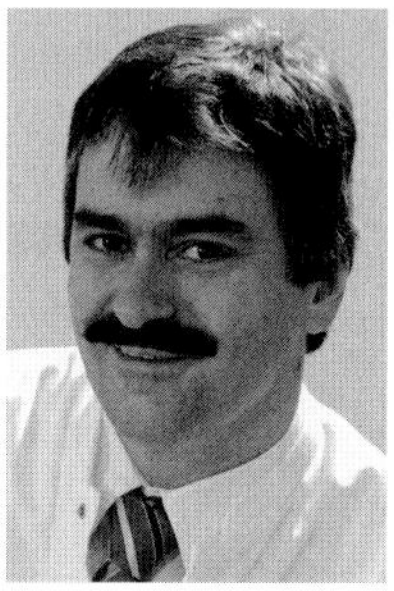

Carsten Perka, MD
Charité Universitätsmedizin Berlin
Centrum für Muskuloskeletale Chirurgie
Chariteplatz 1
10117 Berlin
Germany

Senior Editor

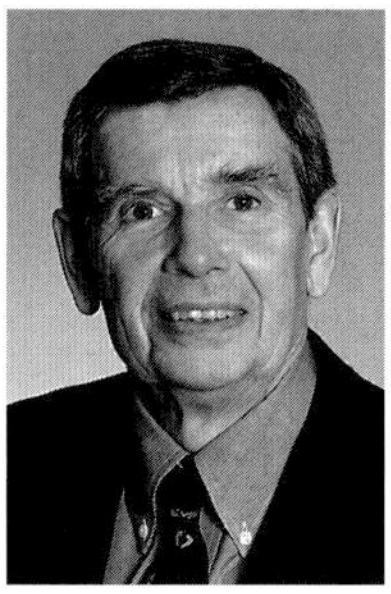

Thomas P Rüedi, Prof, MD, FACS
Founding and honorary member of the AO Foundation
Im Brisig
7304 Maienfeld
Switzerland

Authors

Matthew P Abdel, MD
Mayo Clinic
200 First Street SW
Rochester, MN 55905
USA

Yves Pascal Acklin, Dr med
Kantonsspital Graubünden, Chirurgie
Loëstrasse 170
7000 Chur
Switzerland

David Backstein, MD
Division of Orthopaedic Surgery
Mount Sinai Hospital
University of Toronto
600 University Avenue, Suite 476(A)
Toronto, ON M5G 1X5
Canada

Gregory Bain, MBBS, FRACS, PhD
Department of Orthpaedics and Trauma
University Of Adelaide
Department of Orthopaedic Surgery
Royal Adelaide Hospital and Modbury Hospital
196 Melbourne Street
North Adelaide, SA 5006
Australia

David Barei, MD, FRCSC
Harborview Medical Center
Department of Orthopedics and Sports Medicine
325 9th Avenue
Seattle, WA 98104
USA

Alexej Barg, MD
Clinic of Orthopaedic Surgery
Kantonsspital Liestal
Rheinstrasse 26
4410 Liestal
Switzerland

Marschall B Berkes, MD
Orthopaedic Surgery
Hospital for Special Surgery
535 East 70th Street
New York, NY 10021
USA

Daniel J Berry, MD
Gonda 14
Department of Orthopedic Surgery
Mayo Clinic
200 First Street SW
Rochester, MN 55905
USA

Andrew D Carrothers, MD
19 Ridley Boulevard
Toronto, Ontario M5M 3L1
Canada

John C Clohisy, MD
Campus Box 8233
660 S. Euclid
St Louis, MO 63110
USA

Clive P Duncan, Prof, FRCSC
Diamond Health Centre, 3rd Floor
2775 Laurel Street
Vancouver, BC V5Z 1M9
Canada

Kenneth A Egol, MD
Department of Orthopaedic Surgery
NYU Hospital for Joint Diseases
301 East 17th Street
New York, NY 10003
USA

Emilio Fantin, MD
Hospital Privado de Cordoba
Orthopaedics and Traumatology
346 Naciones Unidas
5016 Cordoba
Argentina

Bernd Fink, MD
Department of Joint Replacement
General and Rheumatic Orthopaedics
Orthopaedic Clinic Markgröningen gGmbH (OKM)
Kurt-Lindemann-Weg 10
71706 Markgröningen
Germany

Jordanna Forman, BS
Department of Orthopaedic Surgery
NYU Hospital for Joint Diseases
280 East 2nd Avenue, Suite 606
New York, NY 10003
USA

Antonio M Foruria de Diego, MD
Shoulder and Elbow Reconstructive Surgery Unit
Orthopedic Surgery Residency Program Director
Department of Orthopaedic Surgery
Fundacion Jiménez Diaz–Capio
Avenida Reyes Católicos, 2
28040 Madrid
Spain

Garbedian Shawn, MD, FRCSC
Division of Orthopaedic Surgery
North York General Hospital
4001 Leslie Street
Toronto, ON M2K1E1
Canada

Emanuel Gautier, MD
Chairman
Cantonal Hospital Fribourg
Department of Orthopaedic Surgery
Bertigny
1708 Fribourg
Switzerland

Allan Gross, MD, FRCSC
Division of Orthopaedic Surgery
Mount Sinai Hospital
600 University Avenue, Suite 476(A)
Toronto, ON M5G 1X5
Canada

Fares S Haddad, MD
The Princess Grace Hospital
42-52 Nottingham Place
London, W1M 3FD
United Kingdom

Beat Hintermann, MD
Clinic of Orthopaedic Surgery
Kantonsspital Liestal
Rheinstrasse 26
4410 Liestal
Switzerland

Pierre Hoffmeyer, MD
Médecin-chef
Hôpital Cantonal de Genève
Service de chirurgie orthopédique
24, Rue Micheli-du-Crest
1211 Genève
Switzerland

Martin Jäger, MD
Department Orthopädie & Traumatologie
Universitätsklinikum Freiburg
Albert-Ludwigs-Universität
Hugstetter Strasse 55
79106 Freiburg im Breisgau
Germany

Richard J Jenkinson, MD, FRCSC
Orthopaedic Surgeon
Sunnybrook Health Sciences Center
Orthopaedic Surgery
2075 Bayview Avenue
Suite MG 321
Toronto, ON M4N 3M5
Canada

Jesse B Jupiter, Prof
Director Orthopedic Hand Service
Massachusetts General Hospital
Department of Orthopedics WAC 527
Yawkey Center, Suite 2100
02114 Boston, MA
USA

Stephen L Kates, MD
Professor, Director of Geriatric Fracture Center
University of Rochester Medical Center
Orthopaedics
8049 Barony Woods
Rochester, NY 14534
USA

Angus Keogh, MBBS, FRACS
Western Orthopaedic Clinic
Suite 213/25, McCourt
St Subiaco, WA 6008
Australia

Peter Kloen, MD, PhD
Chief Orthopaedic Traumatology
Academisch Medisch Centrum
Orthopedic Surgery
Universiteit van Amsterdam
Meibergdreef 9
1100 DD Amsterdam
The Netherlands

Jeffrey S Kneisl, MD
Carolinas Medical Center
Department of Orthopaedic Surgery
1025 Morehead Medical Drive, Suite 300
Charlotte, NC 28204
USA

Hans J Kreder, MD, MPH
Professor
Sunnybrook Health Sciences Centre
Department of Surgery
2075 Bayview Avenue
Toronto, ON M4N 3M5
Canada

Raul Kuchinad, MD, MSc, FRCS(C)
Section of Orthopaedic Surgery
University of Calgary
Rockyview General Hospital
7007 14 Street SW
Calgary, AL T2V 1P9
Canada

Simon Lambert, BSc, FRCS
The Shoulder and Elbow Service
Royal National Orthopaedic Hospital Trust
Brockley Hill, Stanmore
Middlesex, HA7 4LP
United Kingdom

Tak-wing Lau
Department of Orthopaedics andTraumatology
5/F, Professorial block
Queen Mary Hospital
102, Pokfulam Road
Pokfulam
Hong Kong

Jay R Lieberman, Prof, MD,
Chairman, Department of Orthopaedic Surgery
Keck School of Medicine
University of Southern California
Healthcare Consultation Center II
1520 San Pablo Street, Suite 2000
Los Angeles, CA 90033
USA

Dean Lorich, MD
Hospital for Special Surgery
520 East 70th Street
Starr Pavilion, 2nd Floor
New York, NY 10021
USA

Matt C Lyons, MD
North Sydney Orthopaedic and Sport
Medicine Center
Ground Floor
3 Gillies Street
Wollstonecraft, NSW 2065
Australia

Steven J MacDonald, MD
London Health Sciences Centre
430 St. George Street
London, ON N6A 3B4
Canada

Sebastian Manegold, MD
Charité Universitätsmedizin Berlin
Campus Virchow Klinikum
Augustenburger Platz 1
13353 Berlin
Germany

Keith Mayo, MD
Tacoma General Hospital
Department of Orthopedic Surgery
316 Martin Luther King Jr. Way, Suite 200
Tacoma, WA 98405
USA

Christof Meyer, MD
Leiter der Unfall-, Hand- und Wiederherstellung-
schirurgie
Zentrum für Orthopädie und Unfallchirurgie
Klinikum Saarbrücken gGmbH
Winterberg 1
66119 Saarbrücken
Germany

Christopher Morrey, MD
Cairns Orthopaedic Clinic
PO Box 4926
Cairns, QL 4870
Australia

Stefaan Nijs, Prof, MD, PhD
Joint clinical Head Department of Trauma Surgery
UZ Leuven
Campus Gasthuisberg
Traumatology
Herestraat 49
3000 Leuven
Belgium

Akin Önder, MD
Charité Universitätsmedizin Berlin
Klinik für Anästhesiologie mit Schwerpunkt operative
Intensivmedizin
Charitéplatz 1
10117 Berlin
Germany

Natasha O'Malley, MB, BCh, BAO, FRC (Tr&Orth)
15 East Jefferson Road
Pittsford, NY 14534
USA

Joshua C Patt, MD
Carolinas Medical Center
Department of Orthopaedic Surgery
1025 Morehead Medical Drive, Suite 300
Charlotte, NC 28204
USA

Stephan Pauly, MD
Charité Universitätsmedizin Berlin
Centrum für Muskuloskeletale Chirurgie
Charitéplatz 1
10117 Berlin
Germany

Rodrigo Pesantez, MD
Chief of Orthopedic Trauma
Departamento de Ortopedia y Traumatología
Fundación Santa Fe de Bogotá
Avenida 9 # 116–20
Consultorio 820 Bogotá
Colombia

Gregory G Polkowski, MD
New England Musculoskeletal Institute
University of Connecticut Health Center
263 Farmington Avenue
Farmington, CT 06030
USA

Michael Raschke, MD
Direktor
Universitätsklinikum Münster
Klinik für Unfall-, Hand- und Wiederherstellung-schirurgie
Waldeyerstrasse 1
48149 Münster
Germany

William M Ricci, MD
Chief, Orthopaedic Trauma Service
Department of Orthopaedic Surgery
Washington University School of Medicine
Campus Box 8233
660 South Euclid Avenue
St. Louis, MO 63110
USA

Benedict A Rogers, MA, MSc, FRCS (Tr&Orth)
Consultant Orthopaedic Surgeon
Brighton & Sussex University Hospitals NHS Trust
Eastern Road
Brighton, BN25BE
United Kingdom

Oleg Safir, MD
Division of Orthopaedic Surgery
Mount Sinai Hospital
600 University Avenue, Suite 476(A)
Toronto, ON M5G 1X5
Canada

Joaquín Sanchez-Sotelo, MD, PhD
Gonda 14
Department of Orthopedic Surgery
Mayo Clinic
200 First Street SW
Rochester, MN 55905
USA

Michael Sander, Prof
Charité Universitätsmedizin Berlin
Klinik für Anästhesiologie mit Schwerpunkt operative Intensivmedizin
Charitéplatz 1
10117 Berlin
Germany

Takeshi Sawaguchi, MD
Director
Toyama Municipal Hospital
Department of Orthopedic Surgery and Joint Reconstructive Surgery
Imaizumihokubu 2-1
939-8511 Toyama City
Japan

Klaus-Dieter Schaser, Univ.-Prof., Dr. med.
Charité Universitätsmedizin Berlin
Centrum für Muskuloskeletale Chirurgie
Klinik für Orthopädie
Klinik für Unfall- und Wiederherstellungschirurgie
Campus Virchow Klinikum
Augustenburger Platz 1
13353 Berlin
Germany

Inger B Schipper, MD, PhD
Chief, Department of Trauma Surgery
Director of Trauma Center West Netherlands
Leiden University Medical Center
Surgery, D6-39
Albinusdreef 2, PO Box 9600
2300 RC Leiden
The Netherlands

Reinhard Schnettler, Prof, MD
Department of Trauma Surgery
Rudolf-Buchheim-Strasse 7
35385 Giessen
Germany

Philipp Schwabe, MD
Charité Universitätsmedizin Berlin
Centrum für Muskuloskeletale Chirurgie
Klinik für Orthopädie
Klinik für Unfall- und Wiederherstellungschirurgie
Campus Virchow Klinikum
Augustenburger Platz 1
13353 Berlin
Germany

Alexander Y Shin, Prof, MD
Mayo Clinic
Gonda 14
Department of Orthopedic Surgery
Division of Hand Surgery
Mayo Clinic
200 First Street SW
Rochester, MN 55905
USA

Cornel C Sieber, Prof, Dr
Director, Institute for Biomedicine of Aging
Friedrich-Alexander Universität Erlangen-Nürnberg
Heimerichstrasse 58
90419 Nürnberg
Germany

Katrin Singler, MD
Oberärztin Klinikum Nürnberg–Geriatrie
Prof.-Ernst-Nathan-Strasse 1
90419 Nürnberg
Germany

Christoph Sommer, MD
Kantonsspital Graubünden, Chirurgie
Loëstrasse 170
7000 Chur
Switzerland

Karl Stoffel, Prof, MD, FRACS, PhD
Department of Orthpaedics and Trauma
University of Western Australia
Fremantle Hospital and Murdoch Hospital
Fremantle Hospital, Level 6 B Block
Fremantle, WA 6010
Australia

Norbert P Südkamp, Univ.-Prof., Dr. med.
Department Orthopädie und Traumatologie
Universitätsklinikum Freiburg
Albert-Ludwigs-Universität
Hugstetter Strasse 55
79106 Freiburg im Breisgau
Germany

Gabor Szalay, MD
Department of Trauma Surgery
Rudolf-Buchheim-Strasse 7
35385 Giessen
Germany

Shian-Chao Tay, MD, MSc
Department of Hand Surgery
Singapore General Hospital
Outram Road
Singapore 169608
Singapore

Stephan Tohtz, MD
Emil v. Behring Krankenhaus
Department of Orthopedic and Trauma Surgery
Walterhöfer Strasse 11
14165 Berlin
Germany

Ivor S Vanhegan, MD
Division of Surgery and Interventional Science
University College London
4th Floor, 74 Huntley Street
London, WC1E 6AU
United Kingdom

Aart D Verburg, MD
Department of Orthopedic Surgery
Orbis Medical Center
Dr van het Hoffplein 1
Sittard-Geleen
The Netherlands

Philipp von Roth
Charité Universitätsmedizin Berlin
Charitéplatz 1
10117 Berlin
Germany

Michael Wagner, Prof., Dr. med.
Unfallchirurgie Wilhelminenspital
Montleartstrasse 37
1160 Wien
Austria

Arvind G von Keudell, MD
Department of Orthopedic Surgery
Havard Medical School
75 Francis Street
Boston, MA 02115
USA

Rutger G Zuurmond, MD
Isala Clinics Zwolle
PO Box 10500
8000 GM Zwolle
The Netherlands

Abbreviations

ABI ankle-brachial index
ATLS advanced trauma life support
bFGF basic fibroblast growth factor
BMI body mass index
CRP C-reactive protein
CT computed tomography
DSA digital subtraction angiography
ED emergency department
FDA Food and Drug Administration
FGF-2 fibroblast growth factor-2
FTSG full-thickness skin graft
GCS Glasgow coma scale
HFS Hanover fracture scale
HIT heparin-induced thrombocytopenia
HPL high-pressure lavage
IL interleukin
INR international normalized ratio
IV intravenous
LDF laser Doppler flowmetry
LEAP lower extremity assessment project
LISS less invasive stabilization system
LMWH low-molecular-weight heparin
LPL low-pressure lavage
LSI limb salvage index
MESS mangled extremity severity score
MIF macrophage migration inhibitory factor
MRI magnet resonance imaging
MRSA methicillin-resistant *Staphylococcus aureus*
MSC mesenchymal stem cell
NISSSA nerve, ischemia, soft-tissue, skeletal, shock, and age score
NPWT negative-pressure wound therapy
ORIF open reduction and internal fixation
PDGF platelet-derived growth factor
PDS polydioxanone
PLA polylactic acid
PMMA polymethyl methacrylate
PMN polymorphonuclear leukocyte
pO2 partial oxygen pressure
psi pounds per square inch (1 psi = 0.07 atmospheres)
PU perfusion unit
SPARC secreted protein acidic and rich in cysteine
SSRI serotonin reuptake inhibitor
STSG split-thickness skin graft
TGF-β transforming growth factor β
TNF-α tumor necrosis factor α
UFH unfractionated heparin
VAC® Vacuum Assisted Closure
VEGF vascular endothelial growth factor
VRE vancomycin-resistant enterococcus

Table of contents

1

Introduction to periprosthetic fractures

1 Introduction to periprosthetic fractures

Authors **Carsten Perka, Michael Schütz**

Periprosthetic fractures (of bone and/or implant) by definition occur with a prosthesis—or part of it—in situ. They can result from trauma, osteolysis and pathologic bone, fatigue, or wear. They occur in the proximity or around the bed of a component of a joint replacement. The trauma can occur intraoperatively, ie, during the insertion of the prosthetic component, or more frequently postoperatively. In the elderly, periprosthetic fractures are usually caused by a minor trauma and often result in considerable morbidity and disability, or even are fatal.

While practically every joint replacement in the body can be involved in a periprosthetic fracture, those located in the lower extremity are more often involved due to higher mechanical forces. The socioeconomic consequences are considerable. Studies have calculated the average costs of treatment to vary between 20,000 and 200,000 USD. This will rarely be covered fully by insurance **[1]**.

In addition to the general fragility of the aged patient, local biological and mechanical factors can be responsible for a periprosthetic fracture. While a disturbed blood supply to the bone after insertion of a prosthesis may account for a biological deficit, the lack of mechanical stability can be explained by poor quality or loss of bone. Bone deficiency or resorption may also be caused by less than ideal placement and alignment of the prosthesis in the first place. This results in non-physiological loading of the surrounding bone, which in turn may create stress risers.

As every periprosthetic fracture differs from the other, each case has to be considered individually. Nevertheless, it seems possible to categorize or classify most of the fractures according to a simple "Unified Classification System (UCS)", similar to that of the AO/OTA classification (see chapter 4.2). Beside the classification of the fracture, the assessment of the patient and careful decision-making process, the treatment of periprosthetic fractures demands an experienced surgeon. Such a surgeon has not only to be familiar with the different internal fixation techniques and revision arthroplasty procedures but also with the biomechanics of the involved joint as well as with the modern possibilities of anchorage of the different devices in poor quality bone. The many options of surgical approaches must be mastered and their relevance in regard to fracture healing should be understood. To prevent secondary complications due to immobilization of the mostly elderly patients, any treatment should be able to provide adequate stability of fixation allowing immediate or early mobilization of the patient.

Future developments of fracture care should endeavor to be least invasive, provide highest stability, and at the same time be most respectful of the biology of bone and soft-tissue healing. In regard to the technology and design of new prostheses, the risk for periprosthetic fractures to occur should be noted. In view of the increasing incidence of uncontrolled falls and injuries of the steadily growing number of older patients, geriatric medicine should develop better and more effective prevention programs.

References

[1] **Phillips JR, Boulton C, Morac CG, et al.** What is the financial cost of treating periprosthetic hip fractures? *Injury.* 2011 Feb;42(2):146–149.

2

Epidemiology of periprosthetic fractures

2.1 Introduction

Authors **Matthew P Abdel, Daniel J Berry**

By 2030, the demand for primary total hip arthroplasties (THAs) in the United States is expected to grow by 174% to 572,000 procedures annually [1]. Total hip revisions are projected to increase by 137% between 2005 and 2030. During the same period, the demand for primary total knee arthroplasties (TKAs) is expected to grow by 673% to 3.48 million procedures per year, with a concurrent increase in revisions by 601% [1].

As the number of procedures increases, that of periprosthetic fractures occurring intra or postoperatively is also expected to rise [2–5]. The incidence of periprosthetic fractures seems to be increasing due to several factors. Foremost, excellent results with total joint arthroplasty have led to expanded indications for the procedure, both in younger, more active patients as well as in elderly patients [6]. Furthermore, the average life expectancy has increased, leading to a higher number of elderly patients with total joint arthroplasties. This patient population has a higher risk of fracture due to poor bone quality and/or periprosthetic bone loss [6]. Concurrently, an increased population load of patients will have had revision arthroplasty, which in itself is another independent risk factor for periprosthetic fractures [7, 8].

Periprosthetic fractures present a complex situation to the orthopedic surgeon. The challenges in treating such fractures include:

- Poor bone stock, osteolysis, or bone loss
- Altered anatomy
- The requirement to manage issues related to the joint prosthesis and the fracture concomitantly [9].

Furthermore, periprosthetic fractures result in considerable morbidity and dysfunction for patients [10–12]. Therefore, a thorough understanding of the epidemiology and risk factors of periprosthetic fractures is essential for both prevention and treatment.

2.2 Hip

Authors Matthew P Abdel, Daniel J Berry

2.2.1 Acetabular fractures

Intraoperative fractures

Intraoperative periprosthetic acetabular fractures are rare. Almost all occur as a result of impaction forces if press-fit noncemented acetabular components are used [13]. Earlier, a study [14] outlined an incidence of acetabular periprosthetic fracture of less than 0.2% (1 in 5,400) when total hip arthroplasties (THAs) were performed exclusively with cement. Currently, the overall incidence of intraoperative periprosthetic acetabular fractures is unknown. Interestingly, to date only three series discuss the problem. The largest investigation [13] reported on 13 intraoperative fractures from three different institutions using various implants. The majority of patients were women with compromised bone quality. Furthermore, underreaming of the socket was prominent in most patients.

McGrory [15] reported a case of an intraoperative posterior wall fracture in a patient with Paget's disease secondary to underreaming. A recent study by Desai et al [16] reported two acetabular fractures detected, respectively, 2 and 3 weeks postoperatively, in elderly women with osteoporosis after minor trauma. The authors hypothesize that both fractures occurred intraoperatively but were not recognized initially.

In an unpublished review of the experience in the Mayo Clinic to date, 78 intraoperative acetabular fractures of 32,684 primary THAs were identified, corresponding to a rate of 0.24% (2.2-1). Of the 78 fractures, 70 were noncemented components (0.43%) and 8 were cemented (0.05%). In the revision setting, fractures increased to 39 (0.68%) of 5,720 revision THAs, with 31 (0.74%) of 4,201 fractures occurring during noncemented socket placement and 8 (0.53%) of 1,519 occurring during revision to a cemented socket.

Postoperative fractures

While more frequent than intraoperative periprosthetic acetabular fractures, postoperative periprosthetic acetabular fractures are still uncommon. Such fractures can be classified into two categories:

- Those related to an acute traumatic event
- Those related to osteolysis [2].

Miller was the first to describe postoperative acetabular fractures in 1972 [17]. Five fractures were associated with noncemented Ring prostheses, while four involved a cemented McKee cup. Peterson and Lewallen [18] reported eleven acute postoperative acetabular fractures, eight of which were due to trauma. Of these, eight components were radiographically stable (type I), whereas three were loose (type II). There are several other isolated case reports of traumatic postoperative periprosthetic acetabular fractures as well [19–22].

2.2-1 Rate of intra and postoperative periprosthetic fractures around primary and revision total hip arthroplasties (THAs) at the Mayo Clinic, Rochester, MN, USA.*

Variables	Primary total hip arthroplasties (THAs) fracture rate, No. (%)	Revision total hip arthroplasties (THAs) fracture rate, No. (%)
Intraoperative		
Acetabulum		
– Noncemented	70/16,177 (0.43)	31/4,201 (0.74)
– Cemented	8/16,507 (0.05)	8/1,519 (0.53)
– Total	78/32,684 (0.24)	39/5,720 (0.68)
Femur		
– Noncemented	453/9,745 (4.6)	502/2,773 (18.1)
– Cemented	114/22,939 (0.5)	147/2,662 (5.5)
– Total	567/32,684 (1.7)	649/5,435 (11.9)
Postoperative		
Acetabulum		
– Noncemented	81/16,177 (0.5)	64/4,201 (1.5)
– Cemented	105/16,507 (0.64)	19/1,519 (1.3)
– Total	186/32,684 (0.6)	83/5,720 (1.5)
Femur		
– Noncemented	179/9,745 (1.8)	127/2,773 (4.6)
– Cemented	342/22,939 (1.5)	148/2,662 (5.6)
– Total	521/32,684 (1.6)	275/5,435 (5.1)

* Unpublished data

Osteolysis also seems to play an increasing role in postoperative acetabular fractures. One study [23] described three cases of acute periprosthetic fractures of the acetabulum associated with severe osteolytic lesions of the pelvis. In addition, Chatoo et al [24] reported one loose cemented socket associated with a periprosthetic fracture, while Andrews et al [25] described one periprosthetic fracture of the medial wall following a noncemented revision.

Pelvic discontinuity is a separate category of postoperative acetabular fracture in which the superior portion of the pelvis is separated from the inferior portion. This is typically manifested as a transverse acetabular fracture nonunion [2]. While the majority probably occurs as a result of stress fractures due to deficient pelvic bone, acute cases associated with intraoperative complications have been reported [26]. Berry et al [26] identified pelvic discontinuities in 31 of 3,505 acetabular revisions at the Mayo Clinic.

As mentioned earlier, in an unpublished review of the entire Mayo Clinic experience to date, only 186 postoperative acetabular fractures of 32,684 primary THAs were identified, corresponding to a rate of 0.6% (**2.2-1**). However, these figures include geriatric stress fractures and other fractures that did not require surgical intervention. Of the 186 fractures, 81 occurred around noncemented acetabular components (0.5%) and 105 were around cemented acetabular components (0.64%). In the revision setting, the fracture rate increased to 1.5% (83 of 5,720 revision THAs, with 64 (1.5%) of 4,201 fractures occurring after noncemented socket placement and 19 (1.3%) of 1,519 occurring after cemented socket placement.

2.2.2 Femoral fractures

Intraoperative fractures

The rate of intraoperative periprosthetic femoral fractures is difficult to assess accurately given the variation in patient demographics, types of implants used, technique of insertion, and indications for further surgery. However, to assist in the analysis, such fractures can be divided into two general categories: those occurring during primary and those occurring during revision THA. Each category can then be subdivided according to whether the femoral component is cemented or noncemented. A review of the literature reveals that intraoperative fractures occur more commonly during revision procedures [2]. Furthermore, during both primary and revision procedures, fractures occur much more frequently around noncemented stems. This is likely related to the press-fit design—more precisely, the involved impaction forces.

When analyzing intraoperative periprosthetic femoral fractures associated with cemented primary stems, the incidence ranges from 0.1%–2.5% (**2.2-2**) [2, 27, 28]. Taylor et al [29] reported a 1.2% rate of intraoperative fractures in 605 cemented THAs. Looking at the Mayo Clinic Total Joint Registry through 1999, Berry noted [2] an intraoperative fracture in 0.3% of 20,859 cemented primary THAs. However, most intraoperative periprosthetic femoral fractures occur with insertion of noncemented press-fit stems [2]. In the previous Mayo Clinic series, which included the early experience with noncemented implants, the risk of intraoperative periprosthetic femoral fracture increased to 5.4% of 3,121 primary THAs when the stems were press-fitted [2]. Schwartz et al similarly reported a 3.7% intraoperative fracture rate (39 of 1,318) in primary noncemented stems. As such, the incidence of intraoperative periprosthetic femoral fractures associated with noncemented primary stems ranges from 3.7%–5.4% in the earlier literature.

The incidence of intraoperative femoral fractures is higher in the revision setting, with some authors [2] reporting an incidence as high as 20.9%. Such fractures can occur with exposure, hip dislocation, implant removal, cement removal, canal preparation, implant insertion, and hip reduction [31, 32]. Johansson et al [33] reported 22 intraoperative fractures that occurred with revision procedures. Of these, eleven occurred during cement removal. On the other hand, one article [34] reported ten intraoperative fractures during 159 revision THAs, half of which had occurred during hip dislocation.

2.2-2 Rate of periprosthetic fractures surrounding hip arthroplasties.*

Variables	Primary total hip arthroplasties (THAs), range	Revision total hip arthroplasties (THAs), range
Intraoperative		
Acetabulum		
- Noncemented	NA	NA
- Cemented	NA	NA
Femur		
- Noncemented	3.7-5.4%	6.3–20.9%
- Cemented	0.1–2.5%	3.0–3.6%
Postoperative		
Acetabulum		
- Noncemented	NA	NA
- Cemented	NA	NA
Femur		
- Noncemented	0.4–2.9%	2.1–4.2%
- Cemented	0.8–3.5%	NA

* Based on current literature.
NA = not available

A study [35] stated a 17.6% rate of intraoperative periprosthetic femoral fractures with revision procedures compared with 3.5% for primary procedures. Intraoperative fracture is much more common when a revision is completed with a noncemented stem. Morrey et al [36] reported an 18% rate of intraoperative periprosthetic fractures with a noncemented stem compared with 3% with a cemented stem. Likewise, Berry [2] reported a 20.9% (322 of 1,536) intraoperative fracture rate in noncemented femoral revisions compared with 175 (3.6%) of 4,813 in cemented femoral revisions [2]. Of note, this was in the early experience with noncemented implants.

When analyzing the entire unpublished Mayo Clinic experience to date, 567 (1.7%) of 32,684 intraoperative periprosthetic femoral fractures were identified during primary THAs (2.2-1). A total of 453 (4.6%) of 567 fractures occurred during placement of a noncemented stem and 114 occurred during placement of a cemented stem (0.5%). During revision THAs, intraoperative periprosthetic femoral fractures was 649 (11.9%) of 5,435. The majority (502 [18.1%] of 2,773) occurred during placement of a noncemented femoral component, whereas the remaining 147 (5.5%) of 2,662 occurred during placement of a cemented stem.

Postoperative fractures

As previously mentioned, there is an increasing prevalence of postoperative periprosthetic femoral fractures due to various causes [2–6]. Similar to intraoperative fractures, postoperative periprosthetic fractures can be analyzed based on their occurrence following primary or revision THA and whether cement was used (**2.2-1a–b, 2.2-2a–b**). Berry [2] reported a postoperative fracture rate of 1.1% in 23,980 primary stems compared with 4.0% in 6,349 revision stems (**2.2-2**). Likewise, Lindahl et al [37] noted a postoperative periprosthetic fracture rate of 0.4% in primary stems (230 patients) as opposed to 2.1% in revision stems. The same authors noted that the incidence of periprosthetic femoral fractures was increasing in Sweden, with periprosthetic femoral fractures being the second most common reason for revision. Likewise, Kavanagh [38] estimated the incidence of postoperative periprosthetic femoral fractures to be 1% after primary THA and 4.2% after revision THA. Interestingly, in a review of the Swedish National Hip Registry, Lindahl et al [6] found a postoperative complication rate of 18% and a 23% rate of late complications leading to reoperation.

Recently, increased attention has been on early postoperative femoral fractures. In a combined retrospective study from the Mayo Clinic and the Dorr Arthritis Institute, 30

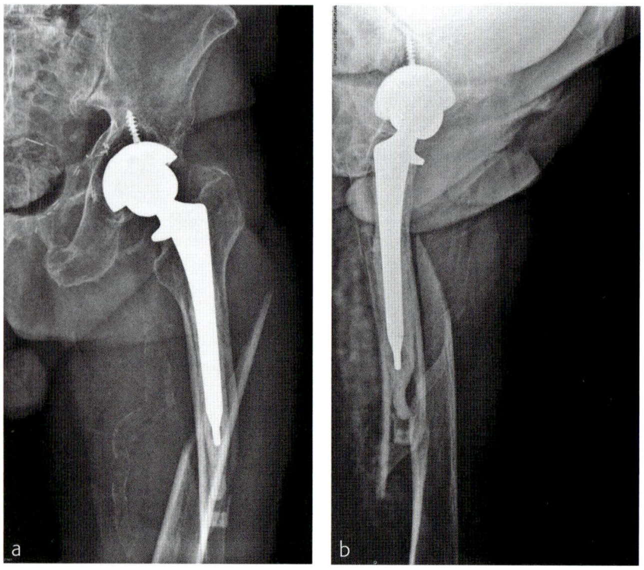

2.2-1a–b X-rays of a 79-year-old male patient with a left-sided periprosthetic femoral fracture of a cemented, well-fixed stem after a fall (UCS type IV.3-B1; Vancouver B1).
a AP view.
b Lateral view.

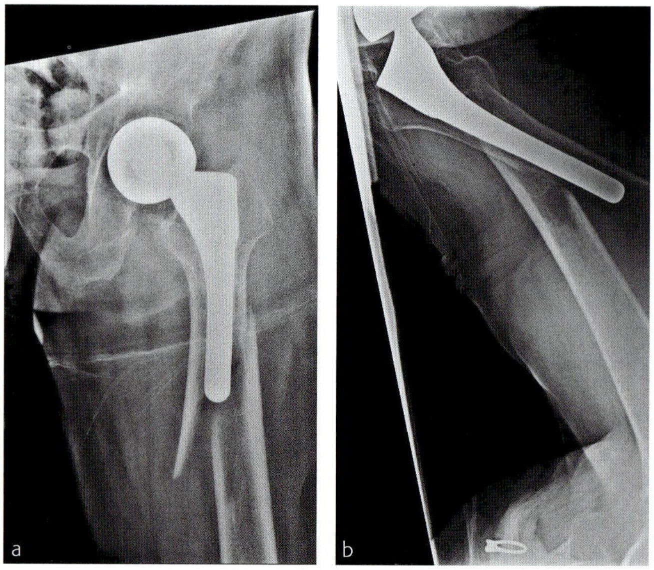

2.2-2a–b X-rays of a 61-year-old female patient with a left-sided periprosthetic femoral fracture of a noncemented but well-fixed stem after a fall (UCS type IV.3-B1; Vancouver B1).
a AP view.
b Lateral view.

early postoperative periprosthetic fractures that occurred within 90 days of an index THA were identified after 7,447 proximally coated, collarless, noncemented implants (0.4%) [40]. Mostly these comprised displaced fractures of the femoral neck, including the lesser trochanter and a variable amount of the proximal medial femoral cortex.

In regard to cemented THAs, Löwenhielm et al [27] noted a 2.5% risk of postoperative periprosthetic femoral fracture when looking at 1,442 primary cemented THAs. Recently, Cook et al reported [10] on 6,458 primary cemented femoral prostheses. The incidence of postoperative femoral fracture was 0.8% at 5 years and 3.5% at 10 years. Park et al [40] found a similar rate of postoperative periprosthetic femoral fractures of 2.9% in 1,270 THA. In 2011, a comprehensive series from the Scottish national database found a 5-year postoperative periprosthetic fracture rate of 0.9% after 52,136 primary THAs and 4.2% after 8,726 revision THAs [41].

When analyzing the entire unpublished Mayo Clinic experience to date, 521 (1,6%) of 32,684 postoperative periprosthetic femoral fractures after primary THAs was found (**2.2-1**). A total of 179 (1.8%) of 521 fractures occurred after placement of a noncemented stem and 342 occurred after placement of a cemented stem (1.5%). Following revision THA, the rate of postoperative periprosthetic femoral fractures was 5.1% (275 of 5,435). Of that 5,435 fractures, 148 (5.6%) of 2,662 occurred after placement of a cemented femoral component, whereas the remaining (127 [4,6%] of 2,773) happened after placement of a noncemented stem.

2.3 Knee

Authors Matthew P Abdel, Daniel J Berry

While generally less common than periprosthetic fractures surrounding THAs, the number of periprosthetic fractures both after primary and revision total knee arthroplasties (TKAs) is rising (**2.3-1**) [2, 42–46]. This is likely due to the increasing number of TKAs performed in combination with higher postoperative activity levels and greater patient longevity [2, 43–46]. When analyzing fractures around TKAs, the majority occur in the femur, either postoperatively or during revision procedures [2, 45].

2.3-1 Rate of periprosthetic fractures surrounding knee arthroplasties.*

Variables	Primary total knee arthroplasties (TKAs), range	Revision total knee arthroplasties (RKA), range
Intraoperative		
– Femur	0.1–0.4%	0.8%
– Tibia	0.07–0.67%	0.36–0.8%
– Patella	NA	0.2%
Postoperative		
– Femur	0.3–5.5%	0.3–38%
– Tibia	0.39–0.4%	0.48–0.9%
– Patella	0.61–1.19%	0.15–2%

* based on current literature. NA = not available.

2.3.1 Femoral fractures

Intraoperative fractures

The occurrence of intraoperative periprosthetic femoral or tibial fractures is less common than of similar postoperative fractures [2, 47]. However, the incidence of such fractures may likely be underestimated as some remain undetected and others have minimal displacement not requiring further intervention [48, 49]. Berry [2] reported an intraoperative periprosthetic femoral fracture rate of 0.1% in 16,906 primary TKAs, as opposed to 0.8% in 2,904 revision TKAs. Lombardi et al [50] noted a 4.4% rate of intraoperative intercondylar fractures if implants with a particular posterior cruciate substituting design were used. This rate was reduced to 0.2% with modifications of implant design and technique related to sizing of the central housing box versus bone preparation to accommodate the box.

In their series of 17,389 primary TKAs, Alden et al [47] found an intraoperative fracture rate of 0.39%. A total of 47 (73%) of the 67 fractures occurred in the femur. The location of the femoral fractures included the medial condyle (20), lateral condyle (11), supracondylar region (8), medial epicondyle (7), lateral epicondyle (2), and posterior cortex (1). Most fractures occurred during exposure and bone preparation (26), whereas the remaining occurred during trial reduction (22), cementation (13), and insertion of the polyethylene spacer (3).

In an unpublished review of the entire Mayo Clinic experience to date, 88 intraoperative femoral fractures of 30,420 primary TKAs were identified, corresponding to a rate of 0.3% (**2.3-2**). All fractures (88 [0.3%] of 29,783) occurred during placement of cemented components. During revisions, the intraoperative fracture rate increased fivefold (74 [1.6%] of 4,749). Again, all fractures occurred during placement of cemented femoral components (74 [1.6%] of 4,688).

Postoperative fractures

The incidence of distal femoral periprosthetic fractures associated with TKAs has been reported to range between 0.3% and 5.5% for primary procedures and up to 38% for revision procedures (**2.3-1**) [2, 41, 44, 45, 51–58]. The majority occurs in the supracondylar region (**2.3-1a–b**) [44]. In a recent comprehensive series from the Scottish national database, Meek et al [41] found a five year postoperative periprosthetic fracture rate of 0.6% after 44,511 primary TKAs and 1.7% after 3,222 revision TKAs. Berry [2] found a postoperative fracture rate of 0.9% in primary procedures (161 of 16,906) and 1.6% in revision procedures (48 of 2,904) of which most occur in women.

In general, postoperative periprosthetic femoral fractures are more common than intraoperative fractures [2, 45]. For instance, Platzer et al reported on 41 periprosthetic fractures, 40 of which occurred postoperatively [45]. In addition, 37 of 41 fractures occurred in the femur, with the remaining four being tibial fractures. In a long term study [59], Vessely et al found a 1.4% rate of femoral fractures, with the majority (8 of 14) occurring after 10 years.

Recent Mayo Clinic data revealed that 345 (1.1%) postoperative periprosthetic femoral fractures occurred out of 30,420 primary TKAs. A total of 11 (1.7%) of these 637 occurred after noncemented stems and 334 (1.1%) of 29,783 occurred after primary TKAs with cemented stems. After revision procedures, the postoperative periprosthetic femoral fracture rate was 97 (2.0%) of 4,749 with 96 (2.0%) of 4,688 fractures occurring after a cemented stem was placed, as opposed to only 1 (1.6%) fracture out of 61 noncemented stems.

2.3-2 Rate of intra- and postoperative periprosthetic fractures around primary and revision total knee arthroplasties (TKAs) at the Mayo Clinic, Rochester, MN, USA.*

Variables	Primary TKA fracture rate, No. (%)	Revision TKA fracture rate, No. (%)
Intraoperative		
Femur		
- Noncemented	0/637 (0)	0/61 (0)
- Cemented	88/29,783 (0.3)	74/4,688 (1.6)
- Total	88/30,420 (0,3)	74/4,749 (1.6)
Tibia		
- Noncemented	0/705 (0)	2/53 (3.8)
- Cemented	37/29,715 (0.12)	62/4,570 (1.4)
- Total	37/30,420 (0.12)	64/4,623 (1.4)
Patella		
- Noncemented	0/268 (0)	0/24 (0)
- Cemented	4/23,732 (0.02)	7/1,927 (0.4)
- Total	4/24,000 (0.02)	7/1,951 (0.4)
Postoperative		
Femur		
- Noncemented	11/637 (1.7)	1/61 (1.6)
- Cemented	334/29,783 (1.1)	96/4,688 (2.0)
- Total	345/30,420 (1.1)	97/4,749 (2.0)
Tibia		
- Noncemented	5/705 (0.7)	0/53 (0)
- Cemented	113/29,715 (0.4)	52/4,570 (1.1)
- Total	118/30,420 (0.4)	52/4,623 (1.1)
Patella		
- Noncemented	9/268 (3.4)	0/24 (0)
- Cemented	228/23,732 (1.0)	53/1,927 (2.8)
- Total	337/24,000 (1.4)	53/1,951 (2.7)

* Unpublished data.

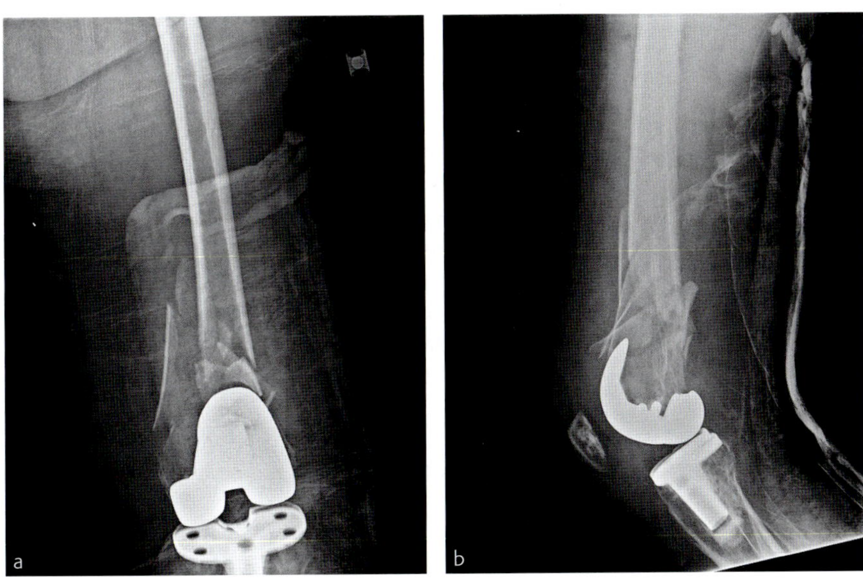

2.3-1a–b X-rays of a 71-year-old female patient with a left-sided periprosthetic distal femur fracture with a well-fixed femoral component after a motor vehicle injury (UCS type V.3-B1; Lewis and Rorabeck type II).
a AP view.
b Lateral view.

2.3.2 Tibial fractures

The incidence of periprosthetic fractures of the proximal tibia ranges from 0.3%–2.5% after primary TKAs and from 1.6% up to 38% after revision arthroplasty [60]. A recent study from the Scottish Arthroplasty Project [41] shows that patients undergoing revision TKA have a threefold higher risk to sustain a periprosthetic fracture around the knee than those having had a primary TKA. Moreover, age (> 70 years) and gender (women) seem to be additional risk factors. Patients aged ≥ 70 years were 1.6 times more likely to have a fracture after TKA than younger patients and women suffered 2.3 times more fractures after TKA than men [41].

Intraoperative fractures

Periprosthetic tibial fractures are the least common type of periprosthetic fracture around a TKA, with reported rates between 0.07% and 0.8% (**2.3-1**) [2, 43, 45, 61]. As previously noted, intraoperative fractures are less common than postoperative fractures, and fractures during primary procedures are less common than during revision procedures [2]. However, such fractures are likely to be underestimated [48, 49]. Of 102 tibial periprosthetic fractures, Felix et al noted 19 intraoperative fractures [43]. This corresponds to a total rate of 0.1% of 17,727 TKAs, with 0.07% pertaining to primary arthroplasties and 0.36% to revision arthroplasties. These fractures occurred at all stages of arthroplasty, including cement or prosthesis removal during revision (4), retraction on bone (1), preparation of the tibia (4), trial reduction (3), and seating of the component (5). In two cases the mechanism was unknown and the fractures were identified on postoperative survey films.

Berry [2] reported an intraoperative periprosthetic tibia fracture rate of 0.67% in 16,906 primary TKAs and 0.8% in revision TKAs. Of 67 intraoperative periprosthetic fractures reported, only 18 occurred in the tibia (0.1%) [47]. Location of the tibial fractures included the lateral plateau (6), anterior cortex (4), medial plateau (3), lateral cortex (3), medial cortex (1), and posterior cortex (1).

In the unpublished review of the entire Mayo Clinic experience, 37 intraoperative tibia fractures of 30,420 primary TKAs were identified, corresponding to a rate of 0.12% (**2.3-2**). All the fractures occurred during placement of cemented components (37 [0.12%] of 29,715). During revisions, the intraoperative fracture rate increased tenfold (64 [1.4%] of 4,623). Of these, two (3.8%) of 53 fractures occurred during placement of a component with a noncemented tibial stem, whereas 62 (1.4%) of 4,570 occurred in association with placement of a component with a cemented stem.

Postoperative fractures

While tibial fractures are certainly the least common periprosthetic fracture, they occur more commonly in the postoperative period (**2.3-1**). In a review [56], only 32 postoperative periprosthetic tibia fractures had been cited in nine reports between 1970 and 1972. Rand and Coventry [62] identified 15 medial tibial stress fractures occurring at an average of 45 months after arthroplasty. Berry [2] reported a 0.4% rate of tibial fractures following primary procedures, but nearly twice that in revision procedures (0.9%). Felix et al found a 0.4% rate of postoperative fracture in 17,727 TKAs, with revision surgery also serving as a risk factor (0.39% versus 0.48%, respectively) [43]. Of the 102 periprosthetic tibial fractures, 61 were type I; 22 were type II; 17 were type III; and 2 were type IV.

The most recent Mayo Clinic data revealed that 118 (0.4%) postoperative periprosthetic tibial fractures occurred out of 30,420 primary TKAs. Five (0.7%) of 705 fractures occurred after noncemented implants and 113 (0.4%) of 29,715 occurred after primary TKAs with a cemented stem. After revision procedures, the postoperative periprosthetic tibial fracture rate was 52 (1.1%) of 4,623. All fractures occurred after placement of a cemented tibial component (52 [1.1%] of 4,570).

2.3.3 Patellar fractures

Intraoperative and postoperative fractures

Periprosthetic patellar fractures are more common than periprosthetic tibial fractures but less common than those occurring in the femur, with reported rates ranging from 0.05–21% (**2.3-1**) [2, 43, 45, 61]. Patella fractures can occur with resurfaced or nonresurfaced patellae. The prevalence of patellar fractures is between 0.2% and 21% in resurfaced patellae, while it is approximately 0.05% in nonresurfaced patellae [2, 48, 61, 63–69]. Berry [2] found no intraoperative patella fractures during primary TKAs but registered 8 during 2,904 revision procedures (0.2%). In the same series, there were 117 (0.7%) postoperative fractures following primary procedures and 53 (1.8%) following revision procedures.

When comparing the incidence of patellar fractures between primary and revision TKAs, Ortiguera and Berry found that periprosthetic patellar fractures were fivefold higher in revision procedures (0.61% versus 0.12%, respectively) [70]. Of these, 44% presented asymptomatically and most occurred within 1–2 years after the index arthroplasty. In another Mayo Clinic series of 1,000 cemented condylar TKAs, Vessely et al found a 2.0% rate of patellar periprosthetic fractures [59]. Unlike femoral fractures, most (15 of 20) patella fractures occurred postoperatively, within the first 5 years.

In a recent systematic review of the literature, a 1.19% rate of periprosthetic patellar fractures in primary cases, with the range being 0.15–12% for revision procedures, was noted [61]. The vast majority (99.1%) occurred in patellae that were resurfaced, with 88.3% occurring without any known trauma.

In an unpublished review of the entire Mayo Clinic experience, 4 (0.02%) intraoperative patella fractures of 24,000 primary TKAs were identified (**2.3-2**). All the fractures occurred during placement of cemented components. During revisions, the intraoperative fracture rate was twentyfold higher: 7 (0.4%) of 1,951. All occurred during placement of a cemented patella.

In regard to postoperative periprosthetic patella fractures, the most recent Mayo Clinic data revealed 337 (1.4%) fractures of 24,000 primary TKAs. Of these, 9 (3.4%) of 268 occurred with noncemented patellae and 228 (1.0%) occurred with 23,732 cemented patellae. After revision procedures, the postoperative periprosthetic patella fracture rate was 53 (2.7%) of 1,951. All fractures occurred after placement of a cemented patellar component.

2.4 Shoulder, elbow, wrist, and ankle

Authors Matthew P Abdel, Daniel J Berry

Similar to fractures surrounding total hip and knee arthroplasties, periprosthetic fractures may occur around any joint that is replaced, including the shoulder, elbow, wrist, and ankle. Moreover, such fractures can occur intraoperatively or postoperatively. The incidence of postoperative periprosthetic humeral fractures associated with shoulder arthroplasty is approximately 0.6–3% [71]. Wright and Cofield [72] noted a periprosthetic fracture rate of 9 (1.8%) of 499 shoulder arthroplasties. While less common, intraoperative fractures of the humerus may also occur. Athwal and Cofield reported on 45 (1.5%) intraoperative humeral fractures of 3,088 shoulder arthroplasties [73]. The authors identified female gender, revision surgery, and press-fit implants as significant risk factors.

The literature describing periprosthetic fractures surrounding total ankle arthroplasties (TAAs) is extremely limited for various reasons. Some authors estimate the prevalence of such fractures around TAAs to be approximately 5%, with nearly all fractures occurring around the tibial component [74]. Risk factors seem to include osteoporosis and inflammatory arthropathies [74–76].

Similarly, the literature about wrist arthroplasties is also rather limited and is discussed in chapter 6.3.

2.5 Conclusions

Authors **Matthew P Abdel, Daniel J Berry**

Periprosthetic fractures involving both hip and knee arthroplasties are increasing in prevalence for a variety of reasons. The incidence of periprosthetic fractures is highest in elderly women with poor bone quality and stock, who are undergoing revision procedures. Risk factors for periprosthetic fractures vary according to anatomical site but include factors related to the host, operative technique, and implants.

References

[1] **Kurtz S, Ong K, Lau E, et al.** Projections of primary and revision hip and knee arthroplasty in the United States from 2005 to 2030. *J Bone Joint Surg Am.* 2007 Apr;89(4):780–785.

[2] **Berry DJ.** Epidemiology: hip and knee. *Orthop Clin North Am.* 1999 Apr;30(2):183–190.

[3] **Garbuz DS, Masri BA, Duncan CP.** Periprosthetic fractures of the femur: principles of prevention and management. *Instr Course Lect.* 1998;47:237–342.

[4] **Lewallen DG, Berry DJ.** Periprosthetic fracture of the femur after total hip arthroplasty: treatment and results to date. *Instr Course Lect.* 1998;47:243–249.

[5] **Younger AS, Dunwoody J, Duncan CP.** Periprosthetic hip and knee fractures: the scope of the problem. *Instr Course Lect.* 1998;47:251–256.

[6] **Lindahl H, Malchau H, Herberts P, et al.** Periprosthetic femoral fractures classification and demographics of 1049 periprosthetic femoral fractures from the Swedish National Hip Arthroplasty Register. *J Arthroplasty.* 2005 Oct;20(7):857–865.

[7] **Haddad FS, Masri BA, Garbuz DS, et al.** The prevention of periprosthetic fractures in total hip and knee arthroplasty. *Orthop Clin North Am.* 1999 Apr;30(2):191–207.

[8] **Learmonth ID.** The management of periprosthetic fractures around the femoral stem. *J Bone Joint Surg Br.* 2004 Jan;86(1):13–19.

[9] **Park MS, Lim YJ, Chung WC, et al.** Management of periprosthetic femur fractures treated with distal fixation using a modular femoral stem using an anterolateral approach. *J Arthroplasty.* 2009 Dec;24(8):1270–1276.

[10] **Cook RE, Jenkins PJ, Walmsley PJ, et al.** Risk factors for periprosthetic fractures of the hip: a survivorship analysis. *Clin Orthop Relat Res.* 2008 Jul;466(7):1652–1656.

[11] **Lindahl H, Oden A, Garellick G, Malchau H.** The excess mortality due to periprosthetic femur fracture. A study from the Swedish national hip arthroplasty register. *Bone.* 2007 May;40(5):1294–1298.

[12] **Schmidt AH, Kyle RF.** Periprosthetic fractures of the femur. *Orthop Clin North Am.* 2002 Jan;33(1):143–152.

[13] **Sharkey PF, Hozack WJ, Callaghan JJ, et al.** Acetabular fracture associated with cementless acetabular component insertion: a report of 13 cases. *J Arthroplasty.* 1999 Jun;14(4):426–431.

[14] **McElfresh EC, Coventry MB.** Femoral and pelvic fractures after total hip arthroplasty. *J Bone Joint Surg Am.* 1974 Apr;56(3):483–492.

[15] **McGrory BJ.** Periprosthetic fracture of the acetabulum during total hip arthroplasty in a patient with Paget's disease. *Am J Orthop (Belle Mead NJ).* 1999 Apr;28(4):248–250.

[16] **Desai G, Ries MD.** Early postoperative acetabular discontinuity after total hip arthroplasty. *J Arthroplasty.* 2011 Dec;26(8):1570.e17–9.

[17] **Miller AJ.** Late fracture of the acetabulum after total hip replacement. *J Bone Joint Surg Br.* 1972 Nov;54(4):600–606.

[18] **Peterson CA, Lewallen DG.** Periprosthetic fracture of the acetabulum after total hip arthroplasty. *J Bone Joint Surg Am.* 1996 Aug;78(8):1206–1213.

[19] **Harvie P, Gundle R, Willett K.** Traumatic periprosthetic acetabular fracture: life threatening haemorrhage and a novel method of acetabular reconstruction. *Injury.* 2004 Aug;35(8):819–822.

[20] **Old AB, McGrory BJ, Peterson CA 2nd, et al.** Locked inferior fracture dislocation after total hip arthroplasty. *J Arthroplasty.* 2008 Feb;23(2):308–310.

[21] **Woolson ST.** Acetabular component migration following traumatic total hip dislocation. A case report. *Clin Orthop Relat Res.* 1984 Jun;(186):42–44.

[22] **Gelalis ID, Politis AN, Arnaoutoglou CM, et al.** Traumatic periprosthetic acetabular fracture treated by acute one-stage revision arthroplasty. A case report and review of the literature. *Injury.* 2010 Apr;41(4):421–424.

[23] **Sánchez-Sotelo J, McGrory BJ, Berry DJ.** Acute periprosthetic fracture of the acetabulum associated with osteolytic pelvic lesions: a report of 3 cases. *J Arthroplasty.* 2000 Jan;15(1):126–130.

[24] **Andrews P, Barrack RL, Harris WH.** Stress fracture of the medial wall of the acetabulum adjacent to a cementless acetabular component. *J Arthroplasty.* 2002 Jan;17(1):117–120.

[25] **Chatoo M, Parfitt J, Pearse MF.** Periprosthetic acetabular fracture associated with extensive osteolysis. *J Arthroplasty.* 1998 Oct;13(7):843–845.

[26] **Berry DJ, Lewallen DG, Hanssen AD, et al.** Pelvic discontinuity in revision total hip arthroplasty. *J Bone Joint Surg Am.* 1999 Dec;81(12):1692–1702.

[27] **Löwenhielm G, Hansson LI, Kärrholm J.** Fracture of the lower extremity after total hip replacement. *Arch Orthop Trauma Surg.* 1989;108(3):141–143.

[28] **Lindahl H.** Epidemiology of periprosthetic femur fracture around a total hip arthroplasty. *Injury.* 2007 Jun;38(6):651–654.

[29] **Taylor MM, Meyers MH, Harvey JP Jr.** Intraoperative femur fractures during total hip replacement. *Clin Orthop Relat Res.* 1978(137):96–103.

[30] **Schwartz JT Jr, Mayer JG, Engh CA.** Femoral fracture during non-cemented total hip arthroplasty. *J Bone Joint Surg Am.* 1989 Sep;71(8):1135–1142.

[31] **Khan MA, O'Driscoll M.** Fractures of the femur during total hip replacement and their management. *J Bone Joint Surg Br.* 1977;59-1:36–41.

[32] **Scott RD, Turner RH, Leitzes SM, et al.** Femoral fractures in conjunction with total hip replacement. *J Bone Joint Surg Am.* 1975 Jun;57(4):494–501.

[33] **Johansson JE, McBroom R, Barrington TW, et al.** Fracture of the ipsilateral femur in patients with total hip replacement. *J Bone Joint Surg Am.* 1981 Dec;63(9):1435–1442.

[34] **Christensen CM, Seger BM, Schultz RB.** Management of intraoperative femur fractures associated with revision hip arthroplasty. *Clin Orthop Relat Res.* 1989 Nov;(248):177–80.

[35] **Fitzgerald RH Jr, Brindley GW, Kavanagh BF.** The uncemented total hip arthroplasty. Intraoperative femoral fractures. *Clin Orthop Relat Res.* 1988 Oct;(235):61–66.

[36] **Morrey BF, Kavanagh BF.** Complications with revision of the femoral component of total hip arthroplasty. Comparison between cemented and uncemented techniques. *J Arthroplasty.* 1992 Mar;7(1):71–79.

[37] **Lindahl H, Garellick G, Regnér H, et al.** Three hundred and twenty-one periprosthetic femoral fractures. *J Bone Joint Surg Am.* 2006 Jun;88(6):1215–1222.

[38] **Kavanagh BF.** Femoral fractures associated with total hip arthroplasty. *Orthop Clin North Am.* 1992 Apr;23(2):249–257.

[39] **Taunton MJ, Berry DJ.** Early postoperative femur fracture after uncemented primarty total hip arthroplasty. *Unpublished.* 2011.

[40] **Park MS, Lee YK, Yang KH, et al.** Management of periprosthetic femoral fractures. *J Arthroplasty.* 2003 Oct;18(7):903–906.

[41] **Meek RM, Norwood T, Smith R, et al.** The risk of peri-prosthetic fracture after primary and revision total hip and knee replacement. *J Bone Joint Surg Br.* 2011 Jan;93(1):96–101.

[42] **McGraw P, Kumar A.** Periprosthetic fractures of the femur after total knee arthroplasty. *J Orthop Traumatol.* 2010 Sep;11(3):135–141.

[43] **Felix NA, Stuart MJ, Hanssen AD.** Periprosthetic fractures of the tibia associated with total knee arthroplasty. *Clin Orthop Relat Res.* 1997 Dec;(345):113–124.

[44] **Kim KI, Egol KA, Hozack WJ, et al.** Periprosthetic fractures after total knee arthroplasties. *Clin Orthop Relat Res.* 2006 May;446:167–175.

[45] **Platzer P, Schuster R, Aldrian S, et al.** Management and outcome of periprosthetic fractures after total knee arthroplasty. *Trauma.* 2010 Jun;68(6):1464–1470.

[46] **Su ET, DeWal H, Di Cesare PE.** Periprosthetic femoral fractures above total knee replacements. *J Am Acad Orthop Surg.* 2004 Jan-Feb;12(1):12–20.

[47] **Alden KJ, Duncan WH, Trousdale RT, et al.** Intraoperative fracture during primary total knee arthroplasty. *Clin Orthop Relat Res.* 2010 Jan;468(1):90–95.

[48] **Parvizi J, Jain N, Schmidt AH.** Periprosthetic knee fractures. *J Orthop Trauma.* 2008 Oct;22(9):663–671.

[49] **Engh GA, Ammeen DJ.** Periprosthetic fractures adjacent to total knee implants: treatment and clinical results. *Instr Course Lect.* 1998;47:437–448.

[50] **Lombardi AV Jr, Mallory TH, Waterman RA, et al.** Intercondylar distal femoral fracture. An unreported complication of posterior-stabilized total knee arthroplasty. *J Arthroplasty.* 1995 Oct;10(5):643–650.

[51] **Culp RW, Schmidt RG, Hanks G, et al.** Supracondylar fracture of the femur following prosthetic knee arthroplasty. *Clin Orthop Relat Res.* 1987 Sep;(222):212–222.

[52] **Delport PH, Van Audekercke R, Martens M, et al.** Conservative treatment of ipsilateral supracondylar femoral fracture after total knee arthroplasty. *J Trauma.* 1984 Sep;24(9):846–849.

[53] **Figgie MP, Goldberg VM, Figgie HE 3rd, et al.** The results of treatment of supracondylar fracture above total knee arthroplasty. *J Arthroplasty.* 1990 Sep;5(3):267–276.

[54] **Rorabeck CH, Taylor JW.** Periprosthetic fractures of the femur complicating total knee arthroplasty. *Orthop Clin North Am.* 1999 Apr;30(2):265–277.

[55] **Ritter MA, Thong AE, Keating EM, et al.** The effect of femoral notching during total knee arthroplasty on the prevalence of postoperative femoral fractures and on clinical outcome. *J Bone Joint Surg Am.* 2005 Nov;87(11):2411–2414.

[56] **Healy WL, Siliski JM, Incavo SJ.** Operative treatment of distal femoral fractures proximal to total knee replacements. *J Bone Joint Surg Am.* 1993 Jan;75(1):27–34.

[57] **Inglis AE, Walker PS.** Revision of failed knee replacements using fixed-axis hinges. *J Bone Joint Surg Br.* 1991 Sep;73(5):757–761.

[58] **Mortazavi SM, Kurd MF, Bender B, et al.** Distal femoral arthroplasty for the treatment of periprosthetic fractures after total knee arthroplasty. *J Arthroplasty.* 2010 Aug;25(5):775–780.

[59] **Vessely MB, Whaley AL, Harmsen WS, et al.** The Chitranjan Ranawat Award: Long-term survivorship and failure modes of 1000 cemented condylar total knee arthroplasties. *Clin Orthop Relat Res.* 2006 Nov;452:28–34.

[60] **Schrøder HM, Berthelsen A, Hassani G, et al.** Cementless Porous-coated total knee arthroplasty: 10-year results in a consecutive series. *J Arthroplasty.* 2001 Aug;16(5):559–567.

[61] **Chalidis BE, Tsiridis E, Tragas AA, et al.** Management of periprosthetic patellar fractures. A systematic review of literature. *Injury.* 2007 Jun;38(6):714–724.

[62] **Rand JA, Coventry MB.** Stress fractures after total knee arthroplasty. *J Bone Joint Surg Am.* 1980 Mar;62(2):226–233.

[63] **Bourne RB.** Fractures of the patella after total knee replacement. *Orthop Clin North Am.* 1999 Apr;30(2):287–291.

[64] **Boyd AD Jr, Ewald FC, Thomas WH, et al.** Long-term complications after total knee arthroplasty with or without resurfacing of the patella. *J Bone Joint Surgery Am.* 1993 May;75(5):674–681.

[65] **Goldberg VM, Figgie HE 3rd, Inglis AE, et al.** Patellar fracture type and prognosis in condylar total knee arthroplasty. *Clin Orthop Relat Res.* 1988 Nov;(236):115–122.

[66] **Grace JN, Sim FH.** Fracture of the patella after total knee arthroplasty. *Clin Orthop Relat Res.* 1988 May;(230):168–175.

[67] **Scott RD, Turoff N, Ewald FC.** Stress fracture of the patella following duopatellar total knee arthroplasty with patellar resurfacing. *Clin Orthop Relat Res.* 1982 Oct;(170):147–151.

[68] **Tria AJ Jr, Harwood DA, Alicea JA, et al.** Patellar fractures in posterior stabilized knee arthroplasties. *Clin Orthop Relat Res.* 1994 Feb;(299):131–138.

[69] **Windsor RE, Scuderi GR, Insall JN.** Patellar fractures in total knee arthroplasty. *J Arthroplasty.* 1989;4 Suppl:S63–67.

[70] **Ortiguera CJ, Berry DJ.** Patellar fracture after total knee arthroplasty. *J Bone Joint Surgery Am.* 2002 Apr;84-A(4):532–540.

[71] **Steinmann SP, Cheung EV.** Treatment of periprosthetic humerus fractures associated with shoulder arthroplasty. *J Am Acad Orthop Surg.* 2008 Apr;16(4):199–207.

[72] **Wright TW, Cofield RH.** Humeral fractures after shoulder arthroplasty. *J Bone Joint Surg Am.* 1995 Sep;77(9):1340–1346.

[73] **Athwal GS, Sperling JW, Rispoli DM, et al.** Periprosthetic humeral fractures during shoulder arthroplasty. *J Bone Joint Surg Am.* 2009 Mar;91(3):594–603.

[74] **Doets HC, Brand R, Nelissen RG.** Total ankle arthroplasty in inflammatory joint disease with use of two mobile-bearing designs. *J Bone Joint Surg Am.* 2006 Jun;88(6):1272–1284.

[75] **Haendlmayer KT, Fazly FM, Harris NJ.** Periprosthetic fracture after total ankle replacement: surgical technique. *Foot Ankle Int.* 2009 Dec;30(12):1233–1234.

[76] **Yang JH, Kim HJ, Yoon JR, et al.** Minimally invasive plate osteosynthesis (MIPO) for periprosthetic fracture after total ankle arthroplasty: a case report. *Foot Ankle Int.* 2011 Feb;32(2):200–204.

3

Causes of and risk factors for periprosthetic fractures

3.1 Age

Authors Katrin Singler, Cornel C Sieber

3.1.1 Orthogeriatric patients with a periprosthetic fracture

Due to the demographic shift within an increasingly aging population, surgeons will be seeing more and more elderly patients with fractures, especially fragility fractures.

Geriatric patients are characterized not only by their higher chronological age (internationally > 65 years) but mainly by their biological age. Higher age often goes hand in hand with osteopenia and sarcopenia (loss of bone and muscle mass) as well as with polymorbidity and subsequent intake of different medications. Polymorbidity means that different chronic conditions exist, such as diabetes mellitus, and that there may also be acute exacerbation of problems linked to trauma. Furthermore, challenges such as thromboembolism, perioperative anemia as well as postoperative mental disorders have to be considered. This is especially true for fragility fractures. The trauma surgeon is, therefore, confronted not only with a broken bone but also with all perioperative problems associated with old age.

3.1.2 Treatment goals in elderly patients

The main aim in treating elderly, more vulnerable patients with a trauma is to prevent a decline of function followed by loss of independence and finally a drop in quality of life. Altogether, a well-orchestrated multidisciplinary approach and understanding of elderly people with fractures will result in improved outcome. Orthogeriatrics is becoming a new specialty.

3.1.3 Preoperative assessment in elderly patients

The preoperative evaluation of a geriatric patient is a crucial step in the future outcome and includes a series of assessments (see chapter 5.2).

One of the key instruments to cover the diversity of elderly people with trauma is the so-called "Comprehensive Geriatric Assessment," (CGA) which includes not only physical but also mental and social aspects of elderly people [1].

Moreover, there are the so-called four "geriatric giants" that surgeons should be familiar with when treating elderly trauma patients:
- Instability
- Immobility
- Incontinence
- Intellectual decline.

Recently, three new items have been added to the list:
- Iatrogenic problems
- Isolation
- Inappetence.

The preoperative assessment of a geriatric patient requires a subtle balance between choosing the essential tests and examinations with the subsequent delay of surgery, which is usually not tolerated as well as in younger patients. Previous medication and the nutritional status together with the patient's preoperative mental status and cognition will determine the postoperative outcome.

Special attention should be given to cardiovascular drugs such as beta-blockers. Pulmonary medication for chronic obstructive pulmonary disease (COPD) should be restarted early after surgery. If corticosteroids are involved, the risk of postoperative adrenal insufficiency must be considered. Diabetes mellitus is the most frequent comorbidity beside arterial hypertension in the elderly, who are prone to hyperglycemic as well as hypoglycemic episodes. With regard to neurological medication, drugs against Parkinson's disease should be given on the morning of surgery and as soon as possible postoperatively. Any antidepressant therapy should also be continued soon postoperatively. Anemia is common in elderly people. Typically, hemoglobin of 9–10 g/dL is considered the minimum level to safely undertake surgery while the electrolytes, platelet count, and coagulation parameters must always be checked. A hidden renal insufficiency with a creatinine level above 2 mg/dL is often accompanied by increased postoperative cardiovascular problems.

To summarize, the important aspects to be checked are:

- Anemia
- Platelets/coagulation
- Metabolic disorders
- Any cardiovascular disease
- Any pulmonary disease
- Diabetes mellitus
- Renal insufficiency
- Malnutrition
- Parkinson's disease
- Neurological disorders
- Polymedication.

Many elderly people have given advance directives about any life support. Patients should be asked and, if they are not able to answer themselves, family members or the family physician should be consulted.

3.1.4 Frailty syndrome

Definition

Frailty has been defined in various ways. It is generally accepted that the frailty syndrome is characterized by an increased vulnerability to external and internal stress factors due to impairment of multiple, interrelated physiological systems. This vulnerability leads to a decline in homeostatic reserve and resilience and implies an increased risk for different adverse health-related problems.

Manifestation

Two main phenotypes of frailty are the "physical" and the "multi-aspect" phenotype.

The physical phenotype is a more one-dimensional concept and most frequently used. It was described by Linda Fried and colleagues [2]. In the physical phenotype, the concept is shaped by clusters of physical impairments, whereas non-physical components are not considered. Criteria include "shrinking" (weight loss), sarcopenia, weakness, exhaustion (poor endurance), slowness, and reduced activity.

The multi-aspect phenotype is characterized by a multifaceted concept, including—in addition to physical components—aspects such as mood, cognition, sensory impairment, chronic diseases, disabilities and social conditions. There is strong evidence that the inclusion of these additional components can be very important [3]. For example, by only looking at the physical criterion of weight loss, prevailing frailty may be underestimated in the obese.

Pathogenesis

Several pathophysiological processes are related to the development of frailty. A predominant role has been attributed to inflammatory mechanisms. Increased C-reactive protein (CRP) values and proinflammatory cytokines are associated with the presence of frailty. In particular, an increase in IL-6 levels repeatedly showed a close association with an increased risk of frailty.

A series of studies have concentrated on the relationship between nutrition and frailty. It was shown that frailty was significantly associated with a daily energy intake below 21 kcal/kg bodyweight as well as a low protein intake. Deficits of micronutrient levels (eg, vitamin B12, D, and E) are considered to be linked to reduced functionality and/or frailty. Changes in body composition, especially a relative and absolute increase in body fat, may be seen as another important aspect in the pathogenesis of frailty. Frail individuals are characterized by higher weight, more truncal obesity, higher insulin resistance and a greater probability for metabolic syndrome. Finally, it appears that sarcopenia plays a central role in this concept [4].

The relationship between frailty and a wide spectrum of clinical diseases like coronary heart disease, Parkinson's disease, stroke, Alzheimer's disease, and venous thromboembolism have been described.

3.1.5 Sarcopenia

Definition

The term "sarcopenia" was coined in the late 1980s in an attempt to increase awareness of age-related muscle loss and its devastating effects on the physical activity and independence of the elderly. Several international consensus conferences were held on this topic, of which the most recent were of particular significance [4, 5]. Muscle mass is an important—but not the only—predictor of muscle strength. It is likely that increased body fat decreases the capacity to generate power (force x speed) and muscle power is more closely related to functional capacity than muscle strength. In addition, increased body fat and age have been associated with increased intramuscular lipid and reduced muscle quality, defined as reduced strength/cross-sectional area. The definition of sarcopenia, therefore, encompasses both the loss of muscle mass and the decline in muscle functionality (eg, gait speed).

Significance

Increasing age is accompanied by several degenerative processes that are superimposed by conditions and illnesses accumulated in the course of life. Apart from diseases often considered as comorbidities that necessitate the intake of multiple drugs, cognitive problems, muscular dysfunction and the tendency to lose one's balance are the hallmarks that threaten an independent lifestyle in older age. While a lot of attention has been paid to osteoporosis during the past decades, the cornerstones of frailty, ie, fatigue, weakness, and reduced physical activity, which clinically point to sarcopenia, require much more attention.

Incidence

The prevalence of sarcopenia in the elderly varies according to the classification used (10–50%). Studies in populations of elderly people using more direct estimates found a value of 12% for people 60–70 years of age and nearly 30% for people older than 80 years. Janssen et al [6], using the large cohort from NHANES III, found the prevalence of sarcopenia (-2SD) in people 60 years and older to be 7–10%.

Pathogenesis

Sarcopenia is a universal phenomenon with a complex, multi-factorial etiology, starting at about the age of 50 years. The major factors playing a causal role are:

- Decreased physical activity
- Age-related endocrine and metabolic dysfunction
- Malnutrition and malabsorbtion
- Neurodegenerative diseases.

The latter are discussed in this section.

Decreased physical activity as a consequence of aging is a principal cause of sarcopenia. The relationship between skeletal muscle mass and the degree of physical activity is complex. Reduced physical activity alters body composition in a number of ways. Muscle mass is decreased while body-fat mass is increased. The loss of bone stock (osteopenia) and sarcopenia are closely linked and directly affected by the degree of physical activity especially in pre and post-menopausal women and in older men. The rate of muscle wasting is accelerated by forced bed rest due to illness. Elderly people are the most likely to be placed on bed rest because of illness, trauma, loss of balance, or increasingly because of a greatly diminished functional capacity. Often, the most frail and medically compromised individuals are on bed rest for devastatingly long periods of time.

Recent studies demonstrate that in older people a prolonged period of bed rest is followed by a far greater loss of skeletal muscle mass than in young people. This muscle-wasting effect due to bed rest is associated with considerably reduced strength and loss of physical activity.

Metabolic changes associated with malnutrition may be caused by a physiological loss of appetite of the aging person (reduced olfactory and taste sensation as well as increased satiating hormones, such as cholecystokinine) or anorexia due to mental depression.

In older people, weight loss results in an increased rate of loss of lean muscle mass. While the rate of muscle protein synthesis is reduced—probably as a result of lower levels of anabolic hormones, such as testosterone, growth hormones, or increased insulin resistance—older, frail people have an increased need for protein (1.0–1.2 g protein per kilogram body weight per day) compared with young people (0.8 g protein per kilogram body weight per day). There also seems to be a correlation between low levels of 25-hydroxyvitamin D (< 30 ng/mL) and the loss of muscle mass and strength, the tendency to fall, and reduction of function [7]. In a longitudinal study of the aging, a low vitamin D status was independently associated with sarcopenia and reduced muscle strength. In addition, in older people with low vitamin D levels, vitamin D replacement improved strength and function, and decreased falls.

Metabolic syndromes are present in approximately 50% of older people, both in the community and in nursing homes. Diabetes mellitus in the elderly has been associated with a decrease in strength, a decline in functional status, and an increase in falls. Increasing body fat, associated with advancing age can also result in increases in proinflammatory cytokines that can directly affect skeletal muscle protein metabolism by stimulating protein degradation.

The proinflammatory cytokines, such as TNF-alpha and IL-6, are associated with muscle loss, decreased strength, and functional deterioration. While a large excess of cytokines, as occurs with cancer or acute infections, may be responsible for the classic signs of cachexia, ie, muscle wasting, lipolysis, hypoalbuminemia, anorexia, and anemia, a lower cytokine excess is so common in older people that IL-6 has become known as the "geriatric cytokine." It has been suggested that there is a cytokine-related aging process, in which cytokines accelerate the rate of aging predominantly by muscle degradation and also by apoptosis.

Atherosclerosis is an almost universal phenomenon in the blood vessels of aging humans and can also lead to sarcopenia. Severe atherosclerosis in the lower limbs results in peripheral arterial disease (PAD) with classic clinical symptoms. PAD of the lower extremities has been reported to occur in as many as 20–30% of older patients. PAD is associated with a loss of muscle mass, decreased strength, and impaired ability to walk. Muscle biopsy studies have suggested that PAD leads to a decrease in the fiber area and proportion of type I muscle fibers as well as a reduction in capillaries in each muscle fiber.

With aging, there is also a loss of motor units in the spinal cord and a decrease in the number of functioning motor units. This progressive denervation plays an important role in the development of sarcopenia. There is a greater loss in fast-twitch fibers which, in part, is compensated by reinnervation by axonal sprouting from slow-twitch motor neurons. Older people have decreased motor-unit discharge rates, however, over six weeks of resistance exercise results in a percentual increase in discharge, compared with younger people. This clearly demonstrates the need for physical exercise even in the frailest elderly people.

Assessment

The measurement of muscle mass in humans is mostly carried out indirectly. The most frequently used and recommended method is the dual-energy x-ray absorption technique (DEXA), but its availability may differ from country to country. Bioelectric impedance analysis (BIA) is a simple, noninvasive and easily performed bedside analysis of body composition. BIA works mainly through the measurement of the body's resistance and reactance to an alternative electrical current and the calculation of Fat-Free Mass (FFM), with predictive equations. Although BIA measurements have limitations in elderly patients due to rapid changes in fluid balance, they are considered to suffice for body-composition analysis. Most indirect measures of fat-free mass incorrectly assume that skeletal muscle remains a constant component of 60% of the fat-free mass. Thus, some authors use only appendicular skeletal mass and correct this for height. Recent studies have demonstrated that not only is muscle mass reduced with advancing age but the quality of muscle may also change [8–12]. Skeletal muscle lipid, assessed by computed tomography, increases with advancing age and contributes to total body fatness. Data shows persistent effects of sarcopenia on strength and functional status as well as the changing quality of skeletal muscle in late life.

Prevention and treatment

Prevention and treatment of sarcopenia always is a combination of physical activity and nutritional intervention. Adequate protein supplementation is often necessary, including protein supplements between meals to meet the daily demands of 1.0–1.2 g of protein per kilogram body weight per day. If caloric intake is below 1,200 kcal per day, one also has to anticipate deficits in micronutrient supply.

Physical exercise should include endurance training. To reduce the risk of falls, power training—the fast development of force—may prove to be even more efficient. It should be stressed once again that muscle mass per se does not directly correlate with muscle strength, which is why the present definition of sarcopenia combines muscle-mass measurement with a functional test. For instance, gait speed with a threshold of < 1 m/s will predict bad outcome.

Disability and mortality as consequences

Sarcopenia is highly correlated with functional decline, disability, and a tendency for falls. Even among middle-aged women (age 34–58 years) almost 9% experience a loss of around 2.5 kg of muscle mass over a 3-year period, which is strongly related to compromised functional capacity. Sarcopenia has also been associated with increased mortality, with weakness as a demonstrably more powerful predictor of mortality in elderly people than the loss of muscle mass.

3.1.6 Malnutrition

Definition

Malnutrition is a condition in which the body does not receive the right amount of nutrients, vitamins, or minerals to maintain its health and organ function.

Incidence and impact of malnutrition

Malnutrition is common in geriatric patients, with two-thirds of the elderly having a prevalence of hidden or overt malnutrition [13]. Overall, protein malnutrition is significant in clinical outcome. After hip fractures, for example, it leads to a worsened outcome, including surgical complications such as impaired wound healing, decubitus ulcers, infections followed by a prolonged postoperative recovery, and an increased rate of mortality [14]. Often, the energy intake during the postoperative period is reduced and the patient's nutritional and functional status deteriorates. Beside poor nutritional intake, other causes for reduced food intake are dental and swallowing problems, depression, pain, and cognitive problems.

Assessment

Screening and, where needed, assessment of malnutrition is vital for the treatment of geriatric patients with fragility fractures. The Mini Nutritional Assessment (MNA) is a short and valid nutritional screening tool for community living as well as for elderly people in acute-care hospitals or long-term care. The MNA covers geriatric-specific items related to nutritional and health conditions, independence, quality of life, cognition, mobility, and subjective health. Recently, the short form with six questions has been reanalyzed and adapted to cases, in which the Body Mass Index (BMI) is not available and can be replaced by calf circumference (CC) (**3.1-1**). A calf circumference of < 31 cm is an indicator of malnutrition/sarcopenia **[15]**. This holds true for people both globally and from different social backgrounds. The MNA short form only requires five minutes and can be adapted and included as part of the comprehensive geriatric assessment (CGA). The test can be carried out by nurse practitioners and other professional groups primarily working on orthogeriatric wards.

Prevention and treatment

Improving food intake in hospitalized elderly patients should be a multidisciplinary effort. Treatable causes of malnutrition, such as pain or delirium, must be detected and addressed. Mobilization of patients and taking meals in a group of patients not only helps to improve socialization but can also lead to an increase in food intake. Oral food intake should be facilitated by the arrangement of meals, providing drinks and snacks in between the main meals, and a comfortable atmosphere.

A	Appetite loss	0–2 p
B	Weight loss	0–3 p
C	Mobility	0–2 p
D	Acute disease	0 or 2 p
D	Depression/ dementia	0–2 p

BMI available?		
F1	BMI < 19	0 p
	19 ≤ BMI < 21	1 p
	21 ≤ BMI < 23	2 p
	BMI ≥ 23	3 p

CC available?		
F2	CC < 31 cm	0 p
	CC ≥ 31 cm	3 p

12–14 p	well nourished
8–11 p	at risk
0–7 p	malnourished

3.1-1 The new Mini Nutritional Assessment Test (MNA-SF) modified according to Kaiser et al [15].

If malnutrition is detected, food supplying a high amount of energy should be offered. Protein intake can be supplemented by liquid oral nutritional supplements between meals.

3.1.7 Osteoporosis

Definition

The definition of osteoporosis as well as the need for specific prevention and treatment strategies is detailed in the regularly updated guidelines of the International Osteoporosis Foundation (IOF). The specific risk for a fracture occurring within the next 10 years can easily be calculated using the FRAX (WHO Fracture Risk Assessment Tool) score as a fast screening tool.

When bone density—measured both at the level of the lumbar spine and the femoral neck—is below a threshold provided by a reference value taken from young adults, this is either referred to as osteopenia (T-score -1.0–2.5) or osteoporosis (T-score > -2.5).

Significance

The major problem associated with osteoporosis is the risk of fragility fractures resulting from low-energy trauma or, typically, falls (eg, hip fractures).

Fractures of osteoporotic bones in the elderly are the most frequent and cumbersome burdens for both patients as well as healthcare resource utilities. Hip fractures in octogenarians, for example, often lead to loss of functionality and, consequently, to loss of independence. Fracture-related costs are, therefore, also increased by the frequent need for institutionalization of elderly (multimorbid) patients.

Pathogenesis

Bone density peaks at about 40 years and then steadily declines. This decline is not only seen in females (especially postmenopausal) but also in males, the only difference is that in males it starts about 10 years later.

Assessment

Bone density is usually measured by osteodensitometry (DEXA, T-score). For details, refer to chapter 4.1.

Prevention and treatment

Preventive strategies are partly the same as for sarcopenia, ie, a balanced, protein-rich diet as well as regular physical exercise. In addition, a daily total intake of 1,000 mg of calcium is recommended. In Europe, most people consume adequate amounts of dairy products and, thus, will maximally need 500 mg of supplemental calcium. In addition, vitamin D in these elderly people is most often clearly below a level of 75 nmol/L (30 ng/mL), significantly increasing the risk for fragility fractures. The recommendations, therefore, advise at least 800 IU vitamin D supplementation per day [16]. In future, this recommended dose will most probably be raised to 2,000 IU per day (based on several ongoing trials).

Once osteoporosis is diagnosed, specific treatments should be set up (in addition to calcium and vitamin D supplementation) to increase bone density either for primary or secondary prevention. Substances to increase bone density include bisphosphonates, selective estrogen receptor modulators (SERM), teriparatide, and strontium ranelate. Bisphosphonates, such as alendronate or risedronate, for example, can be administered orally on a weekly basis. However, medication should not be taken together with calcium due to precipitation. Ibandronate can be administered orally once a month or intravenously every three months but, as yet, no data exists on its influence on femoral fractures. In renal failure, with a glomerular filtration rate (GFR) < 35 mL/min, bisphosphonates are contraindicated. To take bisphosphonates orally, patients must be able to sit upright. Adverse effects are esophageal irritation, heartburn, and rarely acute-phase reactions with fever, weakness, and pain in muscles and bones. If bisphosphonates cannot be taken orally, zoledronate can be administered intravenously once a year. Adverse effects are acute-phase reactions, potential renal toxicity, and hypocalcaemia [17]. There are conflicting results regarding an increased risk for atypical fractures of the femoral shaft associated with bisphosphonate therapy but a recent study shows that the absolute risk is minimal [18].

3.1.8 Problems related to medication

Geriatric patients often suffer from multiple (chronic) diseases, which are treated by a large number of different medications. Adverse side-effects increase with the number of drugs administered. There is, however, no established data base allowing such an evaluation. This increase in adverse effects is nevertheless mirrored by a hypothetical study of a 79-year-old patient with five diseases (type II diabetes mellitus, arterial hypertension, osteoarthrosis, osteoporosis, and COPD). Such a patient was supposed to take twelve different substances at 19 different dosages at five time-points per day, according to evidence-based medical guidelines [19]. This also shows clearly that the geriatric patient depends on a well-organized interdisciplinary team including surgeons and geriatricians or, at least, internists with specific knowledge in geriatric medicine.

The acronym ADME (adsorption, distribution, metabolism, and elimination) can help in searching for reasons of drug-induced adverse effects. Most of the time, adsorption is not diminished in the elderly, whereas most attention should be given to the question of metabolism (eg, liver) and elimination (eg, kidney). The point of distribution has somewhat been neglected in all studies. Nevertheless, sarcopenia and obesity may substantially change the distribution of drugs in the elderly.

Polymorbidity and subsequent multiple medications in geriatric patients are per se a risk factor for the development of a perioperative delirium and are observed in about 50% of the cases. Drugs used most often are those with an anticholinergic and/or dopamine-like action, as well as opioids. With regard to benzodiazepines, prescriptions for patients with an increased risk for delirium should be given with caution.

The treatment goal should always be — "start low, go slowly". Moreover, whenever possible, only one drug should be changed at a time. Eventually, the motto "start low, go slowly" should be changed to "start low, go slowly, but go". Do not refrain from giving the patient important treatment only because of advanced age.

3.1.9 Delirium

Definition

Delirium is an altered state of consciousness, consisting of confusion, distractibility, disorientation, disordered thinking, and memory and facultative defective perception (illusions, hallucinations). Delirium can be hyperactive (prominent hyperactivity, agitation, and autonomic nervous system overactivity), hypoactive (delayed response, lethargic behavior) and, in most cases, showing a fluctuating course. Delirium can be caused by a number of toxic, structural, and metabolic disorders.

Significance

Geriatric patients run a high risk (20–50%) for the development of a postoperative delirium [20]. Delirium is, therefore, a serious complication in older hospitalized patients that is associated with an increased risk of death, need for institutionalization, or developing dementia after discharge. Older people sustaining a fracture and having surgery are subsequently particularly prone to falling into a delirium.

Pathogenesis

Current evidence suggests that neuroinflammatory processes contribute to the development of delirium. Infection, trauma, hypoxia, and surgery are accompanied by increased systemic production of cytokines, which also constitutes a risk for delirium. In addition to the risk factors listed below, a recent review listed additional risk factors among patients in trauma units, such as patients with low Glasgow Coma Scores and multiple blood transfusions.

Strong risk factors in general are preexisting cognitive impairment and polypharmacy.

Even small changes in fluid and food balance may promote delirium in geriatric patients. When delirium is already present, fluid and food intake may become an additional challenge, inducing a vicious circle.

Decline in sight and/or hearing as well as any functional impairment also are predisposing factors for delirium.

Pain is another major risk factor for delirium. Assessment and timely treatment is, therefore, of paramount importance.

Immobility is another risk factor for the development of a delirium. Factors promoting immobilization, such as bladder catheters, infusions, and other physical restraints should be avoided whenever possible. Other reasons also call for an early mobilization (eg, prevention of deep venous thrombosis).

Assessment

Beside the more easily diagnosable hyperactive delirium, hypoactive delirium is often overlooked. Nevertheless, it has the same rate of mortality (up to 50% in the very old).

Delirium is often the first and only sign of an underlying severe disease in a geriatric patient. The most important step for diagnosis is the careful observation of the patient by the entire interdisciplinary team. Criteria to diagnose a delirium are based on the Diagnostic and Statistical Manual of Mental Disorders (DSM IV-TR) and the International Classification of Diseases (ICD-10), respectively. Diagnosis of delirium is easily made by the Confusion Assessment Method (CAM) [21]. Other tools are the Delirium Observation Screening Scale (DOSS) [22], incorporating the observations of nursing staff, and the Delirium Rating Scale (DRS) [23]. The CAM score is a practical tool, only requiring about five minutes. In addition, the CAM has been adapted to special care situations, such as intensive care units (ICU-CAM). It is, therefore, also a valuable tool in patients unable to speak.

Prevention and treatment

By recognizing predisposing and precipitating risk factors, preventive measures can be taken to reduce the risk of delirium. Where delirium is concerned, accurate and timely diagnosis and treatment is essential.

Patients as well as relatives depend on adapted, clear, simple, and repetitive communication, taking into consideration possible language barriers. Active listening, mirroring of feelings, and the presence of nursing staff are helpful. Basal stimulation has also been proven to work. Physical contact should always be announced but is also the basic interpersonal tool for non-communicative interaction. The feeling of loneliness and isolation can be reduced and a degree of safety can be provided.

All means to facilitate orientation of delirious geriatric patients should be undertaken. Orientation aids, such as a calendar and a watch, are especially important for older patients, as their delirium is often multifactorial. Continued use of aids, such as glasses and hearing aids, are both preventive and therapeutic. Preventive measures also include nursing staff and relatives who can provide familiar surroundings to the patient. Their presence is especially valuable to guarantee adequate fluid and food intake.

Psychoactive drugs are most often given in hyperactive delirium. However, drug therapy should only be considered when non-pharmacological intervention fails and/or patients present a danger for themselves or their surroundings. Beside haloperidol, atypical neuroleptics such as risperidone, quetiapine and olanzapine, can be prescribed. In small controlled trials, atypical neuroleptics have been shown to be superior to haloperidol with regard to adverse effects while having equally good effects. The role of acetylcholinesterase inhibitors (eg, rivastigmine and donepezil) are still discussed controversially. Whatever is given, it should be reassessed at regular intervals, as intake of these drugs should be stopped as soon as possible.

3.1.10 Conclusions

The selection of frequently seen problems in the geriatric patient with a fragility fracture discussed above demonstrates the need for well-established orthogeriatric centers. Collaboration of an interdisciplinary team is the prerequisite for the comprehensive treatment of this group of patients prone to frailty. Orthogeriatric units guarantee the orchestrated treatment of geriatric patients, resulting in less morbidity during their stay in hospital as well as a reduced risk of loss of functionality and, therefore, fewer cases of lost independence.

References

[1] **Stuck AE, Siu AL, Wieland GD, et al.** Comprehensive geriatric assessment: a meta-analysis of controlled trials. *Lancet.* 1993 Oct;342(8878):1032–1036.

[2] **Fried LP, Tangen CM, Walston J, et al.** Frailty in older adults: evidence for a phenotype. *J Gerontol Biol Sci Med Sci.* 2001 Mar;56(3):M146–M156.

[3] **Rockwood K, Song X, MacKnight C, et al.** A global clinical measure of fitness and frailty in elderly people. *CMAJ.* 2005 Aug;173(5):489–495.

[4] **Bauer JM, Sieber CC.** Sarcopenia and frailty: a clinician's controversial point of view. *Exp Gerontol.* 2008 Jul;43(7):674–678.

[5] **Fielding RA, Vellas B, Evans WJ, et al.** Sarcopenia: An undiagnosed condition in older adults. Current consensus definition: prevalence, etiology, and consequences. International Working Group on Sarcopenia. *J Am Med Dir Assoc.* 2011 May;12(4):249–256.

[6] **Janssen I, Heymsfield SB, Ross R.** Low relative skeletal muscle mass (sarcopenia) in older persons is associated with functional impairment and physical disability. *J Am Geriatr Soc.* 2002 May;50(5):889–896.

[7] **Bischoff-Ferrari HA.** Vitamin D and fracture prevention. *Endocrinol Metab Clin North Am.* 2011 Jun;39(2):347–353.

[8] **Koster A, Ding J, Stenholm S, et al.** Does the amount of fat mass predict age-related loss of lean mass, muscle strength, and muscle quality in older adults? *J Gerontol A Biol Sci Med Sci.* 2011 Aug;66(8):888–895.

[9] **Delmonico MJ, Harris TB, Visser M, et al.** Longitudinal study of muscle strength, quality, and adipose tissue infiltration. *Am J Clin Nutr.* 2009 Dec;90(6):1579–1585.

[10] **Dey DK, Bosaeus I, Lissner L, et al.** Changes in body composition and its relation to muscle strength in 75-year-old men and women: a 5-year prospective follow-up study of the NORA cohort in Göteborg, Sweden. *Nutrition.* 2009 Jun;25(6):613–619.

[11] **Hughes VA, Frontera WR, Roubenoff R, et al.** Longitudinal changes in body composition in older men and women: role of body weight change and physical activity. *Am J Clin Nutr.* 2002 Aug;76(2):473–481.

[12] **Frontera WR, Hughes VA, Fielding RA, et al.** Aging of skeletal muscle: a 12-yr longitudinal study. *J Appl Physiol.* 2000 Apr;88(4):1321–1326.

[13] **Kaiser MJ, Bauer JM, Rämsch C, et al.** Frequency of malnutrition in older adults: a multinational perspective using the mini nutritional assessment. *J Am Geriatr Soc.* 2010 Sep;58(9):1734–1738.

[14] **Eneroth M, Olsson UB, Thorngren KG.** Nutritional supplementation decreases hip fracture-related complications. *Clin Orthop Relat Res.* 2006 Oct;451:212–217.

[15] **Kaiser MJ, Bauer JM, Rämsch C, et al.** Validation of the Mini Nutritional Assessment short-form (MNA-SF): a practical tool for identification of nutritional status. *J Nutr Health Aging.* 2009 Nov;13(9):782–788.

[16] **Bischoff-Ferrari HA, Shao A, Dawson-Hughes B, et al.** Benefit-risk assessment of vitamin D supplementation. *Osteoporosis Int.* 2010 Jul;21(7):1121–1132.

[17] **Rachner TD, Khosla S, Hofbauer LC.** Osteoporosis: now and the future. *Lancet.* 2011 Mar;377(9773):1276–1287.

[18] **Schilcher J, Michaëlsson K, Aspenberg P.** Bisphosphonate use and atypical fractures of the femoral shaft. *N Engl J Med.* 2011 May;364(18):1728–1737.

[19] **Boyd CM, Darer J, Boult C, et al.** Clinical practice guidelines and quality of care for older patients with multiple comorbid diseases: implications for pay for performance. *JAMA.* 2005 Aug;294(6):716–724.

[20] **Inouye SK.** Delirium in older persons. *N Engl J Med.* 2006 Mar;354(19:1157–1165.

[21] **Wei LA, Fearing MA, Sternberg EJ, et al.** The Confusion Assessment Method: a systematic review of current usage. *J Am Geriatr Soc.* 2008 May;56(5):823–830.

[22] **Schuurmans MJ, Shortridge-Baggett LM, Duursma SA.** The Delirium Observation Screening Scale: a screening instrument for delirium. *Res Theory Nurs Pract.* 2003 Spring;17(1):31–50.

[23] **Trzepacz PT, Mittal D, Torres R, et al.** Validation of the Delirium Rating Scale-revised-98: comparison with the delirium rating scale and the cognitive test for delirium. *J Neuropsychiatry Clin Neurosci.* 2001 Spring;13(2):229–242.

3.2 Arthroplasty

Authors Matt C Lyons, Steven J MacDonald, Matthew P Abdel, Daniel J Berry, Gregory G Polkowski, Jay R Lieberman, Norbert P Südkamp, Martin Jäger, Arvind G von Keudell, Jesse B Jupiter, Ivor S Vanhegan, Fares S Haddad, Alexej Barg, Beat Hintermann

3.2.1 Common surgical hazards

Periprosthetic fractures are increasingly common as joint replacements are more frequently performed and as an increasing number of younger patients with longer life expectancies undergo such surgery. In view of the high number of risk factors related to periprosthetic fractures, it is paramount to know the surgical hazards in order to prevent complications. Therefore, the fundamental principles for surgeons to observe in order to minimize periprosthetic fractures are addressed in this chapter with special focus on preoperative planning, surgical technique, and implant considerations.

3.2.2 Risks due to lack of preoperative planning

The necessity for careful and detailed preoperative planning is an integral part in the prevention of periprosthetic fractures. Effective planning requires extensive assessment of the patient and adequate radiological investigation, which is covered in chapter 4.1, as well as appropriate templating, precise knowledge of the different types of prosthesis, and the contingencies for intraoperative problems.

Recognition of host-related risk factors

It is paramount to recognize specific intrinsic risk factors of periprosthetic fractures such as:

- Inflammatory arthropathy
- Osteoporosis
- Metabolic bone disease (Paget's disease)
- Female gender
- Advanced age
- Osteolysis
- Infection
- Axial malalignment
- Previous surgical interventions.

Other general host-related factors can be obtained from detailed patient histories and are addressed in chapter 3.1. Knowledge of these risk factors allows anticipation of potential difficulties, change of implant choice, and planning for contingencies in case of intraoperative complications.

Diagnostic imaging and its risks

Modern imaging techniques provide essential information in regard to bone quality, quantity, and morphology. X-rays must be recent, of high quality, appropriately centered and in orthogonal planes. Full-length films including adjacent joints are required in order to assess axial alignment and distal pathology, if this is suspected. Osteolysis and remodeling of a deformity may demand further progressive entities, which require recent x-rays to appropriately prepare the surgeon. The assessment of bone stock by advanced imaging techniques—such as computed tomography (CT) or magnetic resonance imaging (MRI)—can be helpful whereas inadequate x-rays may not reveal metaphyseal-diaphyseal mismatching or abnormal morphology in both sagittal and coronal planes.

Native bone is remodeled in response to the transmitted strain in accordance with Wolff's law. In the presence of a prosthesis, strain is preferentially absorbed by the implant and, thus, only a reduced portion is transmitted to the surrounding bone. This mainly occurs because of the different stiffness of the two materials, with the stiffer substance receiving the greater proportion of strain. Note that the stiffness of a material is a function of material modulus and implant geometry. In terms of geometry, stiffness is proportional to the fourth power of the diameter of the implant; therefore, stress shielding is more dominant in larger stems. This process results in severe bone resorption and has been widely documented especially in total hip and total knee arthroplasty [24, 25].

A further consideration for periprosthetic bone loss is the extent of porous coating. Since bone resorption occurs in areas where ingrowth of bone into the implant has taken place, extensively coated devices induce the most pronounced losses in comparison to proximally or partially coated stems [26]. Formation of wear debris, causing aseptic loosening, is the most common mode of implant failure and a further cause of osteolysis.

For more detailed assessment and evaluation of the different radiological imaging techniques, see chapter 4.1.

In 3.2-1a–c a young patient is presented, who had undergone previous varus osteotomy of the proximal femur for developmental hip dysplasia and who subsequently required a THA for osteoarthrosis. The femoral morphology was not fully recognized due to inadequate preoperative x-rays. Despite the use of a modular prosthesis to address the metaphyseal-diaphyseal mismatch in the coronal plane, the degree of sagittal deformity prevented the safe placement of the prosthesis (3.2-1c). An adequate appraisal of appropriate imaging would hopefully have led to a different surgical technique and prevented this cortical perforation.

3.2.3 Risks associated with intraoperative technique

An intraoperative periprosthetic fracture is most often sustained during medullary canal preparation, insertion of the prosthesis, removal of the existing prosthetic stem or cement.

Strategies to reduce intraoperative fractures include:
- Obtaining adequate surgical exposure, which often requires trochanteric/tibial osteotomy
- Overreaming in order to reduce hoop stress and fracture during insertion of noncemented press-fit stems and acetabular cups
- Avoiding eccentric or varus reaming
- Removing cement carefully
- Preventing propagation of the fracture by using prophylactic cerclage cables or wires
- Using the image intensifier during revision surgery.

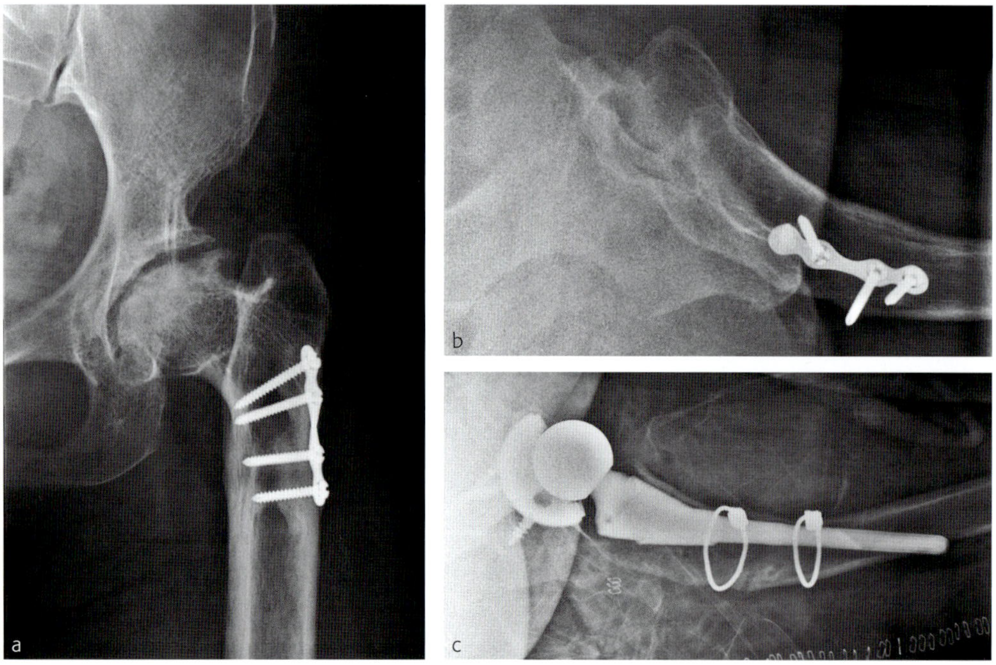

3.2-1a–c Example of an inadequate preoperative assessment and planning in a young patient with earlier hip dysplasia and a proximal varus osteotomy of the femur.

a AP x-ray of a left hip after a previous proximal femoral varus osteotomy.

b Inadequate lateral x-ray of a left hip after a previous proximal femoral osteotomy, which does not allow to fully appreciate the axial deviation.

c Prosthetic malposition and intraoperative fissure or fracture of the femur after inadequate preoperative x-rays and templating. The intraoperative fracture was, however, recognized and fixed with two cerclage bands.

During surgery itself, the surgeon should be aware of the natural anatomy and biomechanics of the joint. Even more important, every effort should be made in order to reduce devascularization and conserve the quantity of remaining bone stock, ie, preserve periosteal blood supply combined with a conservative approach to soft-tissue stripping. Implant size and alignment are crucial due to their effect on joint biomechanics and transfer of stress to surrounding bone. Stress shielding is a major contributor to osteolysis, which arises from the difference in stiffness of implant and bone. Areas of concentrated stress, also called stress risers, can contribute to periprosthetic fracture formation. These most commonly occur in areas of native bone between two prostheses or as a consequence of poor operative technique. Regarding the latter, notching of the anterior femoral cortex can lead to supracondylar fractures following total knee arthroplasty. In this particular example, notching of the anterior cortex significantly lessens the failure load by greatly decreasing both bending and torsional strength.

Distal femoral periprosthetic fractures are not always associated with notching or osteopenia. The proportion of anterior femoral notching associated with periprosthetic femoral fracture is between 7% and 50%; x-ray evidence of osteopenia associated with these fractures ranges between 49% and 100% [27]. A similar process is observed in femoral neck notching with bone-conserving, hip-resurfacing prostheses and can assist in diagnosing susceptible individuals.

3.2.4 Risk of shoulder or elbow fractures

Periprosthetic fractures around the shoulder and elbow (chapters 6.1, 6.2) can occur intraoperatively or postoperatively. Intraoperative periprosthetic fractures of the humerus are probably more frequent than reported. Their incidence can be estimated at approximately 1.5% [28]. Reasons for intraoperative fractures are often due to errors in surgical technique, most of which could have been avoided. Other factors concern poor and thin bone stock, routine use of cemented stems, close association of the major peripheral nerves in the upper limb, and, on occasion, an unstable soft-tissue envelope especially around the elbow.

Reported triggers are the removal of well-fixed stems, excessive external rotation of the arm, especially in stiff shoulders, resulting in spiral fractures, overreaming of the humeral canal, and/or insertion of oversized broaches or stems. Triggers of postoperative periprosthetic fractures are typically simple, low-energy falls. Risk factors are advanced age, female gender, and poor bone quality [29].

3.2.5 Risk of wrist fractures

Periprosthetic wrist fractures are still rare but it is known that intraoperative fractures are more likely to occur in revision arthroplasty than primary interventions (chapter 6.3). Postoperative radius fractures are often caused by a fall.

3.2.6 Risk of acetabular fractures

Intraoperative fractures

Intraoperative acetabular periprosthetic fractures are not very common (chapter 6.4.2).

While there is a paucity of literature surrounding intraoperative periprosthetic acetabular fractures, some risk factors have been identified (**3.2-2**).

Predisposing factors for such fractures include:

- Press-fit, noncemented components
- Oversized components or underreamed sockets
- Poor bone quality
- Metabolic conditions [30].

In 1974, McElfresh and Coventry reported an incidence of periprosthetic fractures of < 0.02% in cemented acetabular prostheses [31]. Noncemented acetabular constructs have become the modern standard. Haidukewych reported an overall 0.4% incidence rate in 5,359 noncemented acetabular components, with elliptical monoblock (0.09%) and hemispherical modular (3.5%) components displaying the highest and lowest rates of fracture, respectively [32]. Noncemented acetabular prostheses rely upon an element of underreaming (press-fit) in order to achieve initial stability and avoid supplemental screw fixation with subsequent risk of neurovascular damage, screw fretting, backside wear, and passage of wear particulate debris along the screw channel [33].

Kim et al [34], using fresh and embalmed cadavers, found that a force of 2,000 N was required to impact a cup with underreaming of 2 mm, while 3,000 N were required for insertion of a press-fit cup with underreaming of 4 mm. Acetabular fractures occurred during insertion of 4 (of 15) cups with 2 mm underreaming, and in 14 (of 15) cups with underreaming of 4 mm. The fracture patterns included peripheral rim and wall fractures, low transverse-type fractures, and anterior column fractures involving the superior pubic ramus. Of the total of 18 fractures, 3 could only be detected after the acetabular component had been removed. In these 3 cases, the AP and lateral x-rays did not show a recognizable fracture of the acetabulum.

3.2-1 Technical and implant-related risk factors for periprosthetic fractures around knee arthroplasties [53, 60, 62, 63, 69–73].

Factors	Femur	Tibia	Patella
Technique-related factors	Revision procedures	Revision procedures	Revision procedures
	Anterior femoral notching	Varus/valgus malalignment	Component malpositioning
	Posterior cruciate stabilizing design	Component malpositioning	Patellar thickness
	Intercondylar box cuts of certain types of prostheses	Previous high-tibial osteotomy	Patellar surface replacement
		Stress risers from previous hardware	Lateral release
		Tibial broaching	Fat-pad excision
		Aggressive retraction	Limb malalignment
		Tibial tubercle osteotomies	
Implant-related factors		Punch instrumentation for keeled implants	Metal-backed patellae
		Keeled tibial components	Large central pegs
		Long-stemmed tibial components	
		Press-fit tibial components	
Overall-Factors	Decreased flexion		

Profound product knowledge of both, tools and implants, is essential in order to understand the relationship of the reamer size to the prosthetic dimensions as each prosthesis varies with respect to peripheral flare, which indeed may change with surface coating and alterations in the size of the implant.

Postoperative fractures

Both, high and low-energy trauma can be expected to lead to postoperative periprosthetic acetabular fractures [35–37]. A number of authors have identified the bone loss associated with osteoporosis as well as osteolysis as additional risk factors [38]. In regard to pelvic discontinuities, Berry et al identified female gender, diagnosis of rheumatoid arthritis, and prior pelvic discontinuity as risk factors [39].

3.2.7 Risk of femoral fractures

Intraoperative fractures

Intraoperative periprosthetic fractures of the femur (chapters 6.4.3, 6.5.2) are more common than acetabular fractures with implant choice being a major risk factor (3.2-1, 3.2-2). The incidence of periprosthetic fractures has been reported as markedly higher in noncemented (5.4%) than cemented (0.3%) stems [30]. Implant design also affects periprosthetic fracture incidence, with comparative studies demonstrating a lower rate with longer, anatomically shaped cemented stems than straight shorter stems [40]. Difficulty in positioning a straight stem with an adequate cement mantle has been described well in reports on the Charnley prosthesis. An inadequate cement mantle, with direct contact between the implant and the inner femoral cortex, has been correlated with long-term loosening, femoral osteolysis, and increased risk of periprosthetic fracture [40]. Noncemented stems require intimate press fitting in order to achieve immediate axial and rotational stability. Lack of primary stability can lead to implant subsidence, retroversion, varus collapse, and lateral femoral cortex impingement, predisposing to subsequent fracture. Achieving a press fit in noncemented stems with sharp edges results in increased interfacial stress [41]. Diaphyseal fixation is associated with significant proximal stress shielding. Proximally coated stems achieve primary stability and bone ingrowth in the metaphysis, while the uncoated distal segment centralizes the stem and provides secondary stability. Metaphyseal fixation may be contraindicated in patients with altered morphology, poor calcar support, metaphyseal-diaphyseal mismatch, and varying corticocancellous ratios. In order to achieve a successful reconstruction, the prosthesis should be chosen in appreciation of patient morphology and understanding the characteristics of the implant, ie, its geometry, fixation, and limitations.

3.2-2 Technical and implant-related risk factors for periprosthetic fractures around hip arthroplasties [52, 60, 62, 63, 69–73].

Factors	Acetabulum	Femur
Technique-related factors	Revision procedures	Revision procedures
	Bone defects (osteolysis)	Bone defects (osteolysis)
	Oversized components	Femoral broaching
	Underreamed sockets	Overreaming
		Aggressive insertion of press-fit component
		Cortical stress risers
		Screw holes
		Previous osteotomy
Implant-related factors	Press-fit noncemented components	Press-fit noncemented components
		Large diameter stems
		Long (especially straight) stems

Following a comprehensive review of high-quality x-rays with suitable scaling, successful reconstruction requires detailed templating in orthogonal planes with the intended and appropriate prostheses. Templating determines the correct size and length of the components in order to achieve reconstitution of the center of rotation, femoral offset, and leg length. Adverse outcome can often be predicted and contingencies planned. Ensuring the availability of the appropriate equipment, time, and staffing completes the preoperative plan.

Postoperative fractures

There are several risk factors for postoperative periprosthetic femoral fractures (3.2-1, 3.2-2). Cook et al recently noted that patients older than 70 years had a 2.9-times greater risk of suffering a periprosthetic femoral fracture [42]. However, they found no association between fracture and gender or implant type. On the other hand, Lindahl et al found a statistically significant increase in the risk of periprosthetic fractures in younger patients possibly due to increased activity resulting in higher risk of loosening [40]. Bethea et al and Beals and Tower also noted that loose implants were a risk factor for periprosthetic fractures [43, 44]. In regard to the type of implant, Lindhal et al found that certain stem designs had an increased risk of fracture [40, 45]. Most fractures occur as a result of minor trauma. Likewise, Lindhal et al revealed that 81% of fractures in the primary THA group and 70% of fractures in the revision THA group were due to trauma [40]. While women seem to be more predisposed for a periprosthetic fracture, study from the Finnish Arthroplasty Register looking at 33,154 primary THAs showed a higher risk of periprosthetic fractures in men after a Cox-regression model was completed adjusting for age [46]. In the most recent comprehensive series from the Scottish national database, age ≥ 70 years, female gender, and revision arthroplasty were all found to be statistically significant risk factors for periprosthetic fractures [27, 47–52].

Biomechanical studies have shown that notching of the anterior cortex significantly lessens the load to failure by decreasing bending strength by 18% and torsional strength by 40%. They also noted that osteopenia was a risk factor. However, surgeons must be aware that some clinical studies have not supported such findings [52].

Other authors have noted that decreased flexion is a risk factor for supracondylar fractures for two reasons [53]. Possible reasons for this observation include:

- Patients are less mobile and agile, increasing their risk of a fall
- Knees with less flexion absorb energy and transfer it to the bone.

In 41 periprosthetic fractures, Platzer et al showed that 39 occurred secondary to trauma [48].

3.2.8 Risk of patellar fractures

Intraoperative fractures

The data for the risk factors of intraoperative periprosthetic patellar fractures is limited compared to that for postoperative fractures. One known risk factor for intraoperative patellar fracture is revision surgery.

Postoperative fractures

There is a set of risk factors more specific to postoperative patellar periprosthetic fractures (chapter 6.5.3) that includes both host- and procedure-related factors. In addition to the host-related risk factors listed in **3.2-1**, male gender, knee hyperflexion, obesity, and high activity level should be mentioned.

Metal-backed noncemented patellae and components with large central pegs have been associated with an increased incidence of patellar fractures [54]. The patellar thickness has an effect on the mechanics of the knee-extensor mechanism and also on patellar bone strength [55, 56]. In a cadaveric study, Hsu et al showed that variation in patellar thickness resulted in smaller contact area and considerably increased joint reaction forces [57]. Furthermore, multiple studies have shown that a thin patella secondary to over-resection compromises the mechanical strength and possibly increases the risk of fracture [58]. Reuben et al showed that patellar thickness of less than 15 mm substantially increased the strain in the anterior patella region and, thus, increased the risk for fracture [55]. In regard to stress fractures, several researchers have noted an increased risk with resurfacing of the patella during TKAs [59, 60].

The manner in which the patella is handled technically during the TKA is also important in determining the outcome. Heat necrosis may increase the incidence of periprosthetic patella fractures. In addition, devascularization of the patella, possibly during lateral release and/or excessive fat-pad excision, may sacrifice the lateral superior geniculate artery and also increase the incidence of such fractures [59,61–64]. Likewise, biomechanical studies have revealed a substantially increased contact force with patellofemoral malalignment, which may also lead to an increased risk of periprosthetic patellar fractures [63].

3.2.9 Risk of tibial fractures

Intraoperative fractures

Intraoperative periprosthetic tibial fractures (chapter 6.5.4) may occur secondary to factors related to the patient, technique, or implant (**3.2-1**). Patient factors are the same as for most other periprosthetic fractures and have been mentioned before. Technique-related factors include tibial broaching and punch instrumentation for keeled implants, removal of well-fixed implants and cement, aggressive retraction, and osteotomy of the tibial tubercle [65]. Design-related features include keeled, long-stemmed, and press-fit tibial components.

Previous surgery such as high-tibial osteotomies may be responsible for intraoperative fractures, while lateral placement of the tibial component or stem may cause perforations of the lateral cortex of the tibia. Stress risers resulting from removal of hardware may increase the risk for intra- as well as postoperative fractures. Finally, revision surgery bears a higher risk for intraoperative periprosthetic fractures.

Postoperative fractures

Beside trauma, varus or valgus malalignment is a potential causative factor for periprosthetic fractures of the tibia [27, 48–52].

3.2.10 Risk of ankle fractures

Intraoperative fractures

The most common reasons for intraoperative fractures (chapter 6.6) include extensive and inaccurate use of the saw blade in combination with limited visualization, insufficient instrumentation, and incorrect sizing of prosthetic components [66, 67]. Furthermore, patients with rheumatoid arthritis and long-term corticosteroid therapy are at higher risk due to reduced bone quality [68].

Postoperative fractures

Fractures may occur in the early postoperative stage, especially medial malleolar fractures. Improper bone resection is often a cause. Altered biomechanics due to incorrect prosthesis positioning may also lead to periprosthetic stress fractures (chapter 6.6).

References

[1] **Stuck AE, Siu AL, Wieland GD, et al.** Comprehensive geriatric assessment: a meta-analysis of controlled trials. *Lancet.* 1993 Oct;342(8878):1032–1036.

[2] **Fried LP, Tangen CM, Walston J, et al.** Frailty in older adults: evidence for a phenotype. *J Gerontol Biol Sci Med Sci.* 2001 Mar;56(3):M146–M156.

[3] **Rockwood K, Song X, MacKnight C, et al.** A global clinical measure of fitness and frailty in elderly people. *CMAJ.* 2005 Aug;173(5):489–495.

[4] **Bauer JM, Sieber CC.** Sarcopenia and frailty: a clinician's controversial point of view. *Exp Gerontol.* 2008 Jul;43(7):674–678.

[5] **Fielding RA, Vellas B, Evans WJ, et al.** Sarcopenia: An undiagnosed condition in older adults. Current consensus definition: prevalence, etiology, and consequences. International Working Group on Sarcopenia. *J Am Med Dir Assoc.* 2011 May;12(4):249–256.

[6] **Janssen I, Heymsfield SB, Ross R.** Low relative skeletal muscle mass (sarcopenia) in older persons is associated with functional impairment and physical disability. *J Am Geriatr Soc.* 2002 May;50(5):889–896.

[7] **Bischoff-Ferrari HA.** Vitamin D and fracture prevention. *Endocrinol Metab Clin North Am.* 2011 Jun;39(2):347–353.

[8] **Koster A, Ding J, Stenholm S, et al.** Does the amount of fat mass predict age-related loss of lean mass, muscle strength, and muscle quality in older adults? *J Gerontol A Biol Sci Med Sci. 2011 Aug;66(8):888–895.*

[9] **Delmonico MJ, Harris TB, Visser M, et al.** Longitudinal study of muscle strength, quality, and adipose tissue infiltration. *Am J Clin Nutr.* 2009 Dec;90(6):1579–1585.

[10] **Dey DK, Bosaeus I, Lissner L, et al.** Changes in body composition and its relation to muscle strength in 75-year-old men and women: a 5-year prospective follow-up study of the NORA cohort in Göteborg, Sweden. *Nutrition.* 2009 Jun;25(6):613–619.

[11] **Hughes VA, Frontera WR, Roubenoff R, et al.** Longitudinal changes in body composition in older men and women: role of body weight change and physical activity. *Am J Clin Nutr.* 2002 Aug;76(2):473–481.

[12] **Frontera WR, Hughes VA, Fielding RA, et al.** Aging of skeletal muscle: a 12-yr longitudinal study. *J Appl Physiol.* 2000 Apr;88(4):1321–1326.

[13] **Kaiser MJ, Bauer JM, Rämsch C, et al.** Frequency of malnutrition in older adults: a multinational perspective using the mini nutritional assessment. *J Am Geriatr Soc.* 2010 Sep;58(9):1734–1738.

[14] **Eneroth M, Olsson UB, Thorngren KG.** Nutritional supplementation decreases hip fracture-related complications. *Clin Orthop Relat Res.* 2006 Oct;451:212–217.

[15] **Kaiser MJ, Bauer JM, Rämsch C, et al.** Validation of the Mini Nutritional Assessment short-form (MNA-SF): a practical tool for identification of nutritional status. *J Nutr Health Aging.* 2009 Nov;13(9):782–788.

[16] **Bischoff-Ferrari HA, Shao A, Dawson-Hughes B, et al.** Benefit-risk assessment of vitamin D supplementation. *Osteoporosis Int.* 2010 Jul;21(7):1121–1132.

[17] **Rachner TD, Khosla S, Hofbauer LC.** Osteoporosis: now and the future. *Lancet.* 2011 Mar;377(9773):1276–1287.

[18] **Schilcher J, Michaëlsson K, Aspenberg P.** Bisphosphonate use and atypical fractures of the femoral shaft. *N Eng J Med.* 2011 May;364(18):1728–1737.

[19] **Boyd CM, Darer J, Boult C, et al.** Clinical practice guidelines and quality of care for older patients with multiple comorbid diseases: implications for pay for performance. *JAMA.* 2005 Aug;294(6):716–724.

[20] **Inouye SK.** Delirium in older persons. *N Engl J Med.* 2006 Mar;354(19:1157–1165.

[21] **Wei LA, Fearing MA, Sternberg EJ, et al.** The Confusion Assessment Method: a systematic review of current usage. *J Am Geriatr Soc.* 2008 May;56(5):823–830.

[22] **Schuurmans MJ, Shortridge-Baggett LM, Duursma SA.** The Delirium Observation Screening Scale: a screening instrument for delirium. *Res Theory Nurs Pract.* 2003 Spring;17(1):31–50.

[23] **Trzepacz PT, Mittal D, Torres R, et al.** Validation of the Delirium Rating Scale-revised-98: comparison with the delirium rating scale and the cognitive test for delirium. *J Neuropsychiatry Clin Neurosci.* 2001 Spring;13(2):229–42.

[24] **Harris WH, Sledge CB.** Total hip and total knee replacement (1). *N Engl J Med.* 1990 Sep;323(12):801–807.

[25] **Harris WH, Sledge CB.** Total hip and total knee replacement (2). *N Engl J Med.* 1990 Sep;323(11): 725–731.

[26] **Wik TS, Foss OA, Havik S, et al.** Periprosthetic fracture caused by stress shielding after implantation of a femoral condyle endoprosthesis in a transfemoral amputee: a case report. *Acta Orthop.* 2010 Dec;81(6):765–767.

[27] **Shawen SB, Belmont PJ Jr, Klemme WR, et al.** Osteoporosis and anterior femoral notching in periprosthetic supracondylar femoral fractures: a biomechanical analysis. *J Bone Joint Surg Am.* 2003 Jan;85–A(1):115–121.

[28] **Athwal GS, Sperling JW, Rispoli DM, et al.** Periprosthetic humeral fractures during shoulder arthroplasty. *J Bone Joint Surg Am.* 2009 Mar 1;91(3):594–603.

[29] **McDonough EB, Crosby LA.** Periprosthetic fractures of the humerus. *Am J Orthop (Belle Mead NJ).* 2005 Dec;34(12):586–591.

[30] **Berry DJ.** Epidemiology: Hip and knee. *Orthop Clin North Am.* 1999 Apr;30(2):183–190.

[31] **McElfresh EC, Coventry MB.** Femoral and pelvic fractures after total hip arthroplasty. *J Bone Joint Surg Am.* 1974 Apr;56(3):483–492.

[32] **Haidukewych GJ, Jacofsky DJ, Hanssen AD, et al.** Intraoperative fractures of the acetabulum during primary total hip arthroplasty. *J Bone Joint Surg Am.* 2006 Sep;88(9):1952–1956.

[33] **Callaghan JJ.** Periprosthetic fractures of the acetabulum during and following total hip arthroplasty. *J Bone Joint Surg Am.* 1997 Sep;79(9):1416–1421.

[34] **Kim YS, Callaghan JJ, Ahn PB, et al.** Fracture of the acetabulum during insertion of an oversized hemispherical component. *J Bone Joint Surg Am.* 1995 Jan;77(1): 111–117.

[35] **Peterson CA 2nd, Lewallen DG.** Periprosthetic fracture of the acetabulum after total hip arthroplasty. *J Bone Joint Surg Am.* 1996 Aug;78(8):1206–1213.

[36] **Harvie P, Gundle R, Willett K.** Traumatic periprosthetic acetabular fracture: life threatening haemorrhage and a novel method of acetabular reconstruction. *Injury.* 2004 Aug;35(8):819–822.

[37] **Old AB, McGrory BJ, Peterson CA 2nd, et al.** Locked inferior fracture dislocation after total hip arthroplasty. *J Arthroplasty.* 2008 Feb;23(2):308–310.

[38] **Andrews P, Barrack RL, Harris WH.** Stress fracture of the medial wall of the acetabulum adjacent to a cementless acetabular component. *J Arthroplasty.* 2002 Jan;17(1):117–120.

[39] **Berry DJ, Lewallen DG, Hanssen AD, et al.** Pelvic discontinuity in revision total hip arthroplasty. *J Bone Joint Surg Am.* 1999 Dec;81(12):1692–1702.

[40] **Lindahl H, Garellick G, Regnér H, et al.** Three hundred and twenty-one periprosthetic femoral fractures. *J Bone Joint Surg Am.* 2006 Jun;88(6): 1215–1222.

[41] **Hu K, Zhang X, Zhu J, et al.** Periprosthetic fractures may be more likely in cementless femoral stems with sharp edges. *Ir J Med Sci.* 2010 Sep;179(3): 417–421.

[42] **Cook RE, Jenkins PJ, Walmsley PJet al.** Risk factors for periprosthetic fractures of the hip: a survivorship analysis. *Clin Orthop Relat Res.* 2008 Jul;466(7):1652–1656.

[43] **Beals RK, Tower SS.** Periprosthetic fractures of the femur. An analysis of 93 fractures. *Clin Orthop Relat Res.* 1996;(327):238–246.

[44] **Bethea JS 3rd, DeAndrade JR, Fleming LL, et al.** Proximal femoral fractures following total hip arthroplasty. *Clin Orthop Relat Res.* 1982;(170):95–106.

[45] **Lindahl H, Malchau H, Herberts P, et al.** Periprosthetic femoral fractures classification and demographics of 1049 periprosthetic femoral fractures from the Swedish National Hip Arthroplasty Register. *J Arthroplasty.* 2005 Oct;20(7):857–865.

[46] **Sarvilinna R, Huhtala HS, Puolakka TJ, et al.** Periprosthetic fractures in total hip arthroplasty: an epidemiologic study. *Int Orthop.* 2003;27(6):359–361.

[47] **Meek RM, Norwood T, Smith R, et al.** The risk of peri-prosthetic fracture after primary and revision total hip and knee replacement. *J Bone Joint Surg Br.* 2011 Jan;93(1):96–101.

[48] **Platzer P, Schuster R, Aldrian S, et al.** Management and outcome of periprosthetic fractures after total knee arthroplasty. *J Trauma.* 2010 Jun;68(6):1464–1470.

[49] **Rorabeck CH, Taylor JW.** Periprosthetic fractures of the femur complicating total knee arthroplasty. *Orthop Clin North Am.* 1999 Apr;30(2):265–277.

[50] **Mortazavi SM, Kurd MF, Bender B, et al.** Distal femoral arthroplasty for the treatment of periprosthetic fractures after total knee arthroplasty. *J Arthroplasty.* 2010 Aug;25(5):775–780.

[51] **Herrera DA, Kregor PJ, Cole PA, et al.** Treatment of acute distal femur fractures above a total knee arthroplasty: systematic review of 415 cases (1981–2006). *Acta Orthop.* 2008 Feb;79(1):22–27.

[52] **Lesh ML, Schneider DJ, Deol G, et al.** The consequences of anterior femoral notching in total knee arthroplasty. A biomechanical study. *J Bone Joint Surg Am.* 2000 Aug;82-A(8):1096–1101.

[53] **Tharani R, Nakasone C, Vince KG.** Periprosthetic fractures after total knee arthroplasty. *J Arthroplasty.* 2005;20(4 Suppl 2):27–32.

[54] **Goldberg VM, Figgie HE 3rd, Inglis AE, et al.** Patellar fracture type and prognosis in condylar total knee arthroplasty. *Clin Orthop Relat Res.* 1988 Nov;(236):115–122.

[55] **Reuben JD, McDonald CL, Woodard PL, et al.** Effect of patella thickness on patella strain following total knee arthroplasty. *J Arthroplasty.* 1991 Sep;6(3):251–258.

[56] **Star MJ, Kaufman KR, Irby SE, et al.** The effects of patellar thickness on patellofemoral forces after resurfacing. *Clin Orthop Rel Res.* 1996 Jan;(322):279–284.

[57] **Hsu HC, Luo ZP, Rand JA, et al.** Influence of patellar thickness on patellar tracking and patellofemoral contact characteristics after total knee arthroplasty. *J Arthroplasty.* 1996 Jan;11(1):69–80.

[58] **Furnes O, Espehaug B, Lie SA, et al.** Failure mechanisms after unicompartmental and tricompartmental primary knee replacement with cement. *J Bone Joint Surg Am.* 2007 Mar;89(3)519–525.

[59] **Grace JN, Sim FH.** Fracture of the patella after total knee arthroplasty. *Clin Orthop Relat Res.* 1988 May;(230):168–175.

[60] **Stulberg SD, Stulberg BN, Hamati Y, et al.** Failure mechanisms of metal-backed patellar components. *Clin Orthop Relat Res.* 1988 Nov;(236):88–105.

[61] **Boyd AD Jr, Ewald FC, Thomas WH, et al.** Long-term complications after total knee arthroplasty with or without resurfacing of the patella. *J Bone Joint Surg Am.* 1993 May;75(5):674–681.

[62] **Goldstein SA, Coale E, Weiss AP, et al.** Patellar surface strain. *J Orthop Res.* 1986;4(3):372–377.

[63] **Parvizi J, Kim KI, Oliashirazi A, et al.** Periprosthetic patellar fractures. *Clin Orthop Relat Res.* 2006 May;446:161–166.

[64] **Le AX, Cameron HU, Otsuka NY, et al.** Fracture of the patella following total knee arthroplasty. *Orthopedics.* 1999 Apr;22(4):395–398; discussion 398–399.

[65] **Burnett RS, Bourne RB.** Periprosthetic fractures of the tibia and patella in total knee arthroplasty. *Instr Course Lect.* 2004;53:217–235.

[66] **Deorio JK, Easley ME.** Total ankle arthroplasty. *Instr Course Lect.* 2008;57:383–413.

[67] **Hintermann B, Valderrabano V.** Total ankle replacement. *Foot Ankle Clin.* 2003 Jun;8(2):375–405.

[68] **Wood PL, Crawford LA, Suneja R, et al.** Total ankle replacement for rheumatoid ankle arthritis. *Foot Ankle Clin.* 2007 Sep;12(3):497–508.

[69] **Chalidis BE, Tsiridis E, Tragas AA, et al.** Management of periprosthetic patellar fractures. A systematic review of literature. *Injury.* 2007 Jun;38(6):714–724.

[70] **Scott RD, Turoff N, Ewald FC.** Stress fracture of the patella following duopatellar total knee arthroplasty with patellar resurfacing. *Clin Orthop Relat Res.* 1982 Oct;(170):147–151.

[71] **Clayton ML, Thirupathi R.** Patellar complications after total condylar arthroplasty. *Clin Orthop Rel Res.* 1982 Oct;(170):152–155.

[72] **Healy WL, Wasilewski SA, Takei R, et al.** Patellofemoral complications following total knee arthroplasty. Correlation with implant design and patient risk factors. *The J Arthroplasty.* 1995 Apr;10(2):197–201.

[73] **Roffman M, Hirsh DM, Mendes DG.** Fracture of the resurfaced patella in total knee replacement. *Clin Orthop Relat Res.* 1980 May;(148):112–126.

4

Diagnosis of periprosthetic fractures

4.1 Assessment

Authors **Ivor S Vanhegan, Fares S Haddad**

4.1.1 Introduction

The key objective in diagnosing a periprosthetic fracture is identifying on which patients to focus available resources and attention. Ultimately, the diagnostic conundrum lies in uncovering the cause of the fracture, deciding on the type of fracture, and the stability of the prosthetic components as well as preventing a refracture after the salvage surgery.

This section aims at raising the index of suspicion based on the history and clinical assessment of the patient, followed by reviewing the merits of the different investigation modalities that are available to establish the correct diagnosis of the fracture. An algorithm (**4.1-1**) is provided to guide the clinician in the use of available diagnostic tools.

4.1.2 Clinical suspicion

A periprosthetic fracture will not be diagnosed unless it is at the forefront of the clinician's mind when assessing such patients. These fractures rarely occur intraoperatively but more often postoperatively, therefore, it is helpful to subdivide them into immediate, early, or late periprosthetic fractures. Patients who are at greatest risk often present with frequent falls, recurrent dislocation or loosening, subsidence, or osteolysis around the prosthesis. A systematic, focused assessment of susceptible individuals is vital to prevent progression to implant failure and further bone loss.

The assessment should focus on patient-related factors on the one hand and the periprosthetic fracture on the other.

4.1.3 Assessment of the fracture

When a periprosthetic fracture is confirmed by imaging (either x-ray or computed tomographic [CT] evaluation), the most important question is about the stability of the prosthetic component, ie, is it well-fixed or loose? The answer will influence decision making, ie, whether internal fixation or revision surgery is the optimal treatment.

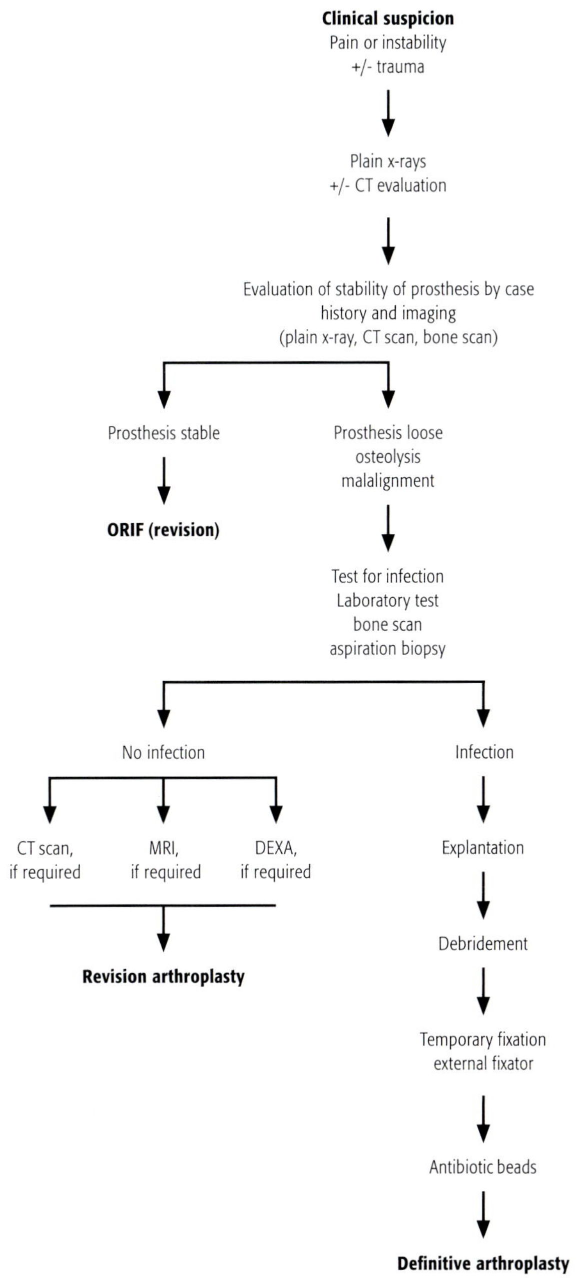

4.1-1 A suggested workflow (algorithm) in the diagnosis of a patient with suspected periprosthetic fracture.

While the patient's history may already raise the suspicion of an unstable or loose prosthesis, the radiological appearance and additional imaging give a more precise answer preoperatively in most cases (chapter 4.1.5). Lastly, if in doubt, the surgeon can check the degree of fixation intraoperatively after exposure of the fracture site.

4.1.4 Assessment of the patient

Analyzing the whole patient

Periprosthetic fractures commonly occur in the elderly where medical comorbidities are more likely. In assessing these patients, a specific geriatric assessment may be indicated (chapter 3.1). In addition, preoperative assessment according to the ASA-Score of the American Society of Anesthesiologists is mandatory for all patients (chapter 5.2).

Analyzing case history

Typical noteworthy features from the case history include insidious onset of pain, instability, deterioration in function, or recent history of trauma (👁 **4.1-2**). The incidence of late periprosthetic femoral fracture is rising because of low-velocity trauma in elderly patients due to falls or, conversely, high-velocity impact traumatic events in the younger population, whose fractures are increasingly treated by insertion of implants. However, there is reliable evidence to indicate that up to half of all patients report no history of a fall or trauma prior to diagnosis [1].

In case of a traumatic periprosthetic fracture without a history of previous pain or other clinical signs of loosening, conventional radiological imaging will suffice when deciding on the most adequate treatment. If, however, the fracture occurred without a clear traumatic event or if the x-ray shows signs of osteolysis around the prosthesis, consider three key factors before embarking on revision surgery:

- Coexisting infection
- Identification of implants to be extracted
- Bone stock.

Identifying underlying infection

The presence of coexisting periprosthetic infection has not been widely published as yet but identifying its presence is vital and its incidence is often underestimated. At the authors' institution 10% of all patients with periprosthetic fractures were diagnosed with concurrent infection. The presence of infection contributing to osteolysis and fracture formation is unequivocal, and failing to diagnose it could have disastrous consequences.

It is the authors' policy that every patient presenting with pain, instability, and suspected fracture be considered infected until proven otherwise. Consequently, each patient undergoes a combination of laboratory blood tests and, if needed, bone scintigraphy. Full blood count checking for leukocytosis and/or neutrophilia, C-reactive protein levels, and erythrocyte sedimentation rate are performed as routine markers of infection and inflammation.

In 2010, Mermans and Haddad [2] compared the efficacy of aspiration and tissue biopsy alone and in combination to improve diagnostic yield in the evaluation of periprosthetic joint infection. They prospectively followed up 120 patients with suspected periprosthetic infection, 56 of whom had a total knee arthroplasty in situ and the remainder had a hip prosthesis. Antibiotic therapy was discontinued for 4 weeks before aspiration/biopsy to minimize the risk of false-negative results. Sensitivity of aspiration alone was 83%, biopsy was 79%, and in combination this rate improved to 90%. The respective accuracies were 84%, 81%, and 90%, prompting

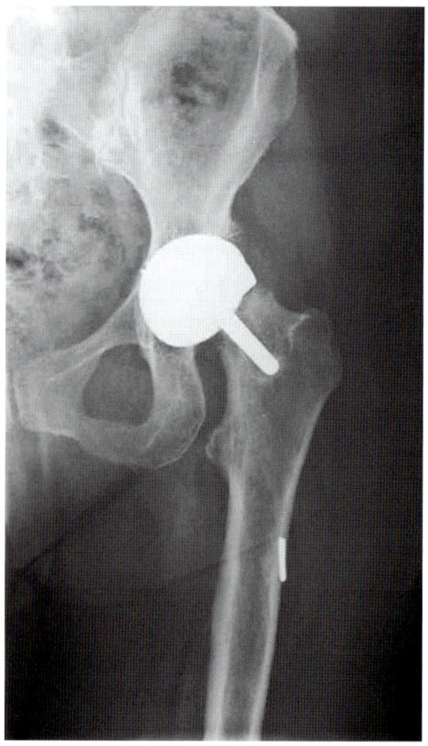

👁 **4.1-2** Patient experienced acute pain following fall on to the right hip. X-rays revealed femoral component failure secondary to femoral neck fracture.

the study to recommend the use of tissue biopsy as an adjunct to joint aspiration to successfully diagnose infection.

Bedair et al [3] investigated the diagnostic test characteristics of white blood cell count, erythrocyte sedimentation rate, differential, and C-reactive protein in synovial fluid aspirates only in the diagnosis of early postoperative infection. In the diagnosis of infection, the optimal cut-off for each parameter was the following:

- Synovial white blood cell count of 27,800 cells/μL (sensitivity 84%; specificity 99%; positive predictive value 94%; and negative predictive value 98%)
- Differential of 89% polymorphonuclear cells
- C-reactive protein: 95 mg/L.

The nuclear medical investigation of choice is triple-phase technetium bone scintigraphy. Although this test has a high sensitivity, it is limited by its low specificity and, therefore, can only aid as a screening tool. Alternative investigations such as a leukocyte bone scan are not popular—despite having 90% specificity in diagnosing infection—because they are technically difficult, time consuming, and expensive. A better perspective appears to be offered by the use of SPECT/CT technology, which combines topographic information from CT and functional information from the bone scan. Early research on its use appears promising but is beyond the scope of this chapter.

Identifying the implants to be removed

Finally, before attempting revision, it is mandatory to be familiar with the index operation, namely what implant system was used, and the exact sizes and fixation method used. It is vital that this information be known, especially if the primary procedure was done elsewhere or by another surgeon. Being prepared allows for adequate planning in terms of explantation instrumentation and avoids unpleasant surprises and difficulties, such as uncovering unexpected cement in the femoral canal. Therefore, it is imperative to know who performed the index operation, the manufacturer and type of prosthesis, the coating method, and type of fixation.

An adjunct to this includes obtaining all x-rays and relevant imaging pertaining to the patient. These images provide an unparalleled insight into the preoperative situation, the immediate postoperative appearance of the prosthesis, and any postoperative changes. These final films offer the most useful information as they indicate changes over time of prosthetic alignment/subsidence, surrounding bone quality, and possible development of osteolysis. They may also indicate previous attempts at repair or reconstruction in the context of an intervention by another surgeon at a different institution.

Entering into such a complex surgery without being fully familiar with all this information is careless and leaves the surgeon at risk of running into serious problems.

Identifying the quality of bone stock

Reduced bone mineral density at the time of primary surgery has been found to correlate closely with the development of osteolysis, placing the patient at an increased risk of fracture. It is recommended to perform dual-energy x-ray absorptiometry (DEXA) scanning as a routine part of the perioperative assessment of patients, unless it would delay treatment. Furthermore, osteopenia at a local and systemic level appears to encourage further periprosthetic bone resorption after joint arthroplasty. Plain film x-rays may reveal reduced bone quality around the prosthesis preoperatively. If there are any concerns, CT can provide a more detailed assessment. Specific examples of periprosthetic fractures around acetabular components in the presence of osteolytic lesions in the pelvis have been reported [4].

Caution should be taken against estimating preoperative osteoporosis on plain x-rays using methods such as the Singh Index. This is now considered an obsolete method of assessing bone mineral density and has been shown to correlate poorly with findings from DEXA [5]. Dual-energy x-ray absorptiometry scanning is a valid investigation and is considered the gold standard in diagnosing osteoporosis. However, it should never delay surgery in a patient with a confirmed periprosthetic fracture. As a preoperative investigation, DEXA shows the quality of the surrounding bone from which the prosthesis is to be explanted most accurately. Furthermore, it influences decision making by indicating the likelihood of adequate fixation of the new revision implant. There is strong evidence to suggest that DEXA is highly sensitive for predicting failure of underlying bone, which could lead to periprosthetic fracture during loading [6]. The key to its use is appropriate timing, which may well be after the revision procedure has been performed.

Identifying subsidence

Axial migration of an implant within its surrounding bone implies inadequate bony ingrowth and fixation, and suggests potential failure. Once diagnosis has been made, information regarding the exact fracture configuration must be sought. Plain film x-ray only provides a 2-D image, which is not sufficiently accurate. The authors advocate the use of cross-sectional imaging with 3-D reconstruction to determine the fracture pattern and plan revision surgery according to this configuration.

4.1.5 Value of diagnostic imaging

General considerations

Diagnostic imaging evaluation of any symptomatic patient after arthroplasty surgery constitutes a fundamental part of the assessment. Typically, this should incorporate a step-by-step approach including the use of plain film x-rays, cross-sectional imaging, bone density measurement, and nuclear medical examination in certain situations. Combined use of these methods can provide information on the underlying bone strength and diagnosis of the fracture itself. The usefulness of cross-sectional imaging has been subject to much debate due to the presence of imaging artifacts caused by the various metallic orthopedic implants used. CT is subject to beam-hardening artefacts and magnetic resonance imaging (MRI) is limited by metal-related susceptibility artefacts.

Value of plain film x-rays

The ready availability, low cost, and relative safety of plain film x-rays make them the first-line investigation of choice. As mentioned previously, these images allow comparison over time to reveal loosening, subsidence, alignment change, and information regarding periprosthetic osteolysis (**4.1-3**). Two separate views of the joint/prosthesis oriented at right angles to one another are a mandatory prerequisite in diagnosing a periprosthetic fracture. In most joints, an anteroposterior and lateral view is all that is required. However, in certain cases an oblique projection may be necessary. These images allow for basic interpretation including fracture location and configuration. Whenever axial malalignment is suspected, the entire extremity (for the leg preferably in an upright, standing position) should be examined radiographically to measure the different axes.

On plain x-rays subtle signs can be detected before the onset of migration and loosening of the prosthesis. In the case of hip resurfacing arthroplasty, this might include the formation of radiolucencies and dense "pedestal lines" around the metaphyseal stem of the prosthesis, densification of the inferior-medial femoral neck, and narrowing of the femoral neck distal to the rim of the prosthesis [7]. A systematic approach to x-ray interpretation reveals these subtle changes and warns of imminent failure.

The value of plain x-rays lies in the possibility to detect and assess the following features:

- Osteolysis
- Subsidence
- Axial alignment.

Value of computed tomography (CT)

Computed tomography is useful to detect implant loosening and to diagnose periprosthetic fractures. It can be valuable to gauge the quality of bone stock preoperatively in order to predict the likelihood of implant stability and longevity. Many studies have shown that bone tissue needs to have a density of approximately 600 Hounsfield units to provide sufficient mechanical stability to an implant [8]. Moreover, a CT scan provides detailed representation of cortical geometry, a further indication of underlying bone strength.

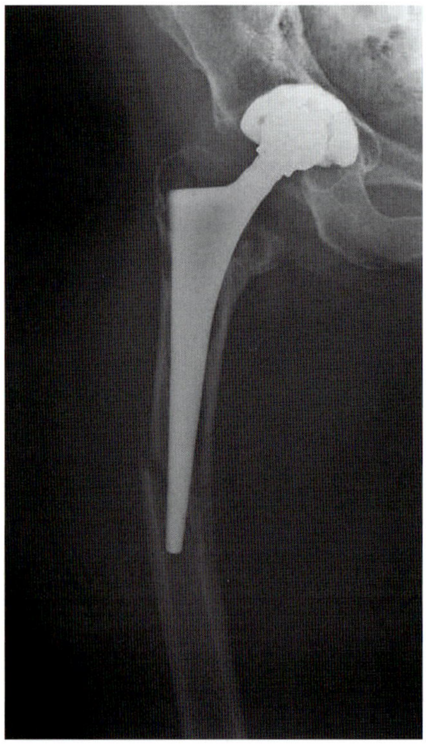

4.1-3 Fall on right hip secondary to fracture around tip of femoral stem. Marked femoral and acetabular osteolysis and horizontal alignment of acetabular component. Cup malpositioning leads to wear that increases fracture risk.

Consequently, CT scans are now readily used in the preoperative analysis of revision cases. It allows better appreciation of possible osteolytic bone loss, occult fractures, and component breakage. Furthermore, the literature confirms the superiority of CT scanning in comparison with conventional x-rays for the evaluation of periprosthetic osteolysis.

A CT scan is now routinely used to assess rotational alignment of components, which is difficult to evaluate on standard orthogonal plain x-ray films. It is highly reproducible in the evaluation of rotational alignment and reveals the presence of osteolysis or an occult fracture (**4.1-4a–f**). The authors advocate the routine use of CT to further assist in diagnosis and management of any patient with a symptomatic joint replacement.

Value of magnetic resonance imaging (MRI)

Much in the same way that CT has evolved over the last decade, MRI now offers the possibility to evaluate the periprosthetic region in greater detail and accuracy. Many investigators have looked into ways of addressing metal-related artifacts from varied orthopedic devices that limit usage.

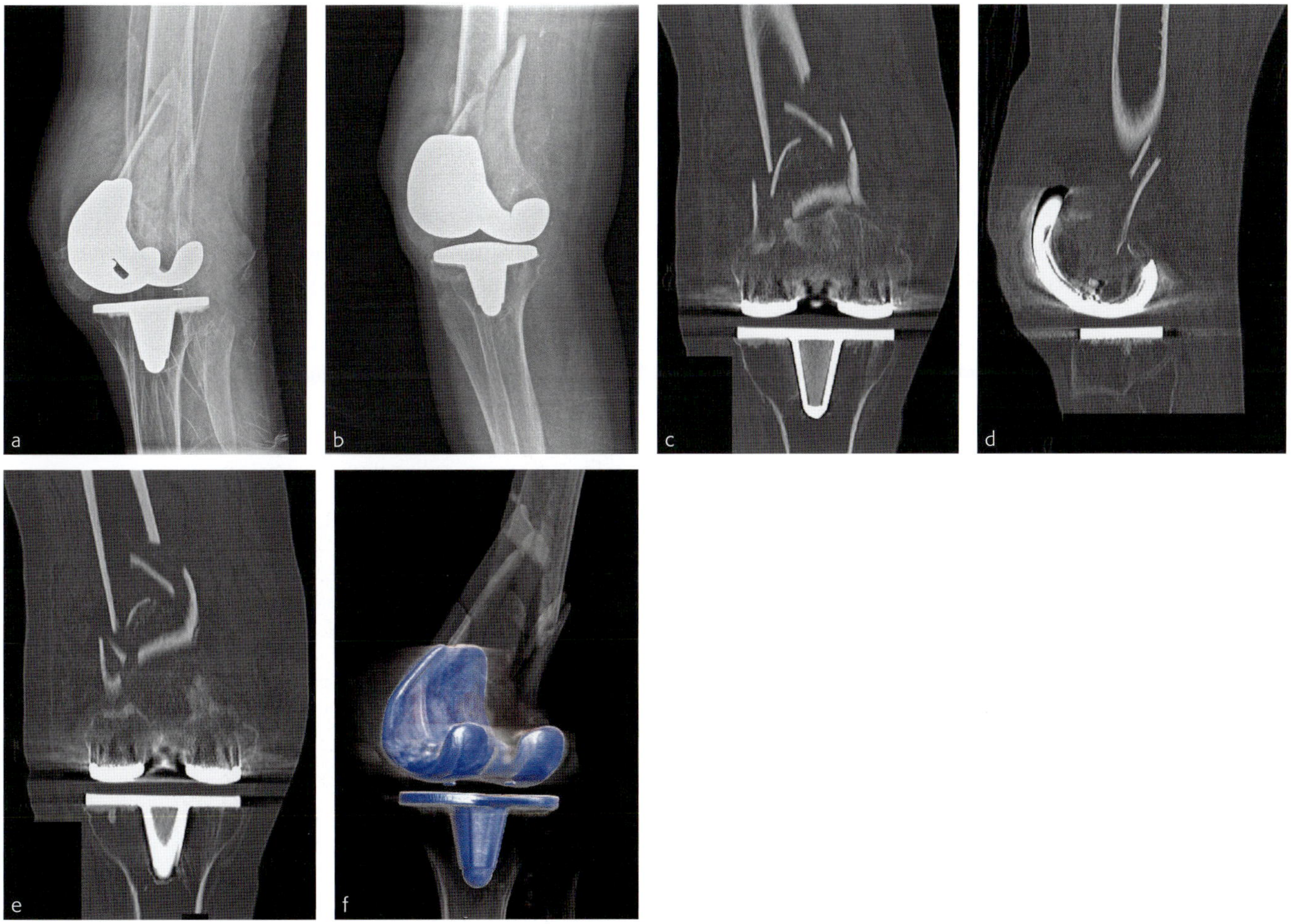

4.1-4a–f Diagnostics workflow of periprosthetic fractures (case provided by M Schütz).
a–b The diagnosis is predominantly achieved by conventional x-rays such as in this patient who sustained a distal femoral fracture.
a Lateral view.
b AP view.
c–f If the conventional x-ray does not provide sufficient information, or for a better understanding of the fracture characteristics for preoperative planning, CT evaluation can be helpful. In this case it was performed with a 256-slice CT scanner for better evaluation of the extension of the fracture in respect to the prosthesis.

Higher magnetic field strengths are associated with increased appearance of artifacts, rendering it difficult to make useful decisions based on the quality of these images. To avoid this situation, useful approaches have included selective orientation of the frequency-encoding direction along the long axis of the device; reduction of the voxel size; increasing the readout gradient strength; using fast-spin echo imaging; and using lower static magnetic field strengths [9].

Currently, MRI is used extensively for evaluating painful hip replacements. An MRI possibly exceeds CT images because the bone, the bone-prosthesis interface, and the soft-tissue envelope can be studied. Through these methods, MRI has proven sensitive and specific for the detection of osseous fractures and provides diagnostic-quality images. Details provided include evidence of implant loosening, penetration of the stem through surrounding cortex, and quality of periprosthetic tissues.

A tremendous advantage of MRI is its ability to provide high-definition images of the prosthesis-fixation interface, specifically its usefulness in detecting bone cement in the femoral canal. This may be helpful when radiolucent bone cement has been used and was not visualized on x-ray. Currently, this is less of an issue as this type of cement is rarely encountered; however, it avoids an unpleasant surprise during surgery. If there is any doubt, an MRI will help to clarify the situation. An MRI can also help to evaluate the extent of any radiolucent cement within bone.

4.1.6 Conclusions

It is important for the orthopedic and trauma surgeon to be aware of periprosthetic fractures as a relatively common complication of arthroplasty surgery—and also to know the typical features exhibited by a patient at risk of imminent periprosthetic fracture. It is much better to preemptively manage the revision situation in the absence of a fracture than wait until one has occurred. The coexisting presence of sepsis must be ruled out by laboratory, aspiration/biopsy, and nuclear medical investigations. Appropriate sequential use of imaging modalities from plain x-rays to cross-sectional imaging should be used in all patients with a prosthesis in situ who complain of a recent deterioration in function—whether it is pain or instability—in the presence or absence of trauma.

Preoperative workup of these patients should include assessment of bone mineral density using DEXA imaging, with attempts to promote bone quality through lifestyle changes and pharmacological means. Surgery should be mindful of blood supply, soft-tissue coverage, and preserve sufficient bone stock for implant stability. Regular patient follow-up needs to include a detailed history of the aforementioned 'red alert' signs and include serial x-rays. These images need to be assessed for evidence of implant loosening, subsidence or malalignment as well as signs of periprosthetic osteolysis. Further radiological evaluation in such cases should include CT and MRI scanning for additional signs of implant loosening and breaching of the surrounding cortex.

4.2 Classification

Authors **Clive P Duncan, Fares S Haddad**

4.2.1 Introduction

Periprosthetic fractures are an increasingly common and potentially serious complication of joint replacement arthroplasty. They can occur intraoperatively as well as in the postoperative period.

The treatment of these fractures is challenging and may be associated with a significant rate of orthopedic and systemic complications. However, the main goals of functional restoration and a painless joint are achievable in the majority of patients.

Based on fracture location and morphology, various host factors as well as the timing of the fracture, a number of treatment options are available to treat this often demanding problem. This chapter will emphasize the core principles that are fundamental to the successful assessment and management of this complication. The authors have assembled these principles in the Unified Classification System (UCS) that can be readily applied to periprosthetic fractures around the shoulder, elbow, wrist, hip, knee, and ankle.

As outlined in the UCS mnemonic and subsequent sections of this chapter, the UCS is alphabetical in its core design for ease of application across all potentially involved bones and joints (Types A to F, with Type B subdivided). The addition of the bone and joint numerical designations is for ease of collection of information for such purposes as data bases and joint registries.

The authors recommend, in the practical clinical setting, where simplicity is key, that the fracture description follow the usual steps of: 1) the fracture type; 2) followed by the bone; 3) followed by the joint replaced.

For instance, the injury illustrated in the x-ray of **4.2-3** would therefore be described as "Type A of the patella associated with knee replacement". The numerical designations outlined in the fracture chart **4.2-3**, and seen in the diagrams to follow, would be added later for the purposes outlined above.

4.2.2 Unified Classification System (UCS)

Background

A number of classification systems already exist that are mostly based on the Vancouver Classification relating to the femur, described by Duncan and Masri in 1995 (**4.2-1**) [10].

Various other classification systems established in relation to other joints, have been combined or unified. Where required, they have been expanded, thereby acknowledging the biological and biomechanical factors that are common to all fractures following joint replacement as well as the

4.2-1 Original Vancouver Classification System for periprosthetic fractures of the proximal femur [10].

Type	Location	Subtype
A	Trochanteric region	A-G Greater trochanter
		A-L Lesser trochanter
B	Around or just distal to the stem	B1 Prosthesis stable (well fixed)
		B2 Prosthesis unstable (loose)
		B3 Implant loose and bone stock inadequate
C	Well distal to the stem	–

important influence of component loosening and bone loss (4.2-3). Where no classification existed, for instance with reference to the wrist and ankle, the principles of the Unified Classification System (UCS) have been applied.

Core principles

The principles on which the modern management of periprosthetic fractures are based include:

- The location of the fracture (whether it involves the bone supporting the implant or is distant to it)
- The fixation of the component (whether or not the bone-implant interface was stable prior to fracture and remained so after the injury)
- The adequacy of the bone stock (**4.2-1a–c**) and bone strength supporting the implant (whether it is sufficient to permit fracture fixation or revision without requiring additional major reconstruction).

These principles apply to all fractures that will be dealt with in this chapter involving hip, knee, ankle, shoulder, elbow, or wrist. For the main part, the guidelines will be demonstrated in the context of fractures that occur after joint replacement but they also apply if the fracture is diagnosed during component implantation.

In the rare circumstance where more than one implant is involved, for instance both the acetabulum and femur after hip replacement, or both the femur and tibia (or patella) after knee replacement, the same core principles apply. This will be dealt with later in this chapter.

Numerical code (anatomical location)

Corresponding to the principles of the AO/OTA Fracture and Dislocation Classification, first the involved joint and then its components should be identified. The authors propose to number the joints I–VI proceeding from the shoulder (I), elbow (II), wrist (III), hip (IV), knee (V), to the ankle (VI) (**4.2-2**). For the identification of the bones, the numbering follows that of the AO/OTA Fracture and Dislocation Classification (**4.2-2**).

Once the anatomical location and bones have been identified, the type of fracture is generally described according to the original Vancouver classification.

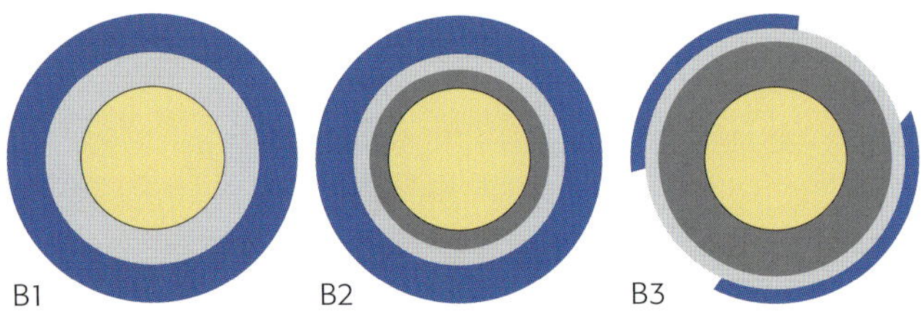

4.2-1 Bone cross sections showing different bone quality.
B1 Good bone, no implant loosening
B2 Good bone with implant loosening
B3 Poor bone or bone defect with implant loosening

Fracture types as a unified concept

Overview

In order to enable the reader to remember the different fracture types of the Unified Classification System (UCS) more easily, the following mnemonic code has been devised:

- Type A: *Apophyseal*
- Type B: *Bed* of the implant
- Type C: *Clear* of the implant
- Type D: *Dividing* the bone between two implants
- Type E: *Each* of two bones supporting one arthroplasty
- Type F: *Facing* and articulating with a hemiarthroplasty.

A more accurate and complete description of the different fracture types can be found in the following paragraphs and in **4.2-3**.

4.2-2 Identification of bone numbering according to AO/OTA Fracture and Dislocation Classification.

Joint	Bone	AO/OTA code
Shoulder	Scapula	14
	Humerus	1
Elbow	Humerus	1
	Ulna	2
	Radius	2
Wrist	Radius	2
	Ulna	2
	Carpus or metacarpals	7
Hip	Pelvis/acetabulum	6
	Femur	3
Knee	Femur	3
	Tibia	4
	Patella	34
Ankle	Tibia	4
	Fibula	4
	Talus (hindfoot)	8

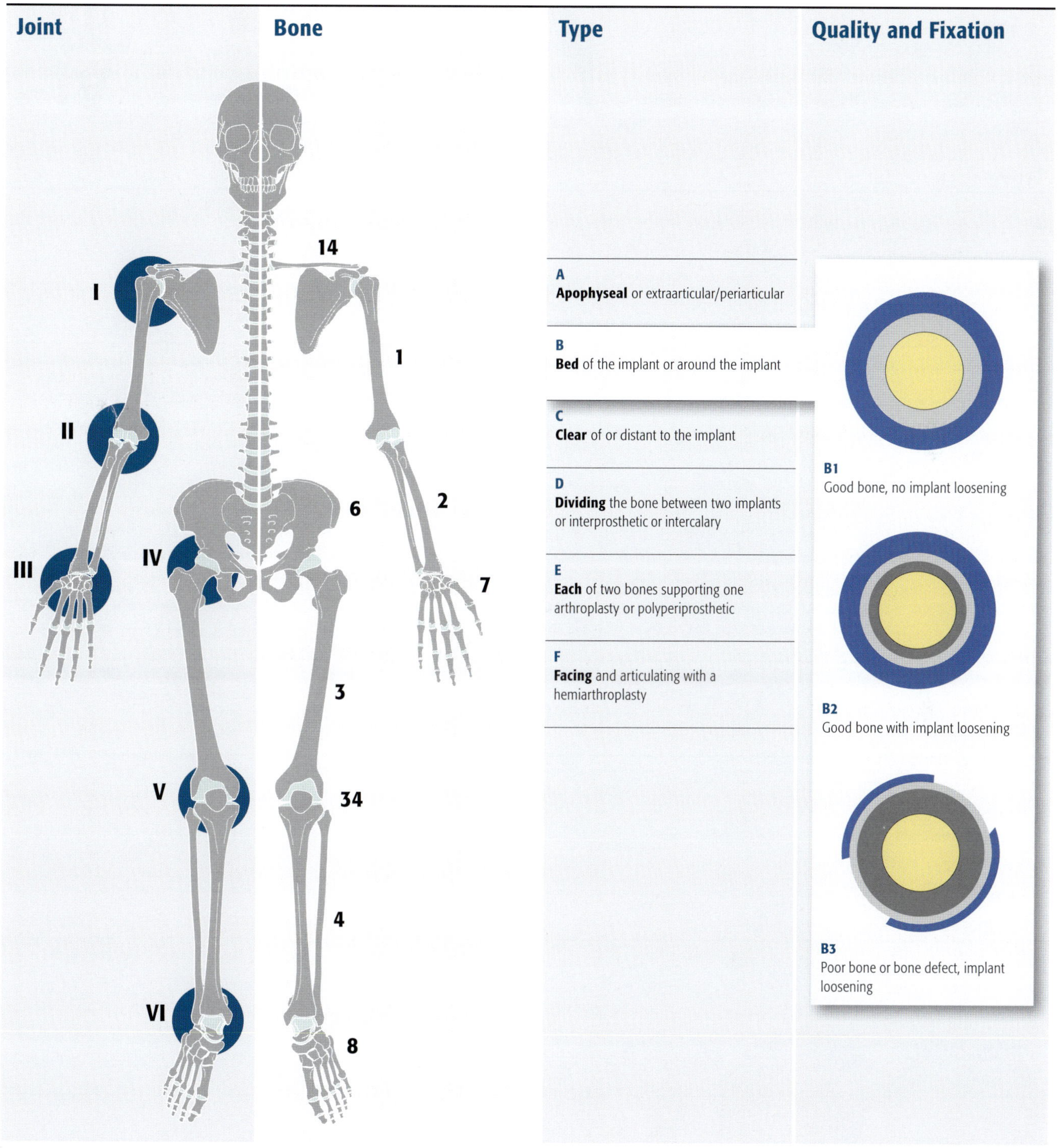

4.2-2 Summary of the Unifed Classification System (UCS).

4.2-3 New Unified Classification System (UCS) applying to all periprosthetic fractures (adaptation and expansion of the original Vancouver Classification System of the proximal femur).

Type		I Shoulder 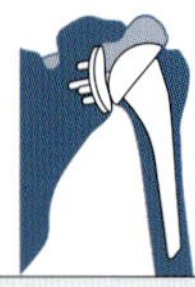		II Elbow 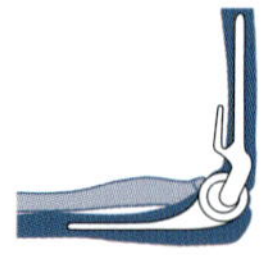		III Wrist 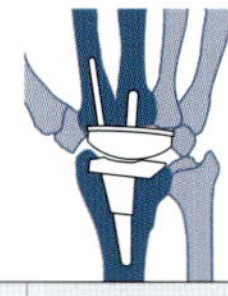	
		I.14	**I.1**	**II.1**	**II.2**	**III.2**	**III.7**
		Glenoid/scapula	Humerus, proximal	Humerus, distal	Ulna/radius, proximal	Radius/ulna, distal	Carpus/metacarpals
A *Apophyseal* or extraarticular/ periarticular	**A1** Avulsion of	Coracoid process	Greater tuberosity	Lateral epicondyle	Olecranon tip	Radial styloid	–
	A2 Avulsion of	Acromion	Lesser tuberosity	Medial epicondyle	Coronoid process, radial tuberosity	Ulnar styloid, if ulna retained	–
B *Bed* of the implant or around the implant	**B1** Prosthesis stable, good bone	Glenoid implant stable, good bone	Humeral implant stable, good bone	Humeral implant stable, good bone	Ulnar implant stable, good bone	Radial implant stable, good bone	Carpal/metacarpal implant stable, good bone
	B2 Prosthesis loose, good bone	Glenoid implant loose, good bone	Humeral implant loose, good bone	Humeral implant loose, good bone	Ulnar implant loose, good bone	Radial implant loose, good bone	Carpal/metacarpal implant loose, good bone
	B3 Prosthesis loose, poor bone or bone defect	Glenoid implant loose, poor bone, defect	Humeral implant loose, poor bone, defect	Humeral implant loose, poor bone, defect	Ulnar implant loose, poor bone, defect	Radial implant loose, poor bone, defect	Carpal/metacarpal implant loose, poor bone, defect
C *Clear* of or distant to the implant	–	Body of the scapula	Distal to the implant	Proximal to the implant	Distal to the implant	Proximal to the implant	Distal metacarpals
D *Dividing* the bone between two implants or interprosthetic or intercalary	–	–	Between shoulder and elbow arthroplasties, close to the shoulder	Between shoulder and elbow arthroplasties, close to the elbow	–	Between wrist and radial-head prosthesis	–
E *Each* of two bones supporting one arthroplasty or polyperiprosthetic	–	Scapula and humerus		Humerus and ulna/radius		Radius/ulna and carpus/metacarpals	
F *Facing* and articulating with a hemiarthroplasty	–	Fracture of the glenoid articulating with the humeral hemiarthroplasty	–	Distal humeral fracture articulating with the radial-head prosthesis	–	–	–

IV Hip 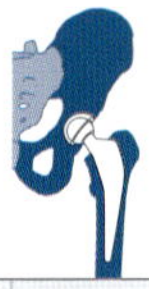		**V** Knee 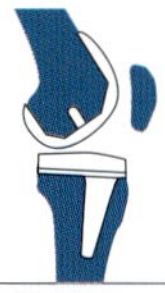			**VI** Ankle 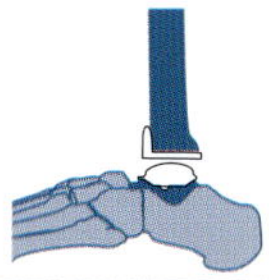		
IV.6	**IV.3**	**V.3**	**V.4**	**V.34**	**VI.4**	**VI.8**	
Acetabulum/pelvis	Femur, proximal	Femur, distal	Tibia, proximal	Patella	Tibia, distal	Talus	**Type**
Anterior inferior and superior iliac spine	Greater trochanter	Lateral epicondyle	Medial or lateral plateau, nondisplaced	Disrupted extensor, proximal pole	Tip of the medial malleolus	–	**A** *Apophyseal* or extraarticular/ periarticular
Ischial tuberosity	Lesser trochanter	Medial epicondyle	Tibial tubercle	Disrupted extensor, distal pole	Tip of the lateral malleolus	–	
Acetabular rim or good bone	Stem stable, good bone; Surface replacement: femoral neck	Proximal to stable stem, good bone	Stem and component stable, good bone	Intact extensor, implant stable, good bone	Transverse or medial malleolus shear, good bone	Body of the talus, good bone	**B** *Bed* of the implant or around the implant
Loose cup, good bone	Loose stem, good bone; Surface replacement: loose implant, no proximal femoral bone loss	Proximal to loose stem, good bone	Loose component/ stem, good bone	Loose implant, good bone	Tibial implant loose, good bone	Body of the talus, loose, good bone	
Loose cup, poor bone, defect; Pelvic discontinuity	Loose stem, poor bone, defect; Surface replacement: loose implant, bone loss	Proximal to loose stem, poor bone, defect	Loose component/ stem, poor bone, defect	Loose implant, poor bone, defect	Tibial implant loose, poor bone, defect	Body of the talus, bone defect	
Pelvic/acetabular fractures distant to the implant	Distal to the implant and cement mantle	Proximal to the implant and cement mantle	Distal to the implant and cement mantle	–	Proximal to the implant	Neck or head of the talus	**C** *Clear* of or distant to the implant
Pelvic fracture between bilateral total hip arthroplasties	Between hip and knee arthroplasties, close to the hip	Between hip and knee arthroplasties, close to the knee	Between ankle and knee arthroplasties, close to the knee	–	Between knee and ankle arthroplasties, close to the ankle	Between an ankle and talonavicular arthroplasties	**D** *Dividing* the bone between two implants or interprosthetic or intercalary
Pelvis and femur		Femur and tibia/patella			Tibia and talus		**E** *Each* of two bones supporting one arthroplasty or polyperiprosthetic
Fracture of the acetabulum articulating with the femoral hemiarthroplasty	–	Fracture of femoral condyle articulating with tibial hemiarthroplasty	–	Fracture of the patella that has no surface replacement and articulates with the femoral component of the total knee arthroplasty	–	–	**F** *Facing* and articulating with a hemiarthroplasty

Type A—*apophyseal* or extraarticular/periarticular

For the purpose of simplicity and reasonable generalization, fractures will be categorized as type A if they involve the bone or apophysis adjacent to the implant but have little influence on implant fixation.

This category would include such examples as:

- The tuberosities of the humerus
- The humeral epicondyles or olecranon tip at the elbow
- The trochanters and epicondyles of the femur
- The spinous extraarticular pelvic fractures
- The poles or tips of the patella
- The tibial tuberosity as well as the malleoli.

The need for surgical management would be based on the location and characteristics of each fracture type and the consequences of nonoperative treatment—irrespective of the presence of an implant.

The guiding principles are based on the importance of the soft-tissue structures attached to an apophysis and whether that apophysis is displaced or not. For example—with reference to musculotendinous attachments—a displaced fracture of the lesser trochanter could be regarded as safe but not a displaced fracture of the greater trochanter. The iliopsoas muscle, for example, is not critical in view of a well-functioning and stable hip replacements, the abductor muscles, however, are. **4.2-3** shows a type A fracture of the patella, ie, a displaced avulsion of the distal pole. Surgical intervention is indicated because of the displacement and importance of the attached tendon for the function of the replaced knee.

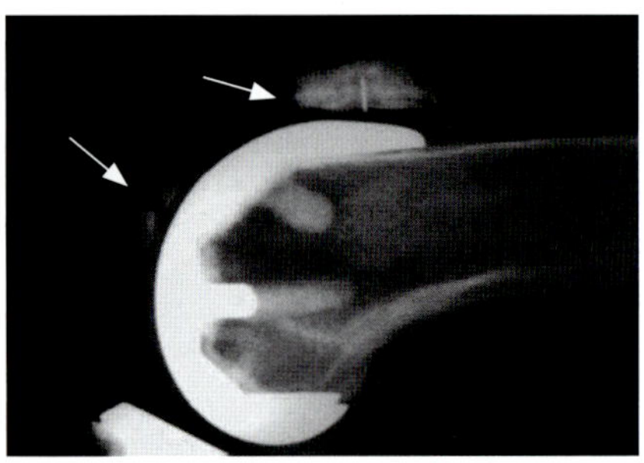

4.2-3 Type A fracture of the patella. There is an avulsion of the inferior pole (arrows) without loosening of the implant. The extensor mechanism has been disrupted.

Similar principles also apply to ligamentous attachments. A displaced fracture of the acromion or coracoid process could be left untreated, but not a displaced fracture of the medial malleolus. The coracoacromial ligament is not important for function after shoulder replacement, while the medial or deltoid ligament of the ankle is important for stability following replacement of that joint.

Type B—*bed* of the implant or around the implant

If the fracture involves the bone-implant interface, which is responsible for the stability of fixation of the implant, this group will be categorized as type B. Typical examples include the shaft of the humerus, femur, or tibia after insertion of a component with a stem, or a fracture of the glenoid, acetabulum, or equator of the patella. In this context two important questions need to be asked in order to further classify the fracture into one of three subcategories:

1) Is the implant well fixed or loose?

- If well fixed: Type B1
- If loose: Type B2.

2) In case of loose implant, is there adequate bone present to successfully support implant revision?

- If yes: Classification remains Type B2
- If not: Type B3.

In some cases the distinction between type B1 and B2 will require further radiological investigation or examination of the bone-implant interface at the time of operation. However, in most cases the distinction will be clear. Moreover, the distinction between type B2 and B3 is one of individual interpretation, without a clear-cut transition. To some extent it will also depend on the reconstruction choice favored by the surgeon. As an example, impaction allografting and cement, with a long stem, would find broad application in expert hands for type B2 and B3 fractures involving the proximal femur after hip replacement, unless bone loss is very severe. A similar approach would apply to the use of tapered, fluted titanium stems, which are gaining in popularity for the management of both B2 and B3 fractures of the femur. There is, however, a blurring of the difference between these fracture types affecting this bone.

As a simple rule of thumb, the authors suggest that the fracture is categorized as type B2 if the loose implant can be revised with a fairly straightforward technique. However, if more specialized techniques or a salvage procedure are necessary, then it should be classified as type B3.

In the majority of cases, the type B fracture will either be type B2 or B3. Implant loosening was either present prior to fracture, or it will have occurred as a consequence of the injury. In the presence of a loose implant (type B2 or B3), reduction and fixation of the fracture alone can have a deleterious influence on the outcome of treatment [11].

In a minority of cases, after critical analysis, the fracture will prove to be a type B1, and osteosynthesis without implant revision can be considered. However, this does not apply to the following situation: After surface replacement of the femoral or humeral head, a fracture of the neck adjacent to the mouth of the implant will inevitably interrupt the remaining blood supply to the head fragment, sooner or later resulting in collapse. Therefore, even with a well-fixed prosthetic stem, which equals a type B1 fracture, revision arthroplasty will be the only option.

4.2-4a–e demonstrates the application of the UCS to just one bone (the femur) following joint replacement. It illustrates periprosthetic fracture types A1, B1, B2, B3, and C (described next) following hip replacement.

In contrast, **4.2-5a–c** demonstrates an application of the UCS to various bones, regardless of the joint involved. The illustrated fractures include: type B1 of the femur, type B2 of the ulna, and type B3 of the tibia. The principles of treatment will be the same although the anatomic sites vary.

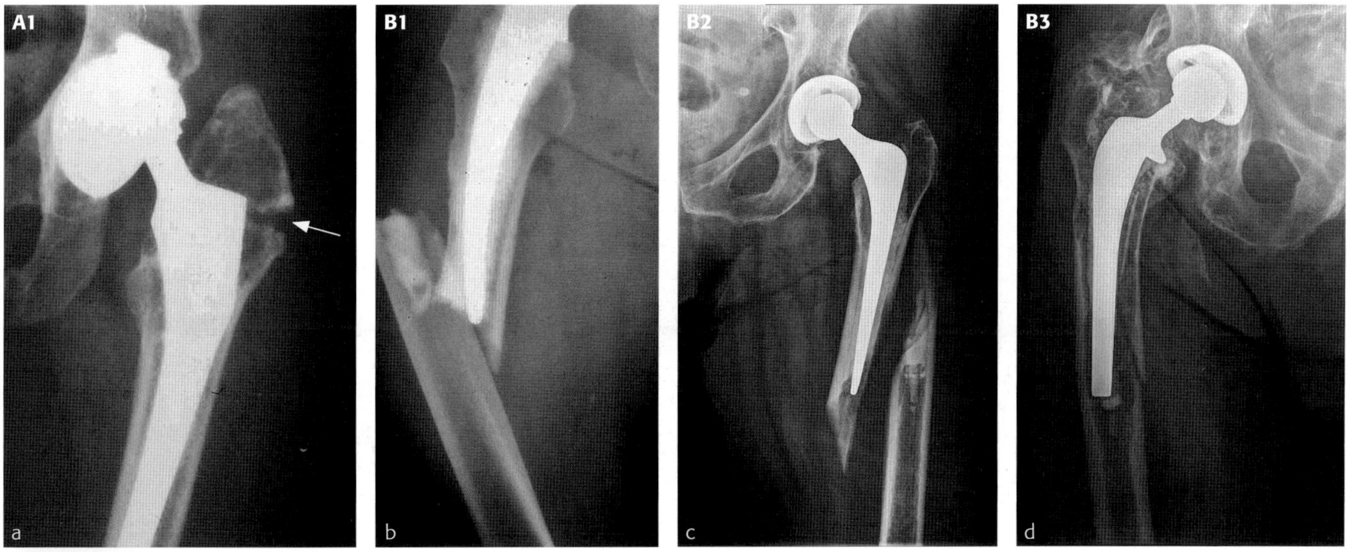

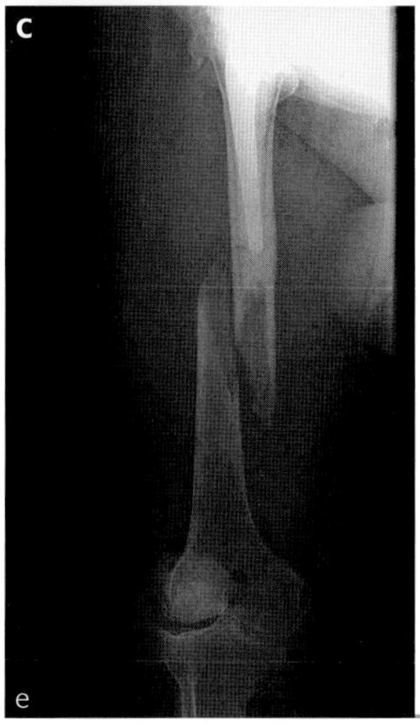

4.2-4a–e Composite application of the UCS to the five most common fractures as they may affect one bone, such as the femur.

- **a** Type A1 fracture.
- **b** Type B1 fracture (cropped to emphasize the stable interfaces).
- **c** Type B2 fracture, which was well fixed before the long spiral fracture destabilized the stem.
- **d** Type B3 fracture, with loosening of the stem and severe bone loss.
- **e** Type C fracture well distant to the stem.

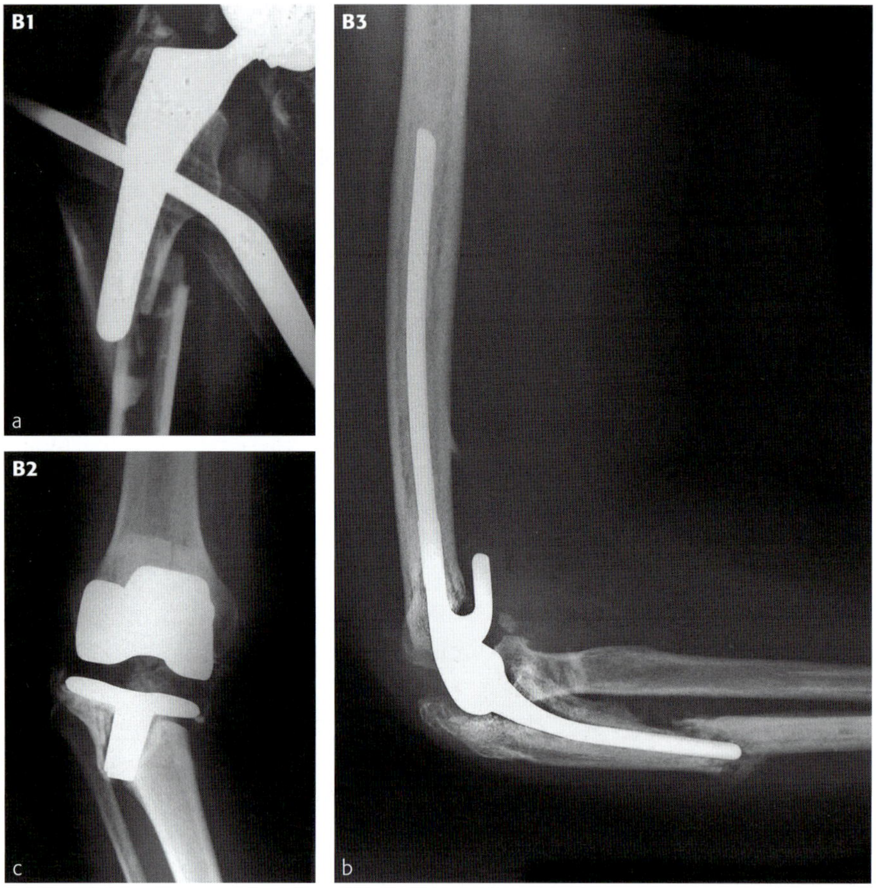

4.2-5a–c Composite application of the Unified Classification System (UCS) across three different joints and bones following joint replacement.

a Type B1 fracture of the femur (confirmed at operation).
b B2 fracture of the ulna.
c B3 fracture of the tibia.

Type C—*clear* of or distant to the implant

If the fracture is quite distant to the arthroplasty, to the extent that the implant can be ignored, it will be categorized as type C. Examples include nonapophyseal fractures of the ilium or pubic rami after hip replacement as well as fractures of the distal femur or of the tibial shaft after knee replacement, if located at a distance from the implant. **4.2-6** illustrates a type C fracture involving the humeral shaft after shoulder replacement.

It is in the setting of a type C periprosthetic fracture that the modern principles of fracture management apply, with little influence brought to bear by the preexisting joint replacement. If the fixation technique must include a part of bone which contains an implant (such as a stem) then some type of modified plate fixation may have to be taken into consideration, such as by cerclage wires, cables, or monocortical screws.

Type D—*dividing* the bone between two implants, interprosthetic or intercalary

These cases are quite uncommon as the fracture involves a long bone that supports two prostheses, both proximal and distal to the fracture site. This is classified as a type D fracture. Most frequently this involves the femur between a hip and a knee replacement. Theoretically, it could involve the humerus, the radius or the tibia, if both, the proximal and distal joints have been replaced. Type D interprosthetic or intercalary fracture, together with the type B3 periprosthetic fracture with severely compromised bone stock and type E polyperiprosthetic fractures represent the three most challenging groups of fractures.

The authors suggest approaching type D fractures by separate analyses of implant stability as well as the available bone stock around each of the implants. Treatment should be based upon those separate analyses. Appropriate treatment may involve revision of one, both, or neither arthroplasty. In 👁 **4.2-7**, separate analyses of the implants suggest a type B3 fracture of the hip and a type C fracture of the knee. The management plan needs to be based on such analyses.

Type E—*each* of two bones supporting one arthroplasty or polyperiprosthetic

In these rare cases, the bones supporting implants on either side of an arthroplasty are both fractured, eg, the acetabulum and femur after hip replacement, the femur and tibia after knee replacement, or the humerus and ulna after elbow replacement. The authors recommend that the fracture, implant stability, and bone stock on each side of the arthroplasty are analyzed separately and dealt with accordingly. If these analyses hold true during intraoperative assessment, then each bone and implant can be managed accordingly. 👁 **4.2-8** illustrates a type E polyperiprosthetic fracture involving the acetabulum and femur. Separate analyses suggest a type B3 fracture affecting the acetabulum and a type B2 fracture of the femur. The management principles involve complex reconstruction of the acetabulum—which are dealt with later—as well as long-stem revision of the femur in combination with fracture reduction and fixation and use of bone grafts. A similar fracture is illustrated by 👁 **4.2-9**, involving an elbow joint. Separate analyses of both fractures reveal type B3 of the humerus and type B3 of the ulna. Complex reconstruction or a salvage procedure must be considered.

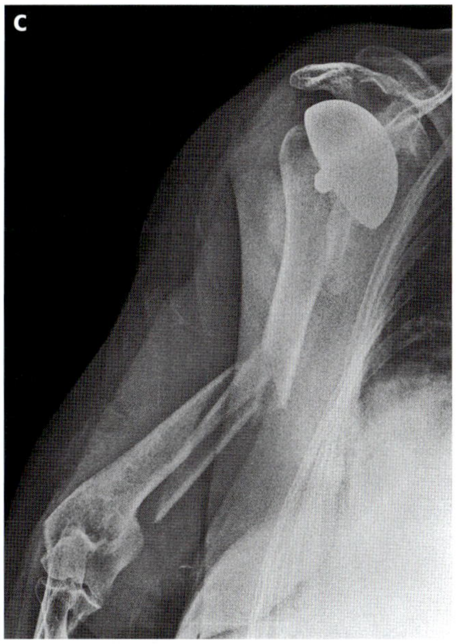

👁 **4.2-6** Type C fracture involving the humerus below a well-functioning shoulder replacement.

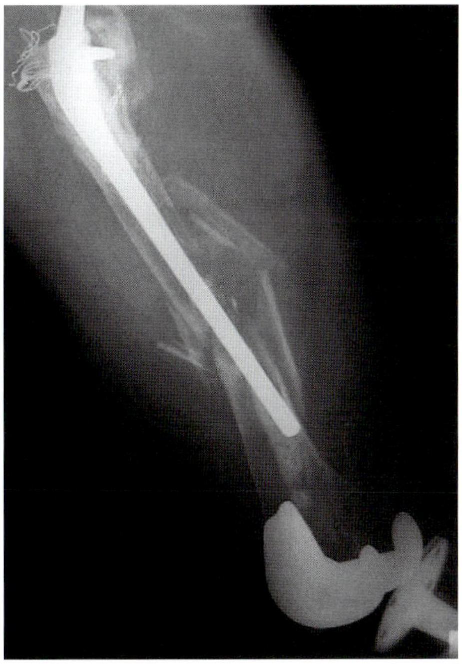

👁 **4.2-7** Type D fracture involving the femur between a hip and knee replacement. Separate analyses of this and other x-rays indicated a type B3 fracture of the femur for the hip arthroplasty (loose stem and severe loss of bone) and a type C fracture for the knee arthroplasty (distant to a well-fixed knee implant).

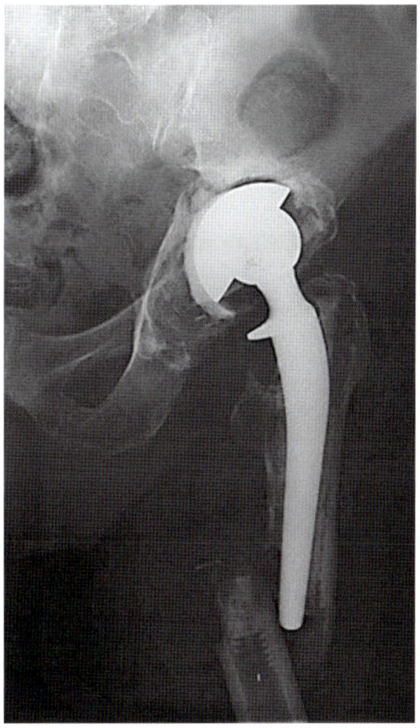

👁 **4.2-8** Type E fracture involving both sides of a hip replacement, with a periprosthetic fracture of the acetabulum and femur. Separate analyses reveal a type B3 fracture of the acetabulum and B2 fracture of the femur.

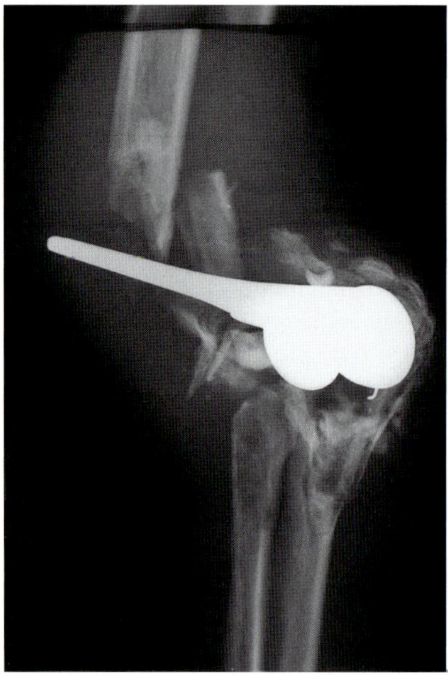

4.2-9 Type E fracture involving both sides of an elbow replacement. Separate implant analysis reveals a type B3 fracture for both components.

Type F—*facing* and articulating with a hemiarthroplasty

Hemiarthroplasty is still used in the treatment of selected injuries, for instance following a displaced subcapital fracture of the femoral neck, a comminuted fracture of the head or neck of the humerus, or a similar injury affecting the head or neck of the radius. Similarly, the patella is commonly not resurfaced during knee replacement but left to articulate with the femoral flange as a hemiarthroplasty.

As a rare event, a subsequent fracture can affect the non-replaced joint surface which faces and articulates with the implant, such as that of the acetabulum, patella, glenoid or lateral humeral condyle (**4.2-10a–b**).

By and large, the principles of management for this category will depend on the degree of fracture displacement and the health of the articulation, ie, whether it was degenerated prior to the most recent injury.

If the displacement is minor, nonoperative management would be reasonable, with the possibility for delayed intervention in case the articulation becomes painful.

If the displacement is substantial and the joint was free of pain before the new injury, then reduction and fixation of the fracture need to be considered. The articulating implant can be left undisturbed. Such a case is illustrated in **4.210a–b**. There is severe medial displacement of a previously painless hemiarthroplasty, with a well-fixed stem. However, if the joint is already degenerated, especially if it was painful before the new injury, revision joint replacement should be considered, soon after injury or after the fracture has healed.

Fracture of the implant

Lastly, there is the issue of fracture of the implant itself, with or without fracture of the supporting bone. The former, without a periprosthetic fracture of bone, is managed as a failed arthroplasty, ie, by revision. The latter can be categorized within the type B subgroups, along the lines that have already been dealt with. The majority will be a type B3 fracture.

4.2-11a–b illustrates two examples of a fracture involving the femoral stem following hip replacement. **4.2-11b** illustrates a combined prosthetic and periprosthetic fracture, which will require evaluation based on the UCS and therapy according to the core principles of treatment as outlined before. It is a type B3 fracture even though the very tip of the broken stem remains fixed.

Reliability and validity of the Unified Classification System (UCS)

The interobserver and intraobserver reliability of this basic classification system as it applies to the femur after hip replacement have been confirmed in studies in North America and Europe [12, 13]. The authors believe it can be applied equally well in order to define fracture treatment in cases pertaining to the replacement of other joints such as the shoulder, elbow, knee, and potentially to the wrist and ankle as well.

As further examples of the versatility and broad generalizability of the UCS, **4.2-12a–c** illustrate the same fracture type (B3) affecting the humerus (**a**, **b**) respectively the patella (**c**) after three types of joint replacement (shoulder (**a**), elbow (**b**), and knee (**c**)).

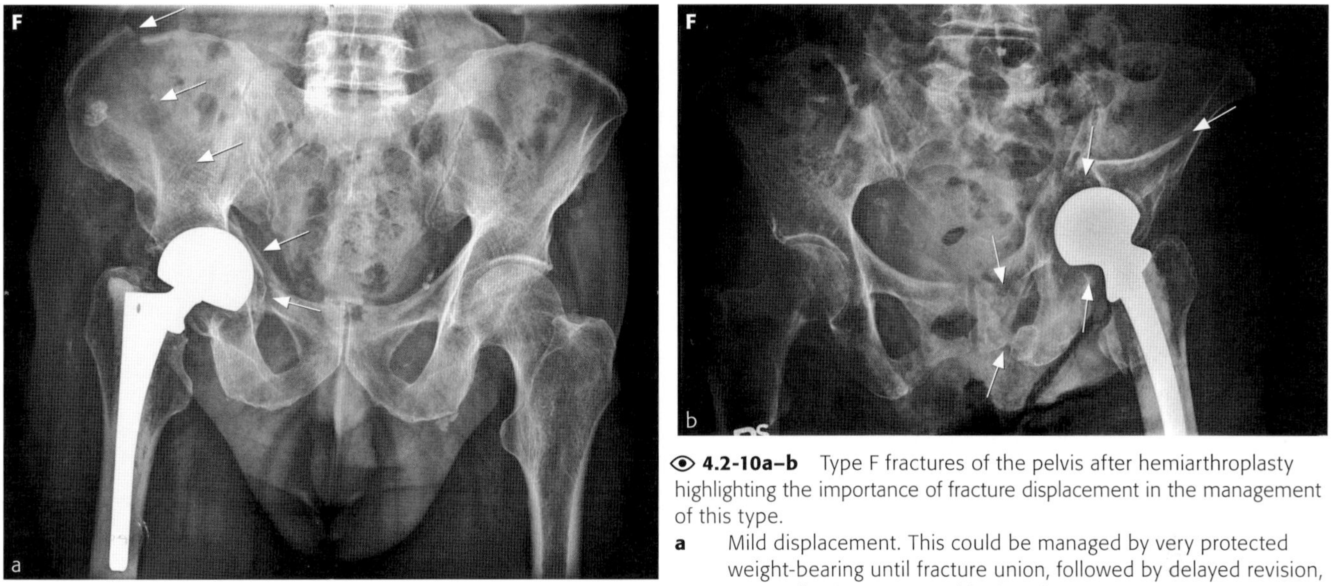

4.2-10a–b Type F fractures of the pelvis after hemiarthroplasty highlighting the importance of fracture displacement in the management of this type.

- **a** Mild displacement. This could be managed by very protected weight-bearing until fracture union, followed by delayed revision, especially if it was painful before the new injury.
- **b** Severe displacement. This requires early fracture reduction and fixation, with early or delayed revision arthroplasty, regardless of the status prior to new injury.

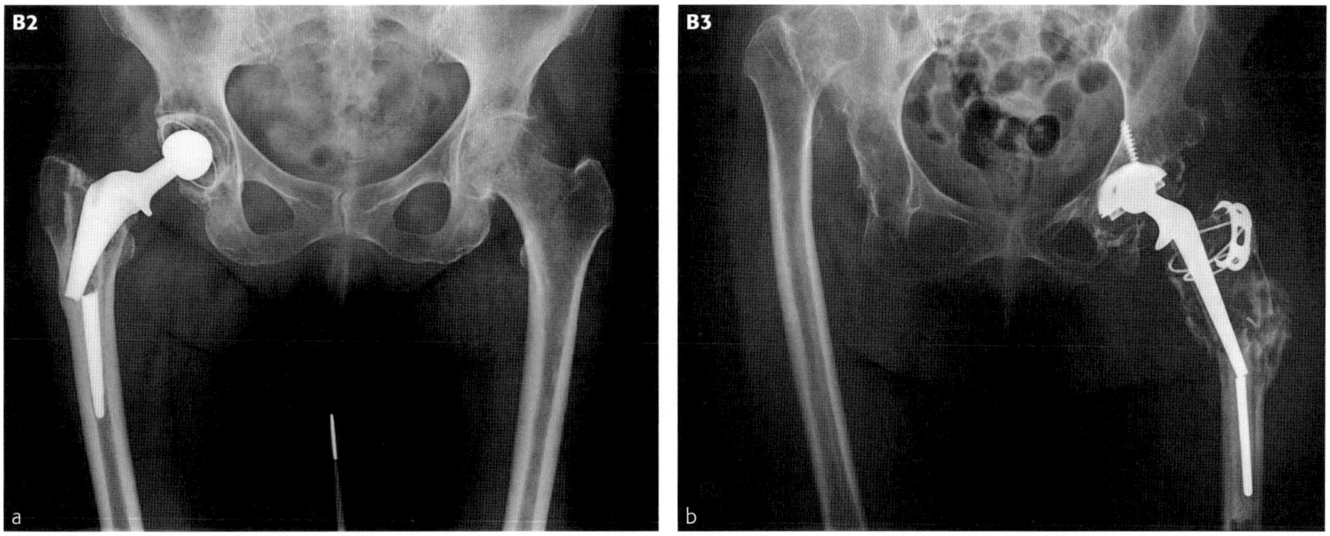

4.2-11a–b Fractures of the implant.

- **a** Only the stem is broken. A revision is required.
- **b** The stem and its supporting bone are fractured along with substantial bone loss. This is a type IV.B3 fracture.

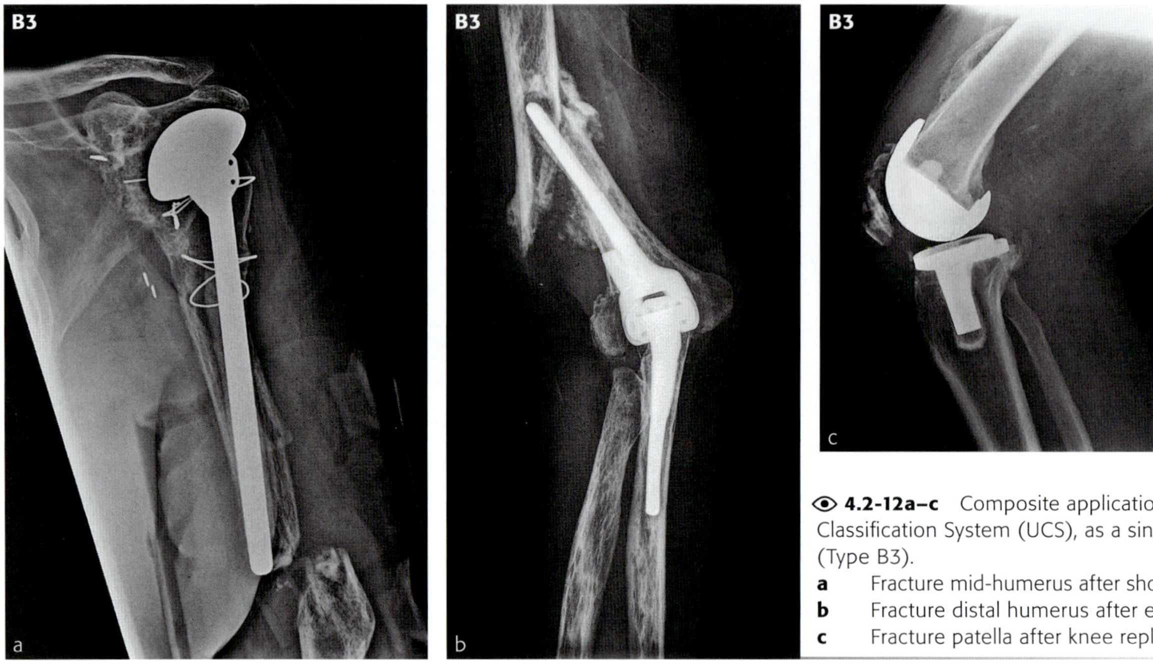

4.2-12a–c Composite application of the Unified Classification System (UCS), as a single fracture type (Type B3).

a Fracture mid-humerus after shoulder replacement.
b Fracture distal humerus after elbow replacement.
c Fracture patella after knee replacement.

4.2.3 Classification of periprosthetic fractures according to anatomical regions

I Shoulder

Existing classification systems

Different authors have proposed a variety of classification systems for fractures of the shoulder (**4.2-4**).

Unified Classification System (UCS)

The Unified Classification System (UCS) and principles of management can be applied to the shoulder.

Scapula (I.14)

Type A
These types of fracture apply to the coracoid and acromion processes of the scapula (**4.2-13a–b**). Any need for surgical management is unlikely.

Type B
These types of fracture apply to the glenoid and are subdivided into type B1, B2, and B3 based on the fixation of the glenoid implant and adequacy of the supporting bone.

Type B1 fractures of the glenoid (👁 **4.2-14**)are unlikely to occur except as an intraoperative event that is amenable to cemented fixation of the component stem. Type B2 fractures (👁 **4.2-15**) will require revision. Extreme cases of bone loss, ie, type B3 (👁 **4.2-16**) may require a salvage procedure.

Type C

In these fractures (👁 **4.2-17**), the body of the scapula is involved. They are also amenable to nonoperative management.

Type D

In practice, this type of fracture will not affect the scapula as the only joint proximal to the glenoid, the acromioclavicular joint, is not amenable to replacement arthroplasty.

Type E

Such fractures would involve the scapula and humerus.

Type F

This type of fractures involves the glenoid after prior replacement of the humeral head (hemiarthroplasty) (👁 **4.2-18**). The principles of management depend on the degree of fracture displacement and the health of the glenohumeral articulation prior to the most recent injury. These have been outlined above in the introductory section to this chapter.

4.2-4 Different classification systems for periprosthetic fractures after shoulder arthroplasty.

Authors	Fracture type	Definition of fracture type
Groh et al [14, 15]	I	Fracture exclusively proximal to the tip of the stem
	II	Fracture at the tip of the stem, running from proximal of the tip to distal
	III	Fracture exclusively distal of the tip of the stem
Wright and Cofield [16]	A	Fracture at the tip of the stem extending proximally more than one third of the length of the stem
	B	Fracture at the tip but with less than one third of proximal extension
	C	Fracture distal to the implant and fractures extending into the humeral metaphysis
Campbell et al [17]	I	Fracture of the greater or lesser humeral tuberosity
	II	Fracture of the proximal humeral metaphysis
	III	Fracture of the proximal humeral diaphysis
	IV	Fracture of the mid shaft and distal humeral diaphysis
Worland et al [18]	A	Fracture about the tuberosities
	B	Fracture around the stem
	B1	Spiral fracture with stable stem
	B2	Short oblique or transverse fracture with stable stem
	B3	Any fracture with unstable stem
	C	Fracture distal to the stem

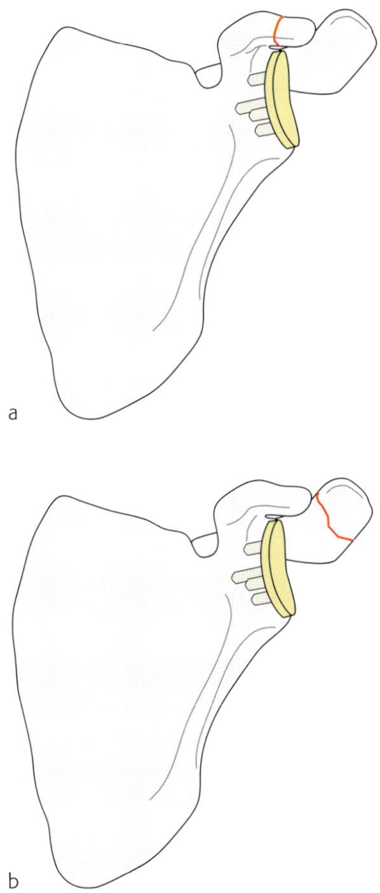

👁 **4.2-13a–b** Periprosthetic fracture types of scapula.
a Type I.14-A1 coracoid process.
b Type I.14-A2 acromion.

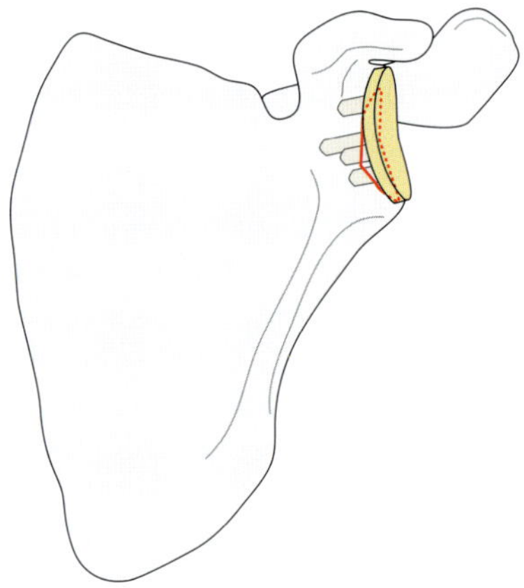

4.2-14 Periprosthetic fracture of glenoid, type I.14-B1.

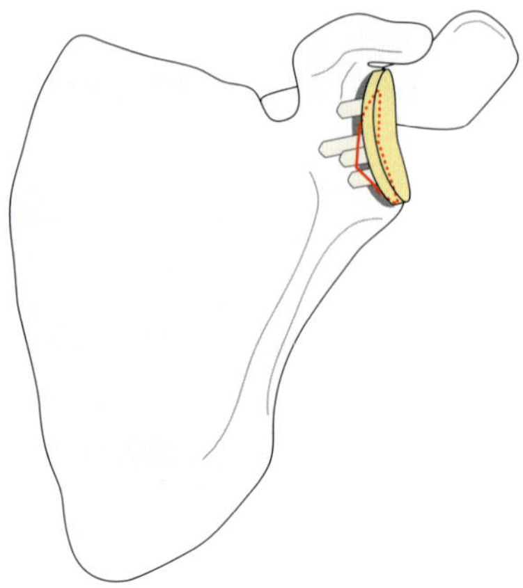

4.2-15 Periprosthetic fracture glenoid, type I.14-B2.

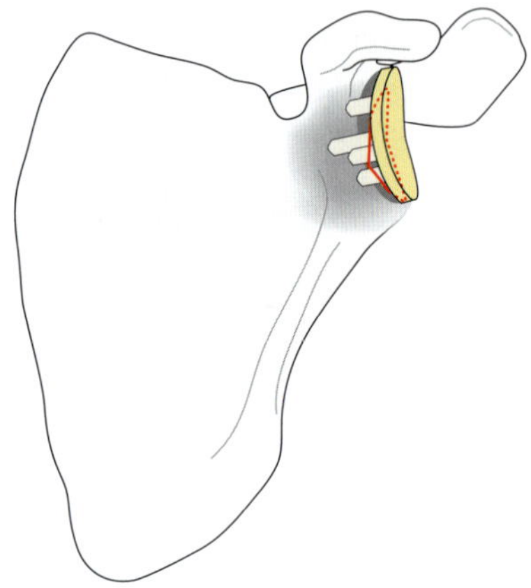

4.2-16 Periprosthetic fracture glenoid, type I.14-B3.

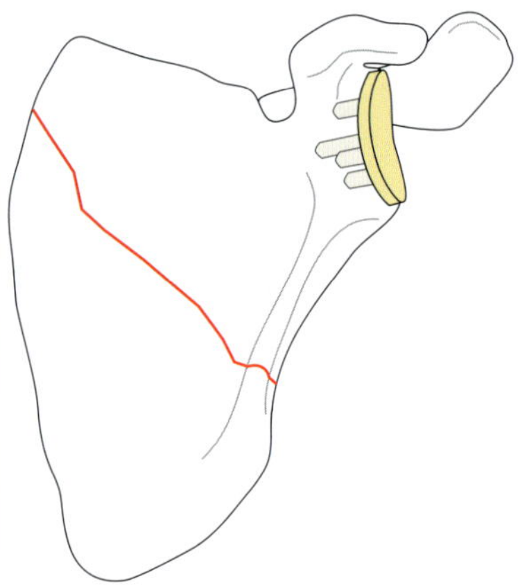

4.2-17 Periprosthetic fracture glenoid, type I.14-C.

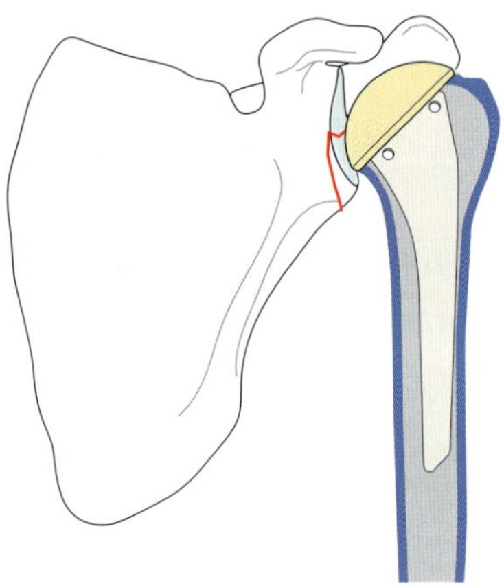

4.2-18 Periprosthetic fracture of glenoid, type I.14-F.

Humerus (I.1)

Type A

These fractures, involving the greater or lesser humeral tuberosity (**4.2-19a–b**), may be managed by observation if minimally displaced. If recognized intraoperatively, simple fixation is a wise choice in order to prevent displacement occurring soon after.

Type B

Type B1 fractures of the humerus (**4.2-20**) may be adequately stabilized by the stem, in which case nonoperative management is feasible. The fracture types B2 and B3 (**4.2-21a–b**) require revision of the stem. The degree of complexity may increase in correlation to the presenting bone deficiency, possibly also requiring an osteosynthesis.

In cases where the humeral head has been resurfaced, instead of replaced, and a type B fracture has occurred, the need to determine subtypes of a type B fracture is insignificant as the fracture will have interrupted the blood supply to the humeral head.

Type C

Such fractures affect the humeral shaft well below the implant (**4.2-6**, **4.2-22**). In selected cases, they may be suitable for nonsurgical management if this is the treating surgeon's usual philosophy of managing such injury in the absence of shoulder replacement. However, reduction and fixation will expedite rehabilitation and may help preserve shoulder mobility.

More distal fractures should be managed following the principles that guide the treatment of juxtaarticular fractures around the elbow.

Type D

These types of fracture involve the humerus between a shoulder and an elbow replacement (👁 **4.2-23**).

Type E

These types of fracture involve bones containing an implant on both sides of a shoulder replacement, ie, both scapula and humerus.

Type F

This category does not pertain to the humerus because replacement of the glenoid alone is not part of standard orthopedic practice.

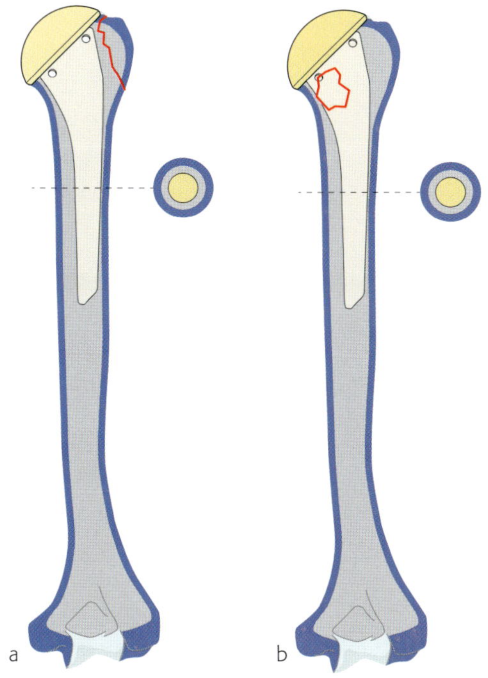

👁 **4.2-19a–b** Periprosthetic fracture of proximal humerus.
a Type I.1-A1 greater tuberosity.
b Type I.1-A2 lesser tuberosity.

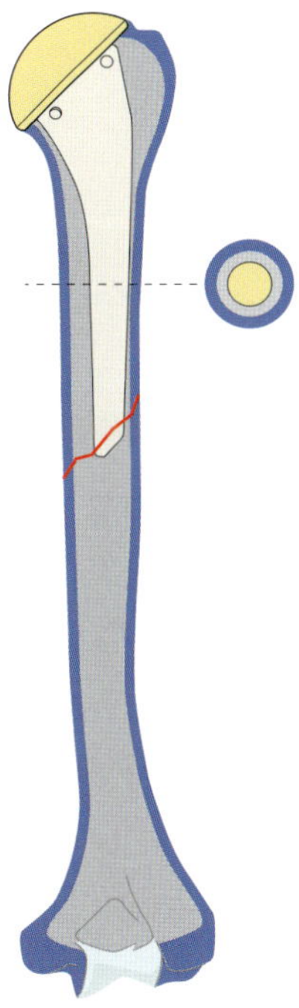

👁 **4.2-20** Periprosthetic fracture of proximal humerus type I.1-B1.

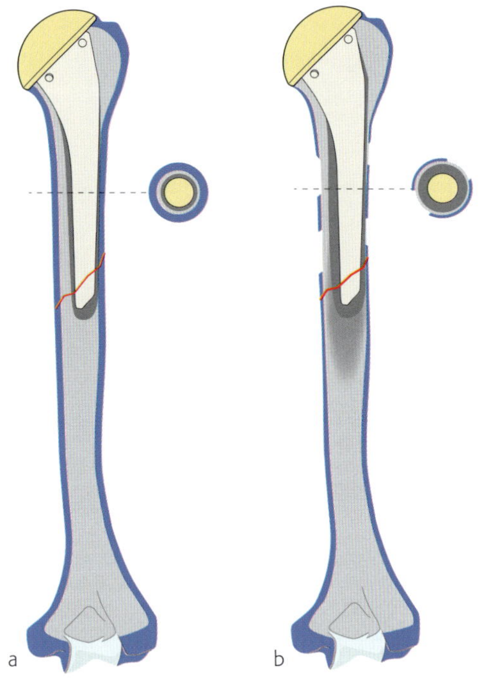

4.2-21a–b Periprosthetic fracture types of proximal humerus.
a Type I.1-B2 loose prosthesis.
b Type I.1-B3 bone defect.

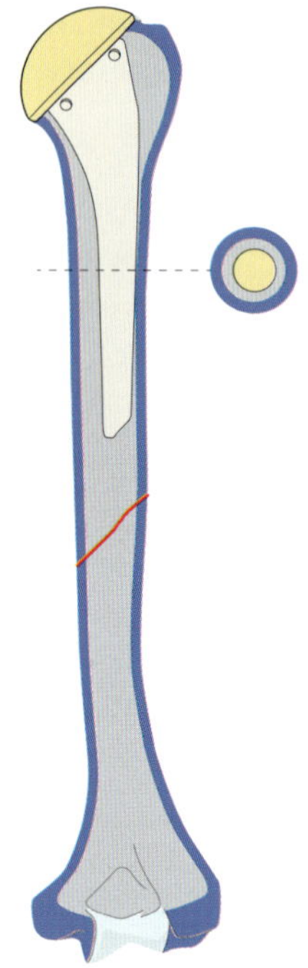

4.2-22 Periprosthetic fracture of proximal humerus type I.1-C.

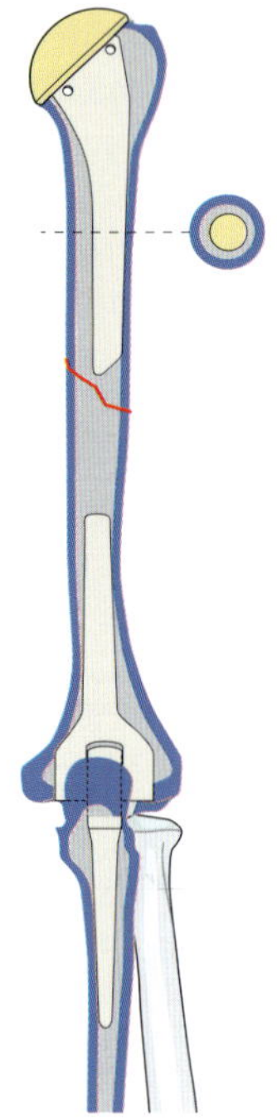

4.2-23 Periprosthetic fracture of humerus distal to prosthesis, type I.1-D.

II Elbow

Existing classification systems

O'Driscoll and Morrey, in applying the Vancouver classification system to the elbow, categorized periprosthetic fractures about the elbow according to the three main factors that determine their prognosis and treatment: the location of the fracture in relation to the stem; the stability of the implant fixation; and the quality of the bone (**4.2-4**, **4.2-5a–b**) [19].

Unified Classification System (UCS)

The Unified Classification System applies to injuries affecting the humerus (II.1), ulna (II.2), and radius (II.2).

Type A

These are periarticular fractures of the humerus (II.1) (epicondyle) (**4.2-24a–b**), ulna (II.2) (olecranon tip or coronoid process), or radius (II.2) (radial tuberosity) (**4.2-25a–b**).

Periarticular fractures are the most common type of fracture and can occur both intraoperatively and postoperatively. Type A1 applies to a fracture of the lateral humeral epicondyle or olecranon tip, while type A2 applies to a fracture of the medial humeral epicondyle or coronoid process/radial tuberosity.

Intraoperative epicondylar fractures occur as a result of stress applied to the thin bone during positioning of the elbow. If the fracture occurs postoperatively, it is usually due to heavy use of the involved muscles or a stress fracture from weakened bone as a result of stress shielding or osteolysis. Such fractures are typically treated symptomatically, without surgery. They usually develop into a stable fibrous nonunion, although sometimes there is bone healing. If the fracture occurs intraoperatively, the surrounding soft tissues are simply sutured together to enable a stable fibrous union.

4.2-5a O'Driscoll and Morrey classification of humeral fractures after elbow prosthesis [19].

Fracture type	Definition of fracture type
HI	Fracture of the columns or condyles
HII	Fracture around the stem
HII-1	Implant well fixed
HII-2	Implant loose with acceptable bone stock
HII-3	Implant loose with severe bone loss
HIII	Fracture proximal to the stem

4.2-5b O'Driscoll and Morrey classification of ulnar fractures after elbow prosthesis [19].

Fracture type	Definition of fracture type
UI	Fracture of the olecranon
UII	Fracture around the stem
UII-1	Implant well fixed
UII-2	Implant loose with acceptable bone stock
UII-3	Implant loose with severe bone loss
UIII	Fracture proximal to the stem

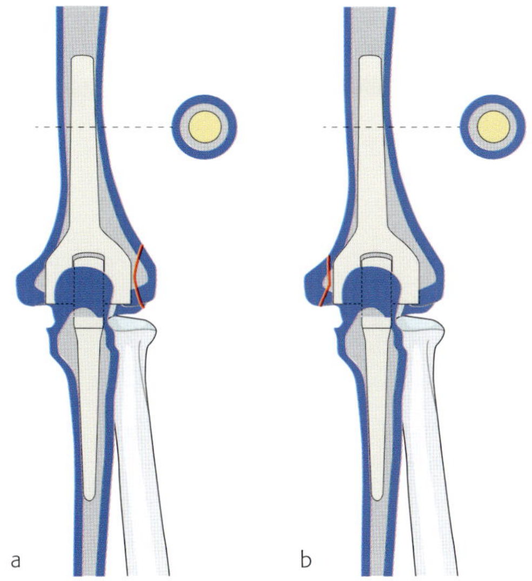

4.2-24a–b Periprosthetic fracture of humeral condyles.
a Type II.1-A1 lateral condyle.
b Type II.1-A2 medial condyle.

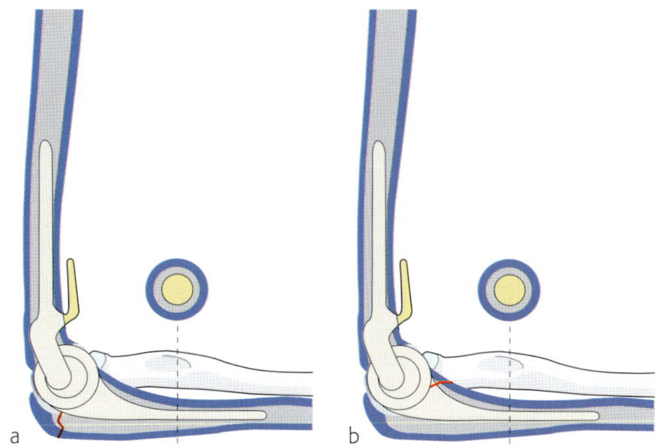

4.2-25a–b Periprosthetic fractures of proximal ulna.
a Type II.2-A1 tip of olecranon.
b Type II.2-A2 coronoid process.

Type B

These are fractures around or at the tip of the stem of the humerus (II.1) or ulna (II.2).

Type B1: Well-fixed implant in humerus or ulna with adequate bone quality (**4.2-26**, **4.2-27**). Fractures in the presence of a well-fixed stem usually occur at the tip of the prosthesis. They are treated by open reduction and internal fixation (ORIF).

Type B2: Fracture in association with a loose implant in the humerus or ulna, with adequate bone quality (**4.2-5b**, **4.2-28**, **4.2-29**). Such fractures usually occur in the presence of component loosening or osteolysis. Combined revision and fracture fixation are required, as with other joints.

Type B3: Fracture in association with a loose implant in the humerus or ulna and severe bone loss (**4.2-12b**, **4.2-30**, **4.2-31**). A complex revision is necessary including the use of allografts or modular oncology-type prostheses; supplementary plating may also need to be considered.

Type B fractures after isolated radial-head replacement for the management of a previous radial-head fracture would follow similar treatment principles. However, simple removal of the implant would be considered more often, resulting in radio-condylar excision arthroplasty.

Type C

These are fractures beyond the tip of the stem in the humeral shaft (II.1) (**4.2-32**), ulna (II.2) or radius (II.2) (**4.2-33**). Fractures beyond the tip of the stem are treated as routine shaft fractures with plate fixation or immobilization and functional bracing.

Type D

These represent fractures of the humeral shaft following both shoulder and elbow replacement, for instance in cases of weakened bone in rheumatoid arthritis (**4.2-34**). It could also affect the radius following radial head and wrist replacement. The principles of analysis and treatment have already been outlined with reference to the femur and tibia.

Type E

These fractures have already been dealt with and a case is illustrated in **4.2-9**.

Type F

This represents a fracture of the lateral humeral condyle, which is articulating with a previously implanted radial-head replacement (**4.2-35**). The principles of management depend on the degree of fracture displacement and the health of the radio-condylar articulation prior to the most recent injury. These considerations have been outlined above in the introductory section to this chapter.

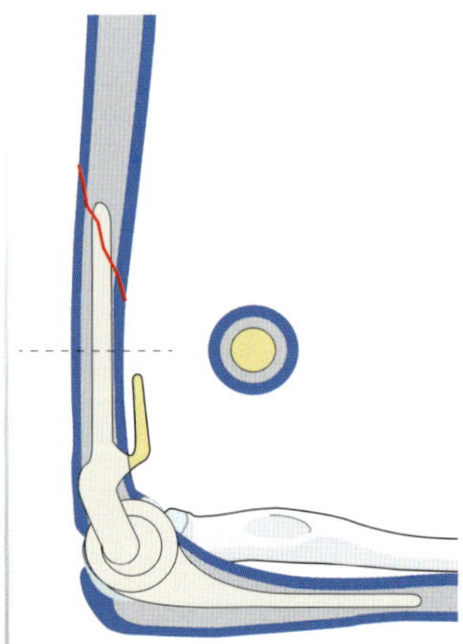

4.2-26 Periprosthetic fracture of distal humerus type II.1-B1.

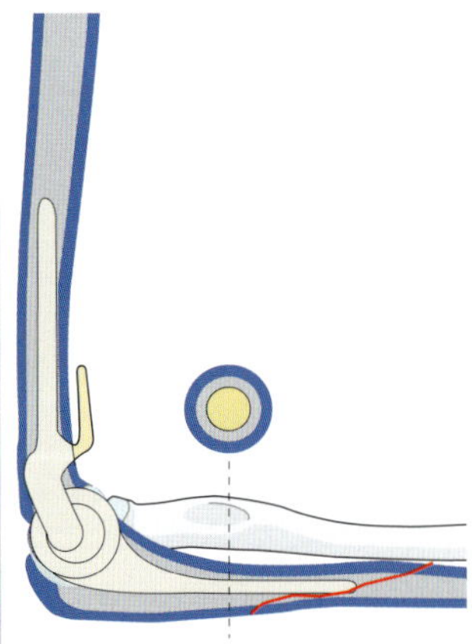

4.2-27 Periprosthetic fracture proximal ulna type II.2-B1.

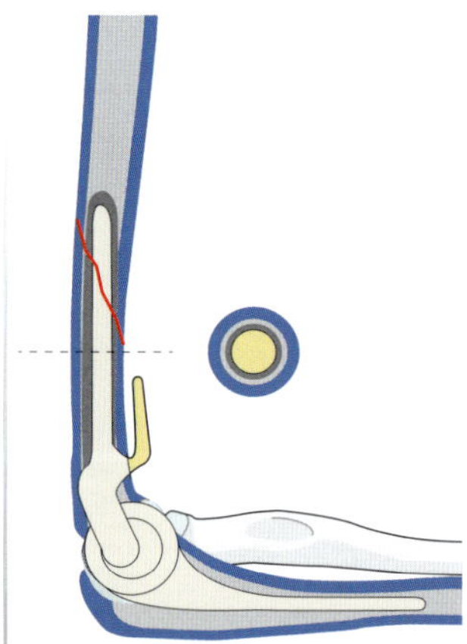

4.2-28 Periprosthetic fracture of distal humerus type II.1-B2.

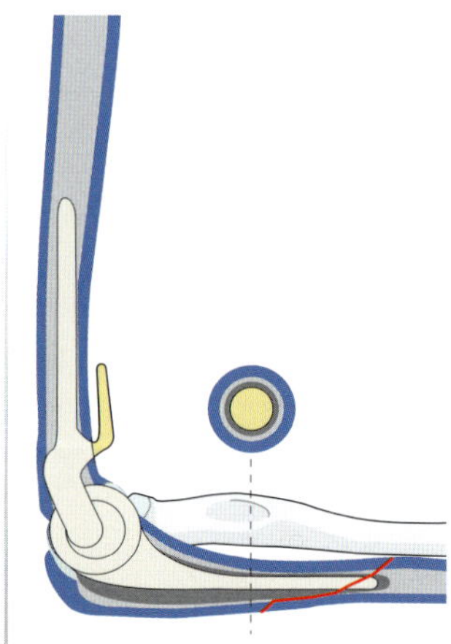

4.2-29 Periprosthetic fracture proximal ulna type II.2-B2.

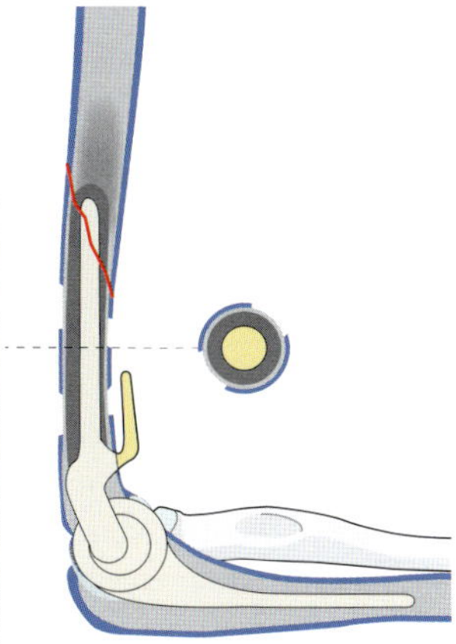

👁 **4.2-30** Periprosthetic fracture distal humerus type II.1-B3.

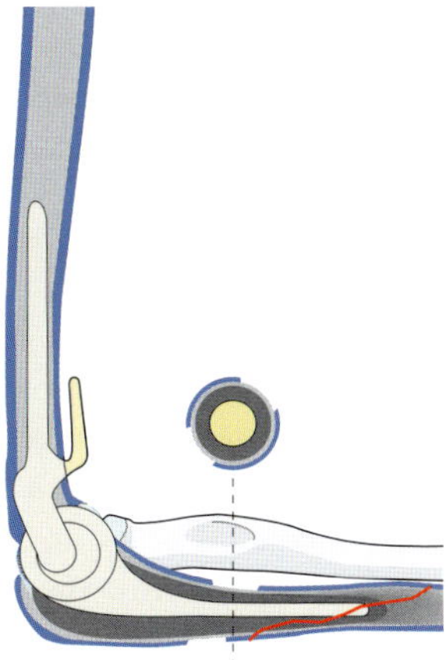

👁 **4.2-31** Periprosthetic fracture proximal ulna type II.2-B3.

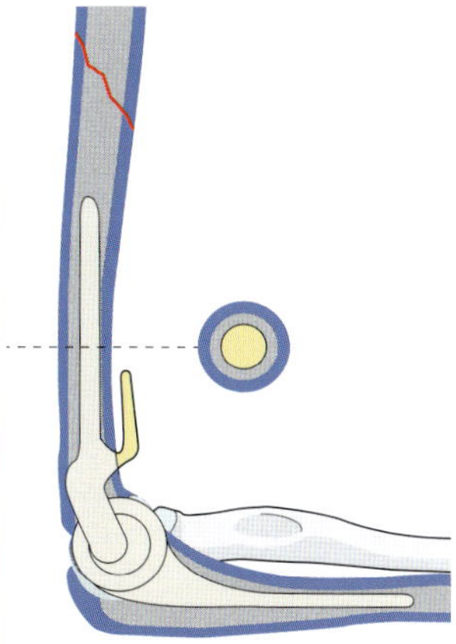

👁 **4.2-32** Periprosthetic fracture of humerus type II.1-C.

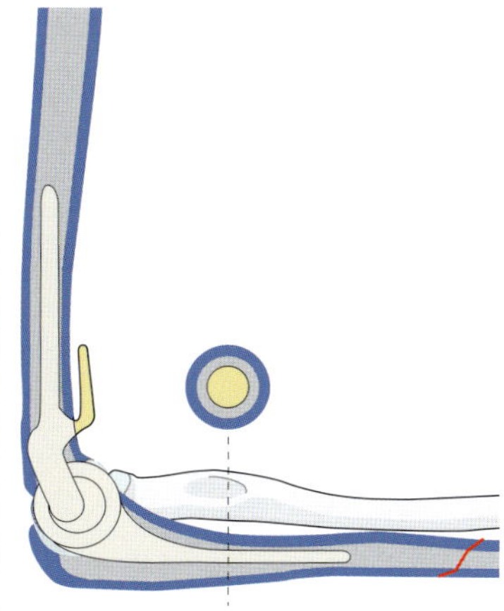

👁 **4.2-33** Periprosthetic fracture of ulna type II.2-C.

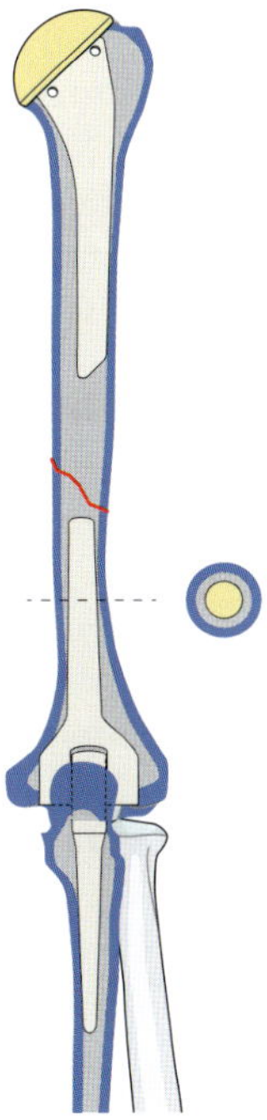

👁 **4.2-34** Periprosthetic fracture of humerus type II.1-D.

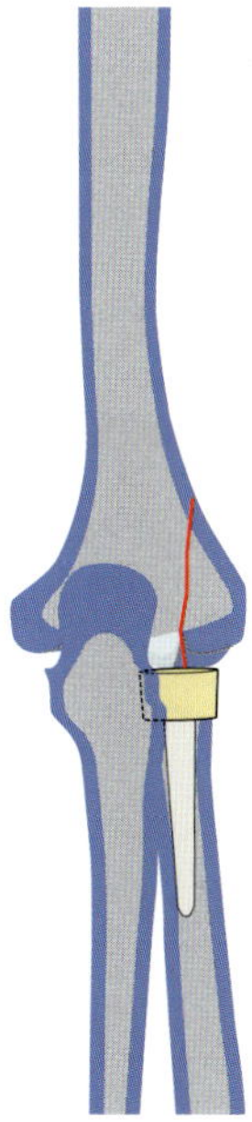

👁 **4.2-35** Periprosthetic fracture of medial condyle opposite to medial head prosthesis type II.1-F.

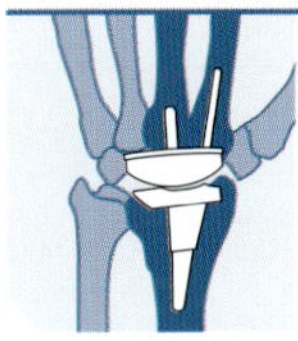

III Wrist

Existing classification systems

Fracture after wrist replacement is a very rare occurrence because this arthroplasty is not commonly used in contemporary practice. Furthermore, to the authors' knowledge, there is no existing classification system. Nevertheless, the principles of management and application of the UCS are the same in such cases.

Unified Classification System (UCS)

The Unified Classification System (UCS) relates to the radius (III.2), ulna (III.2), and carpus/metacarpals (III.7).

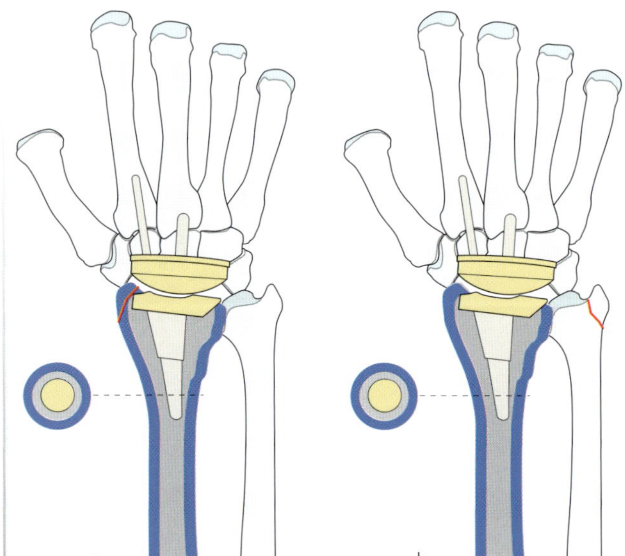

4.2-36a–b Periprosthetic fracture of distal radius/ulna type.
a Type III.2-A1 radial styloid.
b Type III.2-A2 ulnar styloid.

Type A

These types of fracture affect the styloid process of the radius or, if it was retained, the very distal ulna. These fractures are subcategorized as type A1 for the radius and A2 for the ulna (**4.2-36a–b**), which only occur rarely as it is common practice to resect the distal ulna during wrist replacement.

Type B

These fractures affect the radius (**4.2-37a–c**) or carpus/metacarpals (**4.2-38a–c**) around or just adjacent to the implants. They are subclassified as type B1, B2, or B3 based on the stability of implant fixation and degree of bone loss, exactly in accordance to what has already been outlined in context to other bones and joints.

Type C

These fractures affect the implant-bearing radius (**4.2-39**) or metacarpals (**4.2-40**) distant to the implants.

Type D

These fractures affect the radius between a wrist and radial-head replacement.

Type E

These fractures affect both the radius and carpus or metacarpals.

Type F

This category does not pertain to the wrist as replacement hemiarthroplasty of this joint is not part of standard orthopedic practice.

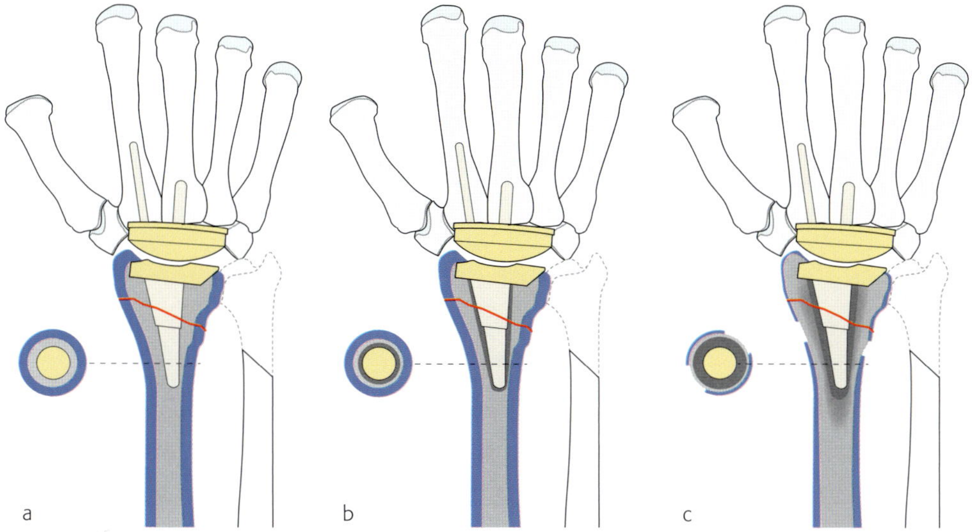

4.2-37a–c Periprosthetic fracture types of distal radius.
a Type III.2-B1.
b Type III.2-B2.
c Type III.2-B3.

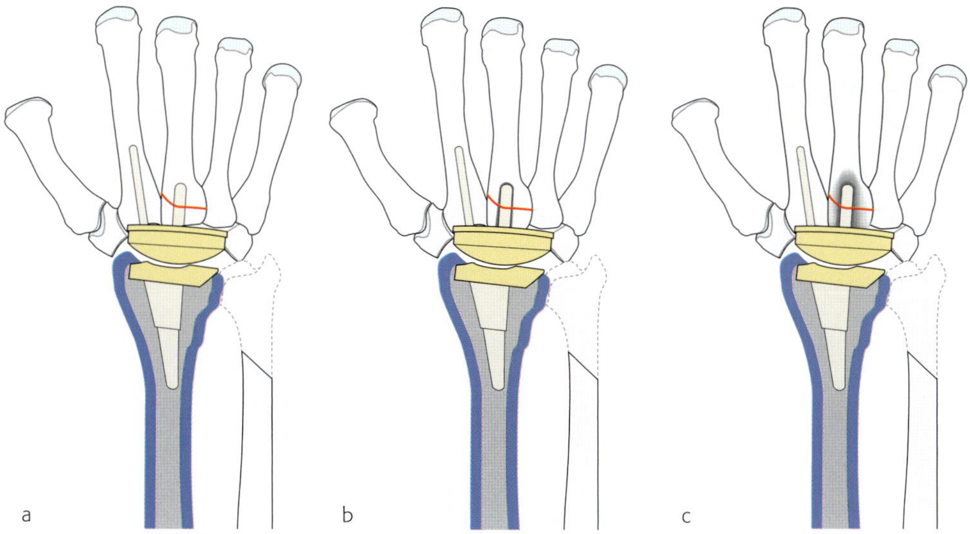

4.2-38a–c Periprosthetic fracture types of metacarpal bone.
a Type III.7-B1.
b Type III.7-B2.
c Type III.7-B3.

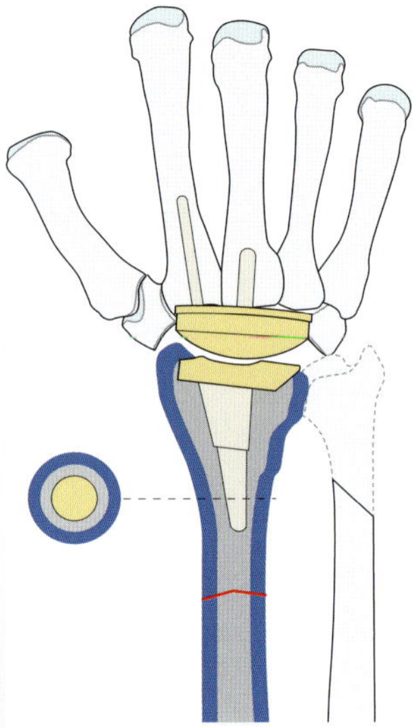

4.2-39 Periprosthetic fracture of distal radius type III.2-C.

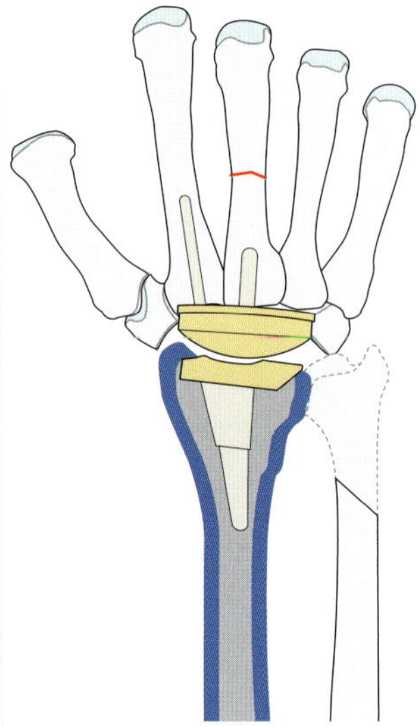

4.2-40 Periprosthetic fracture of metacarpal bone type III.7-C.

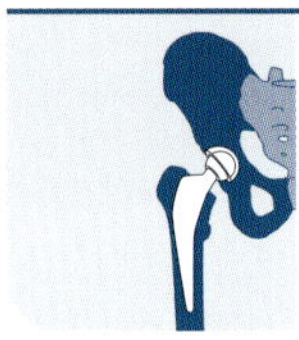

IV Hip

Existing classification systems

For the proximal femur, the Vancouver classification system has already been described (4.2-1).

For periprosthetic acetabular fractures Peterson and Lewallen proposed the most frequently cited classification scheme in 1996 (4.2-6) [20].

A more comprehensive classification system for periprosthetic acetabular fractures was proposed by Della Valle and co-authors (4.2-7) [21].

4.2-6 Modified Peterson and Lewallen classification of the acetabulum [20].

Fracture type	Appearance on x-ray	Pain level	Treatment options
1	Radiographically stable, with no evidence of component loosening or migration	Minimal pain with hip motion	Nonsurgical treatment
2	Obvious radiographic migration or loosening	Painful hip motion	Surgical treatment with open reduction internal fixation and acetabular component revision

Unified Classification System (UCS)

The UCS relates to the pelvis and acetabulum IV.6 and the proximal femur IV.3.

4.2-7 Della Valle classification of periprosthetic fractures of the acetabulum [21].

Fracture type	Definition of fracture type	Fracture subtype	Definition of fracture subtype
I	Intraoperative fractures secondary to acetabular component insertion	IA	Fracture of an acetabular wall recognized intraoperatively; fracture nondisplaced and component stable
		IB	Fracture recognized intraoperatively and displaced; acetabular column or component unstable
		IC	Fracture not recognized intraoperatively
II	Intraoperative fractures secondary to acetabular component removal	IIA	Associated with loss of < 50% of acetabular bone stock
		IIB	Associated with loss of > 50% of acetabular bone stock
III	Traumatic fracture	IIIA	Component stable
		IIIB	Component unstable
IV	Spontaneous fractures	IVA	Associated with loss of < 50% of acetabular bone stock
		IVB	Associated with loss of > 50% of acetabular bone stock
V	Pelvic discontinuity	VA	Associated with loss of < 50% of acetabular bone stock
		VB	Associated with loss of > 50% of acetabular bone stock
		VC	Associated with prior pelvic irradiation

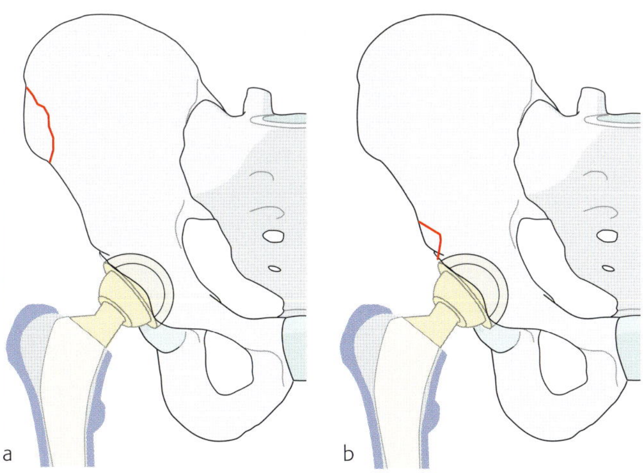

4.2-41a–b Periprosthetic fracture of anterior superior (**a**) and inferior (**b**) spine type IV.6-A1.

Pelvis and acetabulum (IV.6)

Type A

These fractures, eg, an avulsion fracture of the anterior superior or anterior inferior iliac spine (type A1) (**4.2-41a–b**) or the ischial tuberosity (type A2) (**4.2-42**), do not require surgical management.

Type B

The majority of pelvic fractures relevant to this topic belong to type B and involve the acetabulum. These fractures may occur during surgery, although they may not be recognized immediately. The severest variety (type B3) represents pelvic discontinuity or dissociation.

Type B1, such as a fracture of the peripheral lip or rim of the acetabulum or of the floor but with an intact rim (**4.2-43a–b**), is associated with a stable implant interface. Fracture fixation is not required. If a noncemented cup is being used and the fracture is recognized at the time of operation, it is prudent to consider supplementary screw fixation of the shell. If recognized after surgery, protected weight bearing for some weeks is recommended.

Type B2 is associated with an unstable bone-implant interface (**4.2-44a–b**). Regardless whether it is diagnosed at the time of operation, soon after, or much later as a result of injury or osteolysis, cup revision is required. If the fracture and the bone-implant interface cannot be stabilized with screws, separate fixation of the fracture (eg, with a posterior plate) prior to cup insertion must be considered. An example of this principle is the case of a pathological fracture secondary to osteolysis, leading to pelvic discontinuity but with adequate bone stock remaining so that complex reconstruction (eg, with a cage) will not be required. Such a case is illustrated in **4.2-45**.

A type B3 fracture is associated with a loose cup and extensive bone loss due to severe comminution or osteolysis (**4.2-46**). Fracture fixation and new cup insertion with bone graft are not adequate. Instead, more complex reconstruction with an acetabular cage must be considered in order to protect both the fracture and the bone-implant interface during the period in which the fracture heals, the cup stabilizes, and the bone graft is incorporated. An extreme example of this principle in such a unique case is the recently described "cup-cage construct" [22]. **4.2-47** shows an x-ray of such a case.

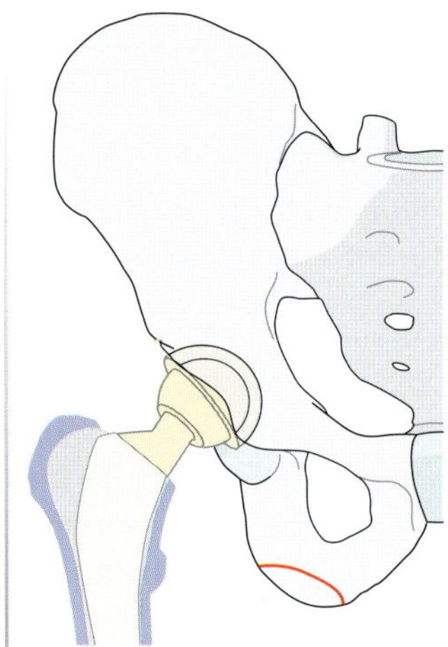

4.2-42 Periprosthetic fracture of ischial tuberosity type IV.6-A2.

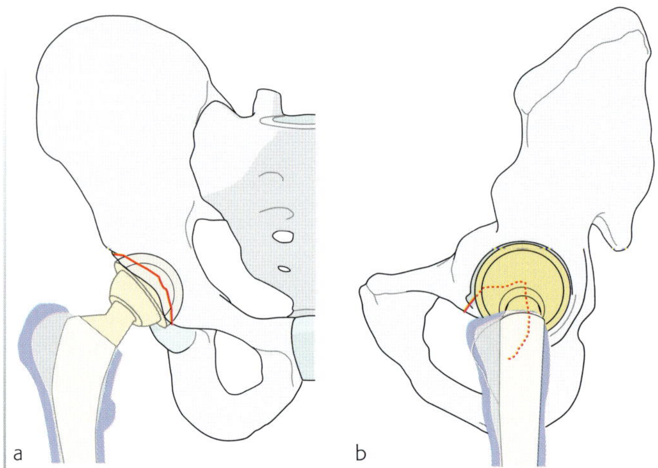

4.2-43a–b Periprosthetic fracture of acetabulum type IV.6-B1.
a Rim.
b Floor.

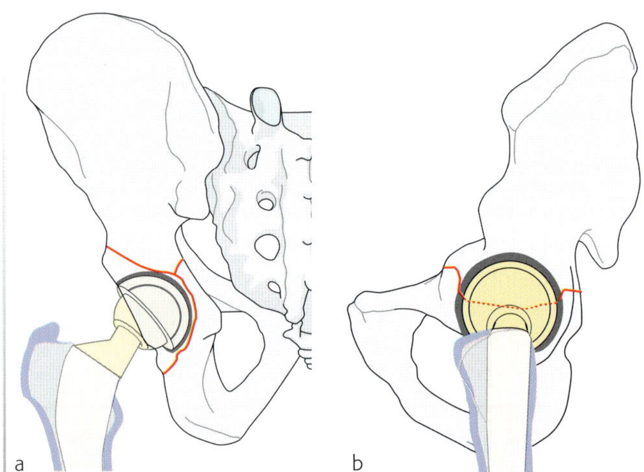

4.2-44a–b Periprosthetic fracture of acetabulum type IV.6-B2.
a AP view.
b Lateral view.

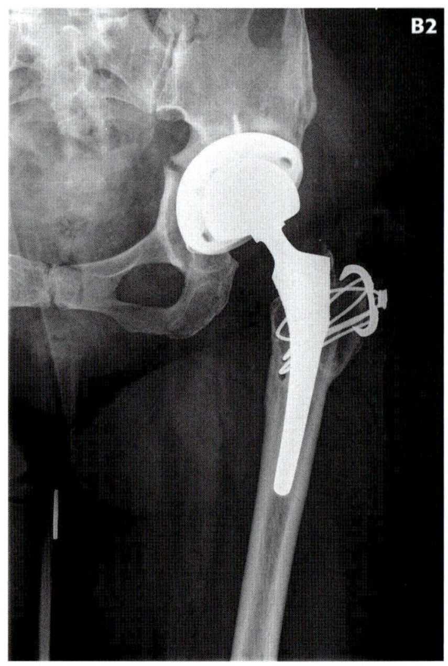

4.2-45 Late onset type B2 fracture of the acetabulum. The cup is loose and there is adequate bone to support a cup revision after fixation of the posterior column.

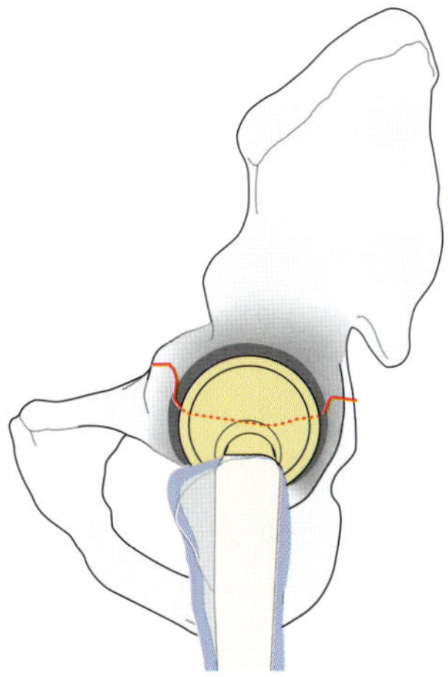

4.2-46 Periprosthetic fracture of acetabulum/pelvic discontinuity type IV.6-B3.

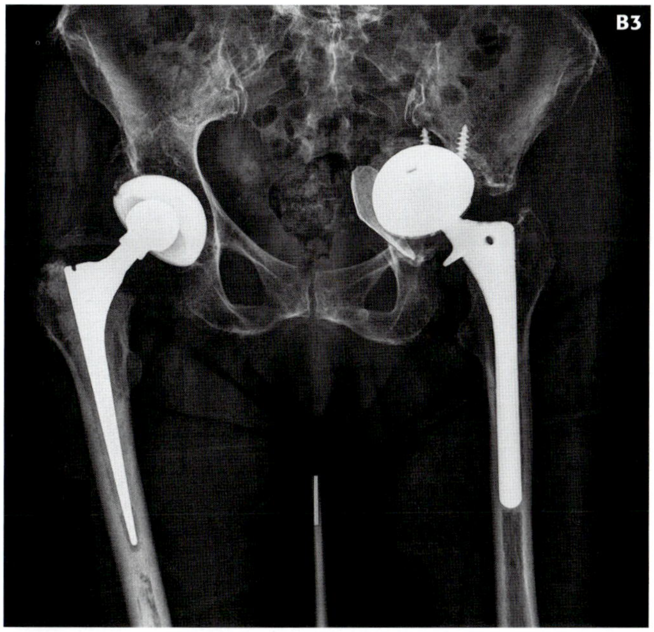

4.2-47 Acute intraoperative type B3 fracture of the acetabulum. The cup is loose and there is severe bone deficiency. More complex reconstruction is required.

A type B3 fracture implies pelvic discontinuity or dissociation, by its very definition. It is very uncommon for this not to be the case.

Pelvic discontinuity or dissociation means that the upper and lower halves of the hemipelvis are discontinuous or separated by a fracture line. While theoretically this could affect any part of the hemipelvis, in practice it involves the floor and columns of the acetabulum in the setting of hip-joint replacement. The fracture orientation may be transverse or oblique, and only rarely it is T-shaped. Regardless of these variants, the effects are similar. The usual cause is a pathological fracture secondary to osteolysis. It can, however, also occur intraoperatively as the result of overzealous reaming or excessive use of force during cup impaction. Moreover, it can occur at any time postoperatively as a result of a traumatic injury.

The principles of management, detailed in chapter 6.4.2, include fracture fixation with stabilization of one or two columns, restoration of missing bone, and achievement of a stable cup construct. In severe cases of bone loss and weakness, it is necessary to utilize a cage in order to protect the construct.

Although it is tempting to separate cases of pelvic discontinuity (dissociation) into those that are acute (as a result of surgical technique or a subsequent traumatic event) and those that are chronic (due to osteolysis), such distinction is not necessary as the same treatment principles apply. It is the extent of bone loss, not the acuity of the event that dictates the surgical principles needed to achieve stable fixation of the cup and the hemipelvis. **4.2-45** shows a case of a chronic type B2 fracture due to osteolysis and motion of the loose cup. It was managed by posterior column fixation and secure cup fixation. **4.2-47** shows a case of acute fracture due to vigorous reaming and excessive insertion force. This intraoperative type B3 fracture required a complex cup-cage construct. The two variants are demonstrated in **4.2-48a–b** and **4.2-49**. In the former, an acute type B2 intraoperative pelvic dissociation, during hip replacement, was managed by posterior column fracture reduction and fixation, along with secure cup fixation. In the latter (**4.2-49**), a chronic type B3 pelvic discontinuity required complex cup-cage reconstruction. These four examples demonstrate the predominance of the available bone stock and strength (B2 or B3) on the decision-making process. The acuity of the event is of secondary importance. Additional imaging is usually required in order to accurately define the degree of bone loss in these cases, such as Judet views of the pelvis, supine false profile views (basically Judet views

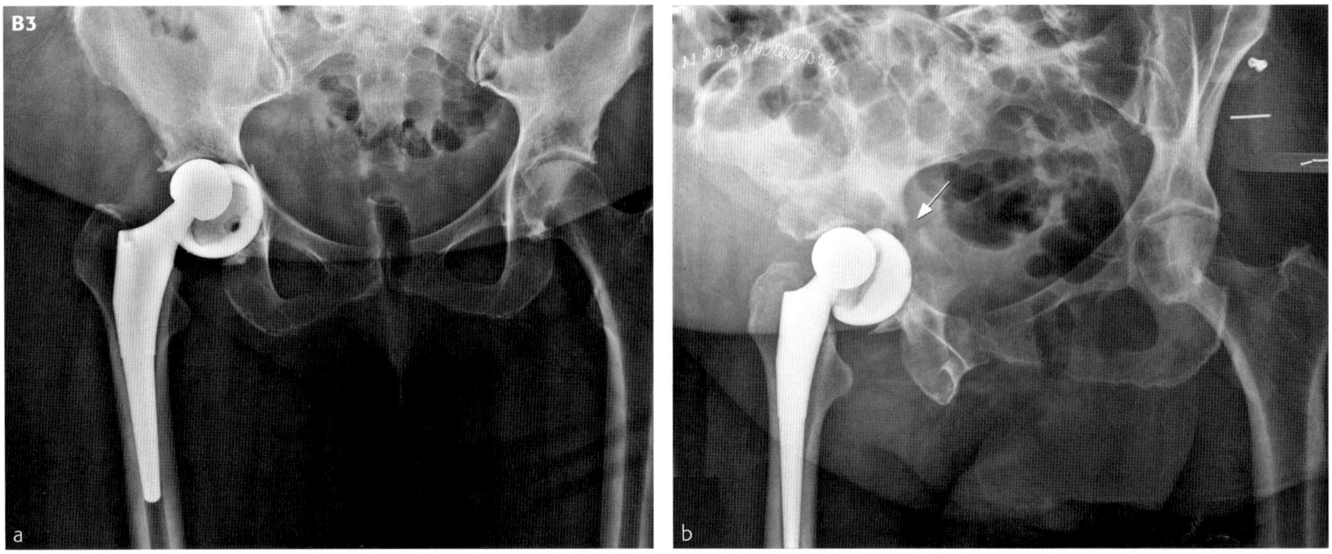

4.2-48a–b Unrecognized, acute intraoperative type B2 fracture of the acetabulum.

a Third postoperative day x-ray revealing the acetabular fracture.

b Judet iliac oblique x-ray confirming the pelvic dissociation. There was sufficient bone remaining to allow posterior column fracture fixation and secure cup fixation, without the need for a cage.

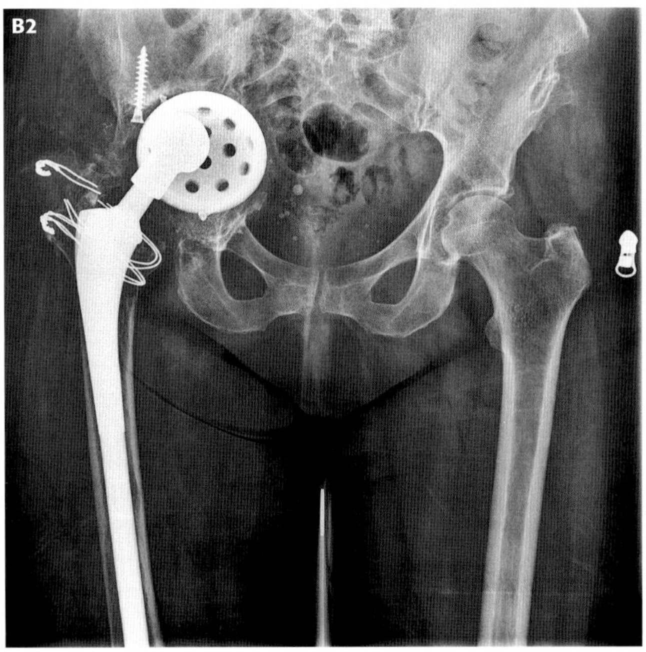

4.2-49 Late onset type B3 fracture of the acetabulum requiring complex cup-cage reconstruction.

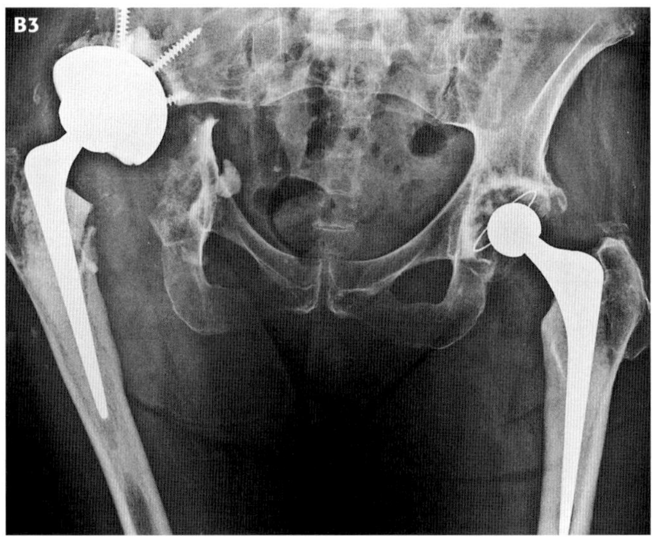

4.2-50 Late onset type B3 fracture of the acetabulum with severe interfragmentary instability. Complex reconstruction will be required.

at 65° rotation instead of 45°), and computerized tomography (CT) with metal suppression. In some cases, CT with three-dimensional reconstruction proves to be valuable.

Rarely, the bone loss accompanying the fracture is so severe it defies any effort at further reconstruction at which point salvage excision arthroplasty must be considered.

It is important to consider a number of additional biological factors when formulating a treatment plan for type B3 fractures of the acetabulum, especially if they are due to chronic bone deficiency. These factors can have a deleterious effect on the ability of the bone to heal and may prompt a more elaborate reconstruction in selected cases. An incomplete list of these factors includes:

- The presence of infection
- The stability of the fragments (**4.2-50**)
- The vascularity of the fracture fragments, for instance, following multiple previous interventions
- The general health of the patient (eg, impairment by diabetes mellitus) and social habits (such as smoking)
- The general health of the skeleton (eg, impairment by severe osteoporosis).

The involvement of reparative biology, in addition to bone stock, is emphasized by a unique and fortunately uncommon type of acetabular fracture, to which the authors have arbitrarily given a type B3 category even though adequate bone stock may be visible on the x-rays. This is a type of fracture that can develop as a result of radiation osteonecrosis before or after joint replacement. Despite the presence of bone, osteogenesis is severely compromised in these cases and specialized methods of management must be considered [23].

Type C

Type C fractures are located distant to the acetabulum and (**4.2-51**) are treated independently of the joint replacement following the principles of pelvic fracture management unless the joint itself has been damaged. Fractures of the ilium and/or the rami represent this fracture type. Such an injury on the pelvic side of the fracture is shown in **4.2-52**.

Type D

This fracture represents a type of fracture of the pelvis between bilateral hip replacements (**4.2-53**). Separate analyses of each joint will guide the surgeon as to which treatment is required. **4.2-54** demonstrates such a case.

Type E

This type of fracture involves both the femur and pelvis as illustrated in **4.2-9** and **4.2-52**. **4.2-9** shows a type B3 fracture involving the acetabulum and a type B2 fracture of the femur. **4.2-52** shows a type C fracture involving the pelvis and a type A1 fracture of the femur. Based on these classifications by separate analyses of each component of each case, treatment can proceed on a rational basis.

Type F

This is a type of fracture of the acetabulum which does not contain an acetabular component but faces and articulates with a previously implanted femoral head replacement or unipolar surface replacement (**4.2-10a–b**, **4.2-55**). The principles of management depend on the degree of fracture displacement as well as the health of the articulation prior to the most recent injury. These aspects have been outlined above in the introductory section to this chapter.

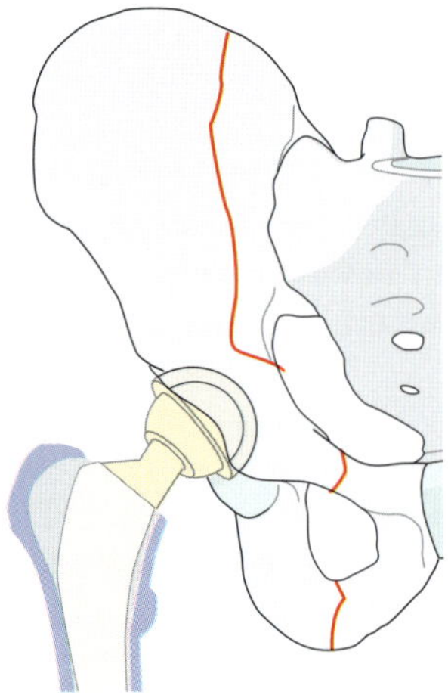

4.2-51 Periprosthetic fracture type IV.6-C.

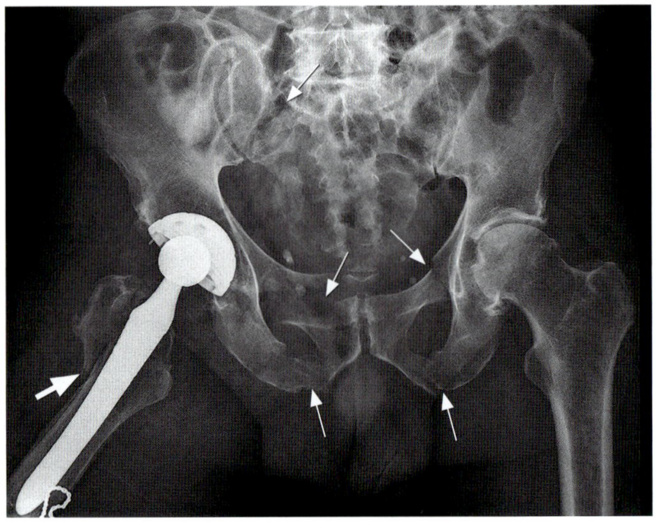

4.2-52 Type E fracture after hip replacement involving both sides of the arthroplasty. Separate analyses reveal a type C fracture of the pelvic ring (including the ala of the sacrum, arrows) and a type A1 fracture of the femur (greater trochanter, arrow).

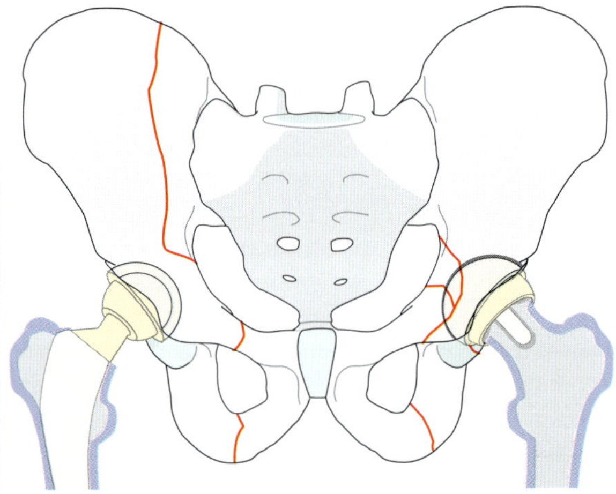

4.2-53 Periprosthetic fractures of pelvis type IV.6-D.

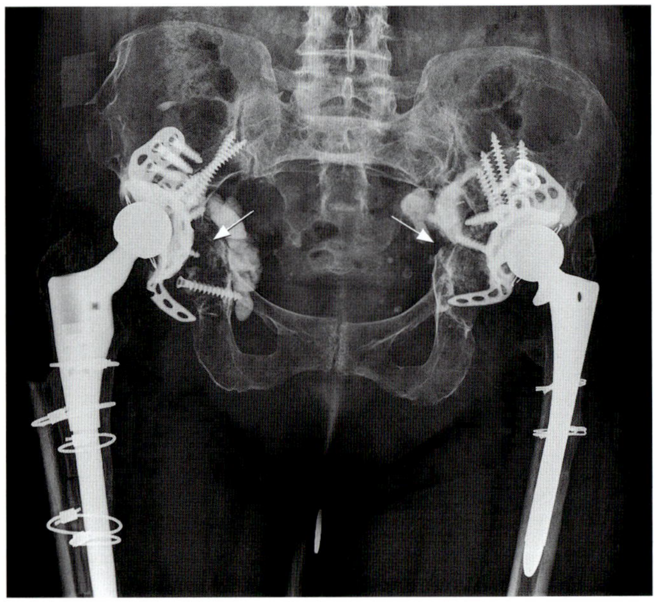

4.2-54 Type D fracture of the pelvis between two hip replacements. Separate analyses of the arthroplasties reveal a type B3 fracture of the acetabulum (pelvic dissociation or discontinuity) on each side (arrows) requiring bilateral complex reconstruction.

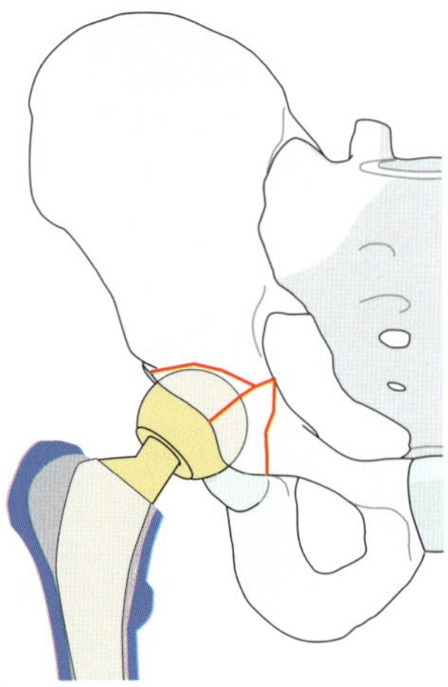

4.2-55 Periprosthetic fracture of acetabulum with hemiarthroplasty of the proximal femur type IV.6-F.

Proximal femur (IV.3)

Type A

Such fractures involve the trochanteric region and require subtyping.

- Type A1 involves the greater trochanter and is most commonly encountered as an avulsion fracture through pathological bone weakened by osteolysis (👁 **4.2-4a**, 👁 **4.2-56a–b**). It typically requires stabilization during revision in order to deal with the failed cup
- Type A2 is a type of fracture of the lesser trochanter and is uncommon to occur as an isolated injury (👁 **4.2-57a–b**).

It is important to distinguish the A2 subtype from a fracture of the lesser trochanter with an attached fragment of the proximal medial cortex. The latter is typically seen soon after implantation of a noncemented tapered stem and leads to destabilization of the implant. This is by definition a type B2 fracture and requires surgical management.

👁 **4.2-58** demonstrates a fracture that could be misinterpreted as a type A2 fracture (pseudo-A2 fracture). However, more is involved than the lesser trochanter being displaced. There is a segment of the proximal medial femoral cortex attached and the stem has become loose. This type B2 fracture requires revision of the stem coupled with reduction and fixation of the fracture.

Surface replacement: Fractures following surface replacement represent a less common variety because of the relative youth of the patients, the better quality of their bone, and the far smaller number of cases worldwide. However, the same classification and principles of management apply, with some obvious differences. Management of femoral type A fractures would be similar, with observation of the A2 subtype (lesser trochanter), and reduction with fixation of type A1 fractures (greater trochanter) unless minimally displaced. A pathological avulsion type A1 fracture through osteolytic bone, as an adverse local reaction to metal, would require management during revision.

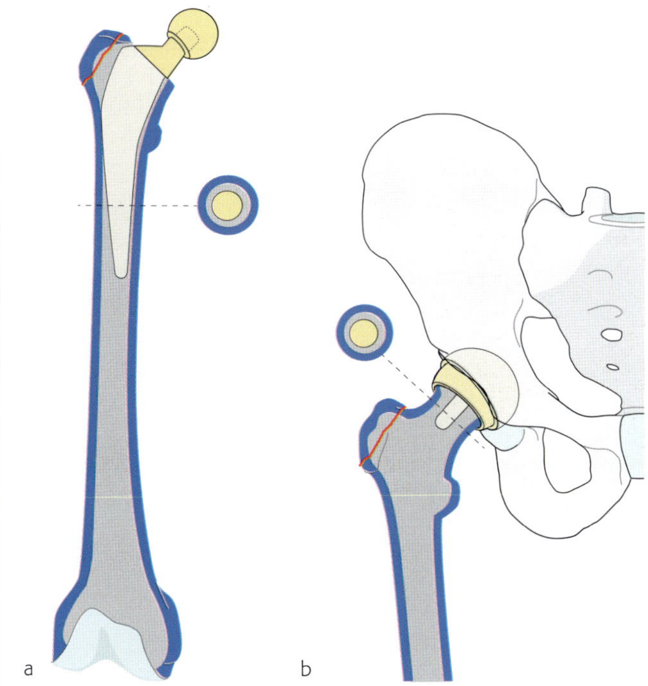

👁 **4.2-56a–b** Periprosthetic fracture of proximal femur, type IV.3-A1 greater tuberosity.
a After THA.
b After surface replacement.

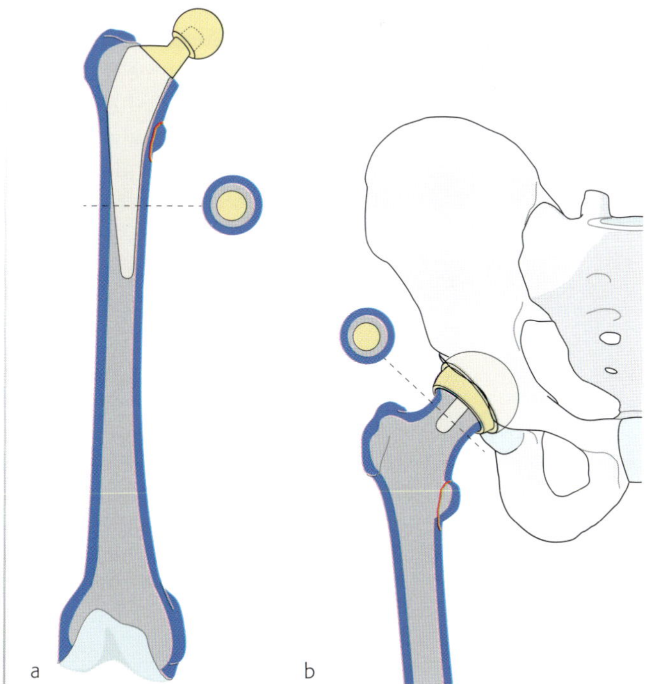

👁 **4.2-57a–b** Periprosthetic fracture of proximal femur type IV.3-A2 lesser tuberosity.
a After THA.
b After surface replacement.

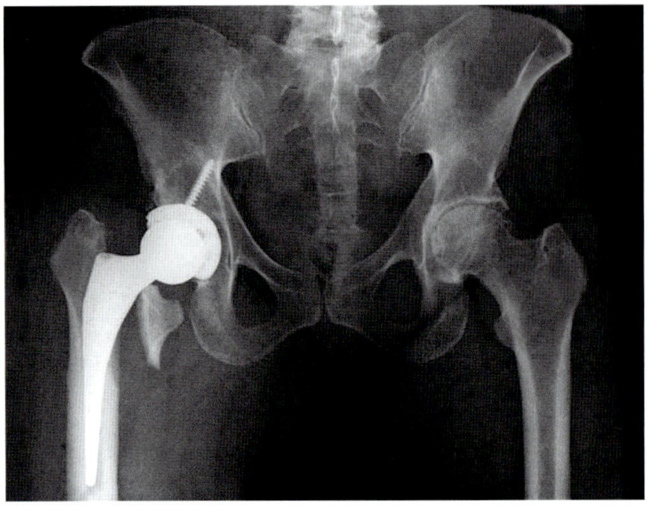

4.2-58 Pseudo-A2 fracture of the femur. There is a segment of cortex attached to the lesser trochanter which has led to destabilization of the stem. By definition this is a type B2 fracture.

Type B

Such fractures occur around or just distal to the stem and involve the bone-implant interface.

Type B1 fractures: The stem of the implant is still well-fixed (**4.2-59a–b**). It is the least common of the three B subtypes (**4.2-4b**, **4.2-5a**). In this circumstance, reduction and fixation without stem revision are appropriate, ideally using the modern techniques of minimally invasive plate osteosynthesis (MIPO) following indirect reduction [24].

Type B2 fractures also involve the femoral shaft around or just distal to the stem. However, in this case the stem is loose (**4.2-4c**, **4.2-60a–b**). Usually, loosening occurred prior to fracture but it can also occur as a result of the injury. Implant revision, along with reduction and fixation of the fracture, are required. Osteosynthesis alone would likely compromise the result, leading to nonunion, progressive bone loss, and the need for further, more complex intervention.

Type B3 fractures involve the same region of the femur, also with a loose stem, but in addition there is also severe preexisting bone loss (**4.2-4d**, **4.2-11b**, **4.2-61a–b**). Often, the patient either had been asymptomatic or had a "silent" impending fracture of the femur and the event occurred after a minor injury. These cases need more complex intervention, in some instances requiring segmental substitution of the proximal femur with a segmental allograft or segmental replacement prosthesis.

Surface replacement: In contrast to hemiarthroplasty and total arthroplasty, the femoral type B fracture after surface replacement always requires revision, even in case of a type B1 fracture (solid fixation of the femoral component). These fractures occur adjacent to the mouth of the femoral component and completely interrupt the blood supply to the femoral head.

4.2-62 illustrates a type B fracture following surface replacement. Although the component was well fixed, it had to be managed by revision hip replacement because the blood supply to the femoral head had been interrupted by the fracture.

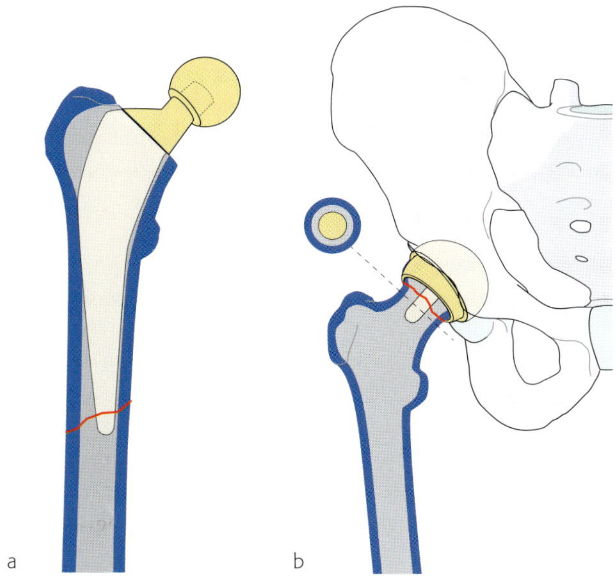

4.2-59a–b Periprosthetic fracture of proximal femur type IV.3-B1.
a After THA.
b After surface replacement.

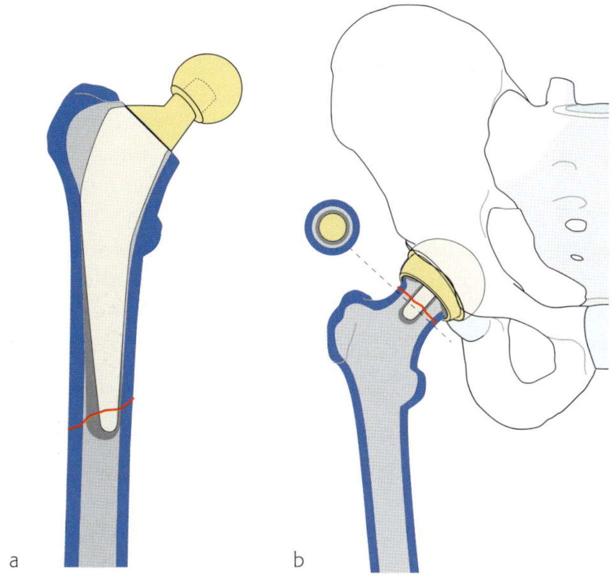

4.2-60a–b Periprosthetic fracture of proximal femur type IV.3-B2.
a After THA.
b After surface replacement.

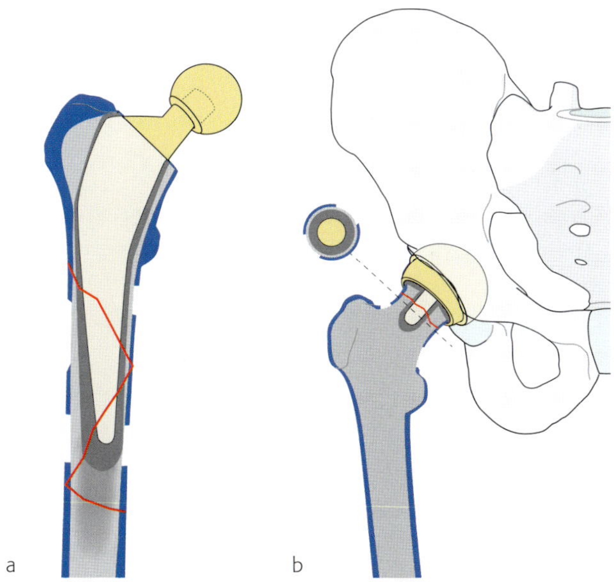

4.2-61a–b Periprosthetic fracture of proximal femur type IV.3-B3.
a After THA.
b After surface replacement.

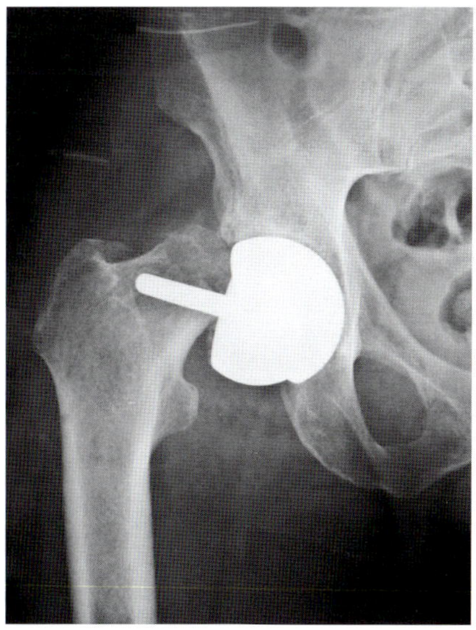

4.2-62 Type B fracture of the femoral neck following surface replacement of the hip. The B subtype is immaterial, even though it is a B1 fracture, because the vascularity of the femoral head has been disrupted. Revision is required.

Type C
Such fractures affect the femur distal to the stem of the prosthesis (**4.2-4e**, **4.2-63a–b**). How far distal is not precisely defined but open to interpretation by the surgical team within the context of the treatment options. Typically, the fractures occur within the distal diaphysis or metaphysis and are best managed according to the contemporary principles of osteosynthesis, without disturbing the stem. In select cases, especially if the stem is loose and the fracture more proximal, the surgeon may elect to deal with the loose implant and the fracture simultaneously, eg, by long-stem revision.

Surface replacement: Type C fractures distal to the base of the femoral neck are amenable to contemporary fracture management. **4.2-64a–b** demonstrates a type C fracture at the basicervical or pertrochanteric region of the femur, which was treated by reduction and fixation. The positive outcome was achieved by taking care to place the fixation lateral to the blood vessels entering the femoral neck.

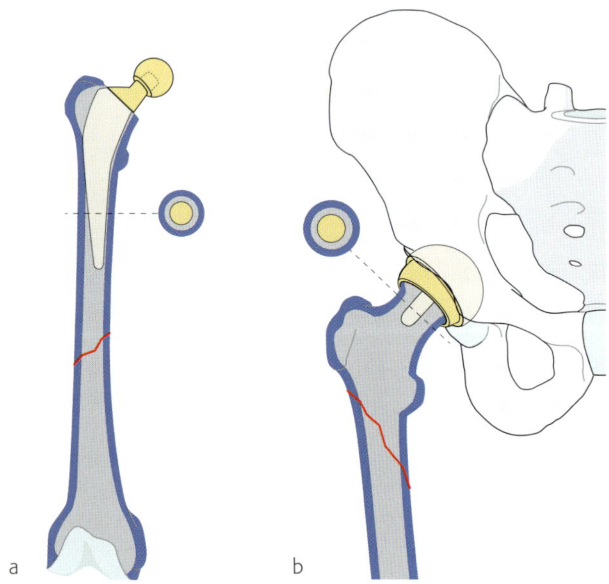

4.2-63a–b Periprosthetic fracture of proximal femur type IV.3-C.
a After THA.
b After surface replacement.

Type D
Most frequently such fractures involve the femur between a hip and a knee replacement (**4.2-7**, **4.2-65a–b**). Type D interprosthetic or intercalary fractures—together with type B3 periprosthetic fractures with severely compromised bone stock and type E polyperiprosthetic fractures—represent the three most challenging treatment groups.

The authors suggest that type D fractures be approached by separate analyses of implant stability and available bone stock around each of the implants and that treatment be based upon these analyses.

Type D fractures after surface replacement are similar to those that may occur after total hip replacement and are managed accordingly.

Type E
Type E fractures represent the rare cases, in which the implant-supporting bones on each side of an arthroplasty are fractured, eg, the acetabulum and femur after hip replacement (**4.2-8**). As with type D periprosthetic fractures, the authors recommend that the fracture, bone stock, and implant stability on each side of the arthroplasty be analyzed separately and dealt with accordingly.

Type E fractures after surface replacement are similar to those that may occur after total hip replacement and are managed accordingly.

Type F
This category does not pertain to the femur because acetabular hemiarthroplasty is not part of standard orthopedic treatment.

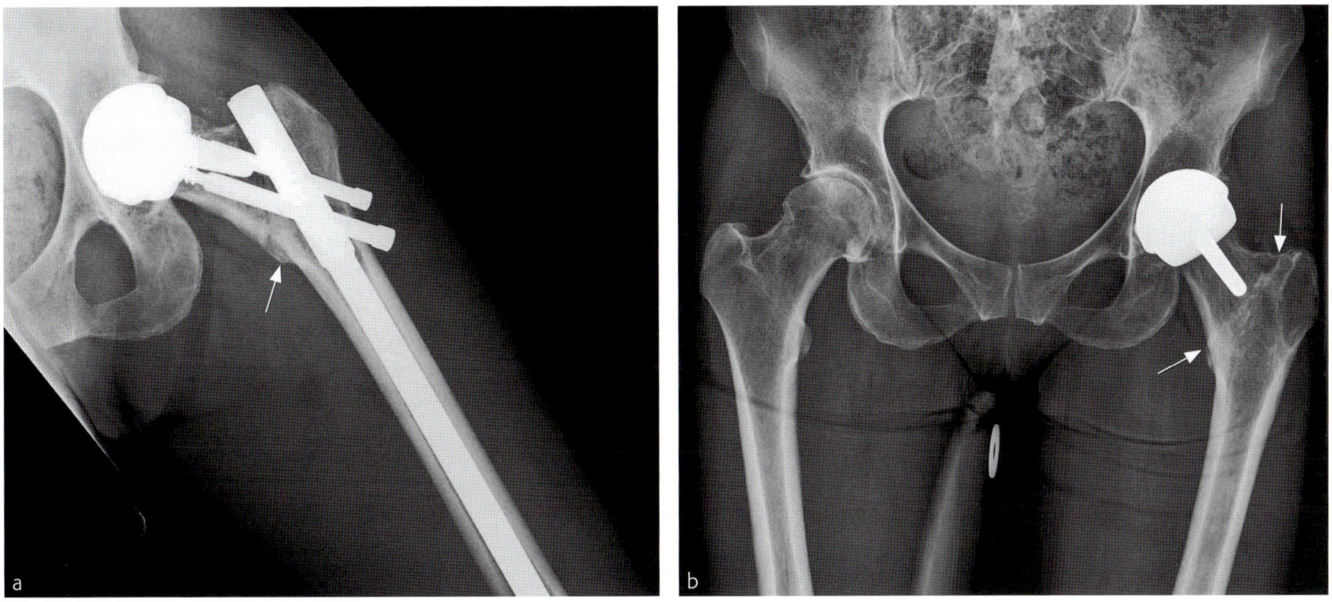

4.2-64a–b Type C fracture of the basicervical or pertrochanteric region of the femur following surface replacement (arrow). Since the fracture was lateral to the femoral-neck blood vessels, management was by reduction and fixation.
a The image reveals the basicervical fracture line (arrow) and fracture fixation.
b The image reveals fracture union (arrows).

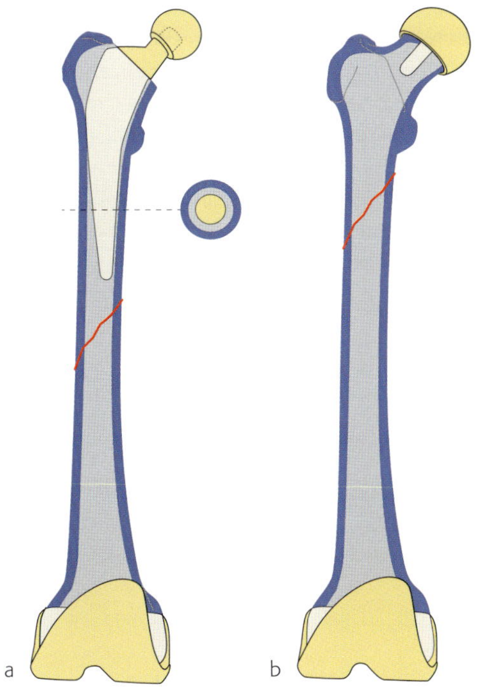

4.2-65a–b Intercalary periprosthetic fracture of proximal femur type IV.3-D.
a THA and TKA.
b Surface replacement and TKA.

V
Knee

Existing classification systems

Several classification systems have been described in the literature to categorize periprosthetic fractures after total knee arthroplasty (TKA). Most of these combine factors such as fracture site, displacement, fixation status of the prosthesis (well fixed or loose), and time of fracture.

For the classification of periprosthetic fractures of the femur the Lewis and Rorabeck system is most commonly used [25]. In this system, fractures are divided into three different types (**4.2-8**). Type I fractures are nondisplaced with stable prosthesis and good bone stock, type II are displaced fractures with a stable prosthesis with or without good bone stock and type III fractures are generally with loose implant with or without displacement of the fracture fragments.

Felix et al classified periprosthetic tibia fractures based on the following three criteria:

- Anatomical location of the fracture in reference to the tibial component
- Whether the fracture occurred intraoperatively or in the postoperative period
- Fixed or loose prosthesis on x-ray [26].

The anatomical location of fractures is further divided into four major anatomical fractures patterns, ie, type I fractures involve the tibial plateau and extend to the interface of the implant, type II fractures are found around the stem in the metaphyseal-diaphyseal junction, type III fractures are distal to the prosthesis, and type IV fractures affect the tibial tubercle. After confirming the anatomic location, these types can be subdivided according to whether the prosthesis is well fixed (A), the prosthesis is loose (B), or whether the fracture occurred intraoperatively (C) (**4.2-9**).

Parvizi et al developed another classification system that also takes into consideration the quality of the bone of the distal fragment (**4.2-10**) [27].

Different classifications for periprosthetic patellar fractures have been described. However, there is no validated classification system that can provide functional outcome measures. At present, the most commonly used classification system is the one published by Ortiguera and Berry [28]. This system classifies the fractures based on the integrity of the extensor mechanism and the fixation status of the patellar component. Type I fractures have a stable implant with intact extensor mechanism. In type II fractures the extensor mechanism has been disrupted, with or without displacement of the implant. Type IIIa fractures refer to loosening of the patellar component with reasonable bone stock and type IIIb fractures are characterized by a loose patellar component and poor bone stock (**4.2-11**).

4.2-8 Lewis and Rorabeck classification of supracondylar femoral fractures [25].

Type of fracture	Characteristics
Type I	Nondisplaced fracture and prosthesis is well fixed.
Type II	Displaced fracture and prosthesis is well fixed.
Type III	Prosthesis is loose, fracture may be displaced or nondisplaced.

4.2-9 Felix et al classification of periprosthetic distal tibia fractures [26].

Major anatomic location	
I.	Tibial plateau
II.	Adjacent to stem
III.	Distal to prosthesis
IV.	Tibial tubercle

Subcategory	
A	Well-fixed prosthesis
B	Loose prosthesis
C	Intraoperative

4.2-10 Parvizi et al classification of postoperative periprosthetic distal femoral fractures [27].

Type	Reducible	Bone stock in the distal fragment	Well-positioned and well-fixed component	Treatment
IA	Yes	Good	Yes	Nonoperative
IB	No	Good	Yes	Surgical fixation
II	Yes/no	Good	No	Revision with long-stem component
III	Yes/no	Poor	No	Prosthetic replacement

4.2-11 Ortiguera and Berry classification of periprosthetic patellar fractures [28].

Type	Integrity of extensor mechanism	Fixation status of the implant
I	Intact	With stable implant
II	Disrupted	With/without stable implant
III	Intact	Loosened implant
IIIa		With reasonable remaining bone stock
IIIb		With poor bone stock

Unified Classification System (UCS)

The UCS relates to the distal femur V.3, the proximal tibia V.4 and the patella V.34.

Distal femur (V.3)

Type A

These fractures represent nondisplaced fractures of the condyles (**4.2-66a–b**) due to varus or valgus injuries. Type A1 classifies a lateral condyle fracture, while type A2 a medial condyle fracture. Both can generally be managed nonoperatively with a brace but may require fixation if displaced.

Type B

Type B1 periprosthetic fractures are such, in which the femoral component remains well fixed and was functioning well prior to injury (**4.2-67a–b**). They are typically managed with fixation devices, depending on the position and configuration of the fracture as well as on the design of the femoral component.

Type B2 periprosthetic fractures are such, in which the implant is loose but there is good bone stock (**4.2-68a–b**). A stemmed femoral revision is usually undertaken with or without additional osteosynthesis.

Type B3 fractures represent the worst case scenario of a loose implant with considerable bone loss (**4.2-69a–b**) . A complex reconstruction is needed, which may include the use of structural allografts, augments, sleeves, and modular oncology implants.

Type C

Such fractures affect the femur proximal to the implant or its stem (**4.2-70**). How far proximal is not precisely defined but open to interpretation by the surgical team within the context of the treatment options. Typically, these fractures are within the distal shaft or metaphysis and are best managed according to the contemporary principles of osteosynthesis, without disturbing the femoral implant or stem. In selected cases, especially if the femoral component is loose and the fracture more distal, the surgeon may elect to deal with the failed implant and fracture simultaneously using a long-stem revision.

Type D

Such fractures—occurring between a hip and knee replacement—are interprosthetic or intercalary in type although the fracture lines may affect one arthroplasty more than the other (**4.2-71**). As already proposed, the fractures should be analyzed separately within the context of each joint replacement and management planned accordingly (**4.2-7**).

Type E

Such fractures involve at least two of the three implant-bearing bones, such as femur and tibia (or patella). As with type E fractures elsewhere, each fracture should be analyzed separately and dealt with accordingly.

Type F

This category does not pertain to the distal femur because neither tibial nor patellar hemiarthroplasty are part of standard orthopedic practice.

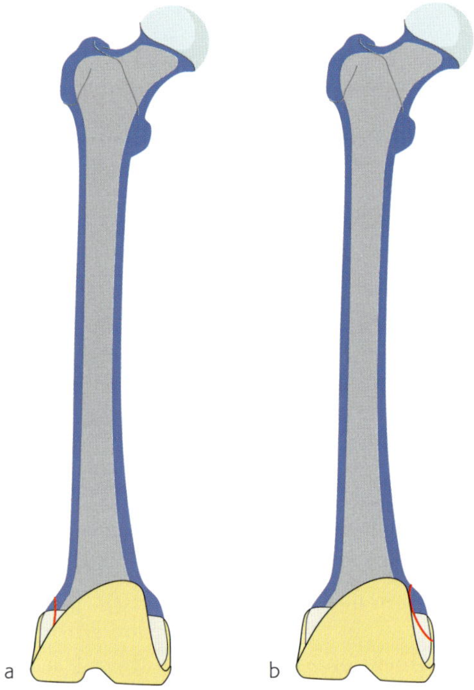

4.2-66a–b Periprosthetic distal femoral condyles fracture types.
a Type V.3-A1 lateral epicondyle.
b Type V.3-A2 medial epicondyle.

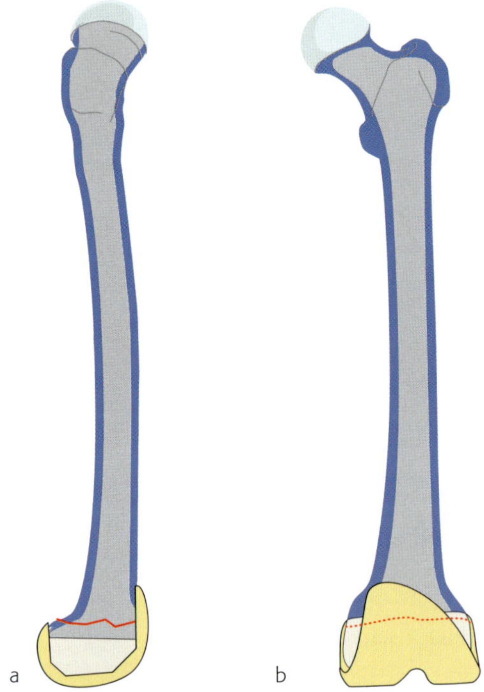

4.2-67a–b Periprosthetic fracture of distal femur type V.3-B1 (closed box).
a Lateral view.
b AP view.

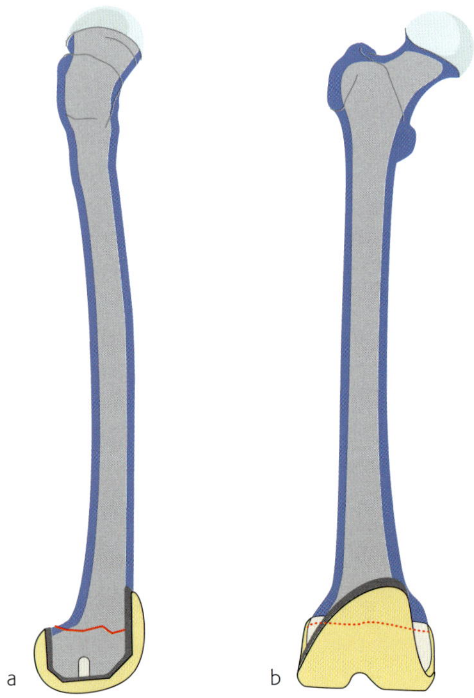

4.2-68a–b Periprosthetic fracture of distal femur type V.3-B2 (open box).
a Lateral view.
b AP view.

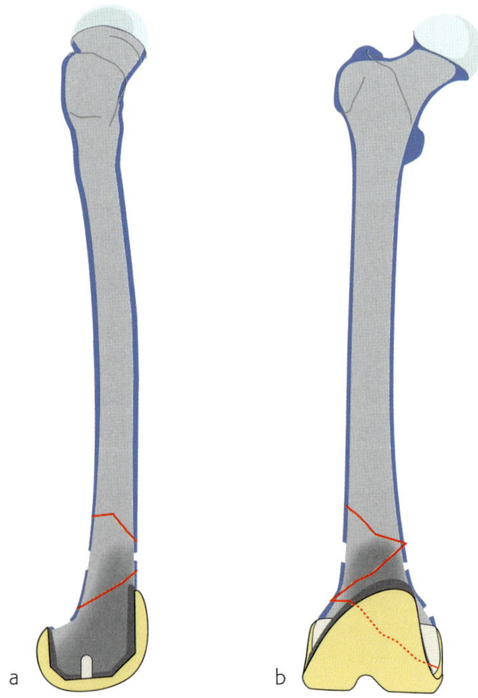

4.2-69a–b Periprosthetic fracture of distal femur, type V.3-B3.
a Lateral view.
b AP view.

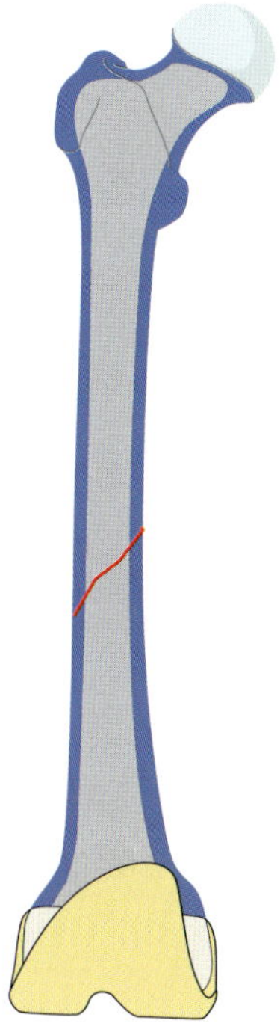

👁 **4.2-70** Periprosthetic fracture of femoral shaft, type V.3-C.

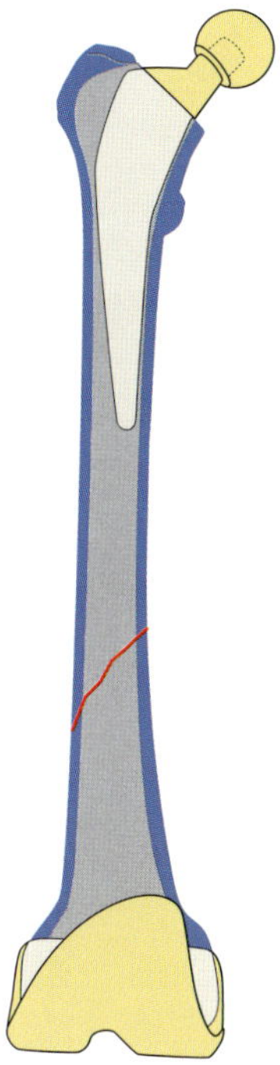

👁 **4.2-71** Intercalary periprosthetic fracture of femoral shaft, type V.3-D.

Proximal tibia (V.4)

Type A

These fractures represent avulsion injuries, eg, of the tibial tubercle (👁 **4.2-72a–c**). These can generally be managed nonoperatively with bracing, but may require fixation if displaced or if the extensor mechanism is disrupted.

Type B

Type B1 fractures are those, in which the implant remains well fixed and was functioning well prior to injury (👁 **4.2-73**). Felix et al recommended conservative management with rigid cast immobilization for nondisplaced or minimally displaced fractures with a well-fixed component [26].The medial tibial plateau is commonly affected and most fractures occur without any history of trauma. These fractures can be treated nonsurgically if nondisplaced. However, if found intraoperatively, open reduction and internal fixation (ORIF) should be considered. Displaced fractures are managed with fixation depending on the position and configuration of the fracture.

Type B2 fractures are those, in which the implant is loose and there is good bone stock (👁 **4.2-74**). A stemmed tibial revision is usually required.

Type B3 fractures represent a loose implant with considerable bone loss (👁 **4.2-5c**, 👁 **4.2-75**). Complex reconstruction is needed, which may include the use of structural allografts, augments, sleeves, and modular oncology implants or plates.

Type C

Such fractures affect the tibia distal to the implant or stem (👁 **4.2-76**). They are best managed with the contemporary principles of osteosynthesis, without disturbing the implant or stem. Generally, these fractures are due to trauma, stress fractures with limb malalignment, tibial tubercle osteotomy, or improper implant orientation. Closed manipulation followed by brace immobilization of the knee is usually successful. However, in cases of displacement or angulation, open reduction and internal fixation combined with a bone graft should be considered.

Type D

This fracture involves the tibia between a knee replacement and ankle replacement (👁 **4.2-77**). The principles of management have already been dealt with above.

Type E

Such fractures involve the tibia and patella or femur. The principles of management have been outlined above.

Type F

This category does not pertain to the tibia because femoral hemiarthroplasty of the knee is not a part of standard orthopedic practice.

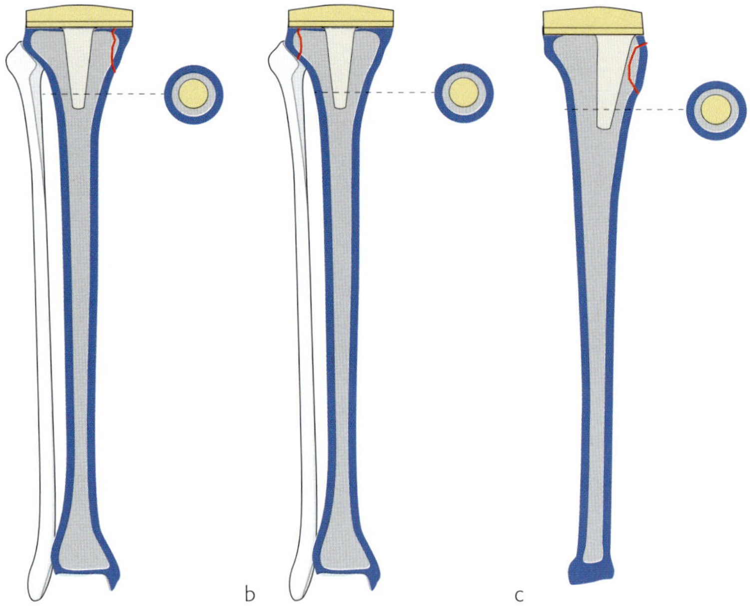

4.2-72a–c Periprosthetic fracture types of proximal tibia.
a–b Type V.4-A1 medial or lateral condyle.
c Type V.4-A2 tibial tuberosity.

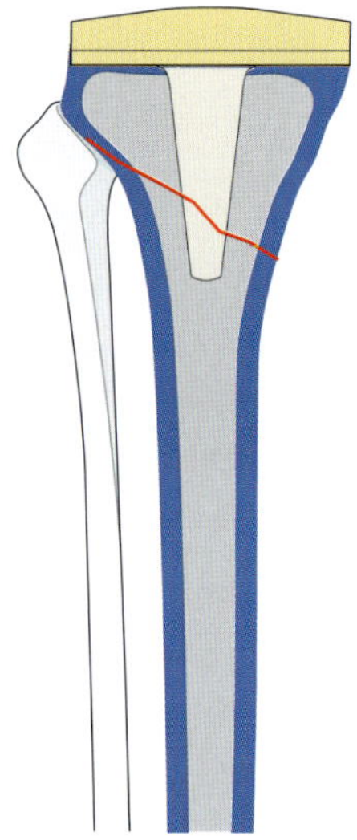

4.2-73 Periprosthetic fracture of proximal tibia, type V.4-B1.

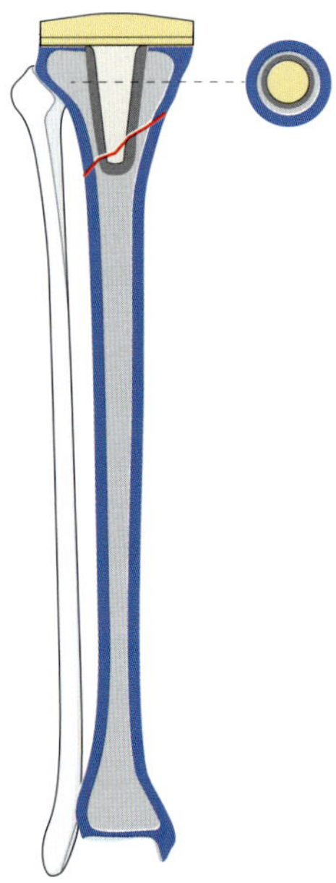

4.2-74 Periprosthetic fracture of proximal tibia, type V.4-B2.

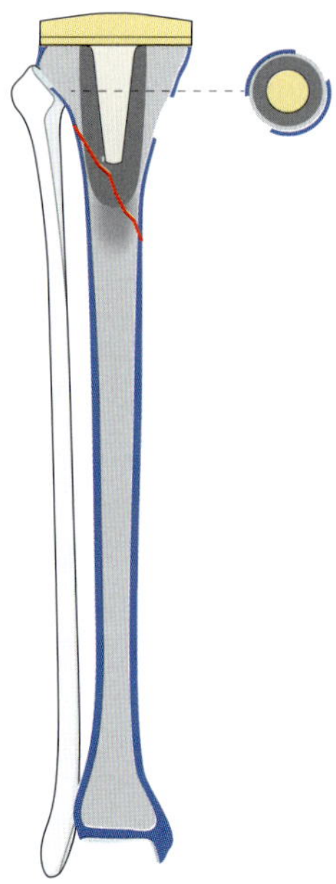

4.2-75 Periprosthetic fracture of proximal tibia, type V.4-B3.

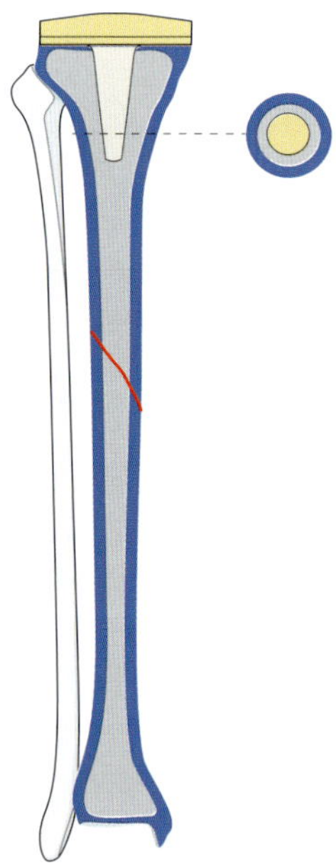

4.2-76 Periprosthetic fracture of tibial shaft, type V.4-C.

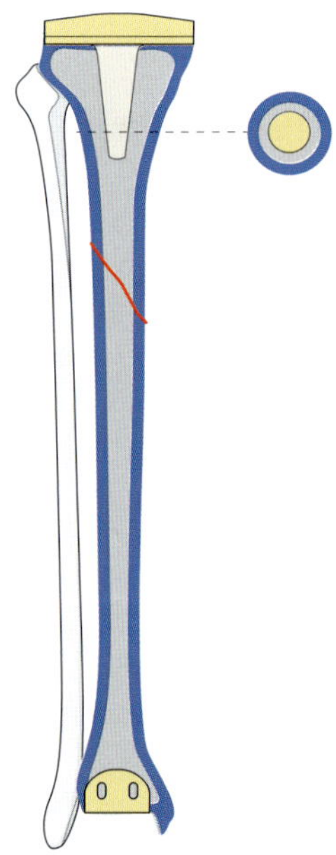

4.2-77 Intercalary periprosthetic fracture of tibial shaft, type V.4-D.

Patella (V.34)

Type A

These fractures are proximal or distal pole fractures without loosening of the patellar component (👁 **4.2-3**, 👁 **4.2-78a–d**). Management depends on the integrity of the extensor mechanism.

If there is an avulsion of the proximal or distal pole of the patella with extensor mechanism disruption, secure repair of the extensor mechanism, with or without partial patellectomy, is recommended; this can be achieved by various surgical techniques ranging from locking stitch to tension-band wiring.

Type B

In type B1 fractures the implant component is well fixed and the extensor mechanism is intact (👁 **4.2-79a–b**). A nondisplaced transverse or vertical patellar fracture with an intact patellar component and an intact extensor mechanism can be treated with a cylindrical cast or locked knee brace in extension for six weeks with immediate weight bearing. Windsor et al [29] recommended nonoperative management for transverse fractures with less than 2 mm displacement and for all vertical and comminuted fractures regardless of displacement. A vertical fracture is usually a stable fracture and rarely affects the extensor mechanism.

In type B2 fractures, the patellar implant component has become loose (👁 **4.2-80a–b**) while type B3 fractures are classified by both loosening of the implant component as well as by substantial bone loss (👁 **4.2-12c**, 👁 **4.2-81a–b**).

A useful protocol suggests that operative treatment is indicated for periprosthetic fractures with ≥ 2 mm displacement together with disruption of the extensor mechanism and loosening or displacement of the patellar implant. If the patellar component is loose, it should be removed in order to facilitate fixation of the fracture and repair of the extensor mechanism. The residual bone stock is generally inadequate to accommodate a new prosthesis, which could increase the risk of nonunion and refracture. If the bone loss is severe, a patellar resection arthroplasty may be needed.

Type C

This does not pertain to the patella because of its small size. The fractures distant to the patellar implant would affect the poles or apophysis of the patella, which already have been classified as a type A fracture.

Type D

This does not pertain to the patella because the bone can support only one implant.

Type E

These fractures pertaining to the patella and femur or patella and tibia have already been dealt with within the context of the femur and tibia.

Type F

This represents a fracture of the patella after partial replacement of the knee without surface replacement of the patella (👁 **4.2-82**). The prior intervention could have been a patellofemoral hemiarthroplasty (rarely used nowadays), a unicompartmental (monocondylar), or bicompartmental (bicondylar) replacement. The principles of treatment will depend on the degree of fracture comminution and displacement as well as the health of the patellofemoral articulation prior to the most recent injury. These aspects have been outlined in the introductory section to this chapter.

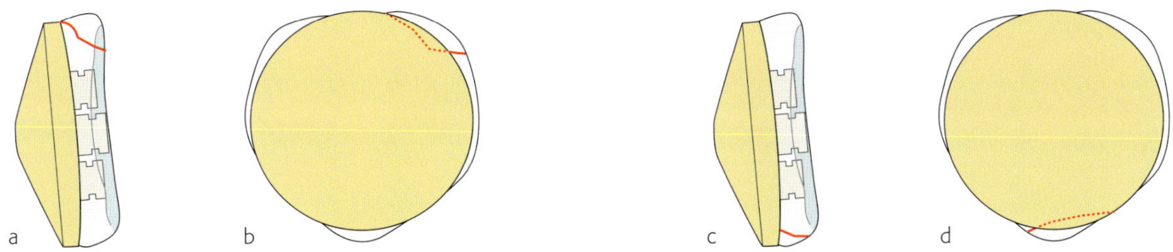

👁 **4.2-78a–d**

a–b Periprosthetic fracture of patella type V.34-A1, disrupted extensor proximal pole.
a Lateral view.
b AP view.
c–d Periprosthetic fracture of patella, type V.34-A2, disrupted extensor distal pole.
c Lateral view.
d AP view.

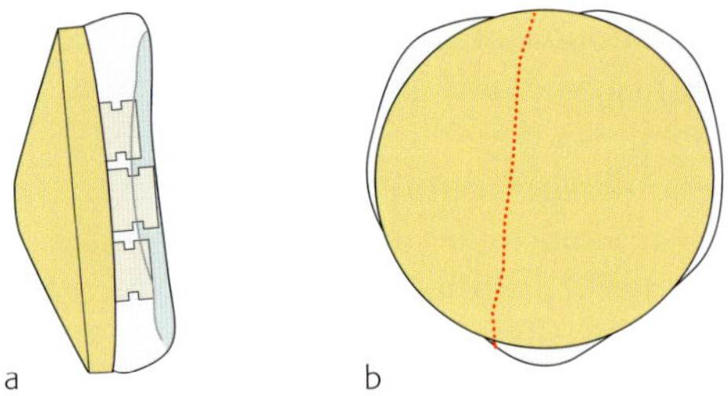

4.2-79a–b Periprosthetic fracture of patella, type V.34-B1.
a Lateral view.
b AP view.

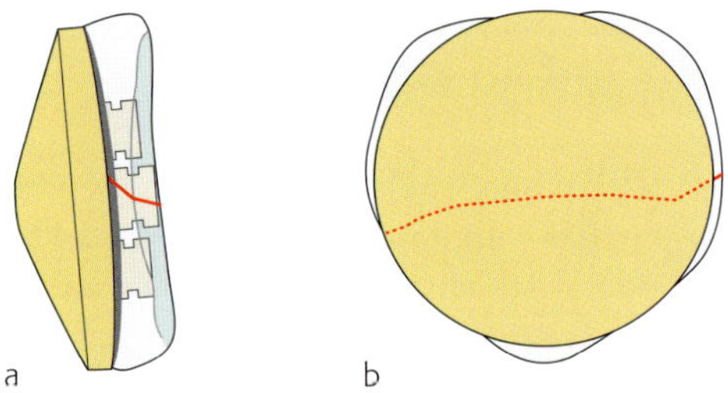

4.2-80a–b Periprosthetic fracture of patella type V.34-B2.
a Lateral view.
b AP view.

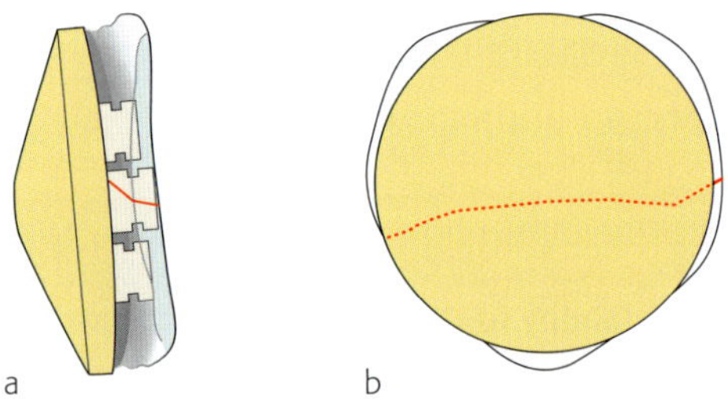

4.2-81a–b Periprosthetic fracture of patella type V.34-B3.
a Lateral view.
b AP view.

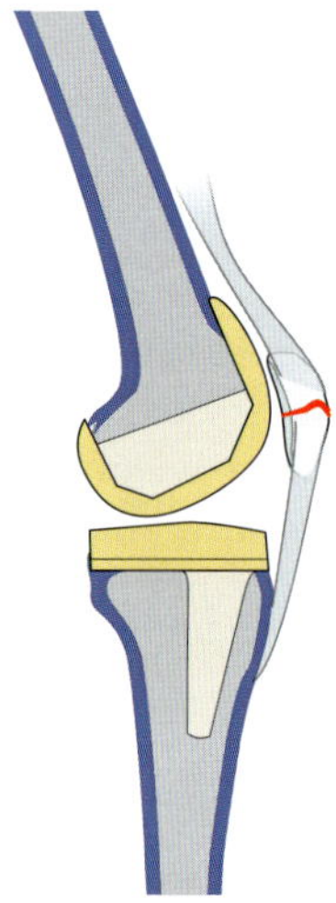

4.2-82 Periprosthetic fracture of patella type V.34-F.

VI
Ankle

Existing classification systems

To the authors' knowledge, no classification system has yet been published.

Ankle replacement is still emerging as a treatment option and it is still evolving in technique and technology. Periprosthetic fractures are, therefore, rarely encountered. But the incidence of such fractures is likely to rise if its use increases. Therefore, a rational approach to treatment will be valuable.

Unified Classification System (UCS)

The Unified Classification System (UCS) applies well to injuries affecting the tibia (VI.4), fibula (VI.4), or talus (VI.8).

Type A
Such fractures affect the tip of the medial (A1) or lateral (A2) malleolus (**4.2-83a–b**). Surgical management will be required if the joint has been destabilized by the injury.

Type B
Such fractures involve the distal tibia, the base of the medial malleolus, or body of the talus. They are subcategorized as type B1, B2, or B3 based on whether the implant is well fixed (B1) or loose (B2), and whether, in the presence of a loose implant, the bone is adequate (B2) or inadequate (B3) to support a new implant. **4.2-84** illustrates a type B1 fracture involving the base of the medial malleolus. Type B1 fractures (**4.2-85a–b**, **4.2-86**) require reduction and fixation, if feasible. Type B2 fractures (**4.2-87**, **4.2-88**) require revision of the implant, combined with reduction and fixation of the fracture.

Type B3 classifies a fracture (**4.2-89**, **4.2-90**) difficult to reconstruct after ankle replacement, which can affect either tibia or talus. Therefore, ankle fusion is commonly chosen as a salvage solution. If salvage options have failed, especially if aggravated by an infection, below-knee amputation may have to be taken into consideration.

Type C
Such fractures involve the tibia proximal to the arthroplasty or, alternatively, the neck or head of the talus (**4.2-91**, **4.2-92**).

Type D
Such fractures involve the tibia between a knee and ankle replacement (**4.2-93**). Theoretically, it could also involve the neck of the talus between an ankle and talonavicular replacement.

Type E
Such fractures are characterized by fractures of both the tibia and talus.

Type F
This category does not pertain to the ankle because replacement hemiarthroplasty of the ankle is not part of standard orthopedic practice.

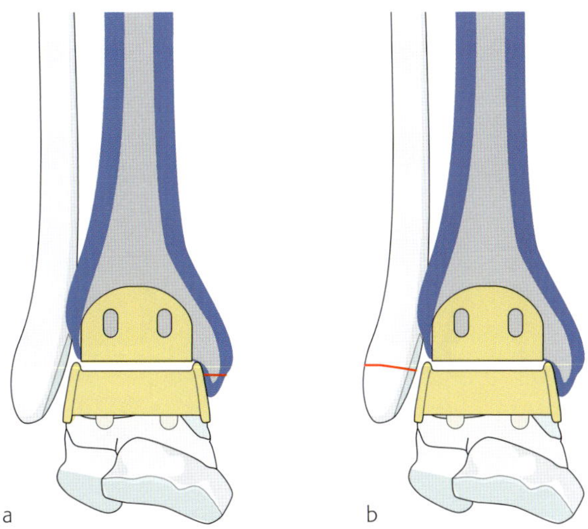

4.2-83a–b Periprosthetic fracture types of distal tibia.
a Type VI.4-A1 medial malleolus.
b Type VI.4-A2 tip of lateral malleolus.

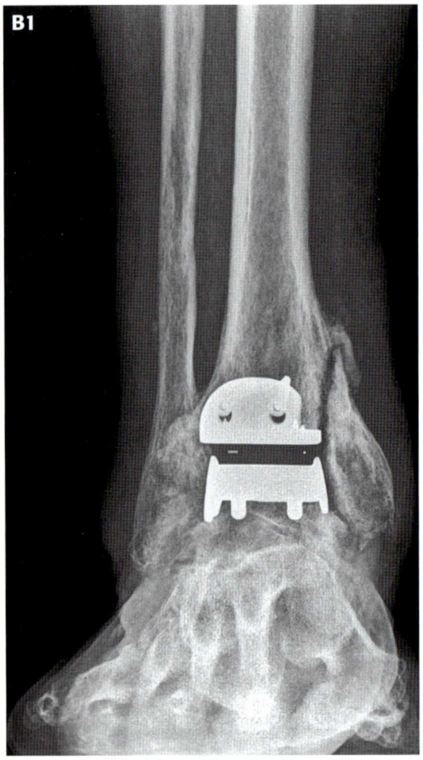

4.2-84 Type B1 periprosthetic fracture of the ankle. The implants are secure. Fracture fixation—but not revision—is required. (Courtesy of Beat Hintermann, Switzerland.)

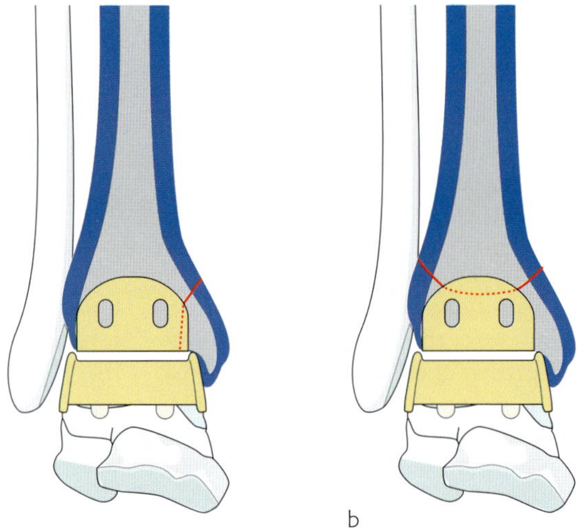

a b

4.2-85a–b Periprosthetic fracture of distal tibia type VI.4-B1.
a Medial malleolus shear fracture.
b Transverse tibia fracture.

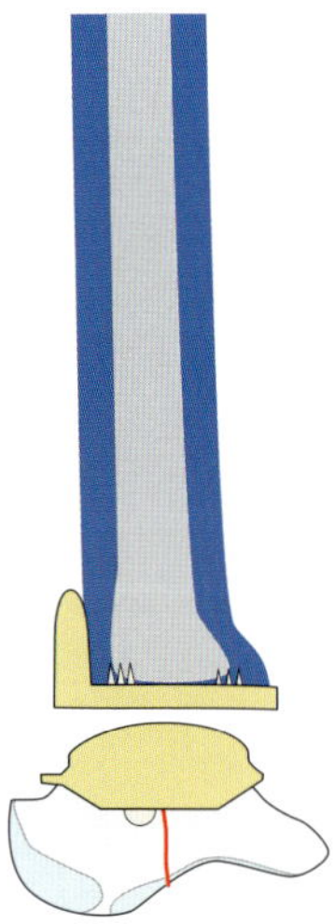

4.2-86 Periprosthetic fracture of talus type VI.8-B1.

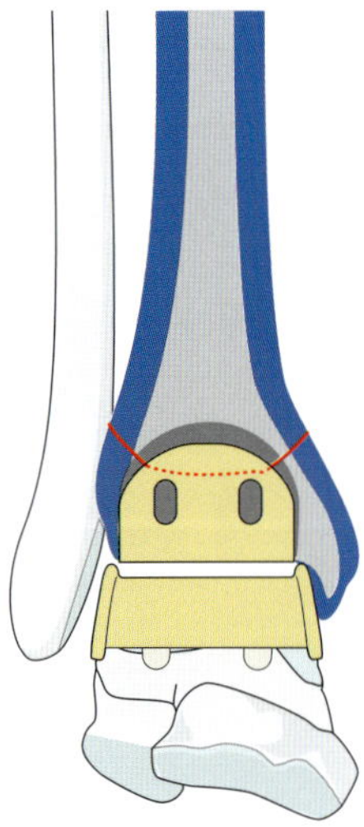

4.2-87 Periprosthetic fracture of distal tibia type VI.4-B2.

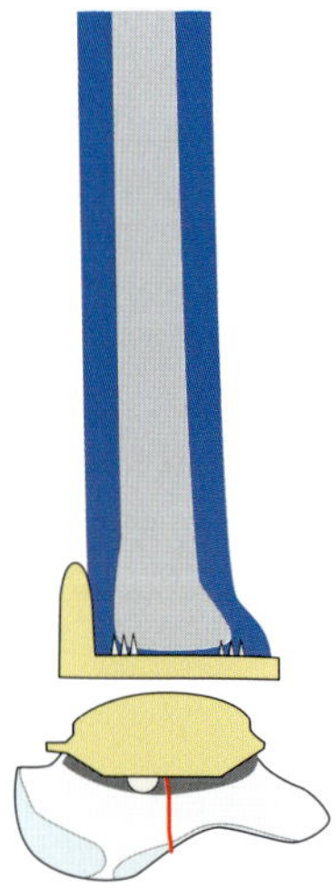

4.2-88 Periprosthetic fracture of talus type VI.8-B2.

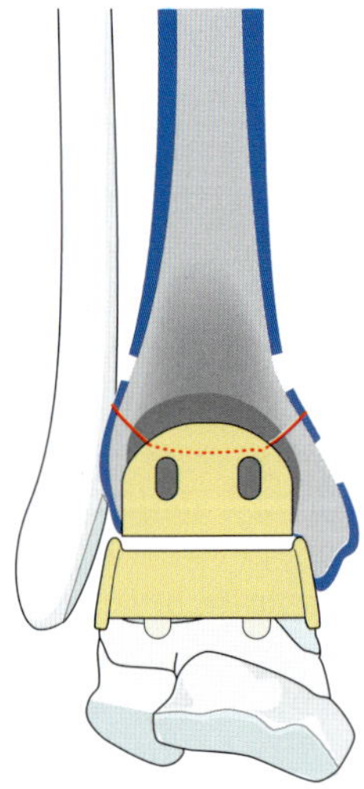

4.2-89 Periprosthetic fracture of distal tibia type VI.4-B3.

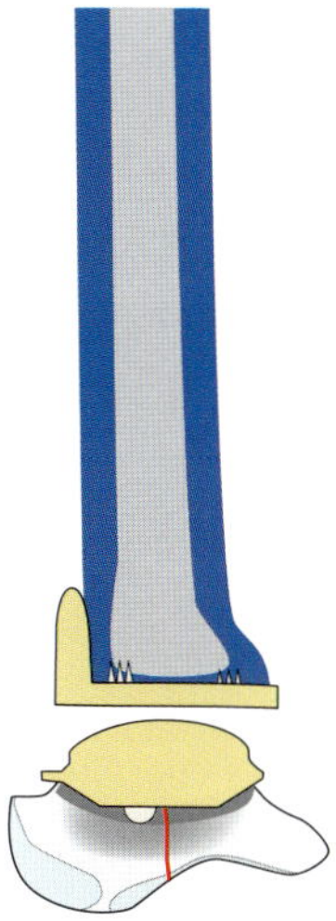

4.2-90 Periprosthetic fracture of talus type VI.8-B3.

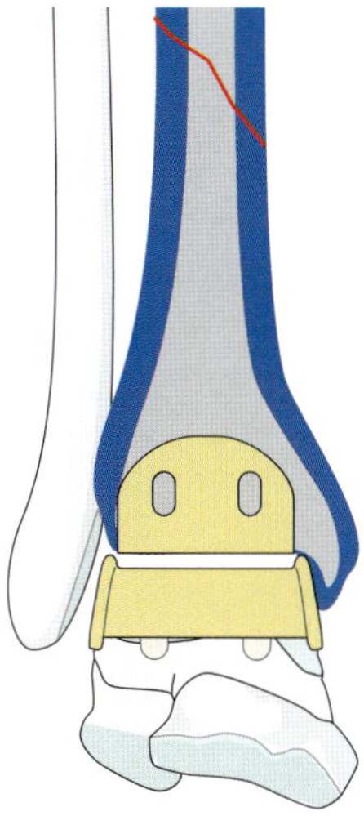

4.2-91 Periprosthetic fracture of tibial shaft type VI.4-C.

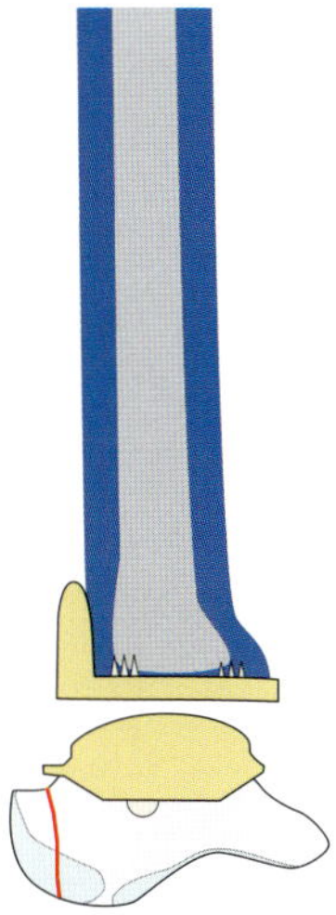

4.2-92 Periprosthetic fracture of talar tuberosity type VI.8-C.

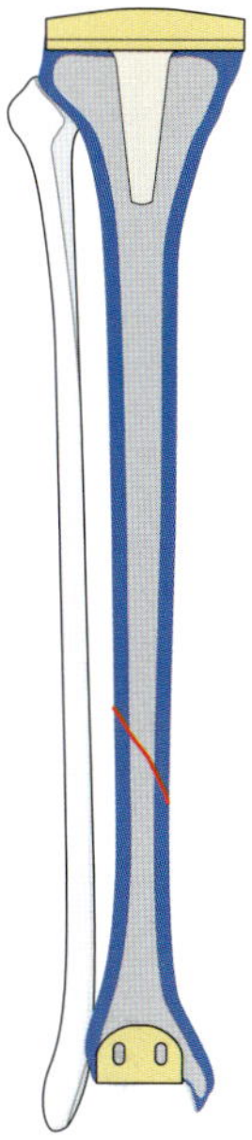

4.2-93 Intercalary periprosthetic fracture of tibial shaft type VI.8-D.

4.2.4 Summary

The number of periprosthetic fractures following joint replacement is rising steadily and, thus, this complication has become the fourth most common reason for revision arthroplasty in several national hip joint registries (after loosening, lysis without loosening, and dislocation). This should not be surprising in view of the fact that the preference for joint replacement as a treatment option is itself rising all over the world, especially notable in the management of hip and knee arthritis. Beside the increasing number of prostheses in service, the incidence of periprosthetic fractures following joint replacement also depends on issues of increasing time in situ (with an increasing risk of fracture with time), deterioration of bone health and strength with advancing age, and the ever present problem of osteolysis.

When presented with such complications, it is essential for the surgeon to understand the core principles that should constitute treatment in order for the outcome to be optimal. It is in this spirit that the Unified Classification System (UCS) is proposed by the authors. Its concern is to highlight the characteristic biomechanical and biological factors which are common to each fracture type, regardless of the actual bone that has been injured and the joint that has been affected. This will help to guide the reader and enhance the results of treatment of periprosthetic fractures.

The Unified Classification System (UCS) has been applied throughout this book.

References

[1] **Lewallen DG, Berry DJ.** Periprosthetic fracture of the femur after total hip arthroplasty: treatment and results to date. *Instr Course Lect.* 1998;47:243–249.

[2] **Meermans G, Haddad FS.** Is there a role for tissue biopsy in the diagnosis of periprosthetic infection? *Clin Orthop Relat Res.* 2010 May;468(5):1410–1417.

[3] **Bedair H, Ting N, Jacovides C, et al.** The Mark Coventry Award: diagnosis of early postoperative TKA infection using synovial fluid analysis. *Clin Orthop Relat Res.* 2011 Jan;469(1):34–40.

[4] **Sánchez-Sotelo J, McGrory BJ, Berry DJ.** Acute periprosthetic fracture of the acetabulum associated with osteolytic pelvic lesions: a report of 3 cases. *J Arthroplasty.* 2000 Jan;15(1):126–130.

[5] **Koot VC, Kesselaer SM, Clevers GJ, et al.** Evaluation of the Singh index for measuring osteoporosis. *J Bone Joint Surg Br.* 1996 Sep;78(5):831–834.

[6] **Shawen SB, Belmont PJ Jr, Klemme WR, et al.** Osteoporosis and anterior femoral notching in periprosthetic supracondylar femoral fractures: a biomechanical analysis. *J Bone Joint Surg Am.* 2003 Jan;85–A(1):115–121.

[7] **Amstutz HC, Le Duff MJ, Campbell PA, et al.** Clinical and radiographic results of metal–on–metal hip resurfacing with a minimum ten–year follow–up. *J Bone Joint Surg Am.* 2010 Nov;92(16):2663–2671.

[8] **Aamodt A, Kvistad KA, Andersen E, et al.** Determination of Hounsfield value for CT–based design of custom femoral stems. *J Bone Joint Surg Br.* 1999 Jan;81(1):143–147.

[9] **White LM, Kim JK, Mehta M, et al.** Complications of total hip arthroplasty: MR imaging—initial experience. *Radiology.*; 215(1):254–262.

[10] **Duncan CP, Masri BA.** Fractures of the femur after hip replacement. *Instr Course Lect.* 1995; 44:293–304.

[11] **Lindahl H, Malchau H, Odén A, et al.** Risk factors for failure after treatment of a periprosthetic fracture of the femur. *J Bone Joint Surg Br.* 2006 Jan;88(1):26–30.

[12] **Brady OH, Garbuz DS, Masri BA, et al.** The reliability and validity of the Vancouver classification of femoral fractures after hip replacement. *J Arthroplasty.* 2000 Jan; 15(1):59–62.

[13] **Rayan F, Dodd M, Haddad FS.** European validation of the Vancouver classification of periprosthetic proximal femoral fractures. *J Bone Joint Surg Br.* 2008 Dec;90(12):1576–1579.

[14] **Groh GI, Heckman MM, Curtis RJ, et al.** Treatment of fractures adjacent to humeral prosthesis [Abstract]. *AAOS Meeting, New Orleans, February 1994.*

[15] **Groh GI, Heckman MM, Wirth MA, et al.** Treatment of fractures adjacent to humeral prostheses. *J Shoulder Elbow Surg.* 2008 Jan–Feb;17(1):85–89.

[16] **Wright TW, Cofield RH.** Humeral fractures after shoulder arthroplasty. *J Bone Joint Surg Am.* 1995 Sep;77(9):1340–1346.

[17] **Campbell JT, Moore RS, Iannotti JP, et al.** Periprosthetic humeral fractures: mechanisms of fracture and treatment options. *J Shoulder Elbow Surg.* 1998 Jul–Aug;7(4):406–413.

[18] **Worland RL, Kim DY, Arredondo J, et al.** Periprosthetic humeral fractures: management and classification. *J Shoulder Elbow Surg.* 1999 Nov–Dec;8(6):590–594.

[19] **O'Driscoll SW, Morrey BF.** Periprosthetic fractures about the elbow. *Orthop Clin North Am.* 1999 Apr;30(2):319–325.

[20] **Peterson CA 2nd, Lewallen DG.** Periprosthetic fracture of the acetabulum after total hip arthroplasty. *J Bone Joint Surg Am.* 1996 Aug;78(8):1206–1213.

[21] **Della Valle CJ, Momberger NG, Paprosky WG.** Periprosthetic fractures of the acetabulum associated with a total hip arthroplasty. *Instr Course Lect.* 2003;52:281–290.

[22] **Kosashvili Y, Backstein D, Safir O, et al.** Acetabular revision using an anti–protrusion (ilio–ischial) cage and trabecular metal acetabular component for severe acetabular bone loss associated with pelvic discontinuity. *J Bone Joint Surg Br.* 2009 Jul;91(7):870–876.

[23] **Rose PS, Halasy M, Trousdale RT, et al.** Preliminary results of tantalum acetabular components for THA after pelvic radiation. *Clin Orth Rel Res.* 2006 Dec;453:195–198.

[24] **Ricci WM, Bolhofner BR, Loftus T, et al.** Indirect reduction and plate fixation, without bone grafting, for periprosthetic femoral shaft fractures about a stable intramedullary implant. *J Bone Joint Surg Am.* 2005 Oct;87(10):2240–2245.

[25] **Rorabeck CH, Taylor JW.** Classification of periprosthetic fractures complicating total knee arthroplasty. *Orthop Clin North Am.* 1999 Apr;30(2):209–214.

[26] **Felix NA, Stuart MJ, Hanssen AD.** Periprosthetic fractures of the tibia associated with total knee arthroplasty. *Clin Orthop Relat Res.* 1997 Dec;(345):113–124.

[27] **Parvizi J, Jain N, Schmidt AH.** Periprosthetic knee fractures. *J Orthop Trauma.* 2008 Oct;22(9):663–671.

[28] **Ortiguera CJ, Berry DJ.** Patellar fracture after total knee arthroplasty. *J Bone Joint Surg Am.* 2002 Apr;84–A(4):532–540.

[29] **Windsor RE, Scuderi GR, Insall JN.** Patellar fractures in total knee arthroplasty. *J Arthroplasty.* 1989;4 Suppl:S63–S67.

5

Management techniques for periprosthetic fractures

5.1 Introduction

Authors Carsten Perka, Thomas P Rüedi

When considering the different treatment options of periprosthetic fractures, it is important to carefully assess the patient and to follow a clear decision-making process.

5.1.1 Decision making

When facing periprosthetic fractures, surgical decision making depends on a number of factors that are similar for all types of fractures, irrespective of their anatomical location. There are different possibilities of treatment for periprosthetic fractures:

- Nonoperative treatment (chapter 5.3)
- Internal fixation of the fracture with osteosynthetic devices (chapter 5.4)
- Revision arthroplasty (chapter 5.5)
- Alternative complex fixation techniques (chapter 5.6).

Besides rather clear indications, such as an evident loosening of the prosthetic component involved in the injury or large bone defects, the surgeon's preference and his/her personal experience also seem to play a decisive role in whether to choose revision arthroplasty or osteosynthesis. A complete history and clinical assessment of the patient as well as detailed information on the original joint replacement procedure (including x-rays and model/manufacturer of the prosthesis), and the acute event has to be obtained. Adequate imaging to determine implant stability and alignment as well as an assessment of the bone quality are crucial to determine the optimal type of treatment (nonoperative or surgical, revision arthroplasty or internal fixation). Last but not least, an infection should be excluded preoperatively as a cause of loosening in order to decide whether to proceed in one or more stages.

Nonoperative management of periprosthetic fractures is generally associated with a prolonged period of inactivity of the involved joint or time on crutches, and a high complication rate. Moreover, timely fracture healing often cannot be achieved, indicating that this option should only be chosen in exceptional cases, preferably in nondisplaced extraarticular type A fractures.

Internal fixation of a periprosthetic fracture should only be performed if the prosthetic component is well fixed in the involved bone segment and the patient's compliance allows an appropriate aftercare on crutches with only partial weight bearing. In all other situations—loose prosthetic implant, suspicion of infection, and poor compliance—the best treatment is revision arthroplasty, which is more invasive and associated with a higher rate of morbidity.

5.1.2 Preoperative planning and patient assessment

Before embarking on surgery, a detailed preoperative plan has to be prepared carefully, including a plan B in case of intraoperative surprises, such as an unexpected infection (chapters 4.1 and 5.2). Except in case of an open or severe injury when immediate stabilization of the injured joint may be crucial, most periprosthetic fractures can be managed in a scheduled manner and should allow for proper planning.

This stage should also be used for a careful general assessment of the patient, including comorbidities, vascular and neurological status, alcohol and smoking habits, drugs and medications as well as mental status and compliance. While waiting for surgery the patient's comfort should be attended to without delay, using temporary immobilization in appropriate splints or traction. Adequate analgesic treatment, such as peripheral nerve blocks and pain medication, should be administered routinely and rapidly. As the rate of morbidity and even mortality from periprosthetic fractures is high in the elderly, special care should be given to the identification of specific general conditions, such as dehydration or organ failure that must be dealt with before surgery is undertaken. It is recommended and important to always confer with a multidisciplinary team involving anesthesiology and geriatric medicine. The peripheral neurological status should be carefully evaluated and special attention should be given to determine the vascular status and in case of doubt the appropriate measures should be taken. These patients are at risk of vascular complications due to plaque emboli or blunt injury to major vessels. Prophylaxis against thromboembolism and infection (short-term antibiotics) are mandatory. Intraoperatively, complications, such as embolization, must be carefully monitored by the anesthesia team.

In the operating room, the necessary instruments and implants including special revision prosthesis should be readily available—in case plan B should come into action—with a team of surgeons and nurses capable and familiar with the complexities of this type of surgery. Having an image intensifier in the operating room is mandatory.

5.1.3 Postoperative management

Postoperatively, and under the surgeon's close supervision, the rehabilitation team should be ready to take charge of the patient. It is not uncommon that in the days following the operation agitation and delirium may occur. Therefore, geriatric consultants should be involved. Getting patients out of bed as quickly as possible and providing the means to regain their mobility and autonomy is of vital importance. It must be kept in mind that much of the success of the rehabilitation efforts depends on the quality of the surgical procedure.

5.2 Patient preparation

Authors **Akin Önder, Michael Sander**

5.2.1 Introduction

Patients undergoing surgery for periprosthetic fractures are usually high-risk elderly patients with a high incidence of comorbidities [1]. Due to the demographic aging of the population, the number of elderly patients (older than 65 years) with multiple, preexisting comorbidities will increase continuously. The average rate of mortality after noncardiac surgery is about 4% [2, 3]. However, the potential risk is higher in the group of patients with periprosthetic fracture.

5.2.2 Influence of preexisting clinical conditions

To guarantee the best possible results after surgery, extremely careful patient preparation is crucial in this group. An important step in the preoperative evaluation is the individual planning of the postoperative course for each patient. Recent research shows that only a third of high-risk patients are admitted to an intensive care unit (ICU) after surgery for postoperative care and monitoring. It was also reported that most patients, who did not survive surgery, died on a standard ward without any intensive care treatment during their stay in an hospital [4]. This fact additionally emphasizes the importance of planning the postoperative allocation to an ICU or a post-anesthesia care unit (PACU), respectively, for patients with increased perioperative risk [2, 5].

Therefore, high-risk patients have to be identified preoperatively to receive appropriate treatment and achieve the best possible preoperative clinical status and postoperative treatment.

Basic steps of patient preparation for patients undergoing surgery for periprosthetic fractures include the evaluation of the patient for severe comorbidities. The goal is to achieve optimal medical control of existing chronic diseases.

All patients should undergo the ASA-Score (American Society of Anesthesiologists Physical Status Classification System) to estimate the risk of surgery and anesthesia. Additionally, the cardiac risk of the individual patient should be checked according to the flowchart provided in **5.2-1**. For patients with stents, acetylsalicylic acid (ASA) should be continuously provided during the perioperative period as this has been shown to decrease cardiac morbidity without increasing transfusion rate. In patients with additional antiplatelet therapy, a bridging therapy should be evaluated. All orthopedic patients should be checked for anemia and coagulation abnormalities.

Additionally, in all patients with existing comorbidities undergoing surgery for periprosthetic fractures, advanced perioperative monitoring technology with pulse contour cardiac output or ultrasound cardiac output should be used to establish optimal goal-directed hemodynamic and volume therapy during the course of surgery and in the postoperative phase.

The overall perioperative risk is influenced by factors such as the medical history of the patient, age, lifestyle habits, the extent and duration of surgery, and perioperative blood loss. Premedication and patient preparation has to establish the existence of important preoperative comorbidities to achieve the best possible outcome in view of these comorbidities and the associated reduction of the patient's physiological resources.

The most important comorbidities in this group of patients are:

- Heart failure
- Coronary heart disease
- Pulmonary disease
- Renal insufficiency
- Diabetes
- Anemia.

Based on the ASA-Score, it is possible to evaluate the perioperative risk for patients (**5.2-1**). The ASA-Score is easy to specify and is based on the comorbidities of the patient. Healthy patients (ASA I) with low surgical risk have a lower risk of complications than patients with comorbidities. The perioperative in-hospital mortality rate for low-risk patients in low-risk surgery is 0.77% versus 35.6% for high-risk patients [6].

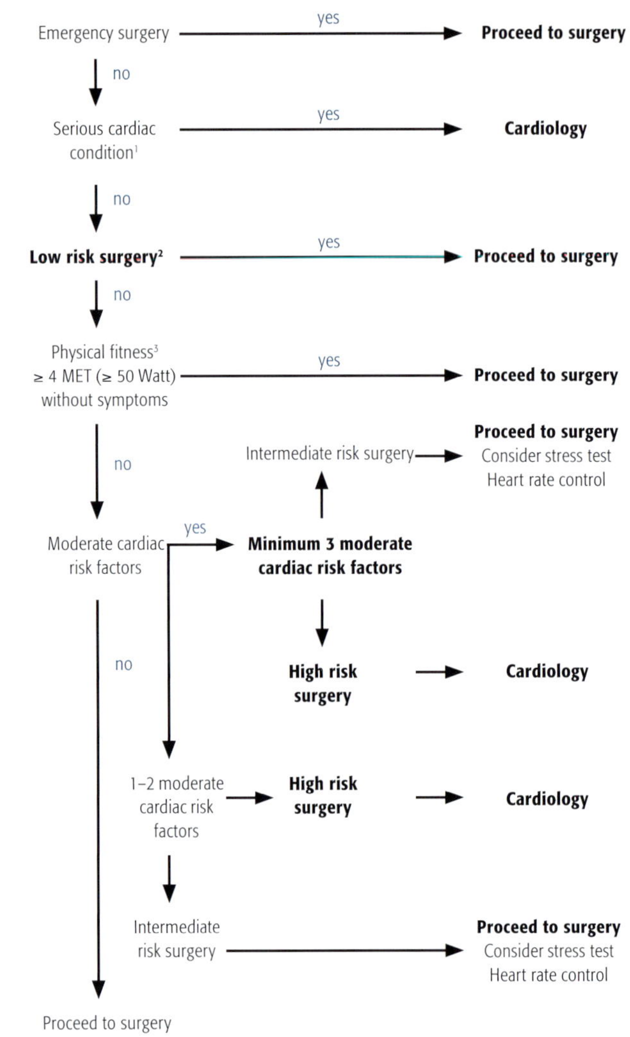

[1] Serious cardiac condition: unstable ischemia, decompensated heart failure, high-grade valve disease, relevant heart-rhythm disturbances.
Cardiac risk factors: history of ischemic heart disease, history of compensated heart failure, diabetes mellitus, renal insufficiency (creatinine level > 2 mg/dL). History of cerebrovascular disease.

[2] Low-risk surgery (<1% cardiac incidents): endoscopic surgery, superficial surgery, cataract surgery.
Moderate surgery risk (1–5% cardiac incidents): intrathoracic or intraabdominal surgery, orthopedic surgery, prostate surgery.
High-risk surgery (> 5% cardiac incidents): surgery on abdominal aorta or peripheral vessels.

[3] Physical fitness in metabolic equivalent of task (MET):
> 4 MET (≥ 50 W): climbing more than one floor, going uphill slowly, slight homework, cycling slowly.
> 6 MET (≥ 150 W): swimming/dancing, going uphill, moving furniture.
> 10 MET: endurance sports.

5.2-1 Flowchart for the identification of patients with high perioperative cardiac risks.

5.2-1 American Society of Anesthesiologists Physical Status Classification System (ASA-Score).

ASA I	A normal healthy patient
ASA II	A patient with mild systemic disease
ASA III	A patient with severe systemic disease
ASA IV	A patient with severe systemic disease that is a constant threat to life
ASA V	A moribund patient who is not expected to survive without the operation
ASA VI	A declared brain-dead patient whose organs are being removed for donor purposes

Cardiac comorbidities and anticoagulation

Patients with cardiac comorbidities usually suffer from complications in the perioperative context. In recent studies, heart failure, arrhythmia, and coronary heart disease have been shown to have a substantial impact on the perioperative course of patients undergoing surgery [5, 7]. These comorbidities, unless controlled properly, were shown to double the mortality rate in orthopedic surgery. Therefore, identification of patients at risk and adequate preoperative therapy are essential for these patients.

Based on the flowchart (**5.2-1**), it is possible to identify patients with high perioperative cardiac risk and, if necessary, initiate preventive treatment before surgery to establish the best medical control and minimize the risk of cardiac complications.

For patients with periprosthetic fractures, the first step should be to identify emergency patients (eg, ongoing bleeding, open fractures, nerve injury). These patients should undergo surgery without delay. However, monitoring and postoperative ICU treatment need to be adapted to the underlying cardiac disease and other comorbidities.

In case of urgent surgery of patients with active cardiac problems, such as acute heart failure, the intervention has to be delayed until the underlying cardiac condition has been treated. The next step in the evaluation of cardiac risks in orthopedic surgery (intermediate cardiac risk) concerns an estimation of physical fitness using the metabolic equivalent of task (MET). Patients with physical activities exceeding 4 MET (can climb a flight of stairs) can undergo surgery without delay. In patients with lower physical activity or whenever—as in some patients with periprosthetic fractures—the physical activity cannot be estimated due to the underlying orthopedic injury, the cardiac risk factors have to be assessed. In accordance to the number of preexisting cardiac risk factors, patients can undergo surgery without delay or, in patients with three or more risk factors, surgery needs to be delayed until a check-up by a cardiologist has been performed. In many cases, a perioperative beta-blockade will be required.

Additional apparative diagnostics are only indicated if they would result in a change of patient management. An exception is echocardiography (ECG) that should be done routinely for all patients with periprosthetic fractures. Combined ECG and stress tests, however, are only indicated in patients with symptoms or risk factors and if no cardiologic diagnostics have been performed within the last 12 months.

Management of patients with cardiac stents

In the last decade, stent implantation in patients with one- or two-vessel coronary heart disease has become the treatment of choice. This has led to great advances in the treatment of coronary heart disease. In contrast, however, it poses some risk for surgical patients. This is because they need to be placed on antiplatelet drug therapy, the duration of the therapy depending on the type of the stent. In their guidelines, various international associations for cardiology recommend that patients with bare metal stents (BMS) need to be given clopidogrel for 4 weeks and acetylsalicylic acid for lifetime. Patients with drug-eluting stents (DES) have to take clopidogrel for 6–12 months and acetylsalicylic acid for lifetime. Clopidogrel may cause intraoperative and postoperative bleeding but its discontinuation increases the risk of vascular events or stent thrombosis in patients with DES, with the potential for fatal outcome. Therefore, patients taking clopidogrel need a bridging of their antiplatelet therapy during the perioperative phase in the first year after DES implantation with a short-acting intravenous glycoprotein IIb/IIIa inhibitor (GP) (eg, eptifibatide or tirofiban) as a bridging therapy [8]. Acetylsalicylic acid should be continued throughout orthopedic surgery in patients with a stent, as this was shown to decrease cardiac complications without increase in transfusion rates.

Antiplatelet bridging procedure for urgent surgery [8]:

- 5–7 days preoperatively: discontinue clopidogrel, continue acetylsalicylic acid
- 3–5 days preoperatively: start with glycoprotein IIb/IIIa inhibitor, continue acetylsalicylic acid
- 8–12 hours preoperatively: discontinue glycoprotein IIb/IIIa inhibitor, one dose of low-molecular-weight heparin
- Day of surgery: no glycoprotein IIb/IIIa inhibitor and monitoring on ICU, one dose of low-molecular-weight heparin 6 hours postoperative
- 1 day postoperatively: continue glycoprotein IIb/IIIa inhibitor
- 1–3 days postoperatively: start clopidogrel (loading dose 600 mg), continue acetylsalicylic acid, stop glycoprotein IIb/IIIa inhibitor, one dose of low-molecular-weight heparin daily until mobilization.

Pulmonary comorbidities

Pulmonary comorbidities increase the risk of perioperative complications.

The major risk factors are:

- Chronic obstructive pulmonary disease (COPD)
- Older than 65 years
- Emergency surgery
- Thoracic surgery
- Length of surgery
- Intraoperative transfusion
- Postoperative reintubation.

Patients with postoperative pulmonary complications have a higher postoperative mortality rate (approximately 20%) than patients without pulmonary complications (> 1–2%) [9, 10]. Such patients need to be identified and it is mandatory to provide a chest x-ray preoperatively. Patients at risk for postoperative pulmonary complications should be treated postoperatively in a PACU or ICU to undergo preventive continuous positive airway pressure (CPAP) or noninvasive ventilation therapy, as this has been shown to decrease the rate of postoperative pulmonary complications and postoperative pneumonia in these patients [11, 12].

Renal insufficiencies

Patients with renal dysfunctions suffer from electrolyte disorders, disorders in their water balance, and secondary diseases. This represents a higher risk for perioperative complications and mortality within 30 days after surgery (9%) compared with elderly patients without renal comorbidities (1%) [13]. This requires identification and planning for advanced intraoperative monitoring for optimal guidance of fluid and volume management with invasive blood pressure recording using dynamic parameters like stroke volume variation, pulse pressure variation, or stroke volume recording [14]. Patients with chronic renal failure with renal replacement therapy should undergo dialysis the day before surgery and enter the operating room without electrolyte disturbances.

Coagulopathy and anemia

Coagulopathies have an influence on the anesthetic and surgical procedure, leading—if not controlled—to increased perioperative blood loss and the need for blood transfusions. A preoperatively existing anemia increases the perioperative risk and has influence on the cardiac and pulmonary function [15]. Blood transfusion itself has been shown to be linked to increased rates of pneumonia and mortality [16]. Anemia in orthopedic patients is also a factor that increases postoperative mortality (hemoglobin 8 g/dL corresponding to a mortality rate of 0% versus hemoglobin 5 g/dL corresponding to mortality rate of 34.4%). Carson et al [17] showed that the in-hospital mortality rate of patients with a restrictive transfusion scheme is 23% lower than in patients with a liberal transfusion scheme in a general surgical population. However, Foss et al [18] reported that the rate of cardiovascular complications and increased mortality was observed in elderly patients undergoing orthopedic surgery with a restrictive transfusion scheme. On the other hand, the results of the FOCUS-study presented no reduction of mortality or in-hospital morbidity in the liberal transfusion strategy in elderly patients at high cardiovascular risk. This data shows that for orthopedic patients a hemoglobin of 8 g/dL can be considered as safe [19]. If possible, anemic patients with delayed surgery should be screened for anemia and, if present, its etiology should be clarified. In case of treatable causes, specific treatment should be initiated (eg, intravenous iron therapy, erythropoietin) [20].

Malnutrition

Patients with periprosthetic fractures are usually elderly or geriatric patients. Malnutrition is an additional risk factor in this patient group and more than half of all geriatric patients in hospitals are malnourished [21]. Del Savio et al [22] showed that baseline nutritional status is an indicator of postoperative complications in elderly patients with hip fractures. The ESPEN guidelines on enteral nutrition suggest that oral nutritional supplements (ONS) can reduce postoperative complications in geriatric patients after hip fracture and orthopedic surgery [23]. However, results of current studies are contradictory. Some other studies could not show a benefit of oral nutritional supplements [24, 25].

The implementation of perioperative ONS and the associated higher daily protein intake may reduce postoperative complications but is not feasible in patients with periprosthetic fractures submitted to emergency or urgent surgery [26]. Here it is only possible to start postoperative administration of ONS after surgery [27]. Symeonidis and Clark [28] demonstrated that the combination of serum albumin level and total lymphocyte count is an independent prognostic factor in patients with hip fracture and can be used as nutritional markers for administration of nutritional supplements.

5.2.3 Postoperative planning

The pathway of postoperative ICU or PACU treatment or return to standard wards should also be based on objective risk stratification. One major point in addition to consequent implementation of evidence-based strategies during and after surgery is careful planning of the postoperative pathway with step-down approaches using recovery ward, PACU and ICUs for patients with different risk profiles. Only the implementation of careful preoperative patient preparation based on the assessment of comorbidities, intraoperative implementation of goal-directed optimization strategies in selected patients, and careful planning of postoperative pathways adjusted to the patient's risk level will lead to a decrease of morbidity and mortality in the high-risk population of patients undergoing surgery for periprosthetic fractures.

References

[1] **Walsh TS, Palmer J, Watson D, et al.** Multicentre cohort study of red blood cell use for revision hip arthroplasty and factors associated with greater risk of allogeneic blood transfusion. *Br J Anaesth.* 2012 Jan;108(1):63–71.

[2] **Pearse RM, Moreno RP, Bauer P, et al.** Mortality after surgery in Europe: a 7 day cohort study. *Lancet.* 2012 Sep;380(9847):1059–1065.

[3] **Pearse RM.** Another inconvenient truth: meeting the challenge of preventing poor surgical outcomes. *Curr Opin Crit Care.* 2010 Aug;16(4):337–338.

[4] **Jhanji S, Thomas B, Ely A, et al.** Mortality and utilisation of critical care resources amongst high-risk surgical patients in a large NHS trust. *Anaesthesia.* 2008 Jul;63(7):695–700.

[5] **Task Force for Preoperative Cardiac Risk Assessment and Perioperative Cardiac Management in Non-cardiac Surgery, European Society of Cardiology (ESC), Poldermans D, et al.** Guidelines for pre-operative cardiac risk assessment and perioperative cardiac management in non-cardiac surgery. *Eur Heart J.* 2009 Nov;30(22):2769–2812.

[6] **Glance LG, Lustik SJ, Hannan EL, et al.** The Surgical Mortality Probability Model: derivation and validation of a simple risk prediction rule for noncardiac surgery. *Ann Surg.* 2012 Apr;255(4):696–702.

[7] **Hammill BG, Curtis LH, Bennett-Guerrero E, et al.** Impact of heart failure on patients undergoing major noncardiac surgery. *Anesthesiology.* 2008 Apr;108(4):559–567.

[8] **Koscielny J.** [Bleeding and thromboembolic risk. Perioperative strategy in aspirin/clopidogrel]. *Pharm Unserer Zeit.* 2009;38(4):352–358. German.

[9] **Shander A, Fleisher LA, Barie PS, et al.** Clinical and economic burden of postoperative pulmonary complications: patient safety summit on definition, risk-reducing interventions, and preventive strategies. *Crit Care Med.* 2011 Sep;39(9):2163–2172.

[10] **Canet J, Gallart L, Gomar C, et al.** Prediction of postoperative pulmonary complications in a population-based surgical cohort. *Anesthesiology.* 2010 Dec;113(6):1338–1350.

[11] **Pelosi P, Jaber S.** Noninvasive respiratory support in the perioperative period. *Curr Opin Anaesthesiol.* 2010 Apr;23(2):233–238.

[12] **Ferreyra GP, Baussano I, Squadrone V, et al.** Continuous positive airway pressure for treatment of respiratory complications after abdominal surgery a systematic review and meta-analysis. *Ann Surg.* 2008 Apr;247(4):617–626.

[13] **Story DA, Leslie K, Myles PS, et al.** Complications and mortality in older surgical patients in Australia and New Zealand (the REASON study): a multicentre, prospective, observational study. *Anaesthesia.* 2010 Oct;65(10):1022–1030.

[14] **Hamilton MA, Cecconi M, Rhodes A.** A systematic review and meta-analysis on the use of preemptive hemodynamic intervention to improve postoperative outcomes in moderate and high-risk surgical patients. *Anesth Analg.* 2011 Jun;112(6):1392–1402.

[15] **Carson JL, Noveck H, Berlin JA, et al.** Mortality and morbidity in patients with very low postoperative Hb levels who decline blood transfusion. *Transfusion.* 2002 Jul;42(7):812–818.

[16] **Pedersen AB, Mehnert F, Overgaard S, et al.** Allogeneic blood transfusion and prognosis following total hip replacement: a population-based follow up study. *BMC Musculoskelet Disord.* 2009 Dec;10:167.

[17] **Carson JL, Carless PA, Hébert PC.** Transfusion thresholds and other strategies for guiding allogeneic red blood cell transfusion. *Cochrane Database Syst Rev.* 2012 Apr;4:CD002042.

[18] **Foss NB, Kristensen MT, Jensen PS, et al.** The effects of liberal versus restrictive transfusion thresholds on ambulation after hip fracture surgery. *Transfusion.* 2009 Feb;49(2):227–234.

[19] **Carson JL, Terrin ML, Noveck H, et al.** Liberal or restrictive transfusion in high-risk patients after hip surgery. *N Engl J Med.* 2011 Dec;365(26):2453–2462.

[20] **Goodnough LT, Maniatis A, Earnshaw P, et al.** Detection, evaluation, and management of preoperative anaemia in the elective orthopaedic surgical patient: NATA guidelines. *Br J Anaesth.* 2011 Jan;106(1):13–22.

[21] **Pirlich M, Schütz T, Norman K, et al.** The German hospital malnutrition study. *Clin Nutr.* 2006 Aug;25(4):563–572.

[22] **Del Savio GC, Zelicof SB, Wexler LM, et al.** Preoperative nutritional status and outcome of elective total hip replacement. *Clin Orthop Relat Res.* 1996 May; (326):153–161.

[23] **Volkert D, Berner YN, Berry E, et al.** ESPEN guidelines on enteral nutrition: Geriatrics. *Clin Nutr.* 2006 Apr;25(2):330–360.

[24] **Avenell A, Handoll HH.** Nutritional supplementation for hip fracture aftercare in older people. *Cochrane Database Syst Rev.* 2010 Jan 20;(1):CD001880. doi: 10.1002/14651858.CD001880.pub5.

[25] **Brown KM, Seabro NA.** Nutritional influences on recovery and length of hospital stay in elderly women following femoral fracture. *Proc Nutr Soc.* 1992;51:132A.

[26] **Botella-Carretero JI, Iglesias B, Balsa JA, et al.** Perioperative oral nutritional supplements in normally or mildly undernourished geriatric patients submitted to surgery for hip fracture: a randomized clinical trial. *Clin Nutr.* 2010 Oct;29(5):574–579.

[27] **Botella-Carretero JI, Iglesias B Balsa JA, et al.** Effects oral nutritional supplements in normally nourished or mildly undernourished geriatric patients after surgery for hip fracture: a randomized clinical trial. *JPEN J Parenter Enteral Nutr.* 2008 Mar-Apr;32(2):120–128.

[28] **Symeonidis PD, Clark D.** Assessment of malnutrition in hip fracture patients: effects on surgical delay, hospital stay and mortality. *Acta Orthop Belg.* 2006 Aug;72(4):420–427.

5.3 Nonoperative treatment

Authors Stephan Pauly, Philipp von Roth, Klaus-Dieter Schaser, Carsten Perka

5.3.1 General conditions and indications

With the rise in numbers of joint arthroplasties performed and the increase of life expectancy, the incidence of periprosthetic fractures is also expected to increase steadily [1]. In individual cases, the treatment of these fractures can be nonoperative. First, the distinction has to be made between intra and postoperative fractures. In most cases fractures identified intraoperatively should undergo immediate surgical treatment. Fractures occurring or identified postoperatively need to be analyzed in more depth to justify nonsurgical therapy.

Periprosthetic fractures require an exact assessment of the fracture pattern and its classification. An overview of current classifications and the new, Unified Classification System (UCS) for periprosthetic fractures is provided earlier in this book (chapter 4.2). All classification systems precisely describe the respective fracture's localization, type (such as transverse or short oblique fractures), and remaining implant stability, and, therefore, help to select the optimal therapeutic approach.

The treatment of periprosthetic fractures aims at achieving stability, fracture union, and stable implants while restoring joint motion and function. However, treatment decisions cannot be based on classification alone but must also take further variables into account. Several factors influence the subsequent therapeutic management and, in particular, the indication for conservative or operative management. These factors can either be fracture, patient or bone related.

Fracture-related factors

Indication for operative or nonoperative treatment depends on factors such as:

- Fracture type, location, and degree of displacement
- Stability of the fracture
- Stability of the prosthetic implant
- Soft-tissue conditions
- Neurovascular status.

In general, stable fractures with only marginal displacement or with stable joint implants are more likely to be treated conservatively. However, indications for surgical revision are triggered by:

- Fracture pattern (such as short-oblique or transverse fractures)
- Risk of secondary displacement
- Risk of damaging the surrounding soft tissues
- Risk of damaging the neurovascular structures.

Indications for conservative treatment with respect to the affected joint are listed in detail within the respective "anatomical" subchapters (section 6).

Patient-related factors

- Patient's general health status and comorbidities
- Patient's functional demand and anticipated level of postoperative compliance
- Patient's joint function
- Concomitant neurological injuries.

The indication for conservative therapy is usually given by the general medical conditions of the patient rather than by the actual fracture pattern. As for any surgical therapy, the potential benefit of a surgical approach must be counterbalanced with the general perioperative risk. An overview of perioperative patient management and anesthesiology is provided in the preceding chapter (chapter 5.2). Aspects in favor of nonoperative treatment are cardiovascular comorbidities, low functional demand of the patient, or high level of expected postoperative compliance.

Bone-related factors

- Quality of bone stock
- Cortical thinning due to osteolysis or excessive reaming of the medial cortex during prosthesis implantation.

The assessment of quality and quantity of the periprosthetic bone stock is relevant for any treatment decision. Particularly in elderly patients, assessment of bone density may be necessary to determine the extent of osteopenia/osteoporosis.

5.3.2 Shoulder

Shoulder arthroplasties are increasingly more popular and, hence, account for an increasing number of complications. One major complication occurring more frequently is the incidence of periprosthetic fractures. Some reports on their treatment are available. However, there is only limited information on periprosthetic humeral fractures after ipsilateral shoulder and elbow surgeries [2, 3]. Moreover, due to the lack of controlled trials, no consensus exists on how to treat periprosthetic humeral fractures.

According to the general indications listed above, any treatment of periprosthetic humeral fractures depends on fracture location, configuration, displacement, and remaining implant stability [4, 5].

Only certain fracture patterns of periprosthetic humeral fractures allow for conservative therapy. Wright and Cofield [6] recommended conservative treatment for long oblique and spiral fractures but surgical intervention for transverse and short oblique fractures as well as in cases of inadequate reduction. Fractures located at the tip of the prosthesis with proximal extension and a loose stem (type I.1-B2/B3) require revision surgery [2, 9]. In case of a stable prosthesis (type I.1-B1), metaphyseal and spiral humeral fractures may undergo a trial of nonoperative treatment but if this treatment is not successful, they should be fixed by plating in the same manner as ordinary humeral shaft fractures [4, 9, 10].

Minimally displaced fractures around the tuberosities (type I.1-A1/A2) can be treated nonoperatively in most instances. However, in case of greater dislocation, they may require surgical refixation with suture material or a tension band to maintain the rotator-cuff insertions [4, 5].

Fractures distal to the tip of the humeral component (type C fractures) can be considered similar to ordinary closed fractures and be treated conservatively with immobilization by a brace [2, 7, 9, 11].

Overall, rehabilitation during nonoperative treatment may be delayed depending on fracture stability and the functional abilities of the individual patient [8].

Displacement of the greater tuberosity (type I.1-A1) and any loosening of the prosthetic stem require surgical therapy [5, 7, 8]. Furthermore, in obese patients, nonoperative treatment options are limited especially in proximal fractures because it is impossible to stabilize the fracture with a functional brace. Other contraindications for conservative management are irreducible fractures or fractures penetrating the bone and cement mantle as well as in case of recent surgery on the contralateral upper extremity [9]. Surgical management of periprosthetic humeral fractures is discussed in chapter 6.1.

Typically, conservative treatment of periprosthetic fractures is associated with high rates of nonunion or failure. Kumar et al [9] observed 16 periprosthetic humeral fractures. Of those, six were successfully treated nonoperatively: 3 type A, 1 type B, and 2 type C fractures. Healing was observed at an average of 180 days by means of a hanging cast, shoulder spica, or coaptation orthesis, with heterogeneous subjective results (unsatisfactory—excellent). However, five more patients required operative treatment after an average of 123 days of unsuccessful conservative treatment leading to secondary fracture healing. The authors concluded that type A fractures not necessarily require operative treatment. The same applies to well-aligned, minimally displaced type B fractures with a stable humeral component. However, after 3 months of failed union, operative intervention should be considered [9].

Successful conservative treatment of type C fractures distal to the stem of the implant is described by several authors [7, 8, 10, 12]. Only if secondary implant instability and/or nonunion develop, surgical revision may be indicated.

Conservative treatment of periprosthetic humeral fractures can be associated with further complications beyond delayed or nonunion. Radial nerve palsy and soft-tissue irritations were reported [6, 7, 13]. Revision surgery may be indicated following unsuccessful conservative fracture treatment; however, Wright and Cofield [6] concluded that surgery following failed conservative fracture therapy was less successful than immediate surgery soon after fracture.

5.3.3 Elbow

Periprosthetic humeral fractures around elbow arthroplasties are rare and those between ipsilateral humeral and elbow arthroplasties even rarer [2, 3, 14–16]. Assessment of the remaining implant stability is mandatory for further treatment decisions.

Following elbow arthroplasties, humeral fractures proximal to the tip of the implant (type C) can be treated conservatively provided the prosthesis is well fixed. Periarticular fractures of the condyles (type II.1-A1/A2) often result from overuse/tension from the forearm muscles on the relatively weak and thin bone, which makes surgical therapy challenging [2, 17]. These fractures rarely cause clinical symptoms and, therefore, should be treated nonoperatively, even though the nonunion rate is high [18, 19].

Most fracture patterns, however, are located at or around the tip of the stem according to type B and often occur due to concomitant osteolysis (type II.1-B2/B3). These lesions are unlikely to unite with nonoperative treatment, particularly when the implant stem is loose, causing further endosteal erosion [17–19]. The respective surgical approach, revision to long-stemmed implants, or exceptionally an osteosynthesis is described in chapter 6.2.

For periprosthetic fractures of the proximal ulna (types II.2-B and C), nonoperative treatment is only exceptionally indicated, as in regular forearm adult fractures that are usually absolute indications for surgery. The choice—revision or osteosynthesis—will again depend on the stability of the implant.

Little evidence is available on dedicated conservative therapy of these fractures.

Greiner et al [18] reported on one H A (H I) fracture of the ulnar epicondyle leading to painless nonunion and acceptable range of motion 6 months later.

Sánchez-Sotelo et al [19] published the largest series on humeral fractures following elbow arthroplasty. All fractures were associated with loose implants and underwent revision surgery.

5.3.4 Wrist

There is only limited literature on the incidence, management, and results of periprosthetic wrist fractures. To the best of the authors' knowledge, the introduced UCS classification (chapter 4.2) is the first classification available on periprosthetic wrist fractures.

Dawson et al [20] reported four cases of traumatic radius fractures after total wrist arthroplasty (two metal/polyethylene, two silicone). The outcome was associated with the degree of displacement: one fracture with only marginal displacement was successfully treated nonoperatively (ie, by cast immobilization). However, the three other cases—with significant displacement—developed nonunion or malunion, requiring revision surgery. Surgical management of periprosthetic wrist fractures is illustrated in chapter 6.3.

5.3.5 Hip

Fractures of the acetabulum

Fractures of the anterior superior or inferior iliac spine (type IV.6-A1, chapter 4.2) or of the ischial tuberosity (type IV.6-A2) can be treated nonoperatively. If the fracture is dislocated, surgical treatment is recommended. Type IV.6-B1 fractures represent fractures of the acetabular lip or rim and fractures of the floor with intact rim and well-fixed implant, all of which generally do not require fracture fixation. Surgical revision, however, is indicated for all type IV.6-B2 and -B3 fractures. Type IV.6-C fractures are located in the periphery of the acetabulum and independent of the implant. Their treatment follows the principles of acetabular fracture management.

Surgical management of acetabular fractures is described in chapter 6.4.2.

Fractures of the femur

Due to the high reliability and validity, the Vancouver Classification was previously used for the classification of periprosthetic fractures of the femur [21]. The Unified Classification System (UCSs is an adaptation and expansion of this classification (chapter 4.2). Intraoperatively identified trochanteric fractures are usually displaced and, therefore, have to be treated surgically. Postoperatively identified fractures of the greater (type IV.3-A1) or lesser (IV.3-A2) trochanter can be treated nonoperatively if the degree of dislocation is less than 2 cm, if the bone stock is good and the prosthesis stable. Dislocated type IV.3-A1 fractures exceeding 2 cm should be treated surgically to avoid instability and impairment of abduction force [22].

Type IV.3-A2 fractures of the lesser trochanter are rare and often affect only a small bone fragment. However, if the fracture involves a large bone fragment, an unstable prosthesis can be expected and, therefore, has to be revised according to a type IV.3-B2 [23]. All other femoral fractures are best treated surgically (chapter 6.4.3) [23]. In case of hip resurfacing prosthesis, Cossey et al [24] recommended a nonoperative treatment for nondislocated periprosthetic fractures of the femoral neck (type IV.3-B1). Jacobs et al [25] reported a successful nonoperative treatment of periprosthetic femoral neck fractures after hip resurfacing arthroplasties in 13 cases. Nondisplaced fractures can be treated conservatively. In these cases, the group proposes protected weight bearing for 8 weeks followed by weight bearing of 50% body weight for 6 weeks. However, Jacobs et al [25] recommend conventional total hip arthroplasty revision surgery if the components are displaced.

5.3.6 Knee

Fractures of the distal femur

Nonoperative treatment of periprosthetic fractures of the distal femur is a rare option and reserved for nondisplaced, stable fractures with a well-fixed implant and for patients with severe comorbidities [1, 26]. The principles of surgical management are summarized in chapter 6.5.2.

Moran et al described the outcome of 24 cases of dislocated supracondylar fractures, nine of which were treated nonoperatively and had poor clinical outcome due to malunion. Culp et al [27] reported on a series of 61 distal femoral fractures. Patients were randomized into two groups. One group (30 patients) were treated nonoperatively, 43% of whom developed malunion or nonunion, while the remaining patients with surgical intervention showed only 19% of insufficient fracture healing [28].

Fractures of the patella

In periprosthetic fractures of the patella, nonoperative treatment is only recommended if the implant is well fixed and the extensor mechanism is intact (type V.34-B1) with a dislocation of less than 2 mm (chapter 4.2). The authors suggest immobilization in full extension for 4–6 weeks with transition to flexion upon complete union of the fracture fragments [26, 29]. Surgical therapy is presented in chapter 6.5.3.

Conservative treatment of 38 patients with type V.34-A or B1 fractures showed satisfactory results in 97% of the group [29]. Many authors report that surgical treatment could only achieve suboptimal results [29-31]. Thus, Dennis et al [26] recommend nonoperative therapy even for displaced fractures with extensor lag as long as the patella component is well fixed.

Fractures of the tibia

Similar to periprosthetic fractures of the distal femur and the patella, exceptionally nonoperative treatment may be considered for stable, nondisplaced fractures with a well-fixed prosthetic component [1]. Nondisplaced fractures of the tibial tubercle (type V.4-A2; chapter 4.2), in which components are usually well fixed, may be treated successfully with extension immobilization [32]. However, these fractures are associated with a high rate of malunion or nonunion [32]. Surgical management of periprosthetic tibial fractures is illustrated in chapter 6.5.4.

Felix et al [33] reported on 23 fractures of the tibial plateau with a loose prosthesis, corresponding to type V.4-B2/B3, which had initially been treated conservatively with immobilization and restricted weight bearing. Of these patients, 92% later underwent revision surgery. Moreover, five fractures around a loose stem were initially also treated nonoperatively, with 80% undergoing secondary revision. To summarize, the nonoperative treatment of tibial fractures with loose components shows poor results. The nonsurgical management of these fractures should, therefore, only be used for patients who cannot tolerate the surgical intervention due to severe comorbidities [34, 35]. Fractures with well-fixed components, however, may be treated successfully nonoperatively.

5.3.7 Ankle

The incidence of periprosthetic fractures following total ankle arthroplasty (TAA) ranges from 12–22% [36]. To the authors' knowledge, the UCS classification (chapter 4.2) is the first to be published for periprosthetic ankle fractures. Little is known about the therapeutic regimen of periprosthetic fractures after TAA. McGarvey et al [36] point out that the treatment depends on the type of prosthesis because some prostheses rely on three-sided ingrowth and syndesmotic compression of the malleoli. The group concluded that any bony defects that occur around these types of prosthesis require immediate surgical intervention. Again, nonoperative treatment is only an option for nondisplaced fractures with well-fixed components. Krause et al [37] described eight intraoperative fractures of the malleoli and one talar neck fracture, which were treated with internal fixation during the index operation. The group observed three stress fractures postoperatively, which underwent conservative treatment [37]. However, no clinical outcome has yet been reported. Surgical management of periprosthetic ankle fractures is illustrated in chapter 6.6.

References

[1] **Sarmah SS, Patel S, Reading G, et al.** (2012) Periprosthetic fractures around total knee arthroplasty. *Ann R Coll Surg Engl.* 2012 Jul;94(5):302–307.

[2] **Mavrogenis AF, Angelini A, Guerra E, et al.** Periprosthetic fractures of the humerus. *J Long Term Eff Med Implants.* 2009;19(4):305–311.

[3] **Mavrogenis AF, Angelini A, Guerra E, et al.** Humeral fracture between a total elbow and total shoulder arthroplasty. *Orthopedics.* 2011 Apr 11;34(4):315.

[4] **McDonough EB, Crosby LA.** Periprosthetic fractures of the humerus. *Am J Orthop (Belle Mead NJ).* 2005 Dec;34(12):586–591.

[5] **Cameron B, Iannotti JP.** Periprosthetic fractures of the humerus and scapula: management and prevention. *Orthop Clin North Am.* 1999 Apr;30(2):305–318.

[6] **Wright TW, Cofield RH.** Humeral fractures after shoulder arthroplasty. *J Bone Joint Surg Am.* 1995 Sep;77(9):1340–1346.

[7] **Campbell JT, Moore RS, Iannotti JP, et al.** Periprosthetic humeral fractures: mechanisms of fracture and treatment options. *J Shoulder Elbow Surg.* 1998 Jul-Aug;7(4):406–413.

[8] **Groh GI, Heckman MM, Wirth MA, et al.** Treatment of fractures adjacent to humeral prostheses. *J Shoulder Elbow Surg.* 2008 Jan-Feb;17(1):85–89.

[9] **Kumar S, Sperling JW, Haidukewych GH, et al.** Periprosthetic humeral fractures after shoulder arthroplasty. *J Bone Joint Surg Am.* 2004 Apr;86–A(4):680–689.

[10] **Worland RL, Kim DY, Arredondo J, et al.** Periprosthetic humeral fractures: management and classification. *J Shoulder Elbow Surg.* 1999 Nov-Dec;8(6):590–594.

[11] **Wutzler S, Laurer HL, Huhnstock S, et al.** Periprosthetic humeral fractures after shoulder arthroplasty: operative management and functional outcome. *Arch Orthop Trauma Surg.* 2009 Feb;129(2):237–243.

[12] **Wirth MA, Rockwood CA Jr.** Complications of total shoulder-replacement arthroplasty. *J Bone Joint Surg Am.* 1996 Apr;78(4):603–616.

[13] **Bonutti PM, Hawkins RJ.** Fracture of the humeral shaft associated with total replacement arthroplasty of the shoulder. A case report. *J Bone Joint Surg Am.* 1992 Apr;74(4):617–618.

[14] **Hanyu T, Nakazono K, Ishikawa H.** Humeral shaft fracture after a total elbow arthroplasty. *J Shoulder Elbow Surg.* 1998 Sep-Oct;7(5):541–544.

[15] **Gill DR, Cofield RH, Morrey BF.** Ipsilateral total shoulder and elbow arthroplasties in patients who have rheumatoid arthritis. *J Bone Joint Surg Am.* 1999 Aug;81(8):1128–1137.

[16] **Carroll EA, Lorich DG, Helfet DL.** (2009) Surgical management of a periprosthetic fracture between a total elbow and total shoulder prostheses: a case report. *J Shoulder Elbow Surg.* 2009 May-Jun;18(3):e9–12.

[17] **O'Driscoll SW, Morrey BF.** Periprosthetic fractures about the elbow. *Orthop Clin North Am.* 1999 Apr;30(2):319–325.

[18] **Greiner S, Stein V, Scheibel M.** Periprosthetic humeral fractures after shoulder and elbow arthroplasty. *Acta Chir Orthop Traumatol Cech.* 2011;78(6):490–500.

[19] **Sánchez-Sotelo J, O'Driscoll S, Morrey BF.** Periprosthetic humeral fractures after total elbow arthroplasty: treatment with implant revision and strut allograft augmentation. *J Bone Joint Surg Am.* 2002 Sep;84-A(9):1642–1650.

[20] **Dawson WJ.** Radius fracture after total wrist arthroplasty. *J Hand Surg Am.* 1989 Jul;14(4):630–634.

[21] **Duncan CP, Masri BA.** Fractures of the femur after hip replacement. *Instr Course Lect.* 1995; 44:293–304.

[22] **Pritchett JW.** Fracture of the greater trochanter after hip replacement. *Clin Orthop Relat Res.* 2001 Sep;(390):221–226.

[23] **Masri BA, Meek RM, Duncan CP.** (2004) Periprosthetic fractures evaluation and treatment. *Clin Orthop Relat Res.* 2004 Mar;(420):80–95.

[24] **Cossey AJ, Back DL, Shimmin A, et al.** The nonoperative management of periprosthetic fractures associated with the Birmingham hip resurfacing procedure. *J Arthroplasty.* 2005 Apr;20(3):358–361.

[25] **Jacobs MA, Kennedy WR, Bhargava T, et al.** Postresurfacing periprosthetic femoral neck fractures: nonoperative treatment. *Orthopedics.* 2012 May;35(5):e732–736.

[26] **Dennis DA.** Periprosthetic fractures following total knee arthroplasty. *Instr Course Lect.* 2001;50:379–389.

[27] **Moran MC, Brick GW, Sledge CB, et al.** (1996) Supracondylar femoral fracture following total knee arthroplasty. *Clin Orthop Relat Res.* 1996 Mar;(324):196–209.

[28] **Culp RW, Schmidt RG, Hanks G, et al.** (1987) Supracondylar fracture of the femur following prosthetic knee arthroplasty. *Clin Orthop Relat Res.* 1987 Sep;(222):212–222.

[29] **Ortiguera CJ, Berry DJ.** Patellar fracture after total knee arthroplasty. *J Bone Joint Surg Am.* 2002 Apr;84-A(4):532–540.

[30] **Goldberg VM, Figgie HE 3rd, Inglis AE, et al.** Patellar fracture type and prognosis in condylar total knee arthroplasty. *Clin Orthop Relat Res.* 1988 Nov;(236):115–122.

[31] **Hozack WJ, Goll SR, Lotke PA, et al.** The treatment of patellar fractures after total knee arthroplasty. *Clin Orthop Relat Res.* 1988 Nov;(236):123–127.

[32] **Hanssen AD, Stuart MJ.** Treatment of periprosthetic tibial fractures. *Clin Orthop Relat Res.* 2000 Nov;(380):91–98.

[33] **Felix NA, Stuart MJ, Hanssen AD.** Periprosthetic fractures of the tibia associated with total knee arthroplasty. *Clin Orthop Relat Res.* 1997 Dec;(345):113–124.

[34] **Kim KI, Egol KA, Hozack WJ, et al.** Periprosthetic fractures after total knee arthroplasties. *Clin Orthop Relat Res.* 2006 May;446:167–175.

[35] **González Della Valle A, Slullitel G, Vestri R, et al.** No need for routine closed suction drainage in elective arthroplasty of the hip: a prospective randomized trial in 104 operations. *Acta Orthop Scand.* 2004 Feb;75(1):30–33.

[36] **McGarvey WC, Clanton TO, Lunz D.** Malleolar fracture after total ankle arthroplasty: a comparison of two designs. *Clin Orthop Relat Res.* 2004 Jul;(424):104–110.

[37] **Krause FG, Windolf M, Bora B, et al.** Impact of complications in total ankle replacement and ankle arthrodesis analyzed with a validated outcome measurement. *J Bone Joint Surg Am.* 2011 May;93(9): 830–839.

5.4 Internal fixation

Authors Karl Stoffel, Christoph Sommer, Christof Meyer, Reinhard Schnettler

5.4.1 Plate fixation

Authors Karl Stoffel, Christoph Sommer

Introduction

While not frequent, periprosthetic fractures can be severe injuries and represent a serious clinical challenge as well as economic and social concern for the future (chapter 1). The management of these fractures is particularly demanding, complex, and expensive as the surgeon often is confronted with the simultaneous issues of aseptic loosening, poor quality bone or bone loss, and a frail, elderly patient [1–8].

Decision making

For decision making, one of the first questions to be answered is whether the prosthetic implant is stable and well-fixed or loose within the bone socket.

Loose prosthesis

Radiological expertise is essential for the classification of a periprosthetic fracture. Lindahl et al [1] indicated that 47% of all fractures initially classified as "stable" type B1 fractures on closer evaluation were "loose" type B2/3 fractures. Surgeons must, therefore, be prepared to adapt their treatment plan in case the intraoperative situation is different from radiological diagnosis. To achieve a better classification, the new Unified Classification System (UCS) proposed and applied in this book (chapter 4. 2) presents the classification for the different joints and locations in greater detail.

Signs of a loose prosthesis stem include slowly increasing pain mainly in the thigh area, particularly when walking [9, 10]. In combination with severe osteolysis, migration or subsidence of the prosthesis, a fracture at the level of the primary fixation (in noncemented stems), separation between the interface of the stem and the cement (in cemented composite beam stems), or damage to the cement sleeve (in cemented tapered stems) may occur. If unsure, best practice dictates exchanging the stem, particularly if the stem exhibits varus malposition [11].

Considering the poor overall results obtained after any kind of fracture repair surgery, a better approach would probably be a surgical intervention before a fracture has actually been sustained [1]. However, in view of the economic constraints to such a management strategy, revision procedures as first-line treatment generally should be reserved for patients with a loose type B2/3 fracture, especially in case of pronounced bone loss. Adequate fracture reduction and fixation of displaced fragments using cerclage wires or cables is required to allow for the implantation of a new stem, while autogenous bone grafts as well as allograft struts and cables are commonly used to further promote fracture repair and implant fixation [5, 6]. Revision surgery is addressed in chapters 5.5 and 5.6.

Well-fixed prosthesis

Type B1 periprosthetic fractures, where by definition the prosthesis appears well fixed, are observed in 11–29% of the cases [1, 12]. If treated nonoperatively, these fractures are associated with the highest rate of complications, especially nonunion in up to 42% of all cases [13]. Type B1 injuries are the most challenging to manage and remain controversial in regard to the optimal surgical intervention [4, 7, 13]. Given a stable prosthetic component and a simple fracture type, open and anatomical reduction with correct varus/valgus and rotational alignment and internal fixation (open reduction and internal fixation) with plates providing absolute stability can be used to allow early postoperative mobilization [6, 8]. For more complex fractures, a more elastic fixation that bridges the fracture zone, combined with a minimally invasive surgical technique, may be the best way to stabilize the bone. As a wide variety of implants, fixation methods, and support modalities is now available, a thorough understanding of the characteristics of the fracture type, good knowledge and experience with the various fixation devices, and the principles of periprosthetic fracture treatment are vital when trying to achieve safe fracture healing while retaining proper function of the prosthesis and limb [2, 13]. Another prerequisite is careful preoperative planning.

Available plates and screws

Conventional plates

In the late 1950s, the newly developed constructs of conventional plates and screws—following the principles put forth by the AO group—were being applied for periprosthetic fractures. These included direct fracture exposure with anatomical reduction of fracture fragments and rigid internal fixation to achieve direct bone healing [14]. Complications when using these non-locking plates and screws were caused by a loss of fixation due to screw pull-out in poor bone or, in fractures distal to the plate, prosthetic loosening, nonunion, and the possibility of stress risers in the distal fragment caused by bicortical screws.

The Ogden construct, a fixation technique using conventional plates and cables, was developed to overcome pull-out of the proximal screw fixation. The proximal fragment is fixed with cerclage wires or cables and the distal fragment with bicortical screws. This offers both an immediate, stable proximal fixation and the advantage that, since no screw has to be inserted next to the stem, nothing interferes with the cement mantle or compromises the stability of the prosthesis. However, in a small series, Tadross et al [11] reported three failures in seven cases, all of which were due to secondary displacement of the stem into varus. They recommended the use of additional struts or monocortical screws in the proximal fragment. However, monocortical screws alone generally do not have sufficient purchase to provide stable fixation in the metaphysis or in osteoporotic bone with a thin cortex [4, 15].

In general, the effectiveness of fixation of a periprosthetic fracture by open reduction and internal fixation (ORIF) using conventional plates—alone or in combination with cerclage wires, cables, or strut allografts—has been unsatisfactory because of too extensive soft-tissue stripping and inadequate screw purchase in osteoporotic bone, particularly within the proximal fragment [16]. Furthermore, large cortical strut allografts may cause immunological reactions or disease transmission, while delayed or even absent revascularization of the allograft leads to failure of the construct in the long term [5].

Locking plates

The introduction of locking-head screws (LHS), appropriate plates, locking compression plate (LCP) and less-invasive stabilization system (LISS) in the late 1990s, which provides angular and superior axial stability in contrast to conventional plates, has radically changed the use and efficiency of plates in periprosthetic fractures.

The advantages of the so-called internal fixator principle are many [17]:

- Periosteal blood supply is preserved as the plate is not pressed against the underlying bone, which prevents avascular footprints beneath the plate
- The transmission of force between plate and bone no longer relies on friction and preload but passes across the fixed-angle screw-plate construct
- The fixed-angle screw-plate construct proves to be considerably stronger against pull-out forces and deformation [18]
- In osteoporotic bone, plates with LHS provide a more reliable fixation as they are considerably more resistant against pull-out forces.

In combination with minimally invasive approaches and indirect reduction techniques without exposing the fracture site, locking plates may be applied as bridging devices providing relative stability. Fracture healing occurs by secondary intention with callus formation, with reduction of possible incidence of infection and nonunion; although there is no evidence for this yet [3]. For periprosthetic fractures, this system is an attractive option to improve fixation of both the proximal and the distal bone segment, provided that long plates (minimum 10 holes) are used, which are fixed only with a few screws placed in the correct fashion (**5.4-1**). To be successful, this requires experience and understanding of the biomechanics and careful planning [3, 8].

The LISS (chapters 11.2, 11.8, and 11.11) and later the condylar locking compression plate (LCP) were originally developed and introduced for the fixation of fractures of the distal femur. Special sets for periprosthetic fractures (consisting of extra-long, broad, or curved locking plates, short-blunt periprosthetic screws, locking-attachment plates (LAP), and dedicated cable instruments) are now available [3]. The many designs of locking plates and screw systems can be categorized in utilizing fixed-angle LHS or variable-axis locking screws (**5.4-1a–c**, **5.4-2a–c**) [19].

5.4-1 General principles for the use of plates in periprosthetic fractures.

Technique		**Fracture type**		
		Simple		**Complex**
		Oblique/spiral (+/- wedge)	Transverse	
Reduction	Goal	Anatomical	Gap free	Correct alignment
	Technique	Direct or indirect	Direct or indirect	Indirect, "no-touch"
Fixation	Principle	Compression	Bridging or compression[1]	Bridging
	Plate length[2]	8x length of fracture zone (>10 holes)		3x length of fracture zone (>14 holes)
	Screw placement at fracture level	At least 2 empty screw holes		Close to the fracture zone
	Number of screws	Good bone: 8 cortices per main fragment poor bone: 10–12 cortices		
	Type of screws	Good bone: CS[3] open technique / MIPO[4] poor bone: LHS[5]		
	Screw type at level of prosthetic shaft[6]	Unicortical or bicortical polyaxial LHS, or bicortical CS, both anterior and posterior. Augmentation with cerclages and/or LAP[7]		
	Screws at plate end	2 bicortical LHS[5] or 1 CS[3] distally angulated and 1 bicortical LHS just proximal to it		

[1] Add strut graft if fracture is between tip of stem and cement plug.
[2] Distance to next implant: > 6 cm or overlapping of implants/plate > 6 cm to prevent refracture.
[3] CS: conventional screws (cortical or cancellous).
[4] Minimally invasive plate osteosynthesis (MIPO).
[5] LHS: Locking-head screws.
[6] In case of cement mantle: overdrill by 0.1–0.2 mm.
[7] LAP: Locking attachment plate.

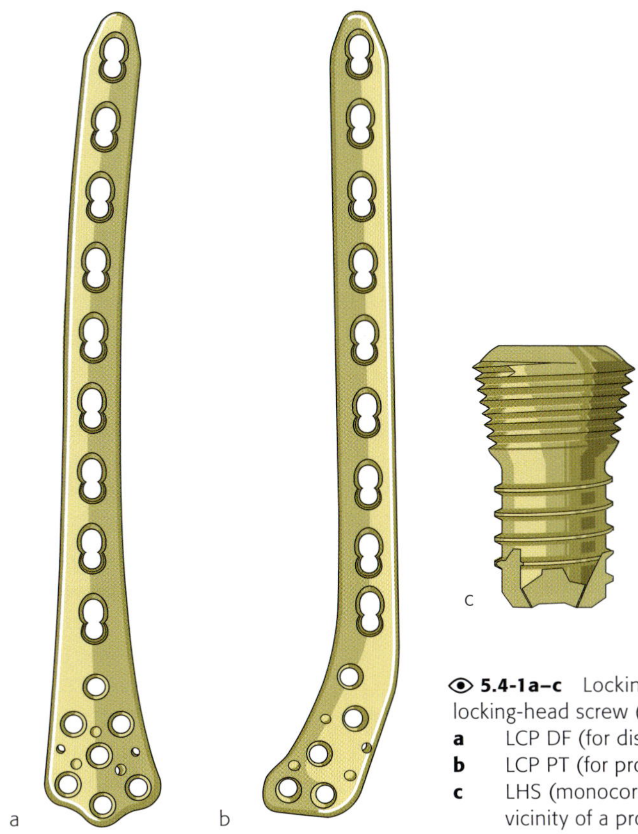

5.4-1a–c Locking-compression plates (LCP) and locking-head screw (LHS).

- **a** LCP DF (for distal femur).
- **b** LCP PT (for proximal tibia).
- **c** LHS (monocortical short) for placement in the vicinity of a prosthetic stem.

However, obstacles to screw placement may appear when using plates with fixed-angle threaded screw holes, particularly when treating periprosthetic fractures. It may be difficult, if not impossible, to insert long bicortical LHS screws in the vicinity of a prosthetic stem or periarticular segment, since the screw trajectory is predetermined by the design of the plate. The surgeon must either use a shorter screw or angle the screw within the threaded locking hole, resulting in significant loss of fixation strength [19]. The use of unicortical screws alone in osteoporotic bone without cement as augmentation can result in fractures of the lateral cortex [20]. Polyaxial or variable-angle locking-plate systems merge variable-angle locking screw technology with conventional plating techniques. They have been designed in particular for fracture fixation in the presence of prosthetic components (**5.4-2a–c**). The variable-angle locking screws can be placed within a range of 30° and allow surgeons to place screws around a stem and adjacent to distal femoral prostheses. While initially the locking mechanism between the screw and the plate was predetermined, later on plates were introduced that allow a screw to be angled first and then locked at end-point tightening. Most of these designs rely on hoop stress and an additional interface between the screw head and the plate rather than a corresponding threaded hole. In some systems, such as the non-contact bridging plate (NCB) angular stability is combined with polyaxial screw placement. The use of locked bicortical screws, either with a monoaxial or polyaxial system, provides improved pull-out strength in osteoporotic bone [21].

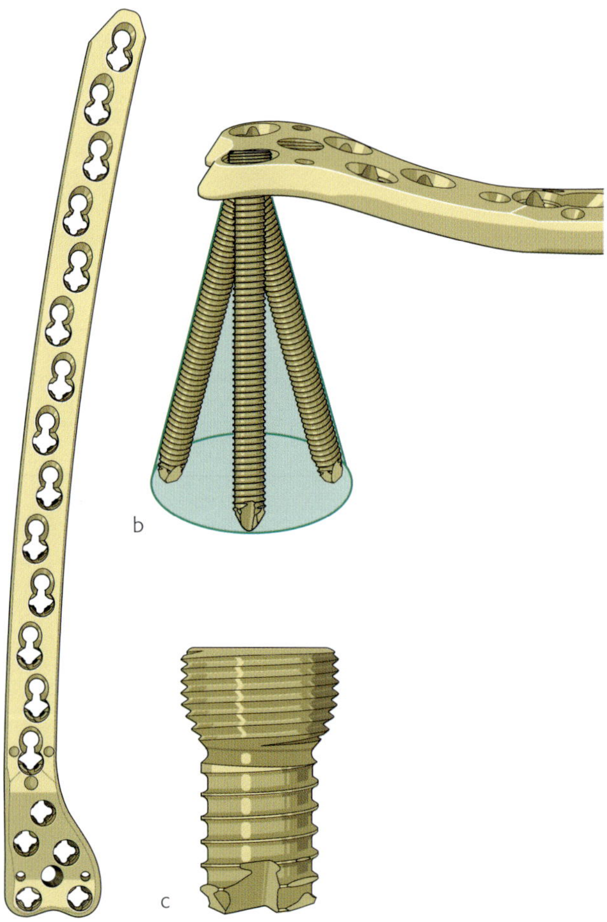

5.4-2a–c Variable-angle locking compression plate (VA-LCP) and locking head screw (LHS).
a VA-LCP (for distal femur).
b Angulations of possible screw directions.
c Design of a VA-LHS screw head.

The LCP system can be further augmented with LAP, which allows the placement of smaller locking screws lateral to the prosthesis stem (**5.4-3**, **5.4-4**) [22, 23]. It could be shown that the LAP is biomechanically superior to a cerclage-LCP construct [22] and the first clinical results are also promising [23]. For most of these implants, however, few data or comparative studies exist regarding their mechanical strength and clinical outcome [19]. Konstantinidis et al [24] used a cadaver model to compare gap displacement under cyclic axial compression between two minimal invasive angle-stable plates (LISS and NCB). Bicortical screw placement provided more stable anchoring compared with monocortical screw fixation. However, in terms of motion at the fracture gap and failure loads, stabilization of periprosthetic femoral fractures was equally well achieved using either the LISS plate with periprosthetic monocortical screws or the NCB plate with polyaxial bicortical screws. Only few studies have compared the biomechanics of different locking-plate constructs in the treatment of periprosthetic fractures. Fulkerson et al [20] found the locked plates to be stiffer in axial and torsional modes compared with an Ogden construct. Torsional failure loads were similar in both groups. Talbot et al [8] found no biomechanical advantage in locking plates compared with non-locking plates if additional allografts were used.

The LAP was developed to improve the fixation of a LCP in the area where the plate overlaps the stem of a prosthesis and where monocortical screws cannot be inserted or would have poor purchase in osteoporotic bone (chapters 7.5, 7.6, 10.16, and 11.5) [22,23]. Up to now, in these situations cerclage wires were applied, which, however, are often mechanically insufficient and biologically questionable. The LAP is designed to be placed over any threaded hole of an LCP (**5.4-3a–b**), where it is fixed to the plate with a special connecting-screw system (**5.4-4a–b**). The lateral extensions

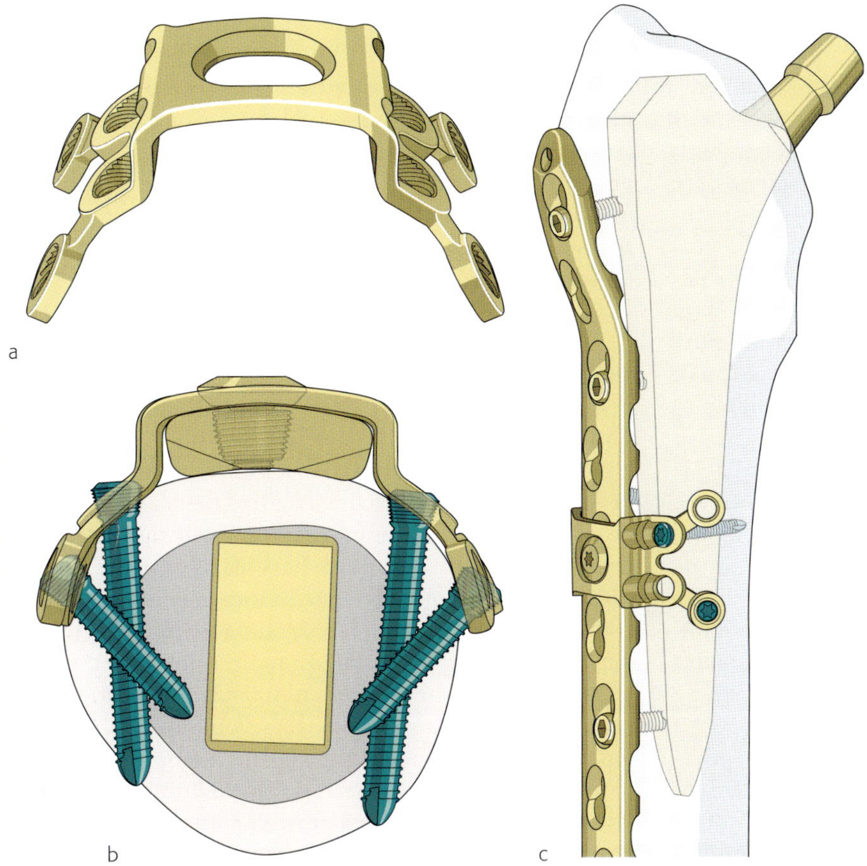

5.4-3a–c Locking-attachment plate (LAP).

- **a** Low profile, anatomically contoured LAP. There are two-plate versions available: one fitting onto a large-fragment LCP and a second version for a proximal femur LCP. Crossed arms on each side of the plate accept 3.5 mm locking screws (or 3.5 mm cortex screws) that will avoid the prosthesis stem.
- **b** Cross-section shows the direction of the screws ventral and dorsal of the prosthetic stamp.
- **c** AP view of proximal femur with LAP applied to LCP.

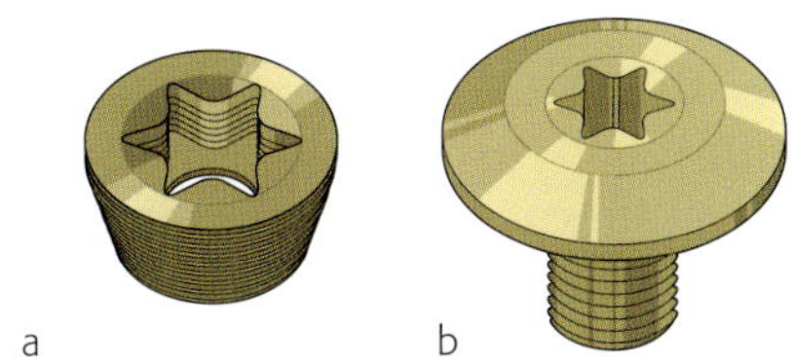

5.4-4a–b Locking-attachment plate (LAP) connecting screw, consisting of two parts (**a** and **b**). The conical part (**a**) is first inserted into the threaded hole of the LCP with the torque-limiting screwdriver. After placement of the LAP over the LCP and adjusting its position, the second component of the connecting screw (**b**) is used to fix the LAP to the first part of the connecting screw.

on each side of the device allow the insertion of 2–4 3.5 mm locking-head screws, which avoid the stem of a prosthesis but are anchored within the cortex around it (**5.4-3b**).

Locking-head screws

For locked plates, the question of how many screws are needed proximal and distal to a periprosthetic fracture remains debatable [14]. A biomechanical study by Stoffel et al [25] recommended up to four screws (eight cortices) per segment, with screws placed closer to the fracture for large fracture gaps (> 2 mm). Wood et al [3] advocated a minimum of ten cortices of fixation above and below the fracture in osteoporotic bone and cited the need for revised guidelines because at present these are based on isolated fractures in younger non-arthroplasty patients. They recommend fixation with a cable, bicortical, conventional, locked screws, or unicortical locking screws applied next to the stem of a well-fixed implant. Distally in the cancellous bone of the femoral condyles, large locking screws are preferable. This hybrid fixation technique has been shown to be mechanically similar to locked constructs and significantly better than non-locked constructs [14].

A specific concern regarding the use of screws in the proximal fragment is the violation of the integrity of the cement mantle. Theoretically, screw insertion could lead to cracks and eventual loosening of the prosthesis [8]. The long-term effects of drilling and inserting screws into the cement mantle around a femoral component are unknown. Monocortical fixation may lower the risk of compromising the cement mantle or a stable femoral stem during the treatment of a periprosthetic femoral fracture with internal fixators, such as the LCP [4, 12]. Kampshoff et al [21] tested the effect of predrilling holes of different sizes for bicortical screws. By increasing the drill diameter, the onset of cracks decreased but so did the screw pull-out resistance. They recommended overdrilling of 0.1–0.2 mm when using a 5 mm bicortical locking screw.

Screw type and distribution have a significant impact on the resistance of locking plates to load. Monocortical screws used alone, ie, without cement, in osteoporotic bone can result in lateral cortex fractures [20]. The use of locked bicortical screws, either with a polyaxial system or with LAP, provides improved pull-out strength in osteoporotic bone [21]. Bottlang et al [18] used an in vitro model to demonstrate that compared with a conventional plating construct a locked plate was 15% stronger in axial compression and equally strong in torsion but 22% weaker in bending. Under bending loads, the focused load transfer of locking plates through fixed-angle screws can increase the risk for a periprosthetic fracture in the osteoporotic diaphysis. The use of fixed-angle locking screws at the end of the plate presents a clinical challenge as the plate often diverges from the midline of the bone, resulting in single-cortex fixation. Using a conventional screw in the outermost screw hole allows angulation of the screw toward the diaphyseal midline, thus avoiding this potential problem and increasing the strength of the construct by 40% in bending with no negative impact on torsion or compression-load resistance (**5.4-1**) [25].

Techniques

Choice of plate length

Next to the anatomical situation, the number and distribution of the screws determines the length of the plate used in periprosthetic fracture fixation. Several recent studies reporting on failures of LCP constructs have attributed the failure to inadequate implant length [3]. Gautier and Sommer [26] discussed the concept of the plate-spanning-width ratio (fracture length to implant length ratio) and recommended that this be greater than 2 or 3 in comminuted fractures and 8–10 in simple fractures. Stoffel et al [25] recommended to use "the longest" plates whenever possible: for a simple periprosthetic fracture a 10-hole plate is considered minimum length, while for a comminuted fracture with an additional number of screw holes lying over the comminuted area, the minimum length should be a 14-hole plate (**5.4-1**).

Fracture reduction

For the reduction of periprosthetic femoral fractures, two surgical techniques are available: direct or indirect reduction.

Direct reduction is recommended whenever the injury involves a simple fracture type (spiral/butterfly, short oblique, or transverse) with two large main fragments that are best fixed rigidly with interfragmentary compression and a neutralization plate.

Indirect reduction is the preferred technique whenever moderate to severe comminution is present. There the goal is to restore correct length, alignment, and rotation, and to bridge the fracture zone with a long plate with few, well-spaced locking screws providing relative or elastic stability. This requires closed fracture reduction without exposure and direct view of the fracture zone before the percutaneous insertion of the fixation device. The maintenance of the soft-tissue envelope is essential for such a biological fixation [3], while in most cases any complications are attributed to the severity of the trauma and/or the lack of experience when applying the implant [7, 15, 27].

Most locking-plate systems offer a set of instruments to facilitate percutaneous—minimally invasive—plate and screw insertion. A review of patients with periprosthetic fractures around well-fixed total knee arthroplasty or total hip arthroplasty prostheses managed by percutaneous insertion of a first-generation locking plate (LISS) suggest such a fixation technique to be an effective although demanding method of treatment.

Complex fractures

The treatment of some periprosthetic fracture configurations is more demanding than others, even if the stem is stable. For example, transverse fractures at the tip of a cemented stem or just above the cement plug, corresponding to type B1, may require stem revision because of the inherently unstable fracture pattern, despite the implant being well-fixed [5, 7]. If internal fixation of the fracture is chosen, some type of combination of screws and cerclage wires or cables is typically preferred. Cables may control bending and torsional forces while the locked screws control axial and rotational displacement. This arrangement reduces the need for orthogonally placed allograft struts in many patients, although such treatment should always be individualized based on bone quality and construct stability [19]. Wood et al [3] recommended that bone grafting be used if the soft-tissue envelope is violated by extensive dissection, and cortical struts be considered in cases of failed hardware and revision fixation. While some studies have reported promising early results with LCP alone for this type of fracture, including axial and angular stability, preservation of the vascular supply by applying minimally invasive insertion techniques, less periosteal stripping, and reduced blood loss, there is no consensus on this method of treatment [5, 7, 19]. The proximal fixation can be improved with the new LAP, which is placed over the principal plate and allows the insertion 3.5 mm LHS without interfering with the prosthetic stem.

Hybrid techniques

Hybrid fixation methods, which allow using conventional screws (eg, lag screws) and LHS in the same plate, are increasingly accepted and available. For example, the LCP with combination holes can be used, depending on the fracture pattern, either as compression plate (interfragmentary compression principle), as pure internal fixator (bridging technique), or as an internal fixation system combining both techniques ('hybrid' technique) (👁 **5.4-5a–b**) [28]. Several biomechanical and clinical studies on large bones have shown that the combination of locking and non-locking fixation methods offers the possibility to achieve a useful synergy of both internal fixation methods.

If LCP is applied as neutralization or compression plate, the surgical technique is much the same as in conventional plating, such that existing screws can be used. As internal fixator, the LCP can be applied through an open, less or minimally invasive (MIPO) approach. An indirect, closed reduction is recommended when using LCP as an internal fixator bridging the fracture zone. Biomechanical testing on cadaver femora with comminuted distal fractures demonstrated that an

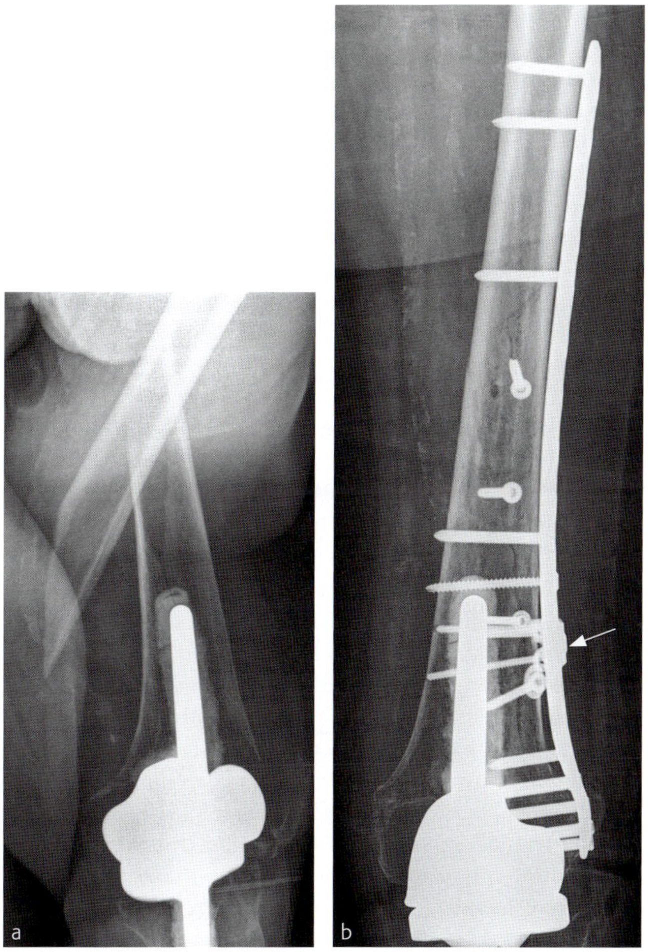

👁 **5.4-5a–b** Type V.3-C periprosthetic fracture of the distal femur treated in a 'hybrid' technique using plate-independent interfragmentary compression screws to achieve primary stability. In the distal fragment, a plate-to-bone compression screw increases rotational stability and a locking-attachment plate (LAP) was added to bypass the need for locking screws around the stem.

- **a** AP view of the periprosthetic fracture of the distal femur, type V.3-C.
- **b** Postoperative AP view of the same fracture fixed in a "hybrid" fashion combining interfragmentary compression with bridging technique and LAP (arrow).

internal fixator provides a significantly higher stiffness, less plastic deformation, and a higher load to failure than a conventional compression plate. The capacity to resist torsional forces was significantly higher when the locking plate was applied in a 'hybrid' technique, first fixed distally to the condyles with a compression or lag screw, then augmented with locking screws [29]. It has been argued that the broad, anatomically preshaped part of the plate would give additional torsional stability through the enlarged geometrical contact area when pressed against the bone. Similar results were reported by Staubli et al [30] on patients undergoing a medial high-tibial osteotomy with a lateral hybrid plate.

Hybrid plating systems do, however, run the risk of failing to achieve either absolute or relative stability, and/or of creating an environment with high strain on the implant. The result is implant failure and delayed or nonunion due to large gaps, respectively [14]. Optimal interfragmentary or plate-to-bone compression must be achieved before the application of the locked screws. The success of LISS in the clinic has provided evidence that lag screws can be used in the metaphyseal area without compromising the metaphyseal-diaphyseal fixation.

Plating combined with bone struts

Plates can be used exclusively or in combination with strut graft augmentation (chapters 10.12, 10.13, and 11.6). Studies using both osteoporotic and healthy bone surrogates have shown significant differences in stiffness between combined lateral/anterior plate constructs and that of a single-locked plate [13, 31]. Zdero et al [13] compared the Ogden construct with a strut graft, a locking-plate construct, and a conventional plate construct, both with or without additional cables, the Ogden construct with an additional strut graft exhibited the highest stiffness. Talbot et al [8] also found an allograft strut-plate construct to be stiffer in bending and have a higher load to failure than a stand-alone locking plate. Fulkerson et al [20] compared locking-plate fixation with an Odgen-type construct and found the first to be superior in stiffness. Clinically high union rates were reported whenever a metal plate on the one cortex was combined with a strut graft on the opposite cortex [16].

Clinical outcome

Despite their clinical usage for more than a decade, there is little information in the literature regarding clinical results from the usage of locking plates. Some early results are promising, with a 90% union rate in patients with osteoporosis reported from early clinical studies using polyaxial locking plates for treatment of periprosthetic fractures [6]. A review by Haidukewych et al [19] indicates high union rates have been achieved with locked plates for fixation of periprosthetic fractures above total knee arthroplasty and below total hip arthroplasty prostheses, with higher rates of union and lower rates of secondary surgery compared with previous controls. In a series of 34 Vancouver B1 fractures, Ricci et al [27] reported a healing rate of 100% and emphasized the importance of preserving the vascularity at the fracture site. Wood et al [3] reported 16 cases of Vancouver B1 and C fractures treated with locking plates, with a radiological healing of 14 cases after 6 months. They recommend bone grafting if the soft-tissue envelope is violated by extensive dissection and, in cases of failed hardware and revision fixation, cortical struts should be taken into consideration. Xue et al [4] presented 12 type B1 periprosthetic femoral fractures treated by LCP and cerclage bands, and all fractures united within an average of 4.8 months.

Summary

The high rate of major complications, revision surgery, and early mortality add up to a considerable morbidity among patients with periprosthetic fracture and a high price for society. While interfragmentary compression by plates and lag screws promote primary bone healing because of anatomical reconstruction and reduction of the strain within the fracture gap to less than 2%, locking plates functioning as internal fixators that bridge the fracture site and provide relative stability with a strain in the gap of 2–10% show healing by secondary or indirect ossification. The choice of fixation must be tailored to the fracture pattern, location, bone quality, and location of plate placement dictated by the anatomy.

Locked plates may prove to be most appropriate for:

- Indirect fracture reduction, as they can tolerate imperfect reduction and do not need to be contoured precisely
- Diaphyseal/metaphyseal fractures in osteoporotic bone
- The bridging of severely comminuted fractures to minimize soft-tissue damage
- The plating of fractures where, due to anatomical constraints, a compression plate may not be placed on the tension side of the fracture.

Most locking-plate systems provide instrumentation to facilitate percutaneous plate insertion and to allow traditional open fixation techniques. They usually allow either nonlocking or locking screws be inserted through the plate hole as well as the use of monocortical or bicortical screws [13]. The theoretical advantage of improved stability offered by locked constructs and the biological advantages afforded by less periosteal stripping and muscle-sparing plate insertion have generally been borne out with reportedly higher union rates. Malalignment, nonunion, implant failure, and periprosthetic fractures as well as a considerable learning curve still present challenges but most recent studies demonstrate lower complication rates with increasing experience of the surgeon and better instrumentation [8]. Early data on current polyaxial screw designs and various anatomically designed plates are encouraging, but further research is needed to define the role of these new technologies.

References

[1] **Lindahl H, Malchau H, Herberts P, et al.** Periprosthetic femoral fractures classification and demographics of 1049 periprosthetic femoral fractures from the Swedish National Hip Arthroplasty Register. *J Arthroplasty.* 2005 Oct;20(7):857–865.

[2] **Giannoudis PV, Kanakaris NK, Tsiridis E.** Principles of internal fixation and selection of implants for periprosthetic femoral fractures. *Injury.* 2007 Jun;38(6):669–687.

[3] **Wood GC, Naudie DR, McAuley J, et al.** Locking compression plates for the treatment of periprosthetic femoral fractures around well-fixed total hip and knee implants. *J Arthroplasty.* 2010 Sep;26(6):886–892.

[4] **Xue H, Tu Y, Cai M, et al.** Locking compression plate and cerclage band for Type B1 periprosthetic femoral fractures preliminary results at average 30-month follow-up. *J Arthroplasty.* 2011 Apr;26(3):467–471.

[5] **Tsiridis E, Krikler P, Giannoudis PV.** Periprosthetic femoral fractures: current aspects of management. *Injury.* 2007 Jun;38(6):649–650.

[6] **Erhardt JB, Grob K, Roderer G, et al.** Treatment of periprosthetic femur fractures with the non-contact bridging plate: a new angular stable implant. *Arch Orthop Trauma Surg.* 2008 Apr;128(4):409–416.

[7] **Buttaro MA, Farfalli G, Paredes Núñez M, et al.** Locking compression plate fixation of Vancouver type-B1 periprosthetic femoral fractures. *J Bone Joint Surg Am.* 2007 Sep;89(9):1964–1969.

[8] **Talbot M, Zdero R, Schemitsch EH.** Cyclic loading of periprosthetic fracture fixation constructs. *J Trauma.* 2008 May;64(5):1308–1312.

[9] **Tower SS, Beals RK.** Fractures of the femur after hip replacement: the Oregon experience. *Orthop Clin North Am.* 1999 Apr;30(2):235–247.

[10] **Bethea JS 3rd, DeAndrade JR, Fleming LL, et al.** Proximal femoral fractures following total hip arthroplasty. *Clin Orthop Relat Res.* 1982;(170):95–106.

[11] **Tadross TS, Nanu AM, Buchanan MJ, et al.** Dall-Miles plating for periprosthetic B1 fractures of the femur. *J Arthroplasty.* 2000 Jan;15(1):47–51.

[12] **Parvizi J, Rapuri VR, Purtill JJ, et al.** Treatment protocol for proximal femoral periprosthetic fractures. *J Bone Joint Surg Am.* 2004;86-A Suppl 2:8–16.

[13] **Zdero R, Walker R, Waddell JP, et al.** Biomechanical evaluation of periprosthetic femoral fracture fixation. *J Bone Joint Surg Am.* 2008 May;90(5):1068–1077.

[14] **Egol KA, Kubiak EN, Fulkerson E, et al.** Biomechanics of locked plates and screws. *J Orthop Trauma.* 2004 Sep;18(8):488–493.

[15] **Fulkerson E, Tejwani N, Stuchin S, et al.** Management of periprosthetic femur fractures with a first generation locking plate. *Injury.* 2007 Aug; 38(8):965–972.

[16] **Zenni EJ Jr, Pomeroy DL, Caudle RJ.** Ogden plate and other fixations for fractures complicating femoral endoprostheses. *Clin Orthop Relat Res.* 1988Jun;(231): 83–90.

[17] **Frigg R.** Development of the Locking Compression Plate. *Injury.* 2003 Nov;34 Suppl 2:B6–B10)

[18] **Bottlang M, Doornink J, Byrd GD, et al.** A nonlocking end screw can decrease fracture risk caused by locked plating in the osteoporotic diaphysis. *J Bone Joint Surg Am.* 2009 Mar;91(3):620–627.

[19] **Haidukewych GJ, Ricci W.** Locked plating in orthopaedic trauma: a clinical update. *J Am Acad Orthop Surg.* 2008 Jun;16(6):347–355.

[20] **Fulkerson E, Koval K, Preston CF, et al.** Fixation of periprosthetic femoral shaft fractures associated with cemented femoral stems: a biomechanical comparison of locked plating and conventional cable plates. *J Orthop Trauma.* 2006 Feb;20(2):89–93.

[21] **Kampshoff J, Stoffel KK, Yates PJ, et al.** The treatment of periprosthetic fractures with locking plates: effect of drill and screw type on cement mantles: a biomechanical analysis. *Arch Orthop Trauma Surg.* 2010 May;130(5):627–632.

[22] **Lenz M, Windolf M, Mückley T, et al.** The locking attachment plate for proximal fixation of periprosthetic femur fractures—a biomechanical comparison of two techniques. *Int Orthop.* 2012 Sep;36(9):1915–1921.

[23] **Dumpies CW, Conrad T, Marintschev I, et al.** [Locking attachment plate—first experience]. *Z Orthop Unfall.* 2012 Jun;150(3):302–308. German.

[24] **Konstantinidis L, Hauschild O, Beckmann NA, Het al.** Treatment of periprosthetic femoral fractures with two different minimal invasive angle-stable plates: Biomechanical comparison studies on cadaveric bones. *Injury.* 2010 Dec;41(12):1256–1261.

[25] **Stoffel K, Dieter U, Stachowiak G, et al.** Biomechanical testing of the LCP—how can stability in locked internal fixators be controlled? *Injury.* 2003 Nov;34 Suppl 2:B11–19.

[26] **Gautier E, Sommer C.** (2003) Guidelines for the clinical application of the LCP. *Injury.* 2003 Nov;34 Suppl 2:B63–76.

[27] **Ricci WM, Borrelli J Jr.** (2007) Operative management of periprosthetic femur fractures in the elderly using biological fracture reduction and fixation techniques. *Injury.* 2007 Sep;38 Suppl 3:S53–58.

[28] **Spitzer AB, Davidovitch RI, Egol KA.** Use of a "hybrid" locking plate for complex metaphyseal fractures and nonunions about the humerus. *Injury.* 2009 Mar;40(3):240–244.

[29] **Stoffel K, Lorenz KU, Kuster MS.** (2007) Biomechanical considerations in plate osteosynthesis: the effect of plate-to-bone compression with and without angular screw stability. *J Orthop Trauma.* Jul;21(6):362–368.

[30] **Staubli AE, De Simoni C, Babst R et al.** TomoFix: a new LCP-concept for open wedge osteotomy of the medial proximal tibia—early results in 92 cases. *Injury.* 2003 Nov;34 Suppl:B55–B62.

[31] **Choi JK, Gardner TR, Yoon E, et al.** The effect of fixation technique on the stiffness of comminuted Vancouver B1 periprosthetic femur fractures. *J Arthroplasty.* 2010 Sep; 25(6 Suppl):124–128.

5.4.2 Intramedullary nailing

Authors Christof Meyer, Reinhard Schnettler

Introduction

Intramedullary nailing (IM) in periprosthetic fractures is practically only applicable in the femur (chapters 10.8, 10.9, 10.11, 10.18, 11.3, and 11.7). As a retrograde technique, it may be considered the gold standard today. It shows consistent and safe fracture healing by callus formation. As a load-bearing construct, it allows early mobilization, which is important especially in elderly patients.

After a periprosthetic fracture, the insertion of an intramedullary nail in the classic way is usually not possible. An in situ coupling of an intact and firmly embedded prosthesis with a tubular intramedullary device is possible, although mentioned in only very few publications (**5.4-2**) [1–4]. An absolute prerequisite of this therapeutic option is precise preoperative planning with assessment of the knee as well as correct measurements of the diameter of the prosthetic stem, and the femoral shaft, and of the length of the distal shaft fragment to commission the appropriate custom-made tubular intramedullary nail. These preparations usually occur under pressure of time, whenever the patient needs to have surgery without delay to minimize the risks of prolonged bed rest as well as pain with the injured leg in traction [2–11].

5.4-2 Overview of the literature of intramedullary nailing techniques for periprosthetic fractures of the femur.

Author	Year	Title	No. of cases
Wenda [4]	2002	In situ connection of a hollow intramedullary nail to the stem of a knee prosthesis in periprosthetic fracture	1
Meyer et al [1]	2007	Treatment of periprosthetic femoral fractures by effective lengthening of the prosthesis	25
Tanaka et al [3]	2007	A new operative procedure using a Küntcher nail for a periprosthetic supracondylar femoral fracture after revision total knee arthroplasty: a case report	1
Meyer et al [2]	2011	Intramedullary nailing of periprosthetic femoral fractures after revision for total knee endoprosthesis. Treatment of periprosthetic femoral fractures by inserted knee endoprosthesis with intramedullary shaft by in situ lengthening of the prosthesis with specially prepared slotted hollow nails	9

Indications

Proximal femoral fractures around a loose prosthetic stem (types IV.3-B2 and IV.3-B3), whether the stem is cemented or not, are best treated with a long-stem revision prosthesis acting as an intramedullary device. Only types IV.3-B1 and IV.3-C femoral fractures with a well-fixed, preferably non-cemented stem may be suited for a retrograde IM nailing procedure. In principle, retrograde IM nailing can also be done in distal periprosthetic type V.3-B1 femoral fractures, if the prosthesis is a stable, open-box knee prosthesis (**5.4-6a–b**). Closed-box prostheses leave no room for the insertion of a retrograde intramedullary nail (**5.4-7a–b**). In exceptional cases of a periprosthetic fracture around stable knee prosthesis with a stem, an antegrade femoral nail may be a good option (chapter 10.18).

Preoperative planning

To perform this fixation technique, an exact history and medical evaluation of the patient before the injury is required, including the degree of mobility, independence, and mental status. Any difference in leg length or rotation compared with the uninjured side has to be investigated as well as clinical signs of loosening.

Further criteria for preoperative planning concern the type and design of prosthesis and its fixation into the bone, which is best done based on CT measurements (**5.4-8**). The ideal situation is a rather wide femoral shaft containing a prosthesis with a conical, tapered end that allows a hollow, slotted, intramedullary nail to be slipped over for a length of about 4 cm. To commission the custom-made intramedullary nail,

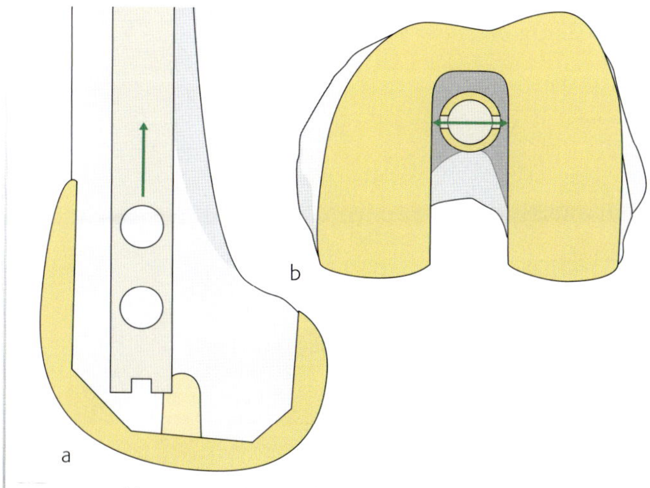

5.4-6a–b In case of a distal femoral fracture type V.3-B1 with stable open-box knee prosthesis, retrograde nail insertion may be possible, provided the intramedullary nail passes through the slot.
a Lateral view.
b Frontal view of knee in flexion.

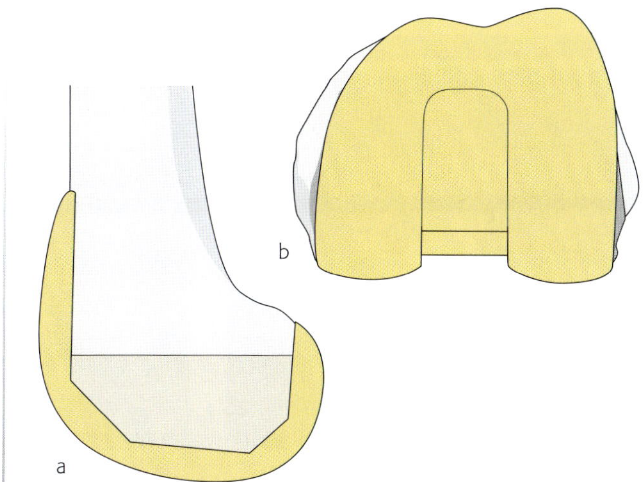

5.4-7a–b Closed-box knee prosthesis that does not allow for the insertion of an intramedullary nail.
a Lateral view.
b Frontal view of knee in flexion.

it is necessary to determine the diameter of the prosthetic stem and that of the intramedullary canal as well as the length of the distal fragment from the point of insertion to the prosthesis.

On the basis of the data obtained, a slotted hollow nail with a means for distal locking and of corresponding length (3–4 cm overlap with the prosthesis stem) matching the internal diameter (**5.4-9**) must be ordered. Manufacturing of the special implant generally takes 2–3 working days.

Surgical procedure

The surgical procedure consists of a custom-made, slotted, hollow, intramedullary nail being inserted with the purpose of lengthening the stem of the prosthesis. The challenge is to obtain a safe and stable coupling between nail and stem (**5.4-10**) [1, 2, 4].

For the most frequently used retrograde insertion of the intramedullary nail, the patient is positioned on a radiolucent operating room table with the knee flexed to about 80°. Two approaches are required—one for the insertion of the nail through the knee, the other for the open exposure of the fracture site.

Tissue samples are taken for histological and microbiological analysis. Any cement has to be removed from around the tip of the prosthetic stem, which must also be freed from any tissue or cement for a length of about 4 cm, while the distal shaft fragment has to be reamed to the nail diameter. The insertion of the intramedullary nail and its coupling to the prosthesis is done under visual control to verify the correct length and rotation. Stable docking between nail and prosthesis can be obtained by a prudent use of a hammer. Depending on the type of fracture and the size of a possible defect, an additional autogenous cancellous bone graft may be indicated. Depending on the type of intramedullary nail, locking of the far end of the nail may have to be done with two locking bolts (**5.4-11**).

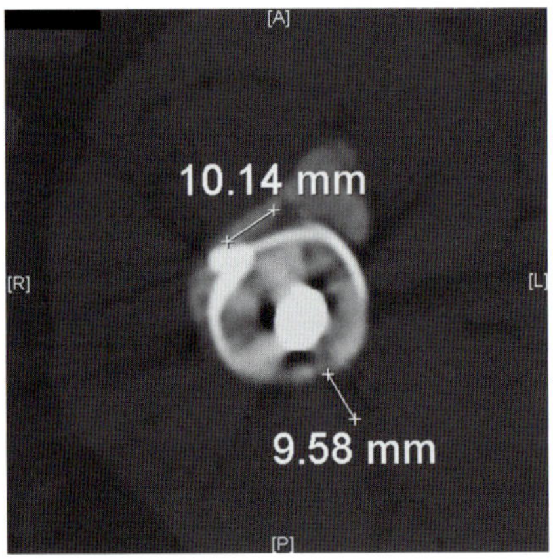

5.4-8 Preoperative computed tomographic measurement of the prosthetic stem 4 cm proximal to the tip (diameter in two planes).

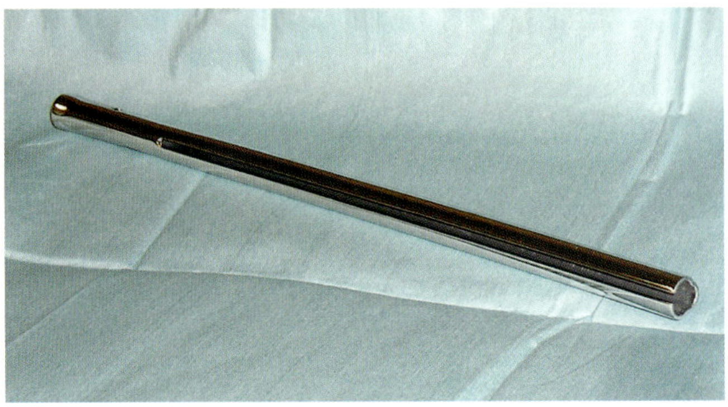

5.4-9 Custom-made, slotted, hollow intramedullary femoral nail for in situ coupling with a prosthetic stem.

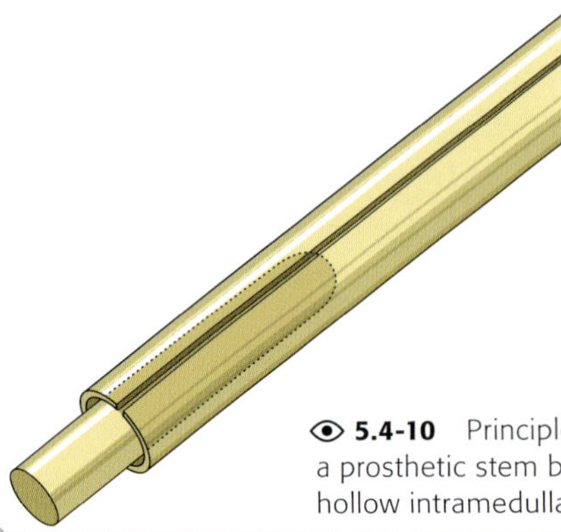

5.4-10 Principle of lengthening a prosthetic stem by coupling it with a hollow intramedullary nail.

Postoperative management

Depending on the postoperative clinical and radiological situation, the patient is mobilized with progressive load bearing over a period of 6 weeks. Thereafter, full weight bearing is allowed as far as the patient is comfortable with it. Exceptionally, immediate full weight bearing may also be permissible if intraoperatively the stability of the coupling was assessed as satisfactory. For the follow-up, clinical and x-ray controls are recommended after 6, 12, and 26 weeks (👁 **5.4-12a–b**).

Outcome

The potential for rapid fracture consolidation using this operative option is remarkable, as also described by other authors (▤ **5.4-2**) [3, 4]. Regarding the need for a bone graft, no demonstrable effect is described in the literature [7]. Among the authors' own patients, the decision was always taken intraoperatively. In case of a bone defect the addition of autogenous cancellous bone (harvested from the ipsilateral tibia head) was done in 7 of the 24 patients. Similarly, the use of debris from reaming seems to promote fracture healing in the manner of an autogenous bone graft.

The operative procedure combines the advantage of a stable intramedullary osteosynthesis as an extension of the embedded prosthesis to a long-stem implant with the possibility of retaining the stable endoprosthesis. Compared with a prosthetic replacement, the surgical intervention is significantly less invasive and clinical experience shows that the achieved stability is clearly superior to that of a plate osteosynthesis [4, 5].

Conclusions

Generally, in situ coupling of an endoprosthesis with a slotted tubular intramedullary nail represents a valuable option for the treatment of periprosthetic fractures of the femur.

In view of the positive experience with this type of treatment—and considering the expected increase in the number of periprosthetic fractures—it is reasonable to ask the manufacturers of prostheses and implants to design and produce prosthetic stems with a distal end terminating in a standardized cone (similar to the neck of prosthesis) as well as manufacture nails to fit them. Thus, an operative procedure that is demanding and costly due to the need for custom-made implants could be developed further to become a safe, standardized method of treatment.

Between 1994 and 2010, the authors treated 33 patients with periprosthetic femoral fractures with a custom-made intramedullary slotted hollow nail, thereby achieving an effective, in situ lengthening of the femoral stem of a hip (24 patients) or knee (9 patients) prosthesis. There were 8 men and 25 women with an average age of 78 years (ranging from 47–90 years). Of these 33 patients, 12 previously had undergone one or more prosthesis revisions. In 18 patients, the authors' stem-lengthening procedure was first used to treat periprosthetic fractures, whereas in the remaining 15 patients, the procedure was performed as revision intervention after failed plate fixation. In all, 24 femoral shafts of the hip, respectively, knee prostheses were cemented and 9 were noncemented. Of the 33 patients, 22 were followed up for a minimum of 6 months (average: 27 months; range: 6–41 months).

In 20 patients available for follow-up, the fractures had healed. In 19 of these 20 patients, proper length and rotation of the femur was restored. In one female patient, loosening of the femur component of a total hip arthroplasty was seen after 8 weeks, which most likely was related to the coupling procedure of the intramedullary nail. Revision prosthesis with a long femoral stem was necessary. In another patient a nonunion resulted. However, while revision surgery was planned, the patient died of renal disease. Finally, one septic nonunion was treated by removal of both implant and prosthesis, followed by secondary complete femur replacement.

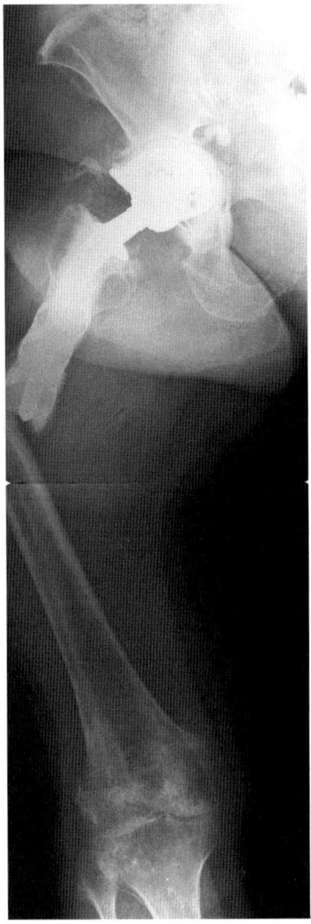

5.4-11 Periprosthetic femoral fracture type IV.3-B1 with a well-fixed stem.

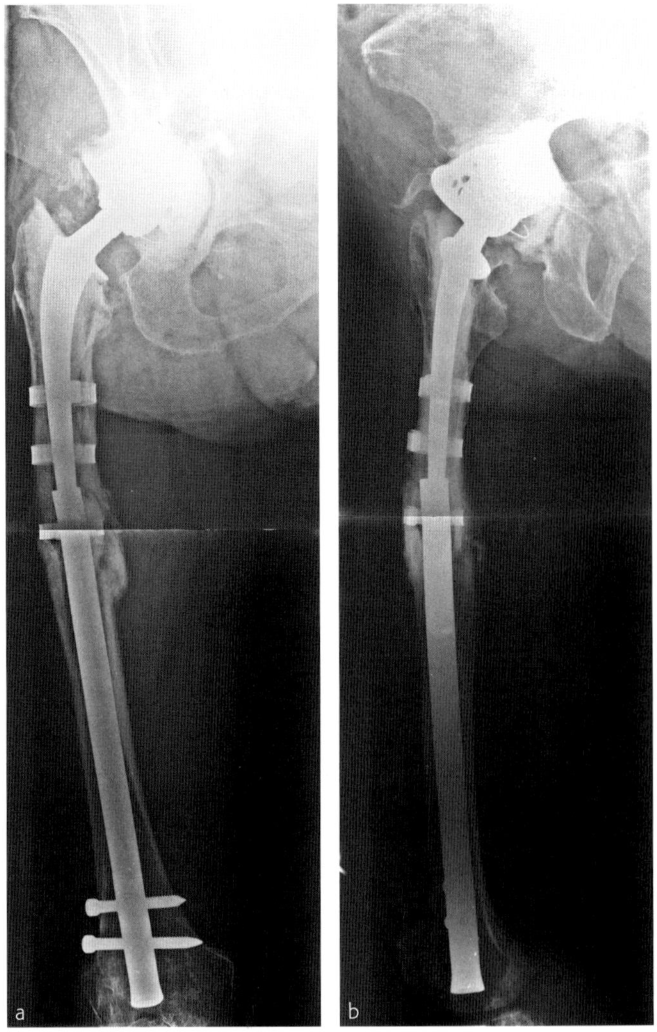

5.4-12a–b Follow-up x-rays of a patient 7 months after insertion of an intramedullary nail, showing callus formation and a consolidated fracture. To prevent any splitting of the femur, cerclages had been placed around the bone.
a AP view.
b Lateral view.

References

[1] **Meyer C, Alt V, Schroeder L, et al.** Treatment of periprosthetic femoral fractures by effective lengthening of the prosthesis. *Clin Orthop Relat Res.* 2007 Oct;463:120–127.

[2] **Meyer C, Alt V, Heiss C, et al.** [Intramedullary nailing of periprosthetic femoral fractures after revision for total knee endoprosthesis. Treatment of periprosthetic femoral fractures by inserted knee endoprosthesis with intramedullary shaft by in situ lengthening of the prosthesis with specially prepared slotted hollow nails.] *Unfallchirurg.* 2011 Mar;114(3):241–247. German.

[3] **Tanaka Y, Kobayashi T, Ohashi M, et al.** A new operative procedure using a Küntcher nail for a periprosthetic supracondylar femoral fracture after revision total knee arthroplasty: a case report. *Knee.* 2007 Jan;14(1):59–62.

[4] **Wenda K.** [In situ connection of a hollow intramedullary nail to the stem of knee prosthesis in periprosthetic fracture.] *Unfallchirurg.* 2002 Jan;105(1):19–22. German.

[5] **Beals RK, Tower SS.** Periprosthetic fractures of the femur. An analysis of 93 fractures. *Clin Orthop Relat Res.* 1996;(327):238–246.

[6] **Gruner A, Hockertz T, Reilmann H.** [Periprosthetic fractures: classification, management, therapy.] *Unfallchirurg.* 2004 Jan;107(1):35–49. German.

[7] **Jukkala-Partio K, Partio EK, Solovieva S, et al.** Treatment of periprosthetic fractures in association with total hip arthroplasty—a retrospective comparison between revision stem and plate fixation. *Ann Chir Gynaecol.* 1998;87(3):229–235.

[8] **Mittlmeier T, Stöckle U, Perka C, et al.** [Periprosthetic fractures after total knee joint arthroplasty.] *Unfallchirurg.* 2005 Jun;108(6):481–496. German.

[9] **Park MS, Lee YK, Yang KH, et al.** Management of periprosthetic femoral fractures. *J Arthroplasty.* 2003 Oct;18(7):903–906.

[10] **Probst A, Schneider T, Hankemeier S, et al.** [The prosthesis nail—a new stable fixation device for periprosthetic fractures and critical fractures of the proximal femur.] *Unfallchirurg.* 2003 Sep;106(9):722–731. German.

[11] **Su ET, DeWal H, Di Cesare PE.** Periprosthetic femoral fractures above knee replacements. *J Am Acad Orthop Surg.* 2004 Jan-Feb;12(1):12–20.

5.5 Revision of prosthetic components

Author Carsten Perka

In periprosthetic fractures, the revision of a prosthetic component is considered the second most important therapeutical option beside osteosynthesis. Compared with a surgical fracture fixation, the revision procedure is by far the more invasive intervention. The indication for a revision must, therefore, be absolutely clear, while the techniques for both revision surgery and fracture fixation must be mastered.

The most frequent indication for revision arthroplasty in a periprosthetic fracture is the evident loosening of the prosthesis combined with resorption of the surrounding bone. Revision surgery may also be indicated if the original prosthesis had been malpositioned or in case of a biomechanically critical fracture pattern (eg, a transverse fracture at the tip of the stem) in a patient who is not able to ambulate without full weight bearing. Furthermore, there are types of prosthesis that are known to have a limited "lifespan" and should be replaced anyway, sooner or later. Finally, if there is an infection associated with the periprosthetic fracture, salvage usually is only obtainable by revision of the prosthetic implant, irrespective of a one- or two-staged procedure.

While in most cases the strategy on how to proceed—revision or osteosynthesis—can be based on the preoperative evaluation, the final decision will always need to be taken during surgery. In case a fracture fixation is planned, it is mandatory to have all appropriate instruments and implants available, including those needed for a revision of the prosthesis. Moreover, surgeons also need to be familiar with the procedure. It should be part of every preoperative plan to be prepared to change from the preferred procedure to a plan B or even C.

For revision surgery in case of a periprosthetic fracture (chapters 7.11, 7.12, 10.2, 10.12, 10.13, and 10.14), it is recommended to use a noncemented implant as otherwise there is a risk that the cement could leak out through the fracture gap, thereby delaying or even preventing bone healing. Furthermore, the high endoluminal pressure required to achieve a firm anchorage of the cemented prosthesis may not be reached in case of fracture. To obtain a satisfactory long-term result it would, therefore, be necessary to reconstruct the tubular bone anatomically by internal fixation beforehand and afterwards introduce the cement and revision prosthesis.

A cemented implant has the advantage of immediate stability, allowing full weight bearing. Furthermore, antibiotics can be added to the cement. The advantages of the noncemented anchorage of the prosthesis are better long-term stability after fracture healing and bony integration.

Mega implants (total femur, intramedullary femur replacement with preservation of the femoral diaphysis) (chapter 5.6) are applicable irrespective of bone stock and quality, and they do not require fracture healing. However, since they are associated with a rather high infection rate and as there is no way to bail out, the indication to use mega prostheses should be restricted to cases when no other possibility of salvage is possible. Nevertheless, such salvage procedures may be the only way to regain an acceptable function in situations of long-standing bone defects or tumors associated with a complex fracture (chapter 11.4).

In all revisions where only one component of the prosthesis is to be replaced (eg, the stem in a hip prosthesis), it is mandatory to identify the type and size of the implant as well as the manufacturer, otherwise the situation may arise that the stem and the head component do not fit.

For every revision procedure, a complete set of appropriate instruments is required including high-speed saws and different sizes of chisels. Different plates and bone reduction forceps may help to stabilize the fracture temporarily. In fractures of the lower extremity, a selection of bone allografts (eg, strut grafts) may prove to be helpful and should also be available.

In conclusion, it should be mentioned that the decisive point in any revision procedure concerns the care of the soft-tissue envelope. Extensive approaches and wide exposure of the bone must be avoided. Additional osteotomies may further reduce the stability of a reconstruction, jeopardize the fixation, and should, therefore, be applied only exceptionally. The removal of firmly fixed implants and cement bears the risk of creating additional multifragmentary fractures. Nevertheless, all cement particles and granulation tissue must be debrided. The use of ultrasonic extraction devices may be helpful.

The length of revision surgery should be reduced to a minimum, which can be achieved by careful planning and ensuring that all necessary instrument sets and implants are readily available. More importantly, the surgeon must be experienced and able to adapt and cope with unexpected situations to ensure that a satisfactory result may be expected.

5.6 Alternative techniques

Authors Joshua C Patt, Jeffrey S Kneisl, Carsten Perka, Stephan Tohtz, Michael Schütz

5.6.1 Indications that require alternatives

Authors Joshua C Patt, Jeffrey S Kneisl

Introduction

Most periprosthetic fractures can be handled with the basic principles of orthopedic and orthopedic trauma management outlined in the preceding chapters. However, a challenging subset of patients will require more creative and innovative solutions. Each individual fracture needs to be assessed in the context of unique patient characteristics, especially in case of a failed first attempt at fracture fixation. For these exceptional situations, decisions need to be based on principles that are adapted to the individual patient rather than a rote "decision tree" with a static fracture classification system or algorithm. This chapter focuses on infrequently encountered, challenging cases that require an innovative application of standard implants, use of novel or unique implants, and, at times, multimodal solutions to complex problems. While the focus is on case examples from the lower extremities, the basic principles can be applied to any other anatomical location.

Failure of conventional internal fixation

Plate osteosynthesis is the gold standard for most periprosthetic fractures with a stable prosthesis. In some circumstances, appropriately applied conventional fixation can fail as manifested by screw loosening, plate breakage, infection, or adjacent bone failure. Prior to embarking on revision fixation, careful analysis of the mode of initial failure must be made. Identified causes of this failure mode include biological and/or biomechanical nonunion, poor fixation due to host-bone deficiency, inappropriate implant selection, or poor surgical technique (👁 **5.6-1a–c**). There is little rationale to support repeating an operation that has already failed once. Before performing a revision operation, the following questions should be asked:

- Which type of blood supply/healing environment exists?
- Which fixation points can be obtained?
- Which sort of soft-tissue coverage can be achieved?
- Which adverse host factors will inhibit success (eg, severe osteoporosis, medical comorbidities, metabolic deficiency, cancer metastasis, or infection)?

In case of reversible factors, treatment may proceed with management of the underlying causative factor (eg, vitamin D deficiency). At other times, systemic factors may be irreversible (metastatic cancer), and an alternative solution should be pursued (👁 **5.6-2a–b**).

Failure of conventional prosthetic implants

Repetitive micro trauma or overloading of an implant can cause mechanical failure of the actual prosthetic implant, corresponding to a type E fracture. Initial implant positioning, excessive size of patient, and improperly selected implants can lead to mechanical failure of the actual implant as opposed to the more commonly encountered failure at the prosthesis-bone interface. In this setting, the opportunity for primary repair or revision internal fixation may not exist, so revision arthroplasty may be chosen. Preoperative planning should anticipate the need for multiple options intraoperatively. This will include having a selection of standard revision implants available as well as oncological-type mega prosthesis to replace anticipated segmental defects. In such exceptional situations, consideration should also be given to transferring the patient to a center where surgeons dedicated to joint revisions or tumor specialists are available for more complex cases (👁 **5.6-3a–b**).

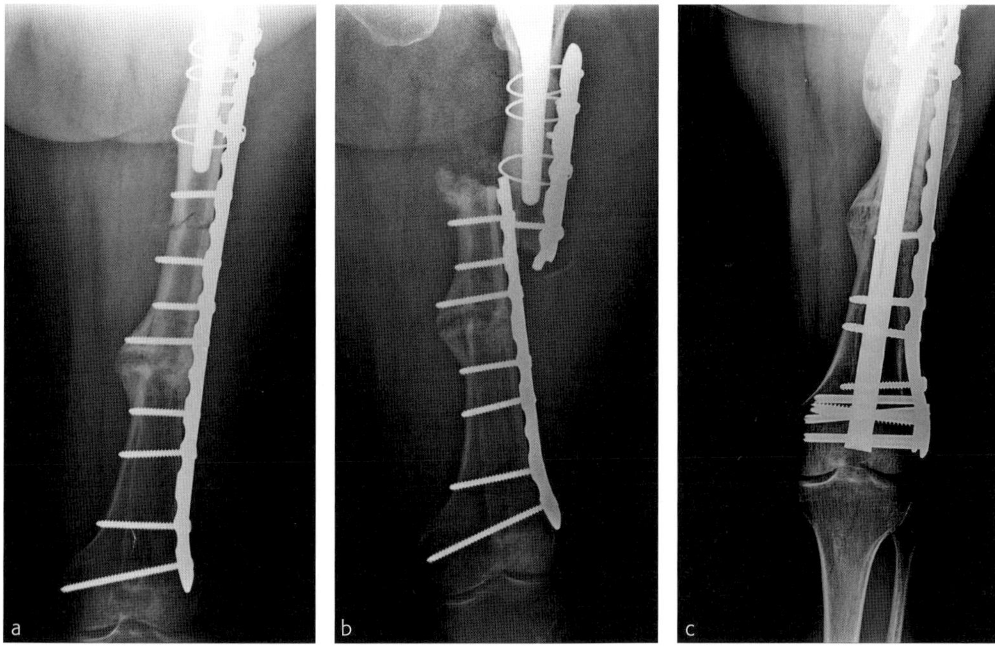

5.6-1a–c X-rays of a 58-year-old woman with failed primary plate fixation.

- **a** Primary open reduction and internal fixation (ORIF) with delayed healing of a proximal fracture.
- **b** Fatigue fracture of the plate at proximal fracture site (distal to tip of stem).
- **c** Repeated ORIF with intramedullary nail and long plate overlapping the nail.

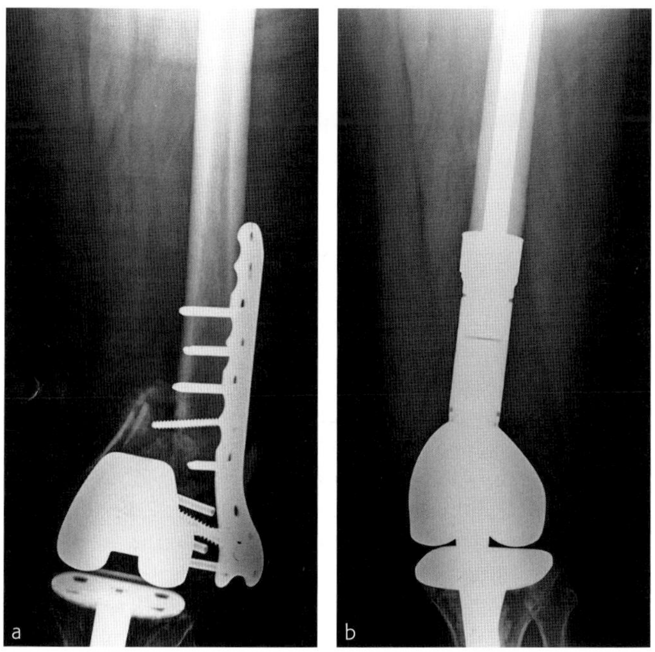

5.6-2a–b X-rays of a 70-year-old woman.

- **a** Failed open reduction and internal fixation (ORIF) with short plate of a distal femoral periprosthetic fracture.
- **b** Revision to replacement prosthesis of the distal third of the femur.

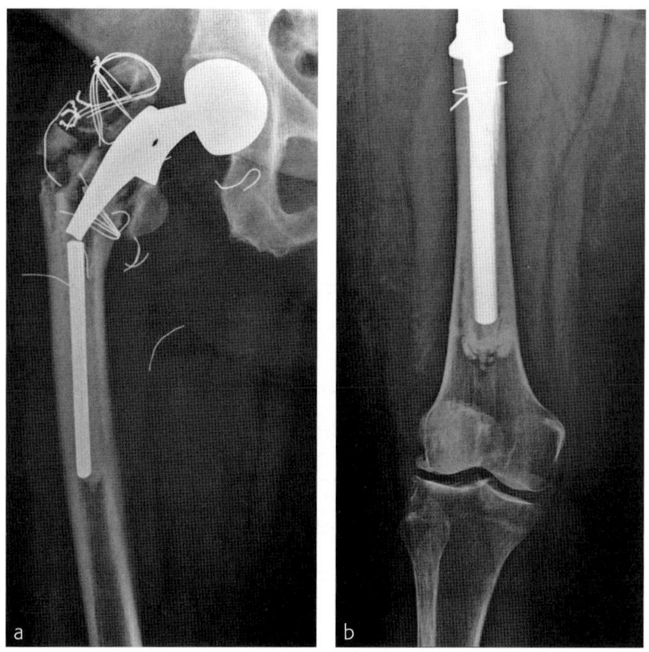

5.6-3a–b X-rays of a 69-year-old woman.

- **a** Failure of calcar replacing hemiarthroplasty after multiple attempts of open reduction and internal fixation (ORIF) for a pathological fracture (renal cell carcinoma).
- **b** Revision to tumor prosthesis with proximal femoral resection and greater trochanteric reattachment.

Bone failure adjacent to an implant

The most common bone abnormality encountered is osteoporosis (chapter 3.1). Even patients with relatively normal overall bone stock can develop relative osteopenia due to stress shielding from the prosthetic joint replacement. Failures due to infection can lead to significant long-term morbidity and treatment must directly address eradication of infection to achieve successful fixation. Another cause of bone failure adjacent to an implant can be a spreading tumor, which can induce a segmental loss of fixation and generally demands prophylactic protection of the entire bone. Finally, the effect of repeated attempts at fixation can weaken the bone through a combination of structural faults (prior screw holes or cement mantles) and nutrient deficiencies causing depleted bone marrow and damaged periosteal vascularity.

Ultimately, internal fixation depends on a well-fixed prosthetic component and multiple host factors. Strategies for optimizing this environment are essential to satisfactory clinical outcome if bone healing is desired. There are pharmacological agents that are considered to prevent bone resorption (eg, bisphosphonates) or to stimulate bone formation (parathormone), which may be helpful to promote the healing process. If these factors are irreversible or otherwise hostile to healing, alternative fixation methods should be considered that do not primarily rely on bone healing. Options include endoprosthetic reconstructions (structured allografts, allograft-prosthetic composites, tumor mega prostheses), novel bone interface options (impaction grafting), and amputation as ultimate solution, particularly in the setting of recalcitrant infections (**5.6-4a–b**). The different alternative solutions are discussed in more detail and case based in part 2 of this chapter.

Soft-tissue repair

The most common host factor that complicates primary and revision fixation is the soft-tissue envelope surrounding the zone of injury. Even low-energy trauma can result in open fractures and soft-tissue loss. Open fracture management should follow established standards of care including timely irrigation and debridement, excision of contaminated and nonviable tissues, temporary stabilization of the fractured limb, and time-appropriate soft-tissue closure. Injuries in certain locations, such as the distal tibia and anterior knee, can predetermine the need for formal soft-tissue coverage. Early consultation with the plastic surgery team may be beneficial if primary closure will be challenging.

Another challenging soft-tissue problem can occur when the fracture line is at or near to the bone-tendon junction. Hip-abductor issues can predetermine hip instability, while critical tendon insertions at the patella can lead to failure of the extensor mechanism. The guiding principle to repair

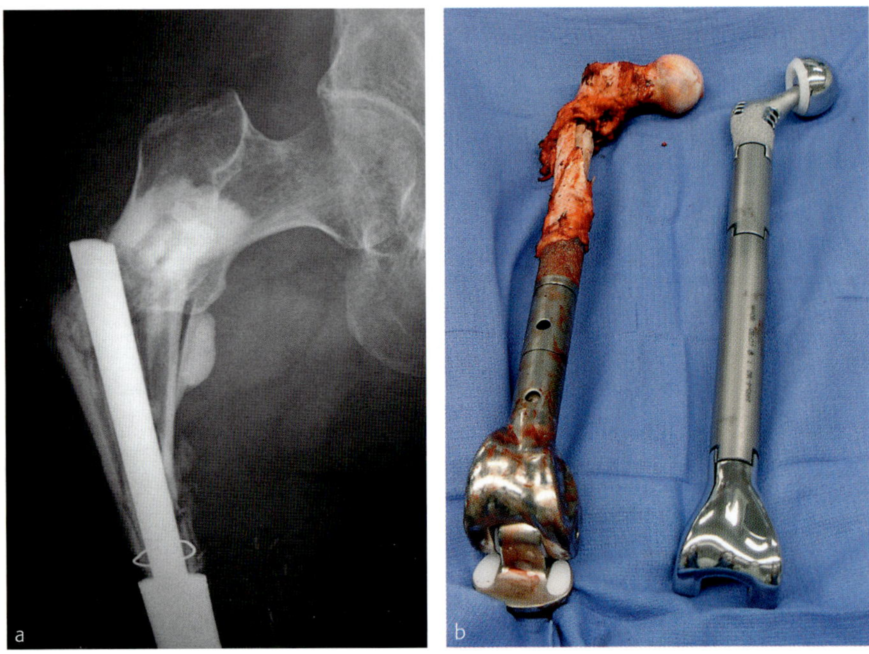

5.6-4a–b 24-year-old woman.
a X-ray of the proximal failure after long-segment endoprosthetic reconstruction for osteosarcoma and multiple revisions.
b Custom-made total femoral resection "mega prosthesis" before implantation.

the high-stress, bone-tendon junctions is to focus on an anatomical reconstruction whenever possible, with adjuvant reinforcement or protection of the repair. For example, when faced with complete detachment of the hip abductors, the authors' favored technique consists of a primary repair with a tension-band wire at the bone-tendon junction. An 18-gauge wire is used to attach the abductors to the prosthesis or, preferably, the bone using a figure-of-eight type weave and cerclage. This is then tightened to maximum tension and, afterward, a trochanteric claw is attached over the top with standard cerclage fixation. While both of these fixation techniques have predictable, independent risk of failure, the authors found that their use in combination in most cases allows sufficient healing to occur without displacement as well as a satisfactory function. A modification of this technique can also be done in the setting of more extensive soft-tissue loss at both the hip and knee with the use of an Achilles tendon allograft.

5.6.2 Alternative solutions for special scenarios

Authors Carsten Perka, Stephan Tohtz, Michael Schütz

Introduction

While the almost "classical" therapeutic principles described above are broadly applicable, not every patient and not every fracture fits neatly into such standard categories. Furthermore, the less invasive nature of an osteosynthesis and the surgeon's preference for a certain technique are most often the reasons why osteosynthesis is performed rather than revision arthroplasty.

In the following paragraphs different scenarios are presented to demonstrate how periprosthetic fractures can be successfully treated using alternative techniques. For this purpose, the hip joint, ie, the joint most heavily loaded, was chosen. In certain cases, the surgeon may even have to deviate from implantation principles prescribed by the implant manufacturer (off-label use).

Scenario 1: Periprosthetic fracture with destruction of the femoral isthmus

Problem

Fractures occurring in poor or pathological bone stock often represent a challenge for stable osteosynthesis or anchorage of a noncemented implant. This situation is particularly challenging when extensive destruction or osteoporosis of the proximal and middle third of the diaphysis—including the isthmus—has occurred and when the medullary canal progressively widens toward the distal end. According to standard practice, the treatment of choice in case of a loosened prosthesis is revision arthroplasty with a standard procedure (noncemented revision stem). However, stable anchoring of the noncemented prosthesis cannot be performed due to the lack of cancellous bone in the medullary cavity.

Solution A

Theoretically, there is the possibility of locking the prosthesis distally. However, the stability provided by locking-head screws is low in osteoporotic bone, especially if there is no additional circumferential support for the prosthetic stem over an adequate length of bone and, even worse, if the patient is not capable of unloading the limb.

Solution B

The so-called push-through prosthesis can be used. However, removal of the old implant is restricted with this option.

Solution C

In the above-described cases, cement is proposed to securely anchor the distal part of a long, noncemented stem or modular stem in the widened medullary canal as an off-label use. In a second step, the proximally located fragments are fixed to the prosthetic shaft with a technique that does not use cement, eg, cerclage wires. The aim is to achieve primary stability in the distal femur by the cemented anchorage and normal force transmission once fragments have been incorporated by healing.

Case example: **5.6-5a–c** illustrates solution C. There is significant damage of the femoral isthmus, so primary fixation of a noncemented stem was achieved with cement in the distal femur. Additionally, noncemented fragment fixation was performed in the proximal femur.

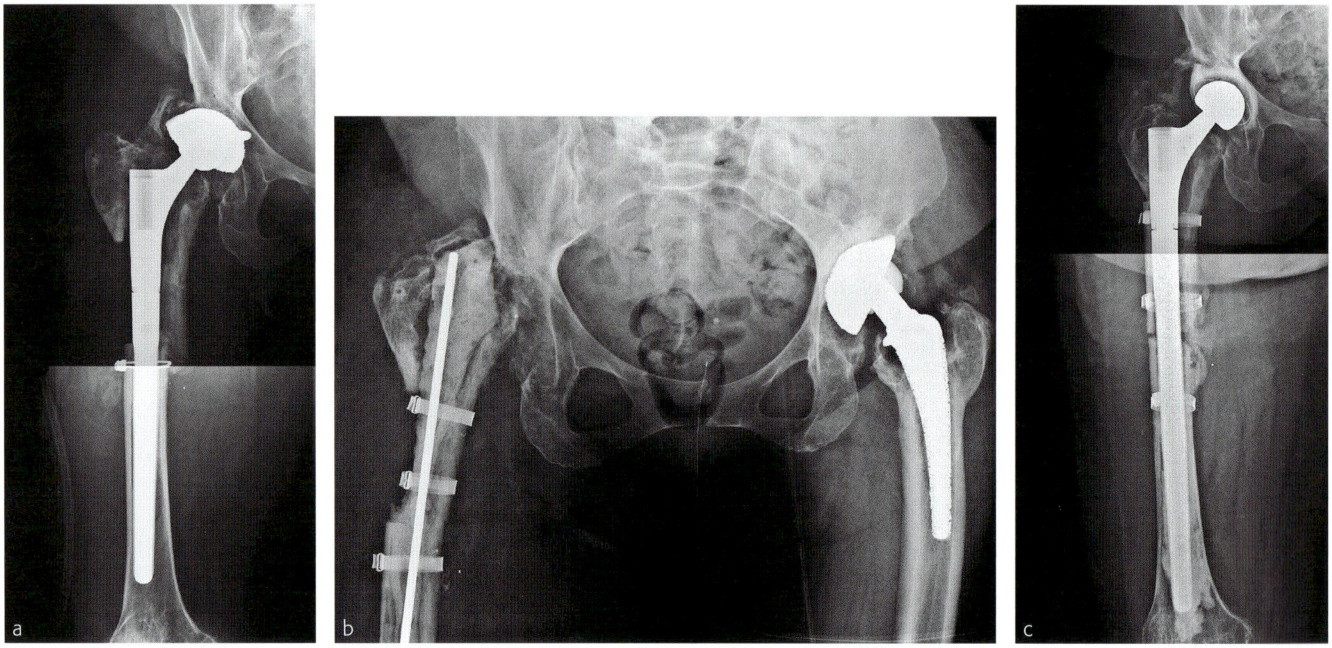

5.6-5a–c A 52-year-old woman with a periprosthetic femoral fracture and infection after stem revision (type IV.3-B3).

a AP view of the infected fracture.

b After removal of the infected total hip arthroplasty (THA), a Girdlestone situation is obtained with a cement spacer that is augmented with antibiotics and a central metal pin as temporary device.

c After reimplantation of a THA with a long, noncemented stem that is distally anchored with bone cement (off-label use), the missing lateral cortex is proximally reconstructed with a structured allograft and fixed with titanium bands.

Scenario 2: Periprosthetic fracture around cemented implants in the proximal femur

Problem

If periprosthetic fractures involve long-shaft prostheses or tumor prostheses that are only anchored in the distal femur and, moreover, if bone stock is poor, repeated anchoring of the prosthesis may be problematic or impossible. There are, however, different options to solve these problems.

Solution A

The standard therapy is revision to a total femoral prosthesis. The advantages of a total femoral prosthesis are immediate full weight bearing and long-term stability. Disadvantages are the difficulty to permanently attach tendons, ligaments, and soft tissues, the increased risk of infection associated with mega prostheses, and the considerable invasiveness of the procedure.

Case example: **5.6-6a–b** illustrates solution A. Periprosthetic fractures in cases with very poor bone stock at all levels of the femur and significant bone defects need treatment with mega prosthesis.

Solution B

In elderly patients whose walking ability had been severely limited even before sustaining the fracture, a minimally invasive procedure should be attempted.

Case example: **5.6-7a–c** illustrates solution B. A severely ill 93-year-old woman was mostly confined to her bed and used to take only a few steps with a walker before the fracture occurred. When it came to fracture fixation, the anesthesiology team considered the risk for a total femoral prosthesis as too high. It was decided to retain the implant and repeat the stabilization by cementing the distal end again. After removal of the loose, accessible cement through the fracture site, the prosthesis was extended by a modified Küntscher nail and reinserted in the medullary canal. This was followed by filling the distal femoral cavity around the "extended" prosthesis with cement. While the cement was still flexible and had not hardened, the fracture was stabilized with two titanium cerclage bands that had been previously placed around the bone. Following this minimally invasive treatment, the patient was free of pain, could get up without difficulty, and was able to reach the toilet independently. The patient died 2 years after surgery of causes not related to the fracture.

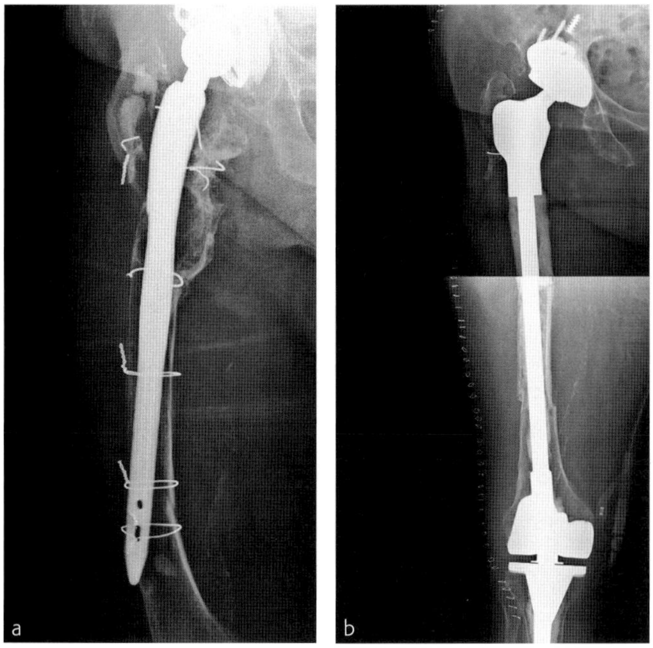

5.6-6a–b An 81-year-old woman with a periprosthetic fracture (type IV.3-B3) after implantation of a noncemented revision prosthesis. Extended proximal and diaphyseal osteolysis with bone defects exists.

a AP view of the fracture distal to the completely loosened revision prosthesis.

b AP view after replacement of the entire femur by a mega prosthesis.

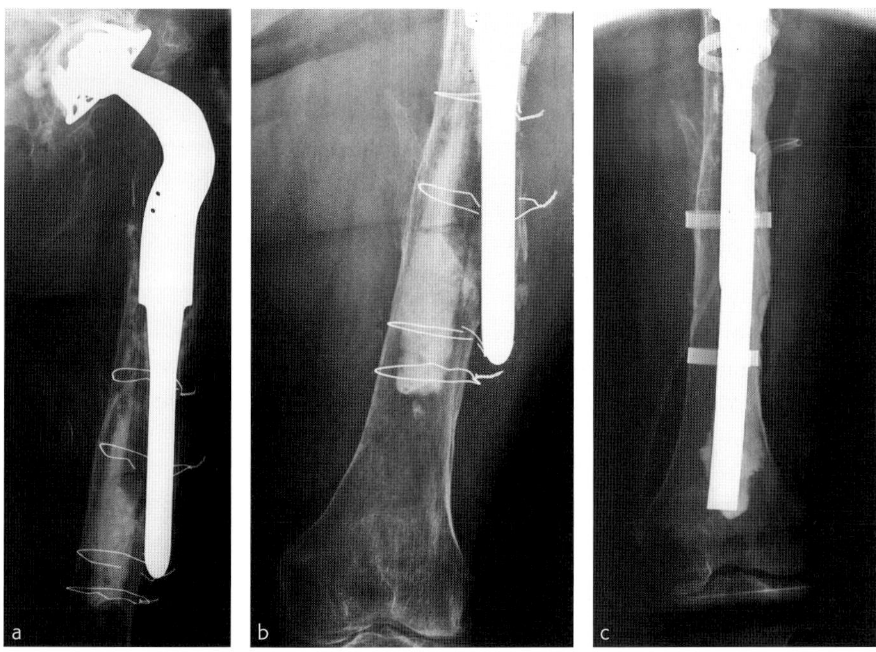

5.6-7a–c A 93-year-old severely ill woman with a periprosthetic fracture (type IV.3-B3) after revision of the proximal femur with a tumor prosthesis.

a AP view of the fracture with displacement of the stem of the prosthesis, bone defects, and severe osteoporosis.

b Lateral view.

c After salvage procedure: loosened cement was removed through the fracture site, while a custom-made, shortened Küntscher nail was placed over the stem to extend it. After adding cement, the titanium cerclage bands were applied to hold the reconstruction. The patient recovered well and lived for another 2 years.

Scenario 3: Severe osteoporosis and/or very poor bone stock in the proximal femur

Problem

The standard treatment of bone defects of the proximal femur is with long, noncemented prosthesis around which the remaining fragments are aligned and fixed. However, whenever there is hardly any bone left in the proximal femur, stabilization in the remaining femur becomes more and more problematic. Definitive treatment without cement cannot be performed in the presence of osteoporosis and a lack of cancellous bone.

Solution A

In this case, the primary recommendation is the implantation of a tumor prosthesis designed to replace the proximal femur. A specific disadvantage of proximal femur replacement is, however, the difficult and non-permanent fixation of the tendons and soft tissues to the tumor prosthesis, which in turn is associated with a high risk of dislocation.

Solution B

A further possible solution in such cases is the reconstruction of the proximal femur with an allograft prosthetic composite (APC), especially in situations with a high risk for dislocation. The technique for preparing the APC is described for the proximal femoral replacement in more detail(**5.6-8a–h**). However, a similar technique can be applied to the distal femur, proximal tibia, humerus, and proximal ulna (see chapters 8.1, 8.2, 8.4, 8.5, and 10.12).

The size of the allograft that is required is estimated by studying x-rays of the contralateral side. A slightly smaller allograft than the host bone is chosen so that the former can be inserted within the prepared "shell" of the host cortex. This allows the muscle or tendon insertions to be preserved. Moreover, the slightly smaller size ensures that the healing process is not endangered and that the soft tissues are not placed under too much strain.

Following the usual approach, the proximal femur is exposed without damaging the different muscle insertions around the greater and lesser trochanter. With the oscillating saw, cuts are placed in the frontal plane. Then the anterior aspect of the proximal femur is elevated and moved proximally like the cover of a coffin (**5.6-8a–b**). After removal of the prosthesis—including the bone cement surrounding it—the dorsal half of the proximal femur is split longitudinally (**5.6-8c–d**). At the fracture site, all free fragments are removed to be able to perform a nice and clear-cut step osteotomy (**5.6-8d**). The allograft is selected and trimmed according to the chosen revision prosthesis and then fitted with the prosthetic stem (**5.6-8e**). If the proximal femur and trochanters show poor bone quality with fragmentation and osteopenia, it is recommended to remove them. The remaining femur and the APC are prepared with as little loss of bone as possible. At this stage, it is important to maintain the original alignment of the joint. The APC is inserted temporarily for fine tuning and adjustment of the fit. The stem of the prosthesis has to be long enough to bridge the graft-host interface by at least two bone widths and should have an overall length of at least 160 mm (**5.6-8f**). Once everything is correctly aligned, the selected femoral component is cemented into the allograft. The process of cementing the component should be undertaken with care to prevent cement from leaking into the interface between graft and host bone, which could inhibit the osseous integration of the allograft. Afterward the composite is implanted into the host bone with good contact between the two fragments, assured by the accuracy of the step osteotomy. In case of a wide medullary cavity, the tip of the stem can be cemented as well. The dorsal slices of the proximal femur are placed around the allograft and held in place with cerclage wires (**5.6-8f**). Finally, the anterior half is placed back onto the graft and fixed with two or more cerclages (**5.6-8g–h**). Autogenous bone (or pieces of resected fragments) can be transplanted to the bone interface, or strut grafts with cerclage can be used to stabilize the interface itself. The advantage of this technique is that early mobilization of the joint is possible. The disadvantages of using allografts arise from the complicated surgical technique—associated with almost twice the risk of infection found normally with standard revision operations—and an increased risk of refracture, nonunion, and bone resorption. Clatworthy et al [1] reported a survival rate of APCs of 72% after 10 years and Kassab et al [2] a union rate of 90%.

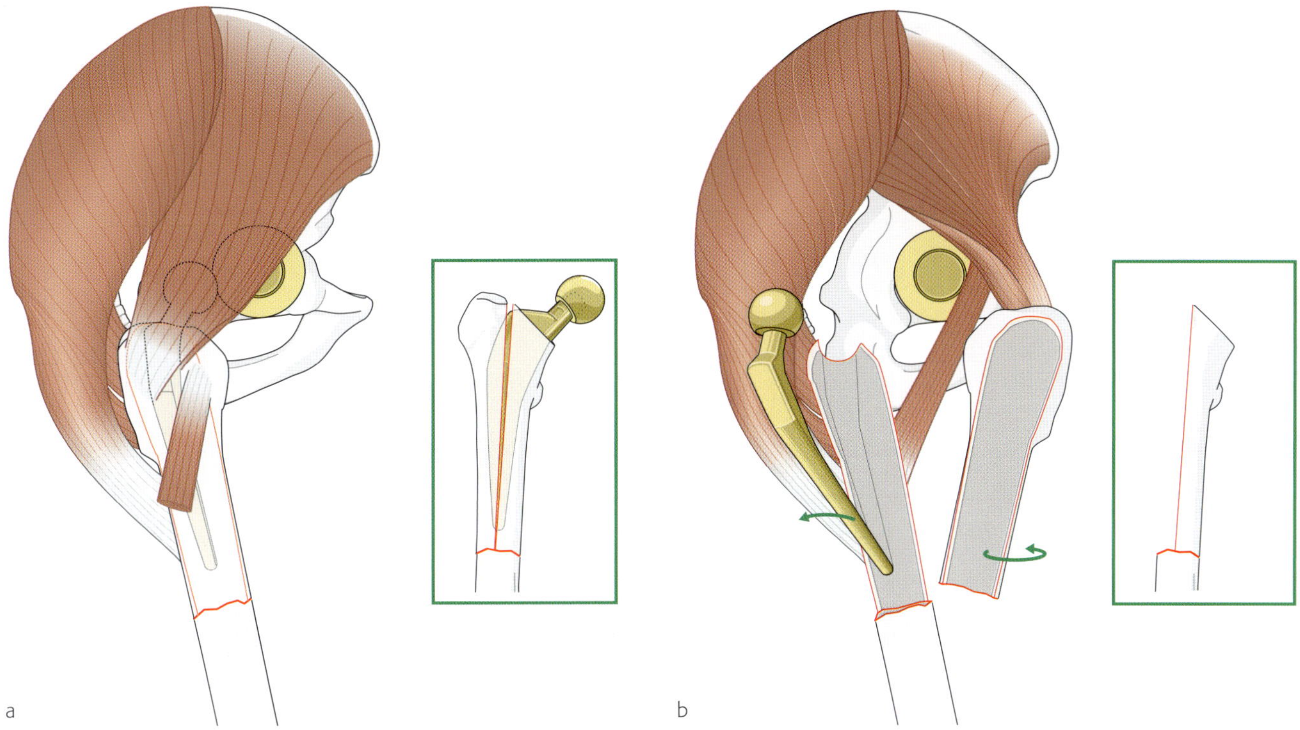

a

b

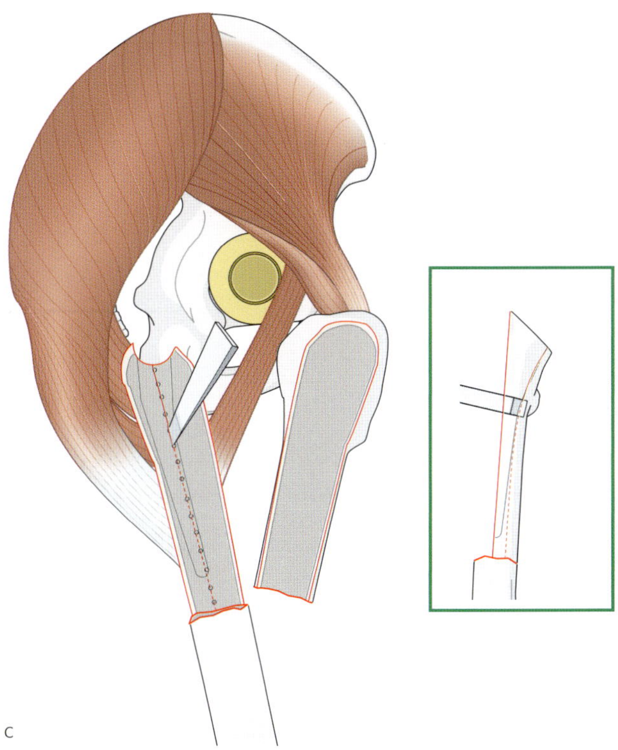

c

5.6-8a–h Allograft-prosthetic composite (APC) in the proximal femur.

a The external rotators are left attached to the femur by leaving the posterior 1 cm of the greater trochanter in contact with the femur.

b Osteotomy of the proximal part of the femur in the frontal plane, which allows removal of the prosthesis and cement while maintaining all important muscle insertions.

c The remaining dorsal half of the cortical sleeve is split with an osteotome or saw, taking care to preserve all muscle insertions.

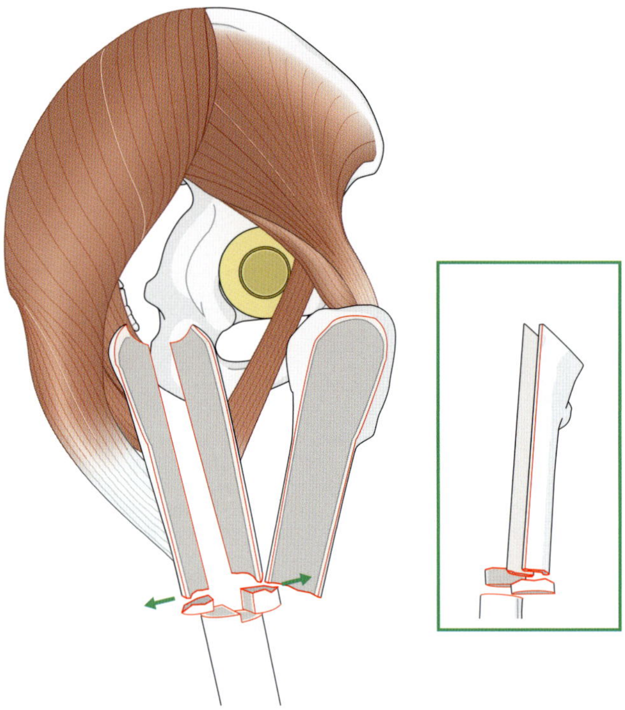

d

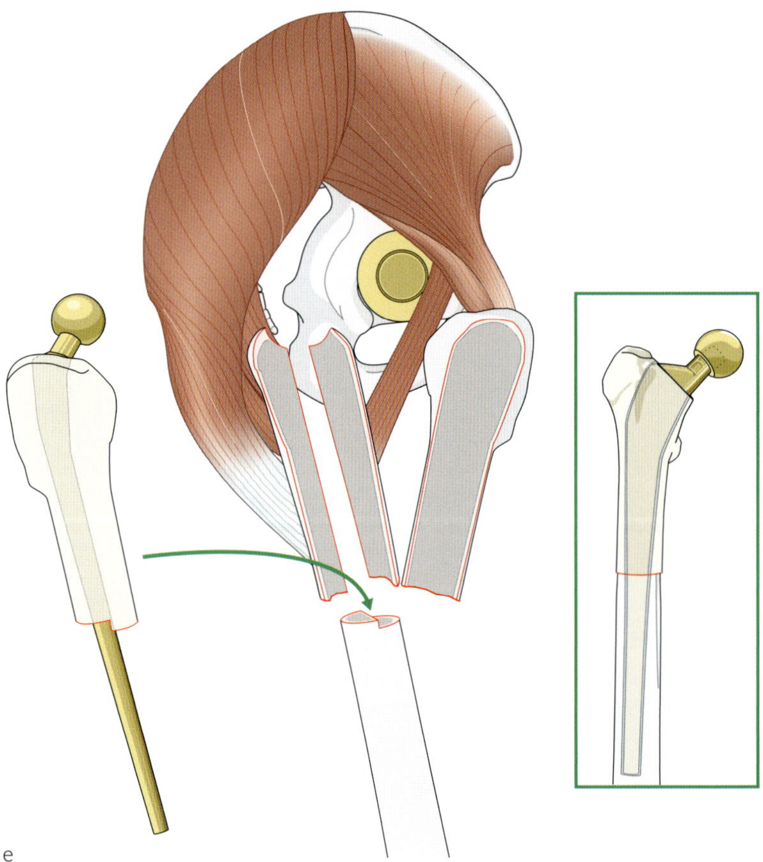

e

5.6-8a–h (cont) Allograft-prosthetic composite (APC) in the proximal femur.

- **d** Any fragments at the fracture site are removed to produce a step-cut osteotomy.
- **e** The slightly smaller APC is inserted into the intact femur with a step-cut osteotomy and fixed distally with cement.

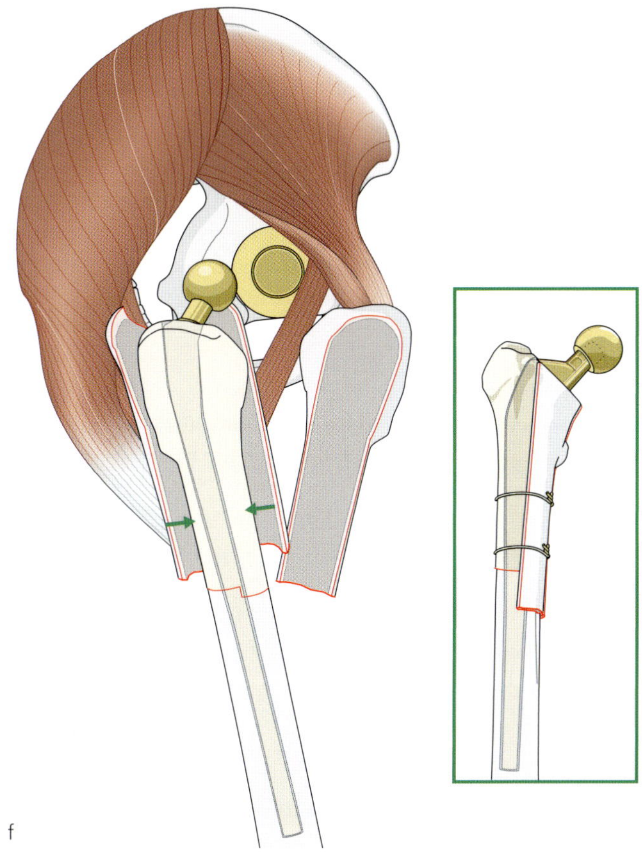

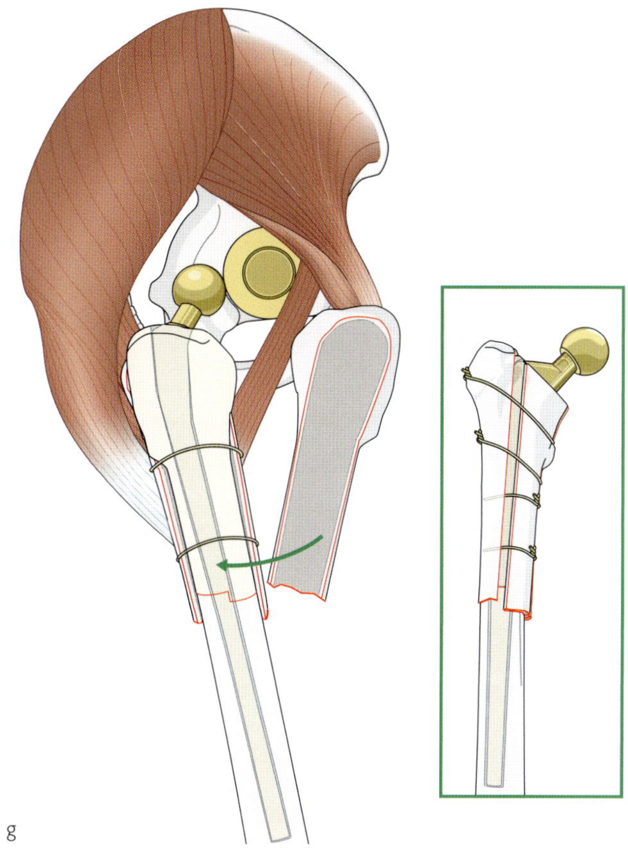

5.6-8a–h (cont) Allograft-prosthetic composite (APC) in the proximal femur.

f The dorsolateral and dorsomedial cortical slices are placed around the allograft and fixed with two cerclage wires.

g The anterolateral fragment with the greater trochanter and the attached small gluteal muscles is placed over the APC and is also fixed with two or more cerclage wires.

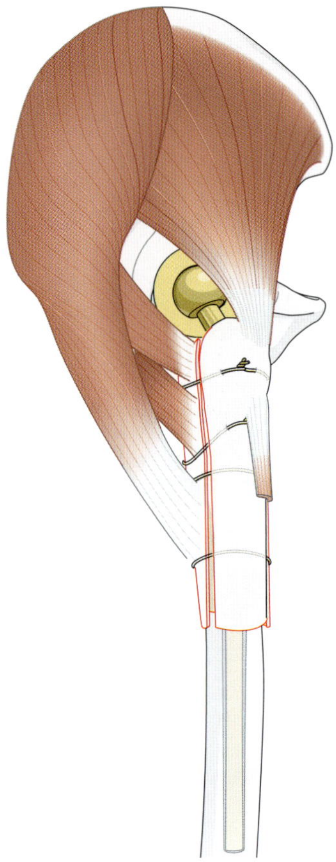

h

5.6-8a–h (cont) Allograft-prosthetic composite (APC) in the proximal femur.
h The prosthesis is reduced and the anatomy of the proximal femur reconstructed.

Scenario 4: Transprosthetic fracture in a cemented prosthesis

Problem

In rare situations, a fracture of the entire femur as well as of the implanted, cemented prosthesis may occur after extensive type E injuries. The standard approach in these cases is the revision to a noncemented stem. Revision with complete removal of the cement may, however, be a problem, particularly in patients with poor health.

Solution

For patients with impaired general health condition in combination with a low-activity level, minimal solutions that deliver mediocre stability but reduce the invasiveness of the operation significantly are indicated. The primary goal in these cases is that the patient survives the operation and starts with weight bearing immediately after the operation.

Case example: For this 86-year-old woman with an impaired general health condition (**5.6-9a**), it was decided to exchange the broken prosthesis, only leaving the surrounding cement mantle in situ. The new prosthesis was fixed again with low-viscosity cement using the "cement-in-cement" technique (**5.6-9b–c**). In addition, the fracture was stabilized with a lateral plate and a medially applied strut graft to reinforce the critical fracture zone and secure the rotation. With this technique it was possible to achieve a simple revision of the prosthesis with a minor surgical intervention. It is, however, mandatory to know the design and size of the previously used implant to achieve a good fit in the cement mantle. The patient returned to full weight bearing and the strut graft was eventually integrated 2 years postoperatively (**5.6-9d–e**).

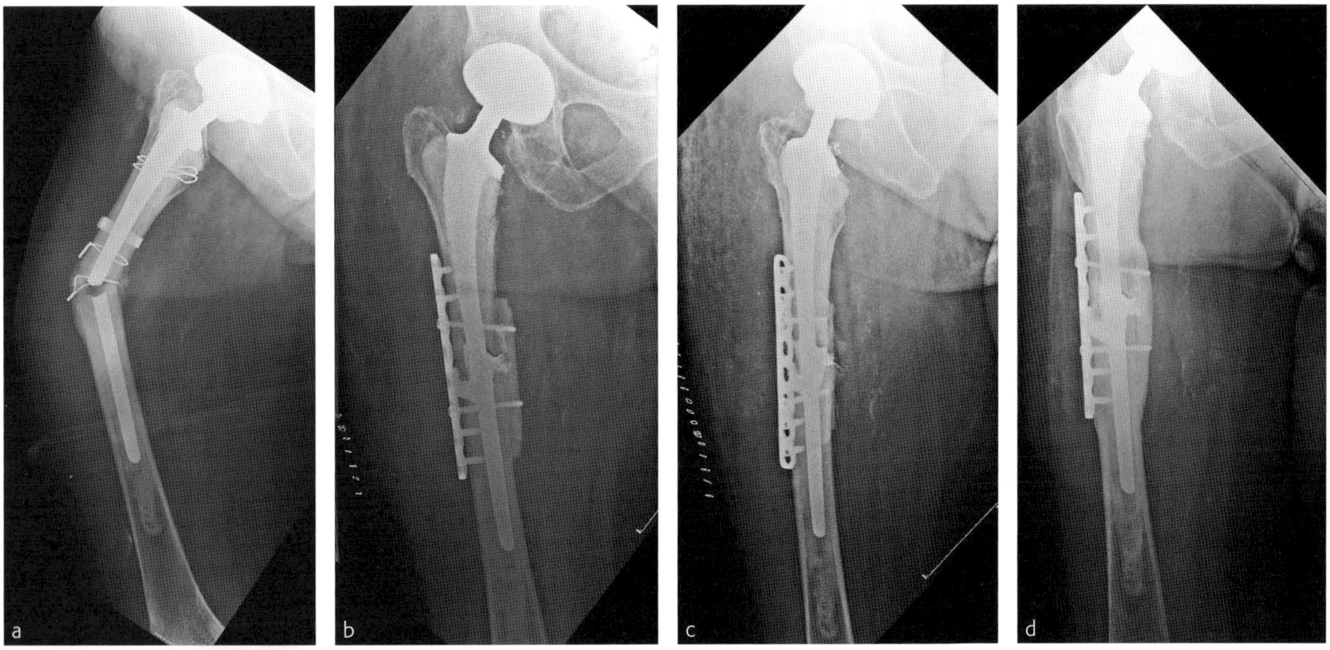

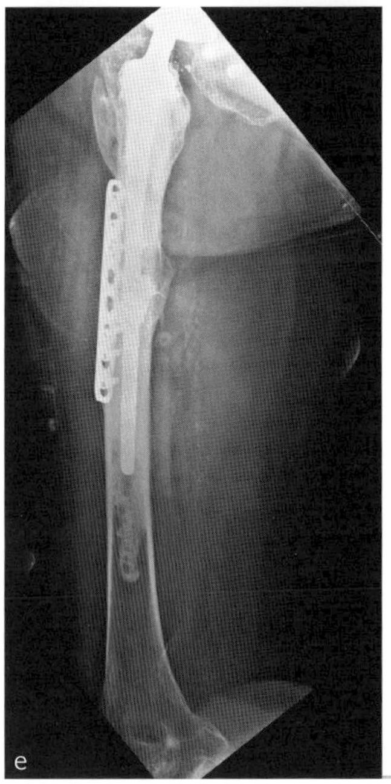

5.6-9a–e An 86-year-old woman with a transprosthetic fracture (type IV.3-E).

a AP view of the transverse fracture of both femur and prosthesis.

b AP view after revision surgery. The broken parts of the prosthesis were removed, conserving the cement sleeve carefully. After reduction of the fracture and fixation with a lateral plate and medial strut graft, a prosthesis of the same design and size was inserted with cement into the existing cement sleeve in the distal fragment.

c Lateral view postoperatively.

d AP view showing a nice integration of the strut graft.

e Lateral view.

Scenario 5: Periprosthetic fracture of the acetabulum

Problem

Fatigue fractures of the bone surrounding the acetabulum after loosening and dislocation of the prosthetic-cup component are usually the result of a delayed revision and not only pertain to an isolated column fracture but rather to a pelvic discontinuity.

Solution

The acetabular roof defect is augmented by metallic tantalum and the fracture is bridged by screw fixation of both the augmented material and the supporting acetabular-ring implant. This simultaneous fracture stabilization and revision of the acetabular-cup component can be performed in a single intervention through one approach, thereby minimizing surgical trauma.

Case example: This 70-year-old woman had a fatigue fracture of the ilium associated with extensive loosening and migration of the entire hip prosthesis (**5.6-10a–c**). The aim of the operative strategy is the stabilization of the fracture as well as the reconstruction of bony defects and stable implant fixation. For defect reconstruction, the tantalum wedge was used in combination with an acetabular-ring implant. The screws for fixation of the implant were also used for stabilization of the fracture. In addition, the stable fixed wedge leads to higher rotation stability of the ring (preventing posterior dislocation) and optimizes the position of the ring in cranial-caudal direction. Thus, the inferior flange of the ring is stably fixed within the ischium.

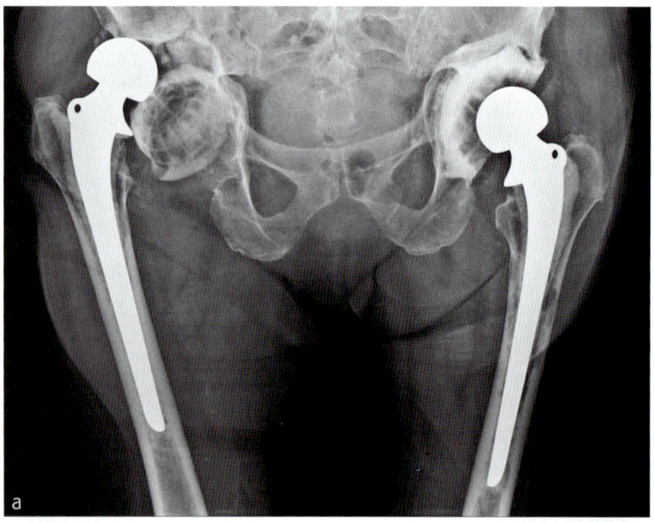

a

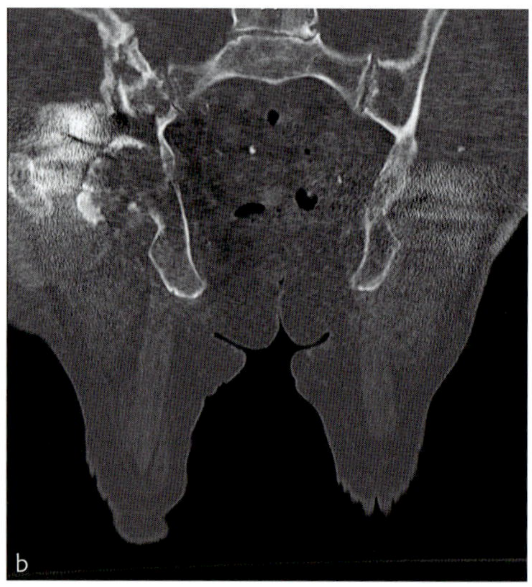

b

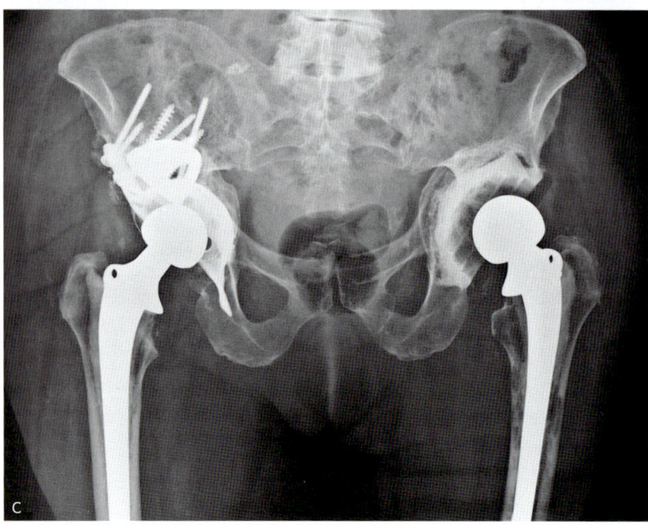

c

5.6-10a–c A 70-year-old woman with a fatigue fracture of the ilium due to dislocation and periprosthetic osteolysis of the acetabulum. The posterior column appears stable (type IV.6-B3).

a AP view of the pelvis showing the dislocated and loosened prosthesis.
b Computed tomographic scan.
c Aspect after augmentation of the bone defect with a tantalum wedge and insertion of an acetabular ring with simultaneous fracture fixation with screws.

Scenario 6: Periprosthetic fractures in cases with poor bone quality and contained defects

Problem

The standard technique to revise a loose prosthesis in a periprosthetic fracture is the use of a noncemented revision implant with press-fit anchorage because a cemented prosthesis would require cancellous bone for adequate purchase. However, in patients with severe osteoporosis a satisfactory press-fit often cannot be achieved.

Solution

In elderly patients with a generally low activity level, cemented anchoring can be obtained technically, although the cancellous bone has usually been destroyed by the previous prosthesis. More importantly, bone cement is not an "adhesive" but needs cancellous bone for stable anchoring. Cancellous bone, however, usually has been destroyed by the previous prosthesis, and cemented revision endoprosthetics of the femoral shaft is known to produce poor results. In these circumstances, the impaction-grafting technique may provide stable anchoring, the aim being to prepare at least the region distal to the fracture for an adequate anchorage in cancellous bone. In the ideal situation of a spiral fracture, the femur can be reduced anatomically with cerclage wires while the closed femoral "tube" is filled with cancellous bone before insertion of the prosthesis.

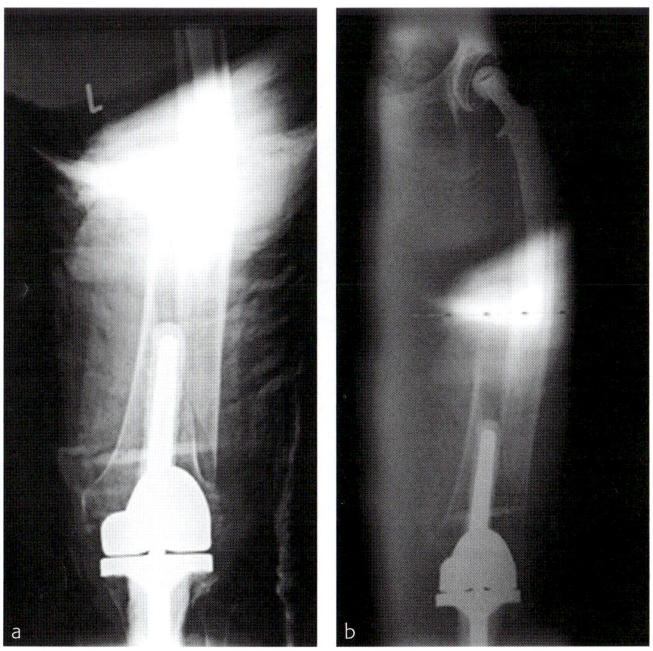

5.6-11a–b A 76-year-old woman sustained an interprosthetic fracture after a fall during the night. The femur prosthesis had been implanted 8 years ago, and the hinged knee prosthesis 6 years ago. Up to the injury the patient was ambulasting independently with a wheel walker.

Scenario 7: Interprosthetic fracture salvaged with double plating

Problem

This 76-years-old—medically fragile—patient sustained an intercalcary femur fracture (V3.-D)—(**5.6-11a–b**). Besides all challenges of an interprosthetic fracture, a hinged knee prosthesis sometimes offers only limited options for a secure fixation of the distal femoral fragment. This may require somehow more unusual fixation techniques with, for example, buttressing from the medial side.

Solution A

A solution for the presented challenging situation could be the exchange of the knee and/or femur prosthesis to a connected prosthesis (custom made) or even a total femur replacement. These suggested surgeries are obviously rather extensive and—in an elderly patient—associated with a clearly increased general risk.

Solution B

After improving the general condition of the patient, a lateral locked plating (open technique) procedure was carried out uneventfully. Intraoperatively it was recognized that due to the shape of the knee prosthesis only monocortical screws (up to 36 mm) could be placed in the distal fragment for fixation (**5.6-12a–c**). Shortly after initial mobilization, the fixation failed distally and a reoperation was required (**5.6-13a–b**). For the preoperative planning a model of the knee prosthesis was used, showing that it should be possible to place 2 long screws in the anterior section in front of the metal shield (**5.6-14**). Furthermore, a locked plate (broad 4.5/5.0 LCP plate—only straight version available at that time) from the medial side was percutaneously inserted to add additional support to the distal fragment. The further course was uneventful and guided by gentle mobilization of the patient. The x-rays after 6 months showed ongoing fracture healing (**5.6-15a–b**) with the implants in an unchanged position.

While this was a case treated in 2002, today the fracture fixation would have been improved with the option of using variable-angled locked plating, additional locking attachment plates and most likely a longer lateral plate up to the trochanter area. For buttressing on the medial side a curved 4.5/5.0 LCP plate would have been chosen today.

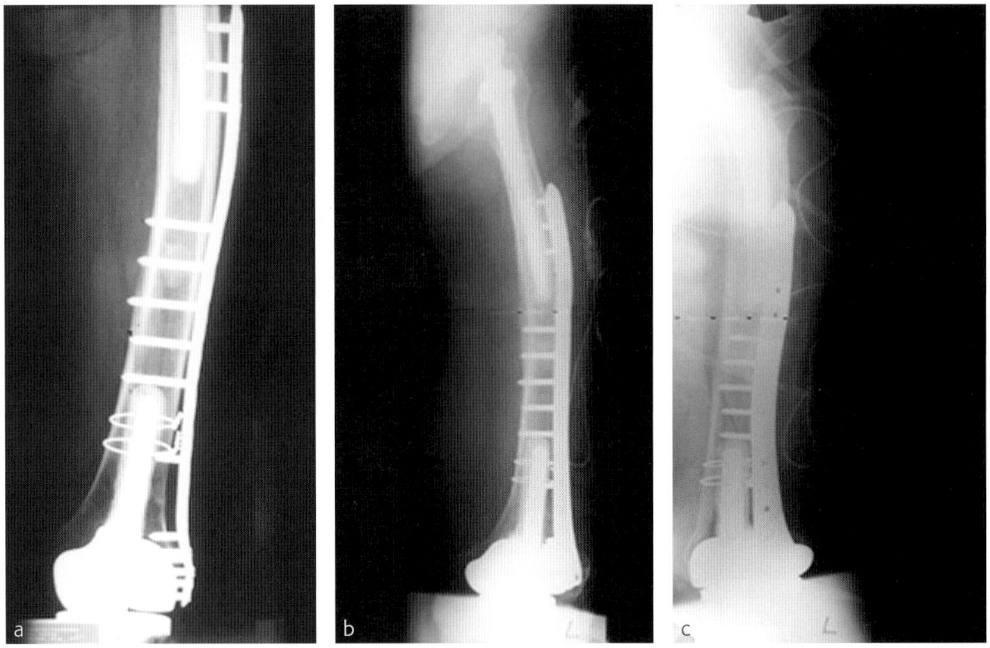

5.6-12a–c The postoperatve films demonstrate the fixation with a LISS plate in a good position. To meet the patient's anatomy, the proximal part of the plate had to be bent to match the pre-exiting varus alignment of the femur, while two cerclages were used to reduce the fracture.

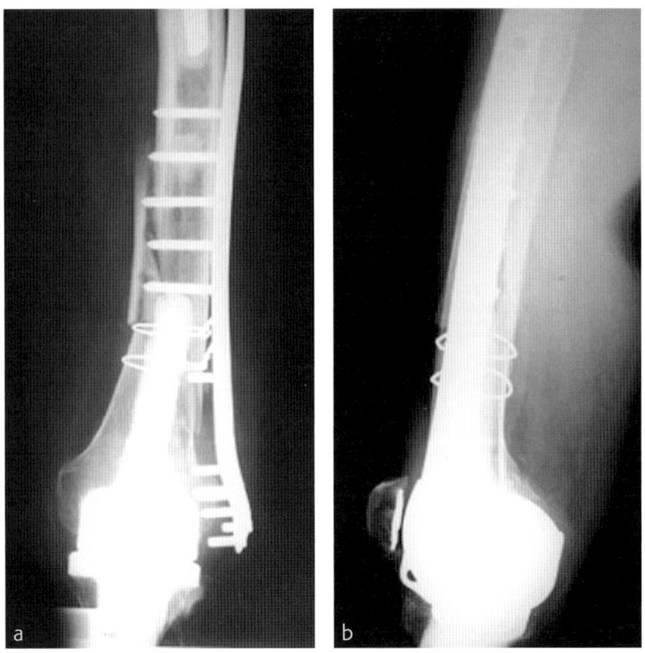

5.6-13a–b Mobilization of the patient was started 4 days postoperatively. Her level of pain had increased significantly due to the failure of the fixation around the knee prosthesis as shown by control x-rays (**a, b**).

a AP view.
b Lateral view.

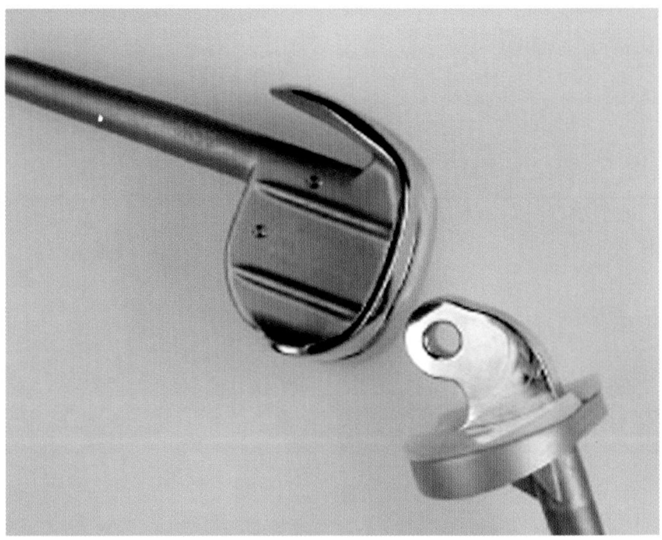

5.6-14 In preparation for the required reoperation a model of the hinged prosthesis was ordered. Measurements showed that between the front and the stem of the knee prosthesis long screws could be placed giving a better anchorage of the plate in the distal fragment.

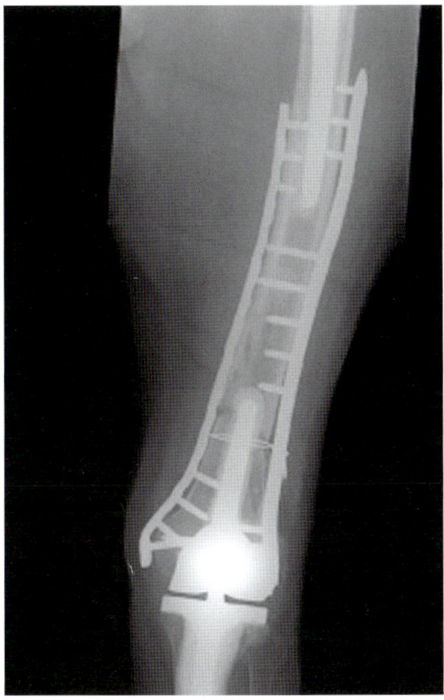

5.6-15 The 6-month follow-up x-ray shows the ongoing healing process with the fixation in place.

References

[1] **Clatworthy MG, Ballance J, Brick GW, et al.** The use of structural allograft for uncontained defects in revision total knee arthroplasty. A minimum five-year review. *J Bone Joint Surg Am.* 2001 Mar;83-A(3):404–411.

[2] **Kassab M, Zalzal P, Azores GMS, et al.** Management of periprosthetic femoral fractures after total knee arthroplasty using a distal femoral allograft. *J Arthroplasty.* 2004 Apr;19(3):361–368.

6

Periprosthetic fractures in specific anatomical locations

6.1 Shoulder

Authors **Norbert P Südkamp, Martin Jäger**

6.1.1 Incidence and risk factors

Periprosthetic fractures of the shoulder, with an incidence of 0.5–3%, are rare and usually involve the humerus [1–3]. Due to the increasing number of shoulder replacements and proximal humeral fractures, the incidence of periprosthetic fractures is also rising. They account for approximately 11% of all complications associated with total shoulder arthroplasty (TSA) and are the third most frequent complication after component loosening and instability [3]. Risk factors are described in chapter 3.2.

6.1.2 Classification

At present different—and yet in many ways similar—classification systems are used. A new Unified Classification System (UCS) has been proposed (chapter 4.2), which can be applied to the shoulder (👁 **6.1-1a–d**). The shoulder joint is numbered "I", the humerus "1", and the scapula "14".

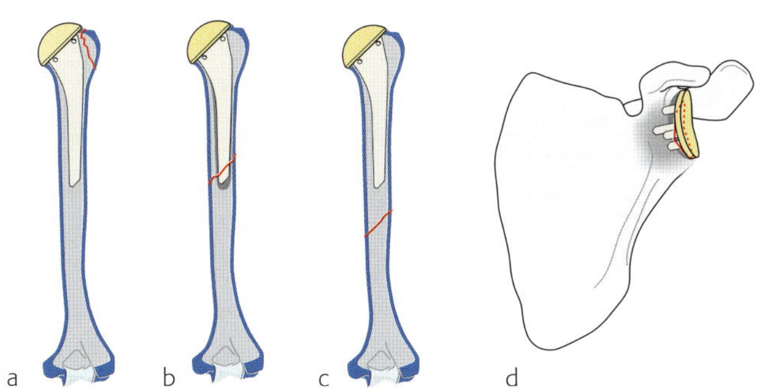

👁 **6.1-1a–d** Examples of periprosthetic fracture types in the shoulder according to the Unified Classification System (UCS).
a Type I.1-A1.
b Type I.1-B2.
c Type I.1-C.
d Type I.14-B3.

6.1.3 Preoperative planning

It is crucial to precisely analyze the fracture. Questions that have to be answered are:

- What is the course of the fracture line
  - In relation to the implant?
  - In relation to the humerus?
- Is the prosthesis still stable?
- Are there any associated fractures?

Plain x-rays generally provide facts about the periprosthetic fracture. However, if any doubt remains about the stability of the prosthesis it is strongly recommended to perform computed tomographic (CT) scans.

If revision arthroplasty is intended, additional aspects have to be addressed. It is crucial to choose the proper type of prosthesis. In any case of superior rotator-cuff insufficiency one should at least think about "reverse" systems. The fixation of glenoid components is usually not a problem. However, it might become challenging if there is severe secondary glenoid arthrosis or after removal of glenoid components in case of conversion of an anatomical into a reversed arthroplasty. In both cases, surgeons should be prepared for bone grafting. Fixation of humeral components might become demanding after removal of a well-fixed stem or if the remaining humerus is short, small, or deviated after prior fractures.

6.1.4 Timing of surgery

Periprosthetic fractures that have occurred postoperatively are typically not an emergency situation. Therefore, they should be planned and scheduled within the first two weeks after trauma. Since these fractures are rare and often challenging, especially if a prosthetic replacement is intended, referral to a specialized shoulder clinic should be considered.

6.1.5 Choice of approach

The choice of approach depends on several factors:
- Fracture location in respect to both the humerus and the prosthesis
- Stability of the implant (fixed or loose)
- Type of intended surgery (osteosynthesis or revision arthroplasty)
- Involvement of radial nerve
- Anatomy of the humerus

Anterolateral approach for internal fixation

A commonly used approach is the anterolateral approach (**6.1-2**), which can be extended from the preexisting anterior approach of the original arthroplasty distally to the radial epicondyle. For this approach, the patient is placed on a radiolucent table in the simple supine position with a hand table to support the forearm. Alternatively, the beach-chair position can be used. The deep dissection proceeds between the biceps brachialis and brachioradialis muscles. The radial nerve is at risk in the distal third of the arm and has to be identified before further dissection. The plate itself can be positioned anteriorly or anterolateral. Sometimes the insertion of the deltoid muscle interferes with plate positioning and has to be released temporarily. The radial nerve is also at risk while drilling the posterior cortex of the humerus in the proximal part of the plate or when applying cerclage wires. A potential benefit of the anterolateral approach is the intraoperative option to convert to revision arthroplasty, if intraoperatively the prosthesis is found to be loose or when a stable osteosynthesis cannot be achieved. The anterolateral approach furthermore allows minimally

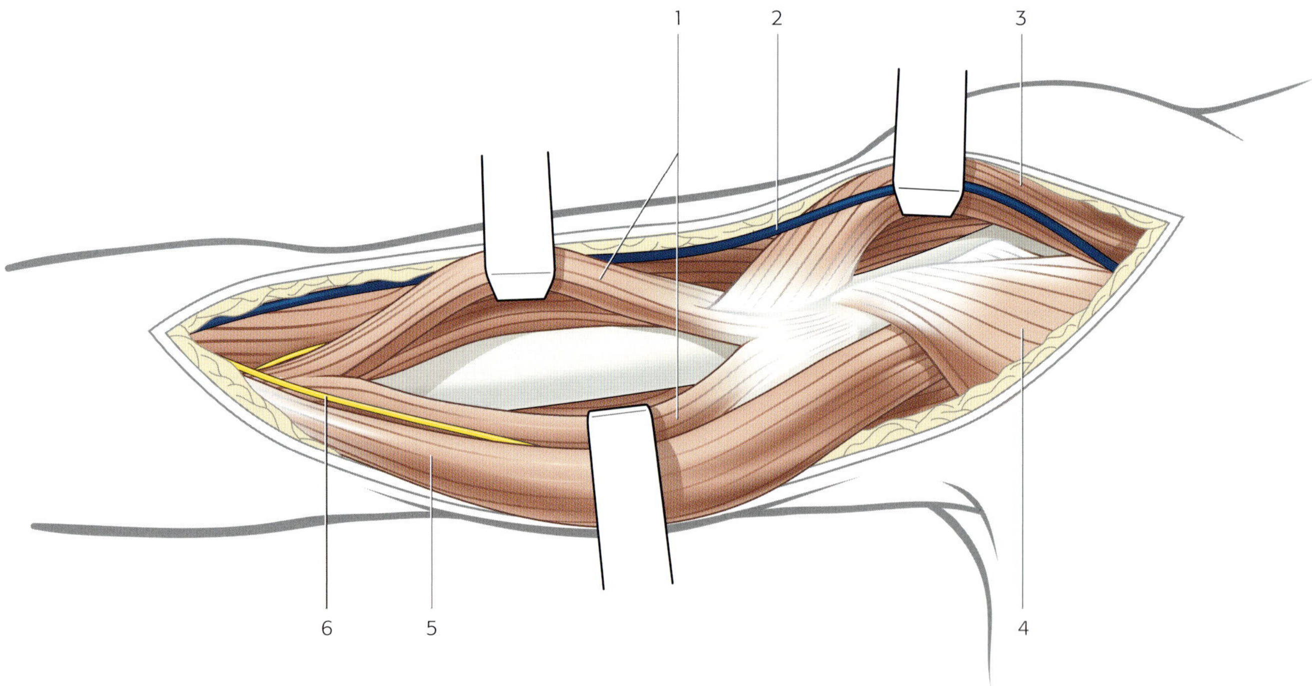

6.1-2 Anterolateral extensile approach. As the incision extends distally, the brachialis muscle is split (the lateral third of the muscle is supplied by the radial nerve and the medial two thirds by the musculocutaneous nerve) to expose the anterior surface of the distal humerus. Two nerves are at risk: the radial nerve where it pierces the intermuscular septum distally; and the musculocutaneous nerve of the forearm as it exits between the biceps brachii and brachioradialis muscle.

1 Brachialis muscle (split).
2 Cephalic vein.
3 Deltoid muscle.
4 Pectoralis major muscle.
5 Biceps brachii muscle.
6 Musculocutaneous nerve.

invasive plate insertion and an additional adhesiolysis of the subacromial and subdeltoideal bursa and/or cuff repair. This might be advisable since mose patients are elderly and usually suffer from compromised shoulder function before the periprosthetic fracture. However, there are only limited possibilities to explore the radial nerve in case of a radial nerve injury.

Posterior, triceps-splitting approach for internal fixation

Alternatively, the posterior, triceps-splitting approach (**6.1-3**) provides excellent access to the midshaft and more distal fractures. It is recommended in case of radial-nerve involvement but it allows only limited access to the proximal third of the humerus due to the overlaying deltoid muscle. The patient is best positioned in a prone or lateral position with the arm placed on a separate support, thereby allowing the intraoperativ use of image intensifier. While the radial nerve can be identified as it circles around the humerus, there is hardly any possibility to explore the prosthesis itself, the glenohumeral joint, or to perform any additional surgery such as subacromial adhesiolysis and/or cuff repair.

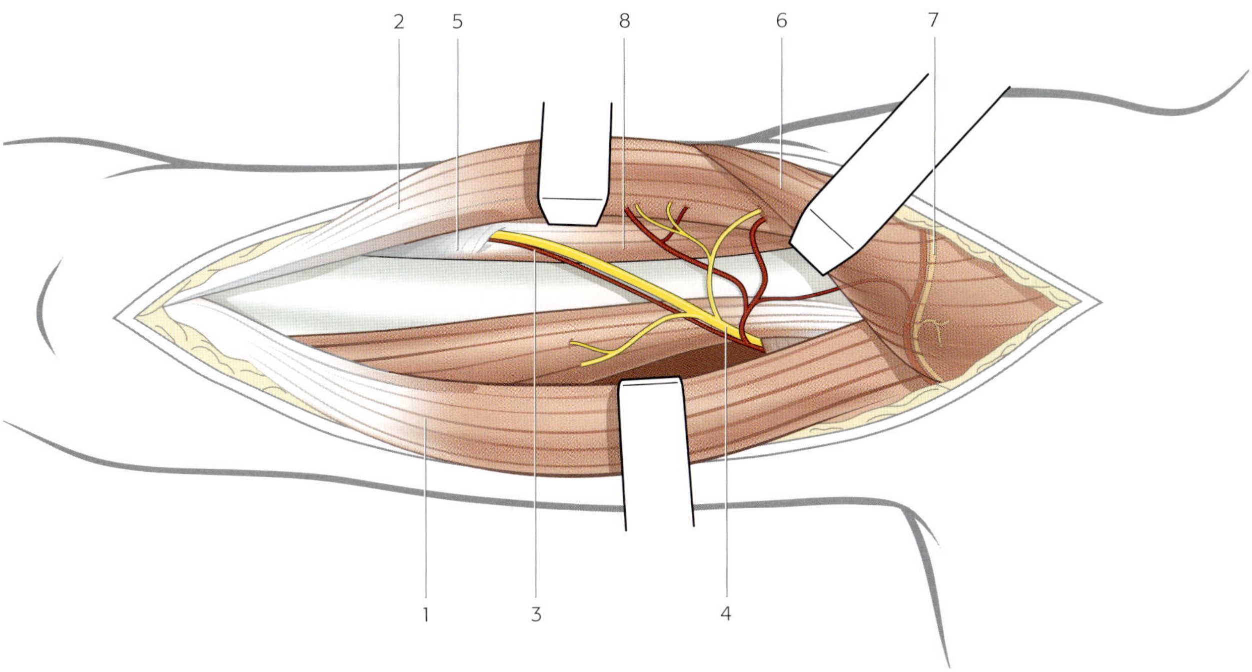

6.1-3 Posterior approach for the distal third of the humeral shaft. The triceps brachii muscle is split bluntly between the long (1) and the lateral (2) head. Distally, in the tendon, sharp dissection is necessary. The profunda brachii artery (3) runs with the radial nerve (4) in the spiral groove and is also at risk of injury. The radial nerve must be identified and traced until it passes into the intermuscular lateral septum (5). The ulnar nerve, though not generally seen, can be injured by careless retraction on the medial side of the distal wound.

1 Triceps brachii muscle, long head.
2 Triceps brachii muscle, lateral head.
3 Profunda brachii artery.
4 Radial nerve.
5 Intermuscular lateral septum.
6 Deltoid muscle.
7 Axillary nerve.
8 Brachialis muscle.

Anterolateral approach for arthroplasty

If an arthroplasty is intended, the standard anterior, deltopectoral approach is the best choice. This approach provides excellent access to the glenohumeral joint and the proximal humerus and can be extended distally without risk of harming the axillary nerve. This approach is strongly recommended if revision arthroplasty has to be done because previous surgery—especially deltoid splitting techniques—may have left scar tissue that places the axillary nerve at high risk. Similarly, lateral or anterolateral approaches should not be used, since the axillary nerve is again at risk, especially if the approach is extended distally.

6.1.6 Treatment

Decision making

Indication for operative or nonoperative treatment depends on many factors, such as

- Patient's comorbidities
- Patient's demands and expectations
- Patient's shoulder situation in terms of function and pain before trauma
- Fracture type, location, and displacement
- Implant stability
- Remaining bone stock and quality of the humerus and glenoid
- Concomitant neurological injury.

While nonoperative treatment (chapters 5.3, and 7.1) may be indicated for sick patients feeling little pain and having few expectations as to function and independent living, there seems to be a high risk of nonunion especially in simple transverse or short oblique fractures at the tip of the prosthesis or cement plug, corresponding to a type B1 injury [4–6]. An acceptable alignment is considered to be 30° in the varus/valgus plane, 20° in the flexion/extension plane, and 20° of rotation [7]. In such cases, functional bracing is recommended [4, 8].

Surgery is the treatment choice for any fracture that is difficult to reduce and stabilize, such as in obese patients. In addition, surgical treatment is indicated in loose prosthesis, significant fracture displacement or in cases of nonunion within three months of non operative treatment [2, 7]. In unstable fractures with well-fixed prosthesis, open reduction and internal fixation (ORIF) may be considered. If the prosthesis is loose, revision arthroplasty is generally recommended [9]. However, due to the low number of periprosthetic fractures and the limited studies, there is still no consensus regarding the best treatment options.

Plate osteosynthesis

Treating periprosthetic fractures is often challenging, especially if osteosynthesis (chapters 7.2–7.10, 7.13, and 7.14) is intended. One reason is that the medullary cavity is filled with a prosthesis stem leaving little space for the placement of screws for plate fixation. Furthermore, there is quite often bad bone quality with fragile bones due to the patient's osteoporosis. Both result in a reduced primary stability of the osteosynthesis. However, it is rarely possible to use bicortical screws. Therefore, locking compression plates (LCPs) are typically placed slightly eccentric to bypass the stem. In addition, cerclages may be used that encircle the whole humerus. To strengthen the stability of these cerclages, fixation using threaded cerclage-positioning caps can be done. These caps are screwed into the threaded hole of the (LCP) and hold the cerclages in place. Cerclages are well-accepted and, according to published literature, show good results. However, the circular interruption of blood supply has been considered a disadvantage. Some surgeons like to combine the application of cerclages with bone struts as grafts. The course of neurovascular structures must also be considered. Especially the radial nerve is at risk because of its proximity to the humerus. The most recent development to improve insertion of locking-head screws is the locking attachment plate (chapter 5.4.1), which is placed over the LCP and has four branches with threaded holes that are oriented to allow screw placement bypassing the stem of a prosthesis.

Intramedullary nailing

From a mechanical point of view, an intramedullary nail provides the best stability. Since a classic intramedullary nail interferes with the stem, the only way to obtain an intramedullary fixation is using a long-stemmed revision prosthesis. The stem should overlap the most distal fracture line by at least 2–3 cortical diameters [8, 10, 11]. This treatment option is elegant and recommended if the implanted prosthesis is loose. If the prosthesis is well fixed, stem replacement is more demanding and typically not necessary. Functional bracing provides the lowest biomechanical stability. Nevertheless, it is well known that most spiral-shaped humeral midshaft fractures heal uneventfully.

Revision arthroplasty

Revision arthroplasty is a highly demanding surgery (chapters 7.11 and 7.12). To achieve optimal results, the decision-making process must carefully include all pros and cons, while preoperative planning is mandatory. Revision arthroplasty is mainly indicated if the prosthesis is loose either before the trauma or due to fracture involvement. In these cases, a long-stemmed implant should be used to bridge the fracture in terms of an intramedullary nail. But it might also prove reasonable if the stem is well integrated, especially in case of preexisting rotator-cuff insufficiency or a symptomatic secondary glenoid arthrosis after hemiarthroplasty.

Typical problems are periprosthetic fractures after anatomical fracture arthroplasty with a well-fixed stem and initial poor shoulder function. It is well known that the outcome of fracture arthroplasty strongly depends on ingrowth of the tuberosities [12–15]. Often malpositioning and migration of the tuberosity with resulting rotator-cuff dysfunction is present. A similar problem is seen in secondary cuff failure after shoulder arthroplasty for degenerative diseases combined with a periprosthetic fracture. As it is not possible to examine shoulder function due to a painful periprosthetic fracture, it is necessary that surgeons look for anamnestic hints and typical radiological findings. These show eccentric prosthetic heads, mainly having migrated upward, subacromial erosions, and/or loosened glenoid components due to a rocking-horse phenomenon. If so, converting a failed anatomical hemiarthroplasty into a reversed TSA may improve the clinical outcome in terms of pain relieve and restoration of function [16–18].

Similar considerations should be taken in case of symptomatic secondary glenoid erosion after anatomical hemiarthroplasty. This might occur in up to 20.6% of all cases and is unique for humeral hemiarthroplasty [9]. Cardinal symptoms are pain and reduced shoulder function. In these cases it might prove to be reasonable to convert the hemiarthroplasty into a long-stemmed TSA. At least an extended soft-tissue release should be performed to reduce the soft-tissue pressure on the glenoid.

In any of these cases, surgeons need to carefully balance the patient's comorbidities and demands on the one side with the necessary extension of the operative trauma on the other. If surgery is intended, it might be reasonable to just fix the fracture (eg, with a plate) and accept poor shoulder function due to rotator-cuff dysfunction. However, removal of the integrated stem by the technique described by Gohlke and Rolf [19] and conversion to a long-stemmed, bridging reversed shoulder arthroplasty not only can restore but also improve shoulder function [20].

The type of prosthesis depends on the integrity of the rotator cuff, the condition of the already implanted components, and the remaining bone stock, especially on the glenoid side. Both, cemented and noncemented revision stems allow good clinical results [2]. However, surgeons must be careful to prevent cement extrusion at the fracture site since this would compromise fracture healing and might violate neural structures, eg, the radial nerve [21].

6.1.7 Complications and outcome

Due to limited reports and the lack of controlled trials, there is still no consensus on how to treat periprosthetic fractures of the shoulder. Literature focusing on nonoperative treatment of periprosthetic fractures is heterogeneous. Many surgeons favor nonoperative treatment [3, 4, 7, 11, 22–24]. However, there are some reports showing a high failure rate of up to 83% [4, 6, 25].

The main goal of operative treatment is to achieve bony healing and to maintain or even improve shoulder function. Therefore, cerclages, screws, plates, or long-stemmed prostheses are commonly used.

Most studies report satisfactory results if displaced fractures with well-fixed implants are stabilized with ORIF using plates [6–28]. Often additional cerclages were used for proximal fixation. Recently, Wutzler et al [27] presented a retrospective analysis of six patients with postoperative periprosthetic fractures with a mean follow-up of 62 weeks. Five of six patients treated by angular-stable plating showed satisfactory functional results with disability of arm, shoulder, and hand and Constant scores comparable with those described after primary shoulder arthroplasty [27]. The sixth patient with the unsatisfactory result had sustained radial nerve damage that was probably caused by severe fracture dislocation and did not recover over time. This patient suffered several episodes of plate loosening and breakage, and was finally treated successfully with a long LCP, additional cable wires, cancellous bone graft, and bone morphogenetic protein.

In 2008, Groh et al [8] published a retrospective study including 6 of 15 patients with perioperative fractures. Of these, one occurred proximal to the tip of the stem four presented a fracture line running from proximal to distal of the prosthesis tip and one was located entirely distal of the tip. Except for one type II fracture, all these postoperative periprosthetic fractures were treated nonoperatively in a fracture orthosis. Open reduction and internal fixation was performed using a compression plate 4.5 secured with cables proximally and screws distally. All fractures healed uneventfully within an average of 11 weeks.

Alternatively, interfragmentary compression cerclages and clamps were used to fix the periprosthetic humeral fracture.

Both implants provided uneventful fracture healing in all reported cases [28–32]. Using cerclages, the cable passer should be passed with direct contact to the bone perpendicular to the humeral shaft around the humerus. In doubt, the radial nerve should be explored to reduce the risk of iatrogenic damage. De Smet et al [29] reports the benefits of broad titanium ribbons. Histological studies have shown the preservation of vital bone underneath these ribbons [4]. However, routinely there seems to be no need for iliac-crest bone grafting [8]. Some authors [31–34] recommend the use of strut allograft augmentation. This might be advantageous, especially if little bone stock is left, compromising both, initial fixation of cables on the medial side and bony healing. Talbot et al [35] were able to demonstrate the biomechanical superiority of strut allograft augmentation after cyclic loading for 100,000 cycles compared with a stand-alone locking plate. Martinez et al [32] reported on six patients treated with strut allograft augmentation. They observed bony union in all cases without any complications. The mean time of union was 5.4 months. However, three patients showed graft-to-host union and in three others the graft had been resorbed.

Jonas et al [36] have provided a recent extension of the spectrum of osteosynthesis in periprosthetic fractures. They described a successful osteosynthesis using a proximal humeral internal locking system plate in a 68-year-old man who had undergone resurfacing TSA due to glenohumeral osteoarthritis. This example may encourage shoulder surgeons to use resurfacing TSAs more often. There are also indications that the incidence of periprosthetic fractures using this type of prosthesis is even lower compared with stemmed implants [37].

References

[1] **Della Rocca GJ, Leung KS, Pape HC.** Periprosthetic fractures: epidemiology and future projections. *J Orthop Trauma.* 2011 Jun;25 Suppl 2:S66–70.

[2] **Steinmann SP, Cheung EV.** Treatment of periprosthetic humerus fractures associated with shoulder arthroplasty. *J Am Acad Orthop Surg.* 2008 Apr;16(4):199–207.

[3] **Bohsali KI, Wirth MA, Rockwood CA, Jr.** 2006 Complications of total shoulder arthroplasty. *J Bone Joint Surg Am.* 88:2279–2292.

[4] **Wright TW, Cofield RH.** Humeral fractures after shoulder arthroplasty. *J Bone Joint Surg Am.* 1995 Sep;77(9):1340–1346.

[5] **Bonutti PM, Hawkins RJ.** Fracture of the humeral shaft associated with total replacement arthroplasty of the shoulder. A case report. *J Bone Joint Surg Am.* 1992 Apr;74(4):617–618.

[6] **Boyd AD Jr, Thornhill TS, Barnes CL.** Fractures adjacent to humeral prostheses. *J Bone Joint Surg Am.* 1992 Dec;74(10):1498–1504.

[7] **Kumar S, Sperling JW, Haidukewych GH, et al.** Periprosthetic humeral fractures after shoulder arthroplasty. *J Bone Joint Surg Am.* 2004 Apr;86-A(4):680–689.

[8] **Groh GI, Heckman MM, Wirth MA, et al.** Treatment of fractures adjacent to humeral prostheses. *J Shoulder Elbow Surg.* 2008 Jan-Feb;17(1):85–89.

[9] **Gonzalez JF, Alami GB, Baque F, et al.** Complications of unconstrained shoulder prostheses. *J Shoulder Elbow Surg.* 2011 Jun;20(4):666–682.

[10] **McDonough EB, Crosby LA.** Periprosthetic fractures of the humerus. *Am J Orthop (Belle Mead NJ).* 2005 Dec;34(12):586–591.

[11] **Campbell JT, Moore RS, Iannotti JP, et al.** Periprosthetic humeral fractures: mechanisms of fracture and treatment options. *J Shoulder Elbow Surg.* 1998 Jul–Aug;7(4):406–413.

[12] **Fialka C, Stampfl P, Arbes S, et al.** Primary hemiarthroplasty in four-part fractures of the proximal humerus: randomized trial of two different implant systems. *J Shoulder Elbow Surg.* 2008 Mar–Apr;17(2):210–215.

[13] **Krause FG, Huebschle L, Hertel R.** Reattachment of the tuberosities with cable wires and bone graft in hemiarthroplasties done for proximal humeral fractures with cable wire and bone graft: 58 patients with a 22-month minimum follow-up. *J Orthop Trauma.* 2007 Nov–Dec;21(10):682–686.

[14] **Kralinger F, Schwaiger R, Wambacher M, et al.** Outcome after primary hemiarthroplasty for fracture of the head of the humerus. A retrospective multicentre study of 167 patients. *J Bone Joint Surg Br.* 2004 Mar;86(2):217–219.

[15] **Boileau P, Krishnan SG, Tinsi L, et al.** Tuberosity malposition and migration: reasons for poor outcomes after hemiarthroplasty for displaced fractures of the proximal humerus. *J Shoulder Elbow Surg.* 2002 Sep–Oct;11(5):401–412.

[16] **Groh GI, Wirth MA.** Results of revision from hemiarthroplasty to total shoulder arthroplasty utilizing modular component systems. *J Shoulder Elbow Surg.* 2011 Jul;20(5):778–782.

[17] **Martin TG, Iannotti JP.** Reverse total shoulder arthroplasty for acute fractures and failed management after proximal humeral fractures. *Orthop Clin North Am.* 2008 Oct;39(4):451–457.

[18] **Boileau P, Watkinson D, Hatzidakis AM, et al.** Neer Award 2005: The Grammont reverse shoulder prosthesis: results in cuff tear arthritis, fracture sequelae, and revision arthroplasty. *J Shoulder Elbow Surg.* 2006 Sep–Oct;15(5):527–540.

[19] **Gohlke F, Rolf O.** [Revision of failed fracture hemiarthroplasties to reverse total shoulder prosthesis through the transhumeral approach: method incorporating a pectoralis-major-pedicled bone window]. *Oper Orthop Traumatol.* 2007 Jun;19(2):185–208. German.

[20] **Greiner S, Stein V, Scheibel M.** Periprosthetic humeral fractures after shoulder and elbow arthroplasty. *Acta Chir Orthop Traumatol Cech.* 2011;78(6):490–500.

[21] **Sherfey MC, Edwards TB.** Cement extrusion causing radial nerve palsy after shoulder arthroplasty: a case report. *J Shoulder Elbow Surg.* 2009 May–Jun;18(3):e21–24.

[22] **Williams GR Jr, Iannotti JP.** Management of periprosthetic fractures: the shoulder. *J Arthroplasty.* 2002 Jun;17(4 Suppl 1):14–16.

[23] **Wirth MA, Rockwood CA Jr.** Complications of total shoulder-replacement arthroplasty. *J Bone Joint Surg Am.* 1996 Apr;78(4):603–616.

[24] **Wirth MA, Rockwood CA Jr.** Complications of shoulder arthroplasty. *Clin Orthop Relat Res.* 1994 Oct;(307):47–69.

[25] **Worland RL, Kim DY, Arredondo J, et al.** Periprosthetic humeral fractures: management and classification. *J Shoulder Elbow Surg.* 1999 Nov-Dec;8(6):590–594.

[26] **Kent ME, Sinopidis C, Brown DJ, et al.** The locking compression plate in periprosthetic humeral fractures. *A review of two cases.* Injury. 2005 Oct;36(10):1241–1245.

[27] **Wutzler S, Laurer HL, Huhnstock S, et al.** Periprosthetic humeral fractures after shoulder arthroplasty: operative management and functional outcome. *Arch Orthop Trauma Surg.* 2009 Feb;129(2):237–243.

[28] **Christoforakis JJ, Sadiq S, Evans MJ.** Use of a Dall-Miles plate and cables for the fixation of a periprosthetic humeral fracture. *Acta Chir Belg.* 2003 Dec;69(6):562–565.

[29] **De Smet L, Debeer P, Degreef I.** Fixation of a periprosthetic humeral fracture with CCG-cable system. *Acta Chir Belg.* 2005 Sep–Oct;105(5):543–544.

[30] **Lill H, Hepp P, Rose T, et al.** Mennen clamp-on plate fixation of periprosthetic fractures of the humerus after shoulder arthroplasty—a report on 3 patients. *Acta Orthop Scand.* 2004 Dec;75(6):772–774.

[31] **Edwards TB, Stuart KD, Trappey GJ, et al.** 2011 Utility of polymer cerclage cables in revision shoulder arthroplasty. *Orthopedics.* 2011 Apr;34(4). doi: 10.3928/01477447-20110228-13.

[32] **Martinez AA, Calvo A, Cuenca J, et al.** Internal fixation and strut allograft augmentation for periprosthetic humeral fractures. *J Orthop Surg (Hong Kong).* 2011 Aug;9(2):191–193.

[33] **Kelly JD 2nd, Zhao JX, Hobgood ER, et al.** Clinical results of revision shoulder arthroplasty using the reverse prosthesis. *J Shoulder Elbow Surg.* 2012 Nov;21(11):1516–1525.

[34] **Kieser DC, Taylor F, Ball CM.** The allograft sleeve: a case report of the surgical management of an interprosthetic fracture between a shoulder and elbow joint replacement. *J Shoulder Elbow Surg.* 2011 Apr;20(3):e4–9.

[35] **Talbot M, Zdero R, Schemitsch EH.** Cyclic loading of periprosthetic fracture fixation constructs. *J Trauma.* 2008 May;64(5):1308–1312.

[36] **Jonas SC, Walton MJ, Sarangi PP.** Management of a periprosthetic fracture after humeral head resurfacing total shoulder replacement: a case report. *J Shoulder Elbow Surg.* 2011 Jul;20(5):e18–21.

[37] **Burgess DL, McGrath MS, Bonutti PM, et al.** Shoulder resurfacing. *J Bone Joint Surg Am.* 2009 May;91(5):1228–1238.

6.2 Elbow

Authors Arvind G von Keudell, Jesse B Jupiter

6.2.1 Introduction

Considerable advance has been made in the designs and applications of total elbow arthroplasty (TEA) since the original description by Venable in 1952 [1]. The indications have also expanded from advanced osteoarthritis or rheumatoid arthritis to nonreconstructable fractures, nonunion of the distal humerus, or following tumor resection. Yet, various complications continue to plague both surgeons and patients and have been reported to vary from 20–45% of all TEAs [2]. Among the complications that prove most challenging are those of periprosthetic fractures. It has been suggested that 5% of all patients with primary TEAs will experience a periprosthetic fracture, with the number occurring after revision surgery not readily known [3]. Revision as well as internal fixation of a periprosthetic fracture about an elbow arthroplasty is much more challenging compared with those in the lower limb because of factors such as poorer and thinner bone stock, the routine use of cemented stems, the close association of the major peripheral nerves in the upper limb, and, on occasion, an unstable soft-tissue envelope.

6.2.2 Classification

Presently different—and yet in many ways similar—classification systems are used. A new Unified Classification System (UCS) has been proposed (chapter 4.2), which can be applied to the elbow (**Fig 6.2-1a–c**). The elbow joint is numbered "II", the humerus "1", and the ulna "2".

6.2.3 Treatment

General considerations

It is recommended to use the previous incision and refrain from forming large skin flaps. The general tactics regarding the repair of a periprosthetic fracture about a total elbow prosthesis starts with identification of the ulnar and radial nerve, evaluation of the stability of the implants, subsequent removal of loose implants, membranes and cement, taking of bacteriological cultures, fracture reduction, and fixation with an allograft strut and/or plate and cables. If the ulnar nerve has not already been transferred anteriorly, this should be performed now, and the nerve should also be freed from scar tissue in case of preexisting neuropathy. Particular care is recommended in the presence of poor bone stock or even osteolysis in order not to injure the radial nerve.

Humeral fractures

Fractures of the condyle of the humerus are the most common among periprosthetic fractures. They occur most often due to poor bone stock during or after surgery. If the quality of bone is sufficient, extraarticular fractures types A1 and A2 can be treated nonoperatively (chapter 5.3) with a low threshold for follow-up x-rays and continuous monitoring. A type B1 fracture, corresponding to a well-fixed prosthetic stem, requires fixation with a plate or cerclage wires, while in types B2 and B3—with a loose implant (chapters 8.1 and 8.2) and frequently poor bone stock—bone-defect revision procedures are recommended using a strut allograft or revision with an allograft-prosthetic composite, or ultimately replacement of the distal segment using a tumor prosthesis [4]. When revising the humeral component, it is mandatory to take care not to penetrate the cortical bone and subsequently injure the radial nerve—even when applying the latest ultrasonic or heat polymerization devices.

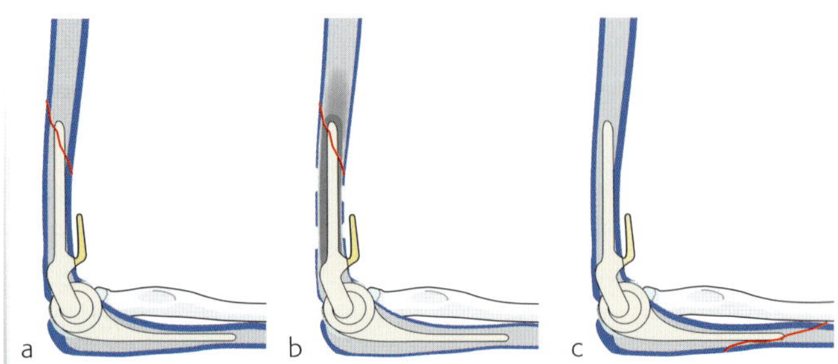

6.2-1a–c Examples of periprosthetic fracture types in the elbow according to the Unified Classification System (UCS).
a Type II.1-B1.
b Type II.1-B3.
c Type II.2-B1.

Ulnar fractures

An ulnar-shaft fracture with a stable prosthesis—type B1 (chapter 8.3)—as well as a displaced olecranon fracture, type A1, can be treated with open reduction and internal fixation. However, this is only successful if bone stock and bone quality are good. If the bone has already thinned out, it should be fixed with cerclages to guarantee a better outcome. In case ulnar revision is necessary (chapters 8.4 and 8.5), it is important to create a sufficiently wide exposure. The osteotomy is usually performed on the medial side and extends through the cement. Following the removal of the cement, the stem is extracted paying meticulous attention to not fracture the ulna. After reinsertion, the new cemented stem is secured with cerclages across the osteotomy site. The addition of a plate may be advisable to increase the stability of fixation.

Impaction grafting

Impaction grafting is usually indicated in case of osteolysis that has not been compromised by a fracture. In case of loss of bone stock in the humerus and ulna, the ulna is approached first. Perforations of the cortical bone, which are believed not to withstand the stress of impaction grafting, should be stabilized with allograft struts and cerclages. Two tubes are inserted into the medullary canal. The inner tube is placed beyond the end of the osteolytic lesion for good component fixation. Subsequently, cancellous allograft bone is finely morselized and pushed into the space between the outer tube and the cortical bone. Cement is then injected into the inner tube, which is slightly retracted until both tubes are at the same level. Now both tubes are withdrawn simultaneously while cement is injected into the empty space. The implant is then cautiously cemented into the cavity within either humerus or ulna.

Struts

Allograft strut composites, although having a high infection rate, still play a crucial role in extensive osteolysis with perforations of the cortical bone (chapters 8.2 and 8.4). After modeling of the two struts, compression is ensured with multiple cerclage wires across the fracture site. Special care should be taken when tightening the wires not to damage either the radial or ulnar nerve. Therefore, wire knots should be placed on the posterior aspect of the humerus or ulna.

6.2.4 Complications and outcome

In a series of 11 patients treated for a periprosthetic fracture around a TEA at the Mayo Clinic, 6 fractures had occurred after the primary TEA, 2 after a revision, and 3 after two revisions [4]. Complications occurred in 6 of the 11 cases, with 2 transient nerve palsies, 1 permanent nerve palsy, 1 olecranon fracture, 1 late humeral stem loosening, 1 humeral nonunion, 1 triceps insufficiency, and 2 of these 6 complication cases developed infections. Of 8 patients seen with a healed fracture, 7 had no or slight pain and 1 moderate pain. The Mayo elbow score overall was 4 excellent, 4 good, and 3 poor. Follow-up x-rays revealed union of an allograft strut with remodeling in 5 patients, union without remodeling in 4, and resorption of the allograft in 1.

References

[1] **Venable CS.** An elbow and an elbow prosthesis; case of complete loss of the lower third of the humerus. *Am J Surg.* 1952 Mar;83(3):271–275.

[2] **Little CP, Graham AJ, Carr AJ.** Total elbow arthroplasty: a systematic review of the literature in the English language until the end of 2003. *J Bone Joint Surg Br.* 2005 Apr;87(4):437–444.

[3] **O'Driscoll SW, Morrey BF.** Periprosthetic fractures about the elbow. *Orthop Clin North Am.* 1999 Apr;30(2):319–325.

[4] **Sánchez-Sotelo J, O'Driscoll S, Morrey BF.** Periprosthetic humeral fractures after total elbow arthroplasty: treatment with implant revision and strut allograft augmentation. *J Bone Joint Surg Am.* 2002 Sep;84-A(9):1642–1650.

6.3 Wrist

Authors **Shian-Chao Tay, Alexander Y Shin**

6.3.1 Introduction

Total wrist arthroplasty (TWA) is an accepted treatment method for low functional demand patients with a painful arthritic wrist who can accept modest wrist motion. Such patients typically suffer from osteoarthritis or rheumatoid arthritis.

Not so long ago, there were only two types of arthroplasty: the first being the resection/flexible implant arthroplasty developed by Swanson; the second, called articulated metal-polyethylene arthroplasty. Articulated metal-polyethylene arthroplasty now supersedes resection-flexible arthroplasty implants due to problems with silicone synovitis and implant fractures in the flexible implants. Common problems associated with metal-polyethylene implants include instability, loosening, subsidence, implant fracture, and bony resorption [1]. Periprosthetic fractures are less common and not much attention has been focused on such fractures [2].

6.3.2 Epidemiology

In a report of 189 wrist arthroplasties, there was no mention of any periprosthetic fractures during follow-up, ranging from 2.6–9.3 years. Prosthetic survival rate was 71% over 10 years with a revision rate of 21%. The most common causes for revision were loosening of components, alignment problems, and pain [3]. Lundkvist et al [4] reported on 30 wrist silicone arthroplasties in 1992. Although there was a high implant-fracture rate of 26%, there were no reported cases of periprosthetic fractures during an average follow-up of 5 years.

According to Dawson [2], the first reported case of periprosthetic fractures of the wrist was by Fatti et al [5], who reviewed their series of silicone wrist arthroplasties. Two periprosthetic fractures were tabulated in radiographic follow-up of 44 of these wrists, ie, a rate of about 5% over 2.5 years of average follow-up. One of the fractures was in the third metacarpal and the other in the radius. There was no further elaboration of these fractures in the article. In 1989, Dawson [2] highlighted the problem when they published a series of four cases of radius fractures that had occurred after TWA (two metal-polyethylene, two silicone). All pateints had suffered fractures of the radius following a fall after having had TWAs performed 2–8 years previously. One had a mildly displaced fracture that did not require reduction and was treated successfully in a cast. However, in the other three patients fractures were significantly displaced and they suffered from problems with nonunion or malunion. Two of these patients eventually required revision arthroplasty; for the third it is under consideration [2]. Silicone wrist arthroplasties are associated with "pathologic" periprosthetic fractures that could occur spontaneously or after minimal trauma. Three cases were reported that showed fractures of the distal radius [2], and third metacarpal [1], in association with significant endosteal scalloping secondary to microparticulate synovitis. One of these patients underwent wrist arthrodesis. The other two were treated conservatively due to advanced age and low functional demand [6]. As silicone wrist arthroplasties are no longer performed, there should be less such cases of pathologic periprosthetic fractures.

6.3.3 Incidence and risk factors

The incidence of intraoperative fractures ranges from 5–38% in revision arthroplasties [7, 8]. Essentially, there are two main types of periprosthetic fractures associated with TWA. The first type is an intraoperative fracture. This occurs during bone preparation or implantation of the arthroplasty components. It usually occurs in the radius but can also occur distally in the metacarpals. Intraoperative fractures occur more likely in revision arthroplasty surgeries—the reported rate was as high as 38%. In Rettig and Beckenbaugh's [8] series of 13 revision TWAs, two fractures occurred in the radius and three in the third metacarpal.

The second type of periprosthetic fractures are postoperative fractures. Postoperative fractures may be an acute posttraumatic fracture that occurs after a fall, usually resulting in a radius fracture. A postoperative fracture may also occur from excessive bony resorption and/or stress risers. These may present as an incomplete fracture such as a radiolucent line or a frank cortical perforation and usually occur in the metacarpal bone. These fractures are generally stable but may become unstable once the fracture line is completed or a pathological fracture occurs through the site of cortical perforation. In the latter cases, the fracture may be missed [6]. Patients typically complain of pain, deformity, and decreased function [2, 6].

The incidence of postoperative periprosthetic fractures ranges from 2% (3.4 years average follow-up) [5] up to 10% for revision arthroplasties performed for patients with bone deficient rheumatoid arthritis (3.8 years average follow-up) [9]. Recurrent postoperative fractures are much more common. These fractures occur a significant period after arthroplasty in bone surrounding the implant. This bone usually shows considerable osteolysis or resorption. The energy required to cause such fractures is significantly less than that for acute postoperative fractures. At an average of 6 years after TWA, the rate of such fractures was 15 (47%) of 32, with 3 (9%) of 32 being obvious cortical perforations. All fractures occurred in the metacarpal bones [7].

6.3.4 Classification

A fracture after wrist replacement is an uncommon occurrence because this type of arthroplasty is not frequently used in contemporary practice. A new Unified Classification System (UCS) has been proposed (chapter 4.2), which can be applied to the wrist (**Fig 6.3-1a–c**). The wrist joint is number "III", the radius and ulna "2", and the metacarpus/metacarpals "7".

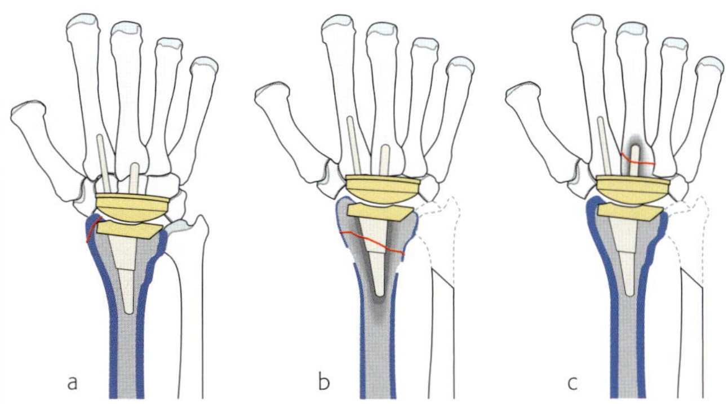

6.3-1a–c Examples of periprosthetic fracture types in the wrist according to the Unified Classification System (UCS).

a Type III.2-A1.
b Type III.2-B3.
c Type III.7-B3.

6.3.5 Treatment

Type A fractures

Type A intraoperative fractures may occur due to poor bone quality during preparation of the distal radius. If the fracture is sizeable and proximal component stability is affected, the fragment may be refixed using sutures, K-wires, tension band wiring, or screws, depending on whatever seems practical.

If the fracture occurs postoperatively, it is usually due to an avulsion-type injury from sudden loading of the wrist. If the joint is stable and not subluxated or dislocated, these fractures may be treated symptomatically, without surgery (chapter 5.3). However, if the injury is extensive, and there is instability, surgery may be required to repair the avulsions using techniques described above.

Type B fractures

The rate of intraoperative type B fractures is about 5% based on a series of 40 TWAs [7]. In this series, all fractures occurred in the third metacarpal bone although fractures also occur in the radius [8]. As mentioned before, intraoperative fractures are most common during revision procedures, particularly during removal of a well-fixed infected prosthesis. The risk is also high when there is significant osteolysis.

Image intensifier is the key to minimizing the risk of intraoperative fractures by ensuring accurate location of the intramedullary canal followed by broaching in the correct alignment. Sizing is also important together with adequate broaching. Inadequate broaching or malalignment, particularly if the cortical bone is weakened or if excessive force is used, can result in fractures or perforations through the cortical bone [8].

If a type B fracture involving the radius shaft occurs during surgery, it should be reduced and fixed with circumferential cerclage wiring to reapproximate and reinforce the shaft and metaphysis. This can be supplemented with additional onlay allograft struts or plates. If the fracture occurs intraoperatively before stem insertion, it is held reduced and a longer stem implant is used to bypass and stabilize the fracture. If this is not possible or available, the fracture can be plated. In some situations when initial solid fixation cannot be achieved intraoperatively, cement fixation should be considered. If solid fixation cannot be achieved, the rehabilitation program will have to be moderated, resulting in a reduced final range of motion due to capsular fibrosis and tendon adhesions [1]. Rettig and Beckenbaugh [8] had two intraoperative fractures involving the radius and three involving the third metacarpal in their series of 13 revision arthroplasties. None of the fractures required additional intraoperative fixation. However, one of the periprosthetic radius fractures never healed despite prolonged immobilization and eventually required arthrodesis.

The carpal component in current implants is typically fixed by a short stem and screws. If an intraoperative carpal fracture occurs, the defect can be augmented by bone graft and the use of longer screws to span the fractured area. Cement should be considered for stem fixation if bony support around the stem is inadequate [1]. Dawson [2] reported on four postoperative type B fractures of the radius following falls in patients with TWAs. Of these, 2 had silicone interposition and 2 articulated metal-polyethylene implants. Almost all, 3 of the 4, were displaced significantly with closed reduction attempted, 1 was mildly displaced. All 4 were initially casted with only the fourth case healing without any significant sequelae. Of the cases, 2 required revision arthroplasty, 1 with a long-stem radial implant, and 1 requiring cementing. The third case took 1 year to heal and was being considered for revision arthroplasty [2].

In a series of ten bone-deficient revision arthroplasties, the rate of postoperative fractures involving the radius was 10% following a fall. This was treated by implant removal and total wrist fusion [9]. In another series, 1 of 12 failed TWAs requiring total wrist fusion was from a postoperative fracture of the third metacarpal following a fall [10]. Apparently, type B postoperative fractures can be seen in both the radius and metacarpal; however, radial periprosthetic fractures seem to be more common.

Type B1 fractures with well-fixed stem

Periprosthetic fractures of the wrist in the presence of a well-fixed stem are usually located at the tip of the prosthesis. They can be treated by splint immobilization or open reduction and internal fixation (ORIF) with plates and screws depending on fracture displacement.

Types B2 and B3 fractures with loose stem

Revision surgery is usually required in such cases for two reasons. First, the fracture is not likely to unite on its own. Second, the loose stem remains symptomatic and causes further endosteal erosion. As such, revision has to address the issues of fracture stabilization as well as stem revision. This can usually be performed by revising to long-stem prosthesis with bone grafting of the fracture site. If cement is used, be careful to ensure that no cement extrusion occurs as this would inhibit fracture healing. Revision surgeries are difficult and require a skilled surgeon familiar with neural anatomy as well as tools for cement removal, the appropriate range of prostheses, and the availability of allografts. Occasionally, internal plate fixation may be needed. Bone grafting may be used in an onlay fashion or impacted into the medullary canal. Alternatively—if revision arthroplasty cannot be performed—conversion to total wrist fusion with internal fixation of the fracture may be performed (chapter 9.1) [10]. In such cases, bone graft requirements will be high and provisions must be made for sufficient allograft availability.

Type C fractures

Fractures well beyond the tip of the stem are treated as routine fractures with ORIF or splint immobilization depending on the characteristics of the fracture.

6.3.6 Complications and outcome

Not much has been published in the English-language literature on the specific complications and outcome of periprosthetic fractures of the wrist. However, due to the complexity of the surgery and the amount of tissue exposure and length of time, infection is a definite possibility and probably higher than in primary arthroplasty, with a reported incidence of 3 (9%) of 32 primary arthroplasties [7]. Correspondingly, the arthroplasty-implant loosening rate should be estimated to be as least 9%. Other possible complications include hematoma formation, wound closure and healing problems, and injury to surrounding neurovascular and tendinous structures. The occurrence of nonunion or malunion should also be expected.

For salvage fusions, the rate of nonunion at the fusion site was 5 (42%) of 12 patients, with 20% of the nonunion cases finally requiring repeat fusion of the wrist due to pain. Due to the large size of the tricortical iliac-crest bone graft used for wrist fusion in this series, the rate of complications at the iliac-crest donor site was 42% and included fractures of the ilium (2), superficial wound infection/dehiscence (2), and pain (10). In the series analyzed by Rizzo et al [11], the union rate was similar at 43% with a revision-surgery rate of 29%. Eventual fusion-union rate was 52%. The procedural complication rate was 38% with hardware problems, such as migration and failures predominating.

The outcome of revision arthroplasties and salvage wrist fusions is well reported. However, these series were not performed exclusively for the management of periprosthetic fractures. It is to be expected that the outcome of periprosthetic fractures managed with revision arthroplasty or wrist fusion will not fare as good.

Revision arthroplasties have a failure rate of 20% with failures being salvaged by total wrist fusions. At an average follow-up of 3.8 years, 60% of patients with revision arthroplasty had no pain and 20% having mild pain. Of all patients, 80% believed that their wrist was better after revision arthroplasty. The average range of motion was 39° and 17° for dorsiflexion and palmar flexion, respectively. The average grip strength was 10 kg [9].

Rizzo et al [11] reported on 21 failed TWAs salvaged by total wrist arthrodesis. The most common cause of failure was aseptic loosening; followed by infection, instability, implant fracture, and silicone synovitis. No salvage was performed as a result of a periprosthetic fracture. The mean time from index arthroplasty to arthrodesis in this series was 7.6 years with a range from 7 months to 20 years. Patient reported satisfaction rate was 82% with 67% of wrists with no pain. In another series, satisfactory outcome was 92%.

References

[1] **Adams BD.** Complications of wrist arthroplasty. *Hand Clin.* 2010 May;26(2):213–220.

[2] **Dawson WJ.** Radius fracture after total wrist arthroplasty. *J Hand Surg Am.* 1989 Jul;14(4):630–634.

[3] **Krukhaug Y, Lie SA, Havelin LI, et al.** Results of 189 wrist replacements. A report from the Norwegian Arthroplasty Register. *Acta Orthop.* 2011 Aug;82(4):405–409.

[4] **Lundkvist L, Barfred T.** Total wrist arthroplasty. Experience with Swanson flexible silicone implants, 1982–1988. *Scand J Plast Reconstr Hand Surg.* 1992;26(1):97–100.

[5] **Fatti JF, Palmer AK, Mosher JF.** The long-term results of Swanson silicone rubber interpositional wrist arthroplasty. *J Hand Surgery Am.* 1986 Mar;11(2):166–175.

[6] **Peimer CA, Taleisnik J, Sherwin FS.** Pathologic fractures: a complication of microparticulate synovitis. *J Hand Surg Am.* 1991 Sep;16(5):835–843.

[7] **van Harlingen D, Heesterbeek PJ, de Vos MJ.** High rate of complications and radiographic loosening of the biaxial total wrist arthroplasty in rheumatoid arthritis: 32 wrists followed for 6 (5–8) years. *Acta Orthop.* 2011 Dec;82(6):721–726.

[8] **Rettig ME, Beckenbaugh RD.** Revision total wrist arthroplasty. *J Hand Surg Am.* 1993 Sep;18(5):798–804.

[9] **Cobb TK, Beckenbaugh RD.** Biaxial long-stemmed multipronged distal components for revision/bone deficit total-wrist arthroplasty. *J Hand Surg Am.* 1996 Sep;21(5):764–770.

[10] **Beer TA, Turner RH.** Wrist arthrodesis for failed wrist implant arthroplasty. *J Hand Surg Am.* 1997 Jul;22(4):685–693.

[11] **Rizzo M, Ackerman DB, Rodrigues RL, et al.** Wrist arthrodesis as a salvage procedure for failed implant arthroplasty. *J Hand Surg Eur.* 2011 Jan;36(1):29–33.

6.4 Hip

Authors Benedict A Rogers, Shawn Garbedian, Raul Kuchinad, Allan Gross, Oleg Safir, David Backstein, Matt C Lyons, Steven J MacDonald, Gregory G Polkowski, Jay R Lieberman, Keith Mayo

6.4.1 Introduction

Authors Benedict A Rogers, Shawn Garbedian, Raul Kuchinad, Allan Gross, Oleg Safir, David Backstein, Matt C Lyons, Steven J MacDonald

Incidence and risk factors

The number of periprosthetic fractures occurring in total hip arthroplasty (THA) has been rising over the last two decades [1]. Given this serious trend, it is important to understand the classification and management of these challenging fractures that are typically associated with advanced age. These fractures can occur intraoperatively or postoperatively, while the incidence of intraoperative fractures varies based on the method of primary implant fixation described in chapter 2.

The numerous risk factors for intraoperative and postoperative fractures around prosthesis have already been described in chapter 3.2.

Although particular care is mandatory throughout the procedure, the most important, high-risk moments are:
- Femoral head dislocation
- Acetabular reaming
- Femoral preparation
- Implantation of the definitive prosthesis
- Fracture reduction.

The combination of force, retraction, and/or torsion on susceptible bone can be deleterious. Extensile approaches and adequate exposure minimize these risks. Knowledge of the anatomy is, of course, mandatory and a highly skilled surgical team is required to undertake the reconstruction and manage potential intraoperative complications.

Diagnosis

Intraoperative periprosthetic fractures may or may not be obvious to discover. With the increasing use of press-fit femoral and acetabular components, greater force is being applied to achieve good stability of the implant. Small cortical cracks, perforations, and distal fractures may go unnoticed until the patient is out of the operating room or begins ambulating. Early postoperative x-rays are recommended for acute diagnosis. Periprosthetic fractures that are noticed intraoperatively are typically found during preparation of the acetabulum or femur, but most often during the final insertion of the implants due to the forces required to achieve good fixation or due to poor bone quality. If a fracture is suspected, intraoperative x-rays or image intensifier may assist the surgeon in determining its extent and exact location. These fractures may be stable enough not to require further stabilization or simply need a modification in the weight-bearing status (chapter 5.3). More significant fractures require definitive management, as discussed later in this chapter.

Postoperative periprosthetic fractures can occur early or late, and may be related to the surgical technique, patient-related factors, or trauma. Increasing pain and loss of function may be signs of osteolysis or infection. While the diagnosis of a postoperative periprosthetic fracture may seem obvious on plain x-rays, additional imaging with Judet views, computed tomographic scans, or bone scans may be required to ascertain the fracture. In the case of acute trauma, the workup is usually straightforward. However, management is less obvious in the presence of infection or osteolysis, or in case of revision arthroplasty.

Classification

The original Vancouver classification introduced by Duncan and Masri in 1995, has been slightly modified and expanded (chapter 4.2). Thus, a new Unified Classification System (UCS) has been proposed (chapter 4.2), which can be applied to the hip. The hip is joint number "IV", the femur is "3", and the pelvis/acetabulum is "6".

Treatment

Except for nondisplaced fractures around the acetabulum/pelvis and nondisplaced avulsions of the trochanter, which can all be treated nonoperatively (chapter 5.3), the majority of periprosthetic fractures around the hip will have to be managed surgically as described in chapters 6.4.2 and 6.4.3. The decision to proceed with an internal fixation technique or with revision arthroplasty depends on the stability of the prosthesis.

Postoperative management

All arthroplasties should be routinely examined radiographically before the patient leaves the operating room to confirm that the reconstruction has followed the preoperative and intraoperative plans. Any complication can be expediently addressed while the patient is still anesthetized.

Physical therapy is focused on building up muscle strength and on achieving a normal gait and confidence while walking. In general, measures are taken to minimize extreme hip motions. If the patient has had a posterior approach, hip flexion of greater than 90° with internal rotation and adduction should be avoided. In case of a direct lateral/anterolateral approach, excessive hip extension and external rotation are prohibited.

For noncemented prostheses, partial weight bearing (50%) for 6 weeks is recommended for both, the soft-tissue reconstruction to heal as well as to prevent any implant subsidence. The use of crutches helps to prevent imbalances and consecutive falls. The surgeon should clearly and carefully document the particulars for postoperative management.

References

[1] **Berry DJ.** Epidemiology: Hip and knee. *Orthop Clin North Am.* 1999 Apr;30(2):183–190.

6.4.2 Pelvis and acetabulum

Authors Gregory G Polkowski, Jay R Lieberman, Benedict A Rogers, Shawn Garbedian, Raul Kuchinad, Allan Gross, Oleg Safir, David Backstein

Introduction

Periprosthetic fractures of the acetabulum remain a fairly uncommon complication following total hip arthroplasty (THA), although their overall incidence has increased. Regardless of their etiology, the surgical management of these fractures is challenging.

Periprosthetic fractures of the acetabulum (chapters 10.1–10.3) can occur in various situations, eg, during insertion of prosthetic components, following a traumatic event, and in association with periacetabular osteolysis. The assessment of acetabular component stability is crucial in determining the appropriate treatment strategy for such fractures. While the initial management of stable periprosthetic acetabular fractures may allow for adequate bone healing, the risk of future acetabular component loosening as a result of altered anatomy is high. The guiding principle for the treatment of unstable periprosthetic acetabular fractures lies in achieving adequate initial component stability to allow for appropriate bony ingrowth of the revision component along with stable fracture fixation of the pelvis. A variety of surgical techniques may be necessary to accomplish success in the management of these highly challenging injuries.

Incidence and risk factors

It is difficult to accurately estimate the incidence of this rare complication. One of the most comprehensive case series describing periprosthetic acetabular fractures was published by Peterson and Lewallen [1], who described 16 fractures in a total of 23,850 primary and revision total hip arthroplasty procedures (THAs) performed at the Mayo Clinic from 1971–1991, corresponding to an overall incidence of 0.07%. Prior to this report, McElfresh and Coventry [2] also described the incidence of a single periprosthetic acetabular fracture at the Mayo Clinic after a total of 5,400 cemented THAs.

Most risk factors contributing to the development of a periprosthetic acetabular fracture are related to poor bone quality. In their multicenter report of 13 cases of acetabular fractures associated with insertion of acetabular components, Sharkey et al [3] noted that 11 of the 13 cases occurred in women, most probably in association with osteopenia as major contributing factor. The other 2 patients of the 13 had rheumatoid arthritis, which also predisposes to osteoporosis. All fractures in this series occurred during insertion of "press-fit" acetabular components that were underreamed by 1–3 mm. The presence of extensive acetabular osteolysis as observed in several cases may contribute to the occurrence of periprosthetic fractures [4, 5]. McGrory [6] reported that the hard sclerotic bone seen in Paget's disease could also play a role in the occurrence of periprosthetic acetabular fractures during insertion of components. More details are presented in chapter 3.2.

Classification

Periprosthetic fractures of the acetabulum may be classified into intraoperative and postoperative fractures or, more specifically, according to the anatomical location and pattern. Furthermore, the stability of the prosthetic implant is essential for the choice of treatment.

At present, several classification systems are in use. A new Unified Classification System (UCS) has been proposed (chapter 4.2) that can be applied to the hip (👁 **6.4-1a–e**). The hip joint is numbered "IV", both pelvis and acetabulum are "6".

Treatment

General considerations

The aims are:

- To recognize the fracture (especially intraoperatively)
- To optimize the stability of the hip joint by restoring the center of rotation and correcting the biomechanics (limb length/offset)
- To restore and/or maintain acetabular bone stock
- To provide stability for the implants.

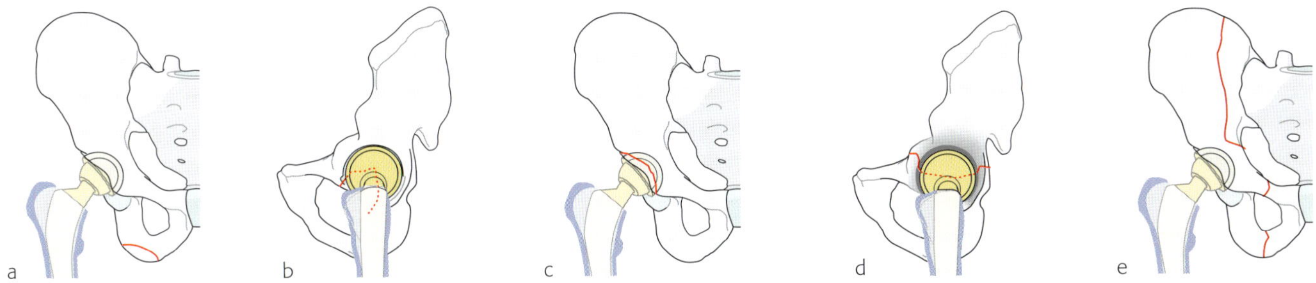

6.4-1a–e Examples of periprosthetic fracture types in the hip according to the Unified Classification System (UCS).
a Type IV.6-A2.
b Type IV.6-B1.
c Type IV.6-B1.
d Type IV.6-B3.
e Type IV.6-C.

The initial, crucial step in the management of periprosthetic acetabular fractures is to recognize that a fracture has occurred. In the case of a perioperative fracture that happens during insertion of a noncemented acetabular component in THA, it may be difficult to make the correct diagnosis. If after impaction of a noncemented acetabular component into an underreamed acetabular bed, "press-fit" does not appear to be satisfactory and stable, there should be a high index of suspicion for a periprosthetic acetabular fracture. The rim of the socket should be inspected and the component should be removed to ensure that no fractures have occurred. This is an important step, as Kim et al [7] found that some acetabular fractures that occurred during their cadaveric study were occasionally missed, even on intraoperative x-rays. Intraoperative plain film x-rays are, therefore, vital to help determine whether any periprosthetic acetabular fractures have occurred.

Once recognized, the strategy for managing these fractures depends on the stability of the acetabular component. If the component is stable, additional screw fixation along with protected weight-bearing postoperatively is recommended until adequate healing is observed.

If the acetabular component is unstable in the setting of a displaced fracture, the component should be removed and the fracture needs to be reduced and fixed with plates and screws as required. The acetabular component should be rereamed in a line-to-line manner and fixed to the acetabular bed with multiple screws.

Fractures that occur as the result of a traumatic event should initially be assessed with AP and oblique plain pelvic x-rays to allow diagnosing the fracture pattern and to assess acetabular component stability. Computed tomography and/or magnetic resonance imaging may be useful to further characterize the fracture pattern and to allow for additional operative planning.

Patients involved in high-energy trauma should be evaluated and given the same consideration as any pelvic ring injury or acetabular fracture in the acute setting, regardless of the presence of previous hip arthroplasty. In the Mayo Clinic series of Peterson and Lewallen, one patient died of complications related to severe hemorrhage following a periprosthetic acetabular fracture after acute trauma.

Patients who sustain periprosthetic acetabular fractures, in which the acetabular component is believed to have remained well fixed, can initially be treated nonoperatively by protected weight bearing (6 weeks are recommended) and gentle joint mobilization. Successful healing occurred in 80% of the cases [1]. However, even though radiological evidence of fracture healing was observed in these cases, all four patients treated in this manner eventually required revision for subsequent loosening of the acetabular component. An initial attempt at nonoperative treatment (chapter 5.3), while it may not ensure long-term success, allows for restitution and healing of the acetabular bone stock that makes subsequent acetabular component revision an easier endeavor.

Periprosthetic acetabular fractures that cause disruption of the fixation of the acetabular component should be treated with immediate ORIF and simultaneous revision of the acetabular component as soon as the patient is considered medically stable. The type of fracture fixation depends on the fracture pattern and, in most cases, plate and screw fixation of the posterior column is indicated. This can usually be achieved through the same posterior approach as the revision arthroplasty, although fractures involving significant portions of the anterior column may require a separate ilioinguinal approach for reduction and fixation. If a lateral approach was used for primary surgery, an additional new approach is required.

The quality of fracture reduction is not as critical in the setting of periprosthetic acetabular fractures as it is in the absence of a prosthesis, where joint incongruities and step off can lead to posttraumatic arthrosis. Imperfections in the reduction can be compensated during reaming and fixation of the acetabular component. Persistent gaps at the fracture site should be treated with supplemental bone grafting, and the fixation of the new acetabular component should include multiple screw fixation in as many planes as possible to ensure adequate component stability. While it is tempting to use the acetabular component as an internal plate construct, this kind of solution was discouraged by Peterson and Lewallen [1] as failure was seen in one case in their series. It is not clear as yet whether the more recent hemispherical acetabular components with enhanced ingrowth surfaces provide a favorable enough environment for initial stability and bony ingrowth to allow for such a strategy to be used in future.

If acetabular revision is undertaken, the femoral component should also be assessed both preoperatively and intraoperatively, especially if there is evidence of wear, loosening, malpositioning, or non-modularity. The option for optimizing head size, offset, and length are all advantages of modular components and aid stability in the revised joint. Due to the risk of intraoperative damage and subsequent excessive wear of the cup, the femoral head should also be replaced in all acetabular revisions using modular stems.

Intraoperative acetabular fractures

Periprosthetic acetabular fractures can occur during cup insertion in THAs. In the era of cemented THA, perioperative acetabular fractures must have been extremely rare—none having been reported in the literature. With the advent of noncemented implants, the initial generation of noncemented acetabular components were typically inserted after reaming the acetabulum to an equal-size diameter as the component to be inserted (line-to-line reaming) and acetabular component fixation was enhanced with screws [8]. This allowed for initial stability until bony ingrowth of the acetabular component had been achieved. Subsequent generations of acetabular-component fixation techniques have relied on underreaming of the acetabulum to a diameter 1–4 mm smaller than the diameter of the implant, achieving greater initial component stability in the absence of screw fixation [9, 10]. These techniques were developed to combat concerns related to potential increases in osteolysis [11], corrosion and fretting between the metal shell and screws [3, 11], and vascular injuries that can occur by drilling and the use of acetabular screws [12, 13].

In the previously mentioned multicenter series of periprosthetic fractures of the acetabulum at four different institutions described by Sharkey et al [3], 9 of 13 fractures were recognized during the insertion of the underreamed acetabular component, while in the remaining cases the fracture was not detected until postoperative x-rays were obtained [3]. In all cases, the acetabular component was inserted with 1–3 mm press-fit. The treatment strategy for these patients varied from the use of additional screws to enhance the fixation of the acetabular component, to bone grafting at the fracture site, and revision surgery at a later date if the component failed to show ingrowth. The authors attributed these fractures to underreaming of the acetabulum in osteoporotic bone.

Postoperative acetabular fractures

The incidence of periprosthetic acetabular fractures after acute trauma is low. An example of a traumatic periprosthetic acetabular fracture is illustrated in **6.4-2**. Several case reports have been published, the most comprehensive

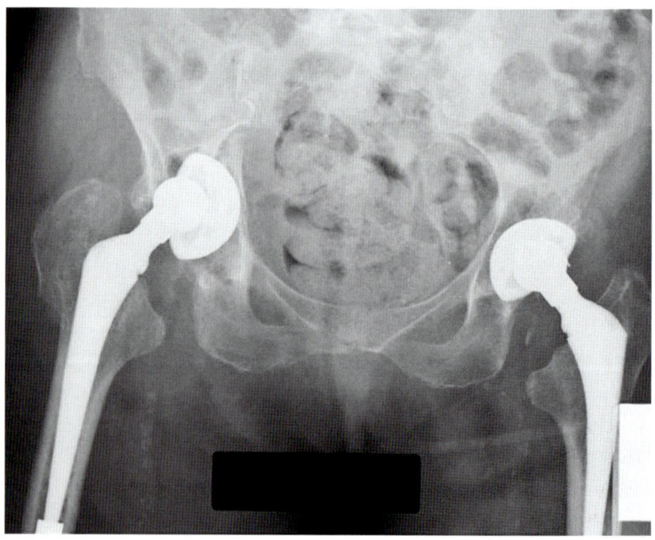

6.4-2 AP x-ray of the pelvis. Bilateral uncemented total hip arthroplasty with periprosthetic fracture of right acetabulum. Transverse fracture involving both anterior and posterior columns of the acetabulum. There is vertical and medial migration of the acetabular component indicating loosening. Type IV.6-B2. The femoral component remained well fixed.

is by Peterson and Lewallen [1]. The authors identified eleven patients with periprosthetic acetabular fractures at an average of 6.2 years following THA. The fracture patterns were variable and included fractures with transverse fracture pattern and fractures of the medial wall, the posterior or the anterior column. Of these eleven patients, one died from acute hemorrhage from a laceration sustained to the posterior branch of the internal iliac artery. The remainder of patients was treated based on the assessment of the stability of the acetabular component. Those with apparently stable, well-fixed acetabular components (Peterson/Lewallen type 1 fracture = UCS type IV.6-B1) were initially managed nonoperatively to allow the fractures to heal, while those with unstable, loose acetabular components as a result of their fracture (Peterson/Lewallen type 2 fracture = UCS type IV.6-B2/B3) were treated with immediate revision THA, one with a cemented and one with a noncemented acetabular component with screws. Of the eight Peterson/Lewallen type 1 fractures (= UCS type IV.6-B1), six patients eventually required revision of their acetabular component. Of these, two developed a delayed union or nonunion, while the remaining four had initial fracture union, with eventual pain and progressive loosening of their acetabular component shown by x-rays. Overall, eight of the ten patients in the series required a revision operation within 15 months of the fracture. The authors concluded that it may be acceptable to begin with nonoperative treatment of stable type 1 (UCS type IV.6-B1) fractures as long as there is no radiological evidence of loosening. However, subtle changes at the interface of the cup may lead to eventual loosening and need revision surgery even in the presence of a healed periprosthetic acetabular fracture.

Acetabular fractures associated with osteolysis

The management of periprosthetic acetabular fractures in the setting of extensive osteolysis (UCS type IV.6-B2/B3) can be especially challenging. Lytic defects can weaken the acetabular bone so extensively that even minor trauma can lead to a pathological periprosthetic acetabular fracture. Frequently, the presence of extensive bone loss makes fracture fixation even more difficult. In cases of contained osteolytic defects with a sufficient rim of host bone providing enough support for the revision acetabular component, morselized bone grafting of the osteolytic defect can provide additional support. With extensive bone loss from osteolysis, a revision cage or structural allograft supplementation of these defects may be necessary for the reconstruction.

Sánchez-Sotelo et al [5] described two cases of periprosthetic acetabular fractures in the setting of acetabular osteolysis: one with a loose cup, the other with a well-fixed acetabular component. Both fractures occurred in the absence of any antecedent trauma, and in both cases the patients were managed with revision THA and bone grafting of their osteolytic defects [5]. Chatoo et al [4] also presented a patient having experienced mild hip pain for 2 years, followed by onset of acute pain and inability to bear weight for 3 weeks. At that point, a fracture of the posterior column and posterior wall of the acetabulum was diagnosed that was associated with pelvic osteolysis. After treatment with ORIF of the posterior column and bone grafting, mesh, and revision with a cemented acetabular component, the patient was pain free at the 18-month follow-up. The x-rays indicated successful healing with incorporation of the bone graft.

Pelvic discontinuity

The management of acute pelvic discontinuity after trauma differs significantly from the chronic form. While the acute form can usually be fixed like any fresh acetabular fracture with plates and a noncemented cup component, the latter, ie, the chronic form is traditionally treated with bone augmentation in the form of a structural allograft or morselized graft in combination with an antiprotrusion cage fixed with screws in different directions.

However, concerns exist regarding the lack of bone ingrowth into an ilioischial cage and the resulting micromotion that limits the functional longevity of the implants. Goodman et al [14] reviewed the complications following acetabular reconstruction using ilioischial rings with either morselized or structural bone graft. Successful outcome—defined as a stable reconstruction with no further revision of the acetabular components and incorporation of the acetabular bone graft—was achieved in 76% of cases at 5 years. There were ten cases of pelvic discontinuity included in this series, of which only five were classified as having a successful outcome at final follow-up. There were four sciatic and two peroneal nerve palsies with partial/full recovery in all cases. Lost fixation of ilioischial rings occurred in four cases; three were revised and one was converted to a bipolar arthroplasty following removal of the reconstruction ring.

These concerns and the arrival of porous tantalum have advanced the treatment of chronic pelvic discontinuity. Hanssen and Lewallen [15] first introduced a technique that utilizes a trabecular metal acetabular component to obtain partial press-fit stability between the superior and inferior portions of the discontinuity. This component is under tension and, therefore, needs to be further stabilized by an antiprotrusion cage into which a polyethylene liner is cemented at the appropriate inclination and version.

The rationale for this technique is that the spanning ilioischial cage endows mechanical stability to the whole construct while biological stability is achieved by bone ingrowth into the trabecular metal. The use of porous tantalum in this situation is attractive as recent reports provide evidence for bone ingrowth even in cases of limited contact with bleeding bone [16]. Kosashvili et al [17] have published a series of 26 consecutive cases of pelvic discontinuity that have been managed using this technique. With a mean follow-up of 44 months, the survivorship of the acetabular components was 88% with significant clinical improvement. Bleeding host-bone contact was less than 50% in all cases.

Pelvic ring fractures not involving the acetabulum

In pelvic ring fractures (type IV.6-C) that do not involve the acetabulum, the principal determinant regarding the treatment pertains to the stability of the pelvis. Stable pelvic ring fractures involving the anterior ring usually do not require any specific treatment, while unstable fractures (anterior or posterior injury) should be handled and fixed in the same way as in any acute trauma. If instability is demonstrated, internal fixation of the pelvic ring is preferable to external fixation because of the inherent risk of pin-track infection.

References

[1] **Peterson CA, Lewallen DG.** Periprosthetic fracture of the acetabulum after total hip arthroplasty. *J Bone Joint Surg Am.* 1996 Aug;78(8):1206–1213.

[2] **McElfresh EC, Coventry MB.** Femoral and pelvic fractures after total hip arthroplasty. *J Bone Joint Surg Am.* 1974 Apr;56(3):483–492.

[3] **Sharkey PF, Hozack WJ, Callaghan JJ, et al.** Acetabular fracture associated with cementless acetabular component insertion: a report of 13 cases. *J Arthroplasty.* 1999 Jun;14(4):426–431.

[4] **Chatoo M, Parfitt J, Pearse MF.** Periprosthetic acetabular fracture associated with extensive osteolysis. *J Arthroplasty.* 1998 Oct;13(7):843–845.

[5] **Sánchez-Sotelo J, McGrory BJ, Berry DJ.** Acute periprosthetic fracture of the acetabulum associated with osteolytic pelvic lesions: a report of 3 cases. *J Arthroplasty.* 2000 Jan;15(1):126–130.

[6] **McGrory BJ.** Periprosthetic fracture of the acetabulum during total hip arthroplasty in a patient with Paget's disease. *Am J Orthop (Belle Mead NJ).* 1999 Apr;28(4):248–250.

[7] **Kim YS, Callaghan JJ, Ahn PB, et al.** Fracture of the acetabulum during insertion of an oversized hemispherical component. *J Bone Joint Surg Am.* 1995 Jan;77(1):111–117.

[8] **Schmalzried TP, Harris WH.** The Harris-Galante porous-coated acetabular component with screw fixation. Radiographic analysis of eighty-three primary hip replacements at a minimum of five years. *J Bone Joint Surg Am.* 1992 Sep;74(8):1130–1139.

[9] **Schmalzried TP, Wessinger SJ, Hill GE, et al.** The Harris-Galante porous acetabular component press-fit without screw fixation. Five-year radiographic analysis of primary cases. *J Arthroplasty.* 1994 Jun;9(3):235–242.

[10] **Curtis MJ, Jinnah RH, Wilson VD, et al.** The initial stability of uncemented acetabular components. *J Bone Joint Surg Br.* 1992 May;74(3):372–376.

[11] **Peters PC Jr, Engh GA, Dwyer KA, et al.** Osteolysis after total knee arthroplasty without cement. *J Bone Joint Surg Am.* 1992 Jul;74(6):864–876.

[12] **Keating EM, Ritter MA, Faris PM.** Structures at risk from medially placed acetabular screws. *J Bone Joint Surg Am.* 1990 Apr;72(4):509–511.

[13] **Kirkpatrick JS, Callaghan JJ, Vandemark RM, et al.** The relationship of the intrapelvic vasculature to the acetabulum. Implications in screw-fixation acetabular components. *Clin Orthop Relat Res.* 1990 Sep;(258):183–190.

[14] **Goodman S, Saastamoinen H, Shasha N, et al.** Complications of ilioischial reconstruction rings in revision total hip arthroplasty. *J Arthroplasty.* 2004 Jun;19(4):436–446.

[15] **Hanssen AD, Lewallen DG.** Modular acetabular augments: composite void fillers. *Orthopedics.* 2005 Sep;28(9):971–972.

[16] **Sporer SM, Paprosky WG.** Acetabular revision using a trabecular metal acetabular component for severe acetabular bone loss associated with a pelvic discontinuity. *J Arthroplasty.* 2006 Sep;21(6 Suppl 2):87–90.

[17] **Kosashvili Y, Backstein D, Safir O, et al.** Acetabular revision using an anti-protrusion (ilio-ischial) cage and trabecular metal acetabular component for severe acetabular bone loss associated with pelvic discontinuity. *J Bone Joint Surg Br.* 2009 Jul;91(7):870–876.

6.4.3 Proximal femur

Author **Keith Mayo**

Introduction

Periprosthetic fractures of the proximal femur are the most frequent and best-known fractures of that kind. They can occur intraoperatively (recognized or not recognized) or, more often, they happen at some interval after surgery for a total hip arthroplasty (THA).

Incidence and risk factors

The epidemiology and risk factors that contribute to periprosthetic fractures are described in detail in chapters 2 and 3.2. The incidence is clearly higher in noncemented (3–5.4%) versus cemented (0.3–1.2%) primary stem insertions [1, 2]. Revision surgery is associated with higher risk than primary prosthesis placement [3, 4]. Here again, the noncemented revision technique is associated with increased fracture rates (19–21%) [2, 5] in comparison with cemented procedures (3%) [2].

The reported incidence of late periprosthetic fractures associated with a total hip prosthesis stem varies between 0.7% and 3.5% [2, 3, 6]. The incidence appears to increase with duration of follow-up [6, 7]. Decreased bone density may be a contributing factor in these conditions. Both clinical and biomechanical studies correlate femoral component loosening with increased fracture risk [7–9]. In both—primary and revision surgery—the incidence of late fracture is higher in noncemented compared with cemented series [10, 11]. With this background of relative risk factors it is not surprising that most (75–84%) late periprosthetic proximal femoral fractures result from low-energy trauma [7, 11].

Classification

Presently different classification systems are used. While the Vancouver classification has been shown to have relatively good reliability and validity for fractures occurring postoperatively [12, 13], this is not necessarily the case for those occurring during surgery [14].

A new Unified Classification System (UCS) has been proposed (chapter 4.2), which can be applied to the proximal femur (**6.4-3a–e**). The hip joint is numbered "IV", the proximal femur "3", and the acetabulum/pelvis "6."

Treatment

General considerations

The entire group of such fractures can amplify even subtle errors in surgical technique. Preservation of the blood supply at the fracture site with careful soft-tissue management is essential. Plating principles must be followed (chapter 5.4.1). Simple transverse fracture patterns are ideally reduced anatomically and then compressed with the plate to create a load-sharing construct. In oblique fracture patterns, interfragmentary fixation is followed by neutralization plating. Fixation should not be concentrated close to the fracture site in order to prevent fatigue fracture of the plate. Segmental (comminuted) patterns are spanned, taking care to completely avoid dissection within the zone of injury. Locked plating can be useful when thoughtfully applied to address issues of deficient bone density. In the frequently observed type B2 or B3 periprosthetic fractures revision arthroplasty (chapters 5.5 and 5.6) is indicated.

The treatment of intraoperative fractures is more straightforward when recognized and treated during the operation itself. In nondisplaced periprosthetic fractures, the treatment often can be limited to a modified postoperative mobilization protocol, augmented with minimal internal fixation, eg, lag screws when appropriate. Lerch et al [15] reported a case-controlled study comparing groups of THA patients with and without intraoperative fractures. The results show no difference in hip scores, SF-36 scores, or postoperative complications. A larger retrospective study by Meek et al [10] also showed no significant difference between fracture and non-fracture groups at a minimum follow-up of 2 years.

For displaced intraoperative metaphyseal or diaphyseal fractures, the surgical indications and techniques are similar to their postoperative counterparts discussed below.

Type A

Fractures in the trochanteric region are frequently nondisplaced or minimally displaced and do not compromise stem fixation. These injuries can be managed nonoperatively with

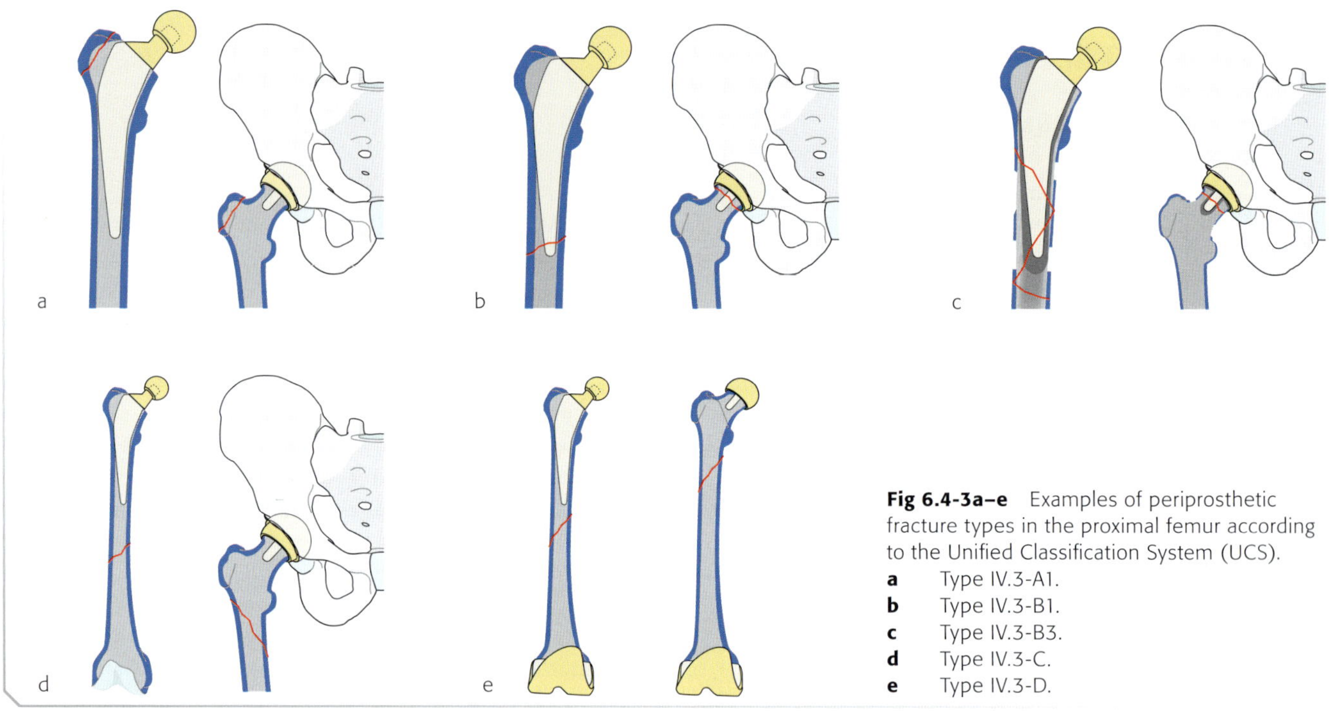

Fig 6.4-3a–e Examples of periprosthetic fracture types in the proximal femur according to the Unified Classification System (UCS).
a Type IV.3-A1.
b Type IV.3-B1.
c Type IV.3-B3.
d Type IV.3-C.
e Type IV.3-D.

protected weight bearing and activity modification. Fractures of the greater trochanter (type IV.3-A1) up to a displacement of 2 cm have been reported to do well clinically [16]. However, detrimental effects on abductor function may warrant intervention within these limits, particularly in younger patients (chapter 5.3). In some cases, fractures of the greater trochanter can be associated with significant osteolysis. When this occurs, removal of wear debris from the bearing surface should be considered as well as acetabular cup or liner exchange. In any case, surgical repair of the trochanteric fracture augmented with bone graft is necessary.

Fractures of the lesser trochanter that involve a large area of the posteromedial buttress (calcar) fortunately are relatively rare but may result in an unstable stem and thus require revision. Therefore, these fractures should be classified as type B2, not as type A2 fractures.

Type B

Type B1

In these fractures (chapters 10.4–10.9) with a well-fixed stem, the fixation usually consists of open reduction and fixation with plate-screw or plate-screw-cerclage constructs. Consideration should be given to long plates that effectively provide an artificial lateral cortex that bridges the entire femur. Proximal and distal fixation should be balanced and not excessive. This type of construct limits the risk of plate failure and subsequent fracture proximal or distal to the plate. Less invasive surgical techniques (MIPO) can be used as long as optimal reduction and fixation is achieved. Locking plates appear to be advantageous in patients with osteoporosis [17]. Fixation adjacent to the stem can be with monocortical or bicortical screws or cerclage systems. Screw purchase in the cement mantle when present is usually excellent but theoretically has the downside of weakening stem fixation [18]. The recently introduced locking-attachment plate (chapters 5.4.1 and 10.16) is placed over the proximal part of the locking plate, while four smaller locking-head screws can be inserted into the cortex around the prosthetic stem. Cortical strut allografts have been used successfully [19]—either as an adjunct to plate fixation—or isolated despite concerns about the biological drawbacks of the additional surgical exposure required for placement [20].

Another option is intramedullary nailing (chapters 5.4.2, 10.8, 10.9, 10.11, and 10.18).

Type B2

Type B2 injuries (chapters 10.10–10.12) require revision of the loose stem whenever the remaining bone stock is considered adequate. A number of revision techniques have been successful. The use of long-stem prostheses will be sufficient in many cases, provided it exceeds the length of the fracture plane by at least 4–6 cm or two diameters of the bone [21]. In other situations, it may be necessary to augment this technique with plate-screw or cerclage constructs. Cemented stems, whose cement mantle is mostly intact, may be reimplanted using the so-called cement-in-cement technique coupled with open reduction and internal fixation of the fracture [22].

Type B3

Type B3 injuries (chapters 10.13 and 10.14) present a major challenge as there is severe loss of bone stock due to osteolysis or fracture comminution. In younger patients, it may be worthwhile to attempt long-stem prosthetic revision supplemented by local allograft to compensate for the osseous deficiencies. A proximal femoral allograft block with long-stem revision prosthesis has also been used in this setting [23]. Authors [24, 25] reported the successful use of an allograft prosthetic composite for the proximal femur in these situations (chapter 5.6). Further options, such as tumor prosthesis or press-fit fixation, are discussed in chapter 5.6.

Type C

These fractures (chapters 10.15 and 10.16) are located well below the prosthesis and can usually be treated without concern about the status of the femoral prosthesis. Asymptomatic loosening may provide the impetus for treatment with long-stem revision prosthesis in some cases but most are managed with open reduction and plate fixation similar to that used with type B1 fractures. However, it seems important that extra-long—preferably locking—plates are used that overlap the end of the stem by several centimeters to prevent any stress risers. Minimally invasive submuscular insertion of such plates is recommended to minimize exposure and devitalizing of the bone.

Type D

Type D fractures include all interprosthetic or intercalary fractures occurring between a total hip and knee arthroplasty. Their treatment again depends on the stability of the prosthetic components, the quality of bone stock, and on the possibility of fixation distally in the condylar area. Locked plates are presently the preferred means of fixation (chapters 10.17 and 10.18).

Type E

Type E fractures describe the rare situation in which fractures involve both components of the prosthesis, eg, acetabulum and proximal femur or distal femur and proximal tibia. The salvage treatment has to follow the principles described above and varies for every single case.

Complications and outcome

The results of treatment of periprosthetic proximal femoral fractures as demonstrated by numerous series have shown higher rates of failure than isolated fractures in a nonprosthetic setting. This has proved true irrespective of implant/prosthetic choice or whether the operating surgeon has a reconstructive or trauma background.

References

[1] **Davidson D, Pike J, Garbuz D, et al.** Intraoperative periprosthetic fractures during total hip arthroplasty. Evaluation and management. *J Bone Joint Surg Am.* 2008 Sep; 90(9):2000–2012.

[2] **Berry DJ.** Epidemiology: hip and knee. *Orthop Clin North Am.* 1999 Apr;30(2):183–190.

[3] **Schwartz JT Jr, Mayer JG, Engh CA.** Femoral fracture during non-cemented total hip arthroplasty. *J Bone Joint Surg Am.* 1989 Sep;71(8):1135–1142.

[4] **Taylor MM, Meyers MH, Harvey JP Jr.** Intraoperative femur fractures during total hip replacement. *Clin Orthop Relat Res.* 1978 Nov–Dec;(137):96–103.

[5] **Malkani AL, Lewallen DG, Cabanela ME, et al.** Femoral component revision using an uncemented, proximally coated, long-stem prosthesis. *J Arthroplasty.* 1996 Jun;11(4):411–418.

[6] **Cook RE, Jenkins PJ, Walmsley PJet al.** Risk factors for periprosthetic fractures of the hip: a survivorship analysis. *Clin Orthop Relat Res.* 2008 Jul;466(7):1652–1656.

[7] **Lindahl H, Malchau H, Herberts P, et al.** Periprosthetic femoral fractures classification and demographics of 1049 periprosthetic femoral fractures from the Swedish National Hip Arthroplasty Register. *J Arthroplasty.* 2005 Oct;20(7):857–865.

[8] **Thomsen MN, Jakubowitz E, Seeger JB, et al.** Fracture load for periprosthetic femoral fractures in cemented versus uncemented hip stems: an experimental in vitro study. *Orthopedics.* 2008 Jul;31(7):653.

[9] **Harris B, Owen JR, Wayne JS, et al.** Does femoral component loosening predispose to femoral fracture?: an in vitro comparison of cemented hips. *Clin Orthop Relat Res.* 2010 Feb;468(2):497–503.

[10] **Meek RM, Garbuz DS, Masri BA, et al.** Intraoperative fracture of the femur in revision total hip arthroplasty with a diaphyseal fitting stem. *J Bone Joint Surg Am.* 2004 Mar;86-A(3):480–485.

[11] **Beals RK, Tower SS.** Periprosthetic fractures of the femur. An analysis of 93 fractures. *Clin Orthop Relat Res.* 1996;(327):238–246.

[12] **Brady OH, Garbuz DS, Masri BA, et al.** The reliability and validity of the Vancouver classification of femoral fractures after hip replacement. *J Arthroplasty.* 2000 Jan;15(1):59–62.

[13] **Rayan F, Dodd M, Haddad FS.** European validation of the Vancouver classification of periprosthetic proximal femoral fractures. *J Bone Joint Surg Br.* 2008 Dec;90(12):1576–1579.

[14] **Franklin J, Malchau H.** Risk factors for periprosthetic femoral fracture. *Injury.* 2007 Jun;38(6):655–660

[15] **Lerch M, Windhagen H, von Lewinski G, et al.** [Intraoperative femoral fractures during the implantation of the cementless BiCONTACT stem: a matched-pair analysis of 84 patients]. *Z Orthop Unfall.* 2007 Sep–Oct;145(5):574–578. German.

[16] **Pritchett JW.** Fracture of the greater trochanter after hip replacement. *Clin Orthop Relat Res.* 2001 Sep;(390):221–226.

[17] **Bryant GK, Morshed S, Agel J, et al.** Isolated locked compression plating for Vancouver Type B1 periprosthetic femoral fractures. *Injury.* 2009 Nov;40(11):1180–1186.

[18] **Kampshoff J, Stoffel KK, Yates PJ, et al.** The treatment of periprosthetic fractures with locking plates: effect of drill and screw type on cement mantles: a biomechanical analysis. *Arch Orthop Trauma Surg.* 2010 May;130(5): 627–632.

[19] **Font-Vizcarra L, Fernandez-Valencia JA, Gallart X, et al.** Cortical strut allograft as an adjunct to plate fixation for periprosthetic fractures of the femur. *Hip Int.* 2010 Jan–Mar;20(1):43–49.

[20] **Chandler HP, Tigges RG.** The role of allografts in the treatment of periprosthetic femoral fractures. *Instr Course Lect.* 1998;47:257–264.

[21] **Fawzy E, de Steiger R, Gundle R, et al.** The management of periprosthetic fractures Oxford trimodular femoral stem. A survivorship study. *J Arthroplasty.* 2009 Sep;24(6):909–913.

[22] **Richards CJ, Duncan CP, Crawford RW.** Cement-in-cement femoral revision for the treatment of highly selected Vancouver B2 periprosthetic fractures. *J Arthroplasty.* 2011 Feb;26(2):335–337.

[23] **Wong P, Gross AE.** The use of structural allograft for treating periprosthetic fractures about the hip and knee. *Orthop Clin North Am.* 1999 Apr;30(2):259–264.

[24] **Kellett CF, Boscainos PJ, Maury AC, et al.** Proximal femoral allograft treatment of Vancouver type-B3 periprosthetic femoral fractures after total hip arthroplasty. Surgical technique. *J Bone Joint Surg Am.* 2007 Mar;89 Suppl 2 Pt.1:68–79.

[25] **Maury AC, Pressman A, Cayen B, et al.** Proximal femoral allograft treatment of Vancouver type-B3 periprosthetic femoral fractures after total hip arthroplasty. *J Bone Joint Surg Am.* 2006 May;88(5):953–958.

6.5 Knee

Authors **Bernd Fink, Pierre Hoffmeyer, Marschall B Berkes, Dean G Lorich, Michael J Raschke**

6.5.1 Introduction

Author **Bernd Fink**

Incidence

The incidence of osteoarthritis of the knee is increasing worldwide with more than 70% of older adults affected. This situation leads to an estimated yearly combined number of primary and revision knee prostheses of over 2 million.

Periprosthetic fractures about the knee are rare after primary total knee arthroplasties (TKAs) (0.3–2.5%). However, they occur more often after revision arthroplasties (1.6–38%) and are also more challenging to treat. Furthermore, a c onsiderable increase in fractures around TKAs is expected in the future as the number of total knee replacements is rising dramatically. More information can be found in chapters 2 and 3.2.

Classification

At present different classification systems are used. A new Unified Classification System (UCS) has been proposed (chapter 4.2), which can be applied to the knee (👁 **6.5-1a–f**). The knee joint is numbered "V", the femur "3", the tibia "4", and the patella "34."

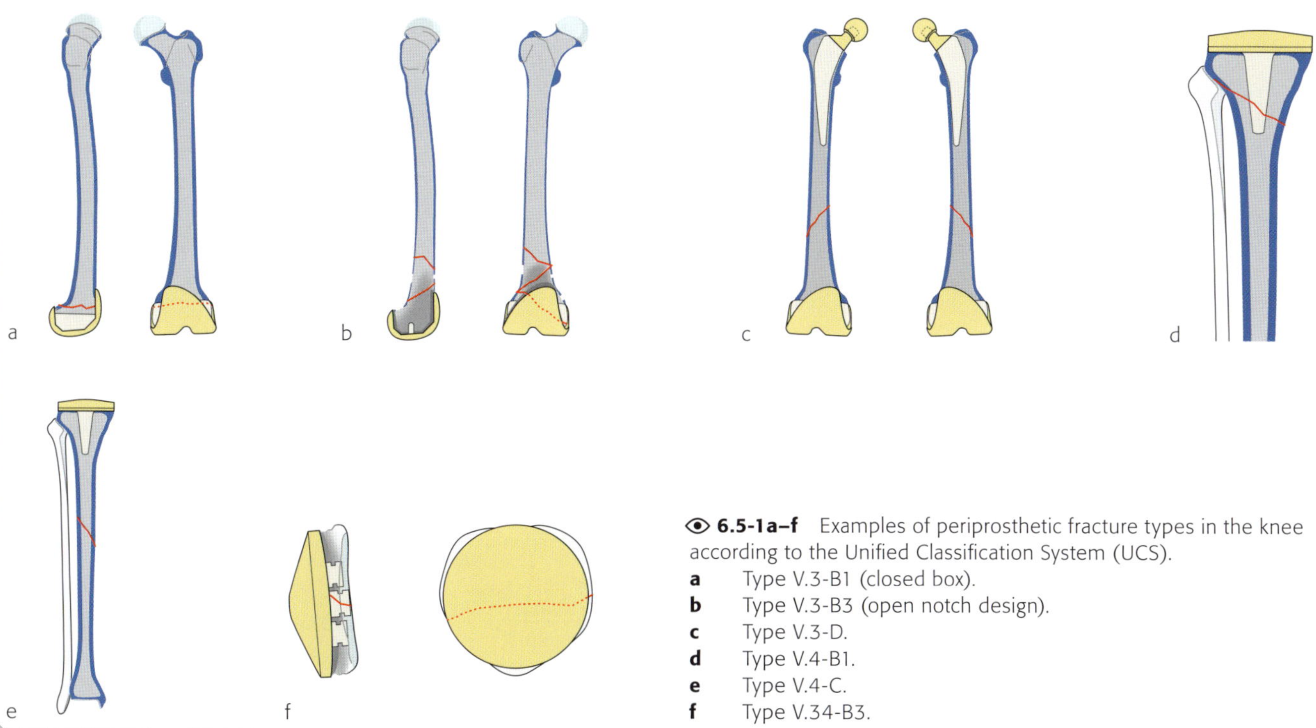

👁 **6.5-1a–f** Examples of periprosthetic fracture types in the knee according to the Unified Classification System (UCS).

- **a** Type V.3-B1 (closed box).
- **b** Type V.3-B3 (open notch design).
- **c** Type V.3-D.
- **d** Type V.4-B1.
- **e** Type V.4-C.
- **f** Type V.34-B3.

Preoperative evaluation

The circumstances that will lead to revision arthroplasty rather than attempting an osteosynthesis are outlined below and necessitate careful preoperative planning and intraoperative assessment of the anchorage of the prosthesis on the one hand and the stability of the knee ligaments on the other. As often this cannot be clarified absolutely before the intervention, a suitable prosthesis should always be available during surgery. Preoperative implant stability is assessed with the aid of adequate x-ray imaging of the femur and tibia in two projections as well as of the patella (including correct axial view if possible to assess the position of the patella). An x-ray of the whole leg is also desirable to assess axial alignment. If loosening of the prosthesis is suspected on the standard x-rays, a comparison with previous x-rays is recommended. More information about imaging procedures is detailed in chapter 4.1.

Treatment

The design and function of the existing prosthesis (unicondylar prosthesis surface replacement, axis constrained stem prosthesis, etc) will influence the choice of treatment, which in exceptional cases can be nonoperative (chapter 5.3) or usually is based on fracture fixation by screws and plates, intramedullary nails, or revision surgery (chapters 6.5.2–6.5.4) (**6.5-1**).

6.5-1 Indications for revision arthroplasty in periprosthetic fractures of the knee.

Type of fracture	Situation	Problems
Periprosthetic fracture with stable implant	ORIF* with uncertain healing/outcome	Severe osteoporosis
	Metastatic lesions	A-L Lesser trochanter
Periprosthetic fracture with loose or failed implant	Aseptic osteolysis	Ligamentous imbalance
	Septic osteolysis	

* ORIF indicates open reduction and internal fixation.

Internal fixation

Internal fixation of periprosthetic fractures about the knee is indicated whenever the prosthetic component appears well fixed and the bone stock is able to provide adequate purchase for the fixation devices. Thus, open reduction and internal fixation is not indicated for severe osteoporosis, in the presence of extensive osteolysis, or if metastatic lesions have been identified. Moreover, as surgical fracture fixation—especially if performed by more or less indirect and closed techniques—is considerably less invasive than revision surgery, the patients' condition, compliance, and ability to use crutches as well as their expectations should also be considered during the decision-making process. If an internal fixation is planned, there are different options for the distal femur, the proximal tibia, and the patella. The rationale and technique preferred for a specific location and fracture type is described in more detail in chapters 11.8 –11.11.

Revision surgery

Revision surgery should always be considered whenever a fracture has occurred and the prosthetic implant has failed as a result of loosening, malposition, wear, or ligamentous instability. In addition, revision of the prosthesis is indicated whenever conservative treatment or osteosynthetic procedures seem contraindicated. This is the case with poor bone quality making fracture fixation unlikely to succeed or if the patient is unable to maintain the necessary partial weight bearing of the operated leg (**6.5-2**). If the implant is malpositioned (approximately > 5° varus/valgus malalignment or malrotation), revision of the prosthesis is necessary even if the implant is still stable. Especially in case of malrotation, the likelihood for progressive loosening and poor function to occur is high, which can be prevented by revision surgery. Nevertheless, surgeons should remember that revision surgery usually is the much more invasive procedure.

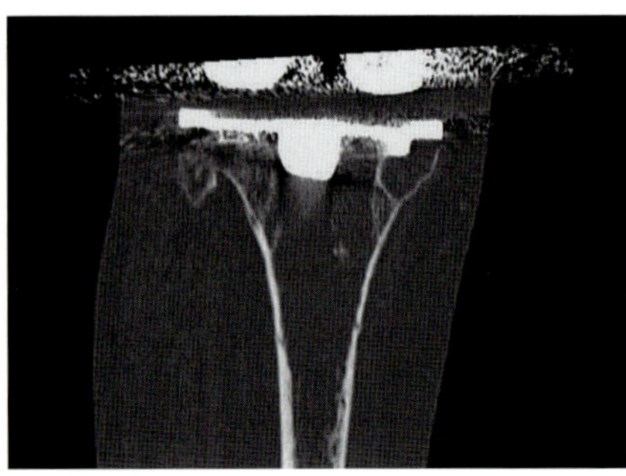

6.5-2 CT scan of a periprosthetic fracture of the tibia with osteolysis due to polyethylene wear in a 68-year-old woman with rheumatoid arthritis.

Ligamentous instability

The trauma causing the fracture can also lead to ligamentous instability of the knee, which in turn may require the insertion of a knee prosthesis that replaces ligament function (= constrained prosthesis) (👁 **6.5-3a–e**). Reconstruction of a bone defect is only one of the features of revision procedures. The restitution of ligamentous stability and the related degree of constraint of the prosthesis is also important in the selection of the type of prosthesis. During surgery, it is vital to check for both valgus/varus instability and a possible mismatch between the gaps during extension and flexion. A semiconstrained prosthesis (👁 **6.5-4**) can be used if valgus/varus instability occurs together with balanced flexion and extension gaps. If there is a mismatch between the flexion and extension gap, a hinged-knee prosthesis (👁 **6.5-5**) must be used because luxation of a semiconstrained prosthesis could occur during flexion whenever the gap becomes too large.

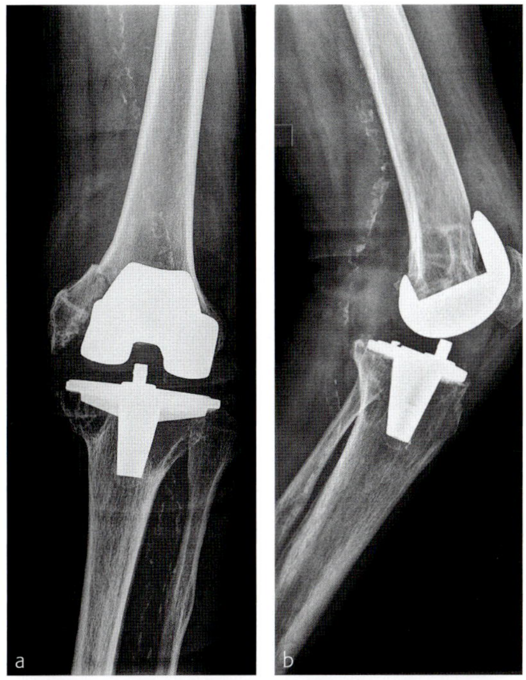
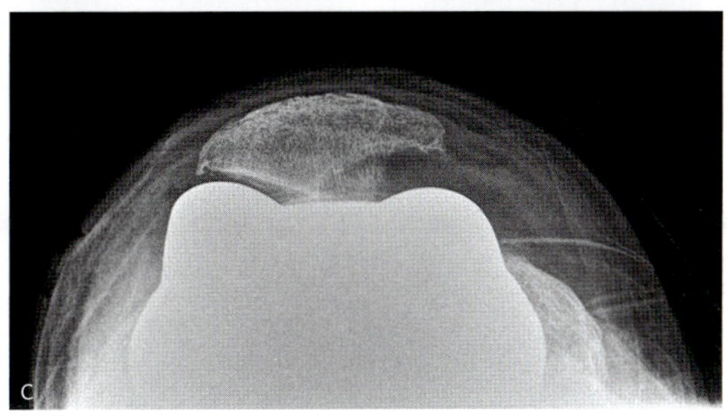
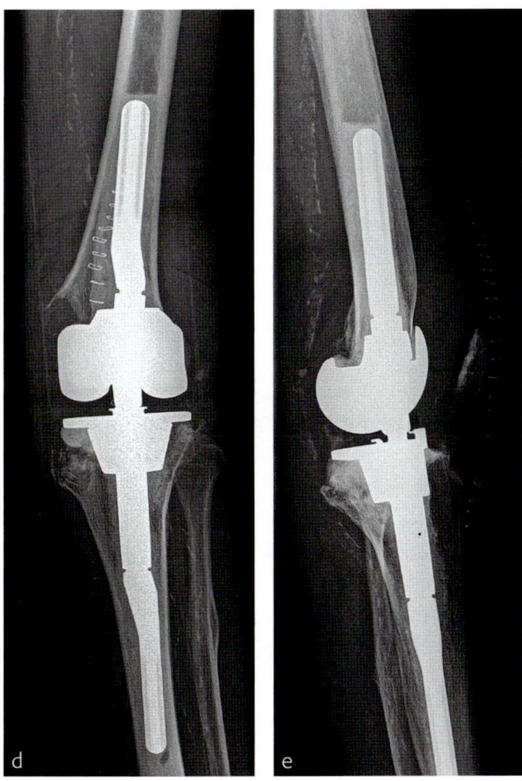

👁 **6.5-3a–e** Periprosthetic fracture of an 82-year-old man with knee arthroplasty 13 years ago.

a–b Periprosthetic fracture of the medial femoral condyle and the medial tibial plateau with osteolytic bone defects due to polyethylene wear.

a AP view.

b Lateral view.

c Tangential x-ray of the patella showing an osteolytic bone defect due to polyethylene wear.

d–e Postoperative x-rays after revision arthroplasty to a hinged modular revision prosthesis and reconstruction of bone defects with trabecular metal cones.

d AP view.

e Lateral view.

The use of ligamentous stabilizers is not advisable for segmental bone loss with the knee joint developing ligamentous instability. Instead, the application of revision prostheses with a higher degree of constraint is recommended—as it is for tumor prostheses—if previous reconstruction of the defect had been performed with sleeves and allografts. If this is not considered sufficiently, the revision prosthesis may become unstable. Replacement of the distal femur or the proximal tibia, together with the attachment sites of the ligaments, by mega prosthesis (chapter 5.6) results in a much higher degree of constraint than that of a hinged prosthesis.

Postoperative management

It is imperative that the knee is passively mobilized daily to avoid adhesions to the articular surfaces. This mobilization can normally be initiated immediately after surgery. If there is any uncertainty regarding fixation of the fracture, knee mobilization should be delayed by 7–10 days, while the knee is stabilized with an orthotic device for mobilization of the patient. The use of an orthotic device during patient mobilization is also recommended if ligamentous stability is questionable or weak after revision surgery.

Periprosthetic fractures fixed by internal fixation around a noncemented stem of the revision prosthesis need 8–12 weeks to achieve solid healing that allows full weight bearing. This period of recovery should be used to gradually—but continually—increase the level of weight bearing starting with 10–20 kg partial weight bearing for the first 6 weeks. Further increase of 10 kg per week is allowed, depending on the clinical outcome.

After fixation of a periprosthetic fracture of the patella, a stepwise increase in the flexion over the next 6 weeks is allowed as tolerated. Once the fracture has healed and the secondary retropatellar replacement has been carried out, a normal rehabilitation course, ie, after implantation of a primary knee prosthesis, can be initiated. Physical therapy to strengthen the muscles and to reduce postoperative swelling as well as lymph drainage and cryotherapy help to shorten the period of rehabilitation.

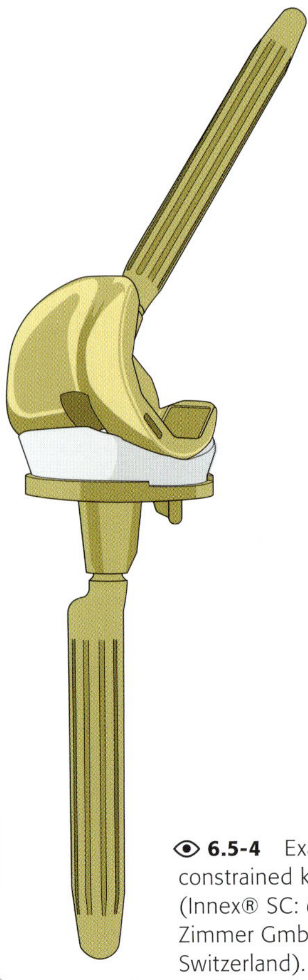

6.5-4 Example of semi-constrained knee prosthesis. (Innex® SC: courtesy of Zimmer GmbH, Winterthur, Switzerland).

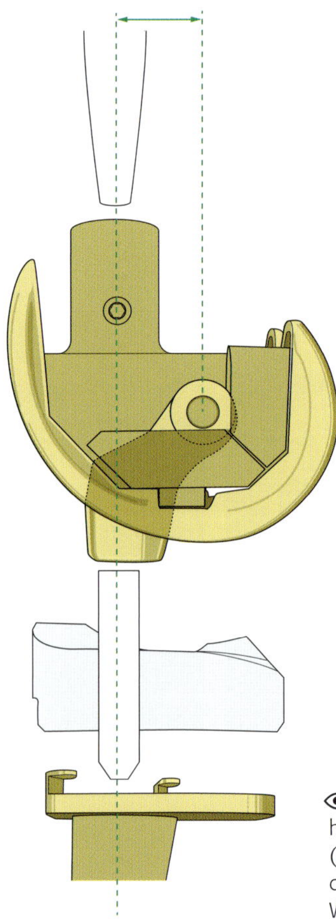

6.5-5 Example of a hinged-knee prosthesis. (Rotating hinge knee design: courtesy of Zimmer GmbH, Winterthur, Switzerland).

6.5.2 Distal femur

Author **Pierre Hoffmeyer, Bernd Fink**

Etiology

Most periprosthetic fractures about the knee occur at the distal femur in the supracondylar region of greatest weakness due to bone fragility, only seldom at the tibia. It may be argued that the presence of a large metallic implant in the metaphysis of the distal femur creates a stress riser favoring the occurrence of a fracture in a location subjected to large flexion and torsion forces.

Because of the magnitude of the moments of force involved at the distal femur, fractures occur even after low-energy trauma, such as a simple fall in a domestic environment. In the tibia, the applied forces tend to occur mainly in compression and the bone is structurally more resistant to this type of stress.

Other causes are related to patient-specific factors and bone quality; some may be of iatrogenic origin while still others may be associated with implant design and make-up. Patient-related causes pertain to bone fragility either due to osteoporosis, disuse atrophy, inflammatory or metastatic diseases (chapter 2).

Well-described iatrogenic causes include surgical technique and, specifically, notching of the anterior cortex during preparation of the distal femur [1, 2]. Prosthesis-related causes involve osteolysis due to metallic or polyethylene wear debris that activates osteoclast activity. Thereby, open spaces are created at the bone-implant interface, which predisposes the bone to break in the vicinity of the prosthesis. The same is true for loosened implants—irrespective of cause—that alter bone mechanics and lead to distal femoral fractures [3]. Other less frequent causes are fractures due to stress risers created by pinholes when using temporary antennae for implant navigation purposes.

Classification

At present different classification systems are used. A new Unified Classification System (UCS) has been proposed (chapter 4.2), which can be applied to the knee (👁 **6.5-6a–c**). The knee joint is numbered "V", the femur "3."

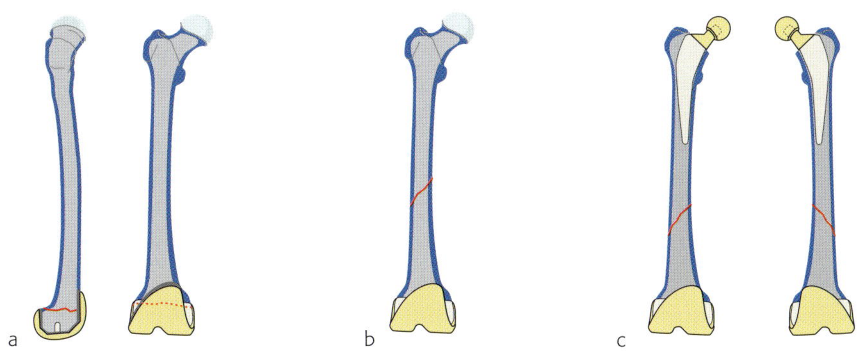

👁 **6.5-6a–c** Examples of periprosthetic fracture types in the distal femur according to the Unified Classification System (UCS).
a Type V.3-B2.
b Type V.3-C.
c Type V.3-D.

Decision making

Surgery is the main treatment option for periprosthetic or interprosthetic fractures involving the distal femur. In exceptional cases of nondisplaced fractures—or if the patient is too frail for surgical intervention—conservative treatment with an immobilizing brace is indicated (chapter 5.3) until callus formation is visible on control x-rays. The patient should be informed of treatment modalities and be prepared for surgery.

Periprosthetic fractures may occur in the presence of well-fixed or loose implants. The implant status must be accurately evaluated because when faced with a well-fixed femoral component (type B1) the goal will be to achieve strong fracture fixation with some type of internal fixation device. However, with a loose implant (types B2 and B3), revision arthroplasty needs to be contemplated. A history of long-standing pain and discomfort along with signs of radiolucency will usually help dispel any doubts as to the choice of procedure. However, infection must first be ruled out.

The prosthetic implant must be identified exactly, and ideally the operation report of the index procedure should be available preoperatively. Cruciate-sparing implants will usually have an open-notch design that may allow the insertion of a retrograde intramedullary nail (IM). This type of fixation will not be possible in posteriorly stabilized or hinged-knee prostheses. Interprosthetic fractures (type D) do not, as a rule, lend themselves to IM unless specially designed custom-made implants are used.

The question of the degree of stability obtained depends on the fracture pattern and on the bone quality. Strong bone even with comminution is amenable to fixation with a laterally placed blade plate or, preferably, with a locking-screw-plate device.

Fragile bone may need an additional medial plate, bone strut, or the use of bone cement.

The degree of osteoporosis will influence the fixation technique. Locked screws and fixed-angle blade plates have been shown to be more effective in this situation than conventional plates and screws. Improved plate and implant technology, however, cannot overcome basic biomechanical facts. Adequate stabilization of a periprosthetic fracture of the distal femur needs a solid medial buttress to avoid failure (with a deformity) or a nonunion due to muscle-force imbalance and varus-bending moment upon weight bearing. If this cannot be achieved or if there is major bone loss in the metaphysis or diaphysis, either due to loosening or to the fracture, some authors recommend the use of cortical strut grafts. These are usually long cortical femoral allografts that are fixed to the diaphysis using cerclage wires or cables. The aim is to obtain incorporation of the allografts, thereby strengthening the weakened femoral cortex.

The application of the strut-graft technique (chapter 11.6) is more popular for periprosthetic fractures around stems of total hip arthroplasties (THAs) but may also be useful in the distal femur. Kumar et al [4] have reported on the use of fibular cortical allografts as an adjunct for the reconstruction of the distal femur.

In rare cases, such as major soft-tissue injury, infection, or patient comorbidities, the fracture may be temporarily immobilized with an external fixator (large or small pin). However, after an interval not exceeding 10–15 days, definitive internal fixation may be undertaken. In some instances, external fixation may be necessary as part of definitive treatment [5].

Treatment

Intramedullary nailing

The biomechanically ideal implant for a comminuted supracondylar fracture, especially with poor possibilities for buttressing and mediocre bone quality, is a retrograde distal femoral locked nail (chapters 5.4.2, 10.11, and 11.7). This IM should be locked both proximally and distally with bicortical screws or distally with a spiral blade. In supracondylar fractures at the level of the femoral component, the nail should reach as far as the middle of the diaphysis. However, the application of a retrograde IM is only possible if the femoral component has an open design, ie, with a minimal aperture diameter that allows nail insertion. Therefore, it is imperative to identify the implant manufacturer and specific model preoperatively. Only in exceptional cases, an antegrade locked IM can be inserted, if the proximal implant is a cephalomedullary nail that can be removed (chapter 10.18).

The approach is essentially the same as that used when the total knee prosthesis was implanted. With the patient supine and using bolsters or a meniscus support to prop up the knee and image intensifier in place, a midline skin incision with a medial parapatellar arthrotomy is the favored technique for approaching the prosthesis. In some situations with a lateral incision and a tibial tuberosity osteotomy the situation must be assessed. It may be necessary to go through the same approach that was used during the first operation especially if less than a year has elapsed since the primary surgery. In other cases, it may be more practical to use a medial parapatellar incision as long as there is a distance between the two incisions leaving a skin bridge of 7 cm. A real problem may arise whenever there are multiple incisions around the knee or in multiple-operated posttraumatic cases. The surgeon is left with the decision which type of incision to use. As a rule it is best to choose the last incision, most likely the one that was used for the implant in place. In rare instances a comminuted fracture of the patella may be associated with the periprosthetic fracture. In this case if a distal femoral nail is contemplated, a transpatellar approach may be used. Patellar reconstruction is then performed after the nail has been successfully inserted [6].

In many situations, however, using a retrograde nail is not an option. This may either be the case because the femoral component has a closed box and will not allow for the passage of a nail or the proximal femur has been fitted with an implant such as a hip arthroplasty or an intramedullary fracture implant (proximal femoral nail or similar). A standard retrograde nail is certainly not the procedure of choice if a proximal intramedullary device is in place because of the inevitable formation of an intense stress riser at the junction zone between the two stems. Some authors have devised retrograde nails that may dock and engage the proximal stem. This may be an answer for certain situations and for this technique to be useful issues such as the presence of cement or bone plugs must be dealt with [7, 8].

Plate osteosynthesis

For most periprosthetic fractures of the distal femur with a well-fixed prosthesis, the use of a long bridging plate with locking-head screws (LHSs; LISS or DF-LCP, etc) has proved to be a satisfactory solution to an otherwise difficult problem (chapters 10.15–10.17, 11.2, 11.3. and 11.5) [9–11]. The plates are inserted either openly in a traditional fashion or by the minimally invasive plate osteosynthesis (MIPO) technique. The traditional open approach entails a large exposure with extensive soft-tissue dissection while the MIPO technique requires some practice as well as a lengthier use of the image intensifier to check reduction and implant positioning. Depending on the fracture pattern of the diaphyseal segment, a bridging technique with relative stability will be chosen for comminuted fractures or anatomical reduction and axial compression for simple fracture types. While the direction of the LHS is "predetermined" in the plate types mentioned above, the screw should not protrude medially as this might create painful irritation upon knee motion. Newer locking plates are available that allow angulation of the locking screws, which facilitates screw placement.

The required principles comprise:

- Restoring the anatomical axes (including rotation)
- Rigid fixation of articular segments
- Relative stability for bridging of diaphyseal comminution
- Atraumatic soft-tissue handling.

Finally, success depends on early motion of the injured limb and mobilizing of the entire patient.

The correct length of the LISS plate is still under debate. Generally, in a transverse fracture at the level of the prosthetic implant, the plate should at least reach the midpoint of the femoral diaphysis. In the distal fragment as many LHSs as possible should be inserted, while proximal to the fracture at least four well-spaced bicortical LHSs should be inserted. According to Gautier and Sommer [12], the plate length should be 2–3 times the length of the fracture zone in a comminuted fracture and 8–10 times the length of the fracture zone in a transverse or short oblique fracture. This rule of thumb is based on empirical data. Precise biomechanical testing still needs to be performed.

When a lateral locking-compression plate (LCP) is considered, the problem of the medial buttress must be addressed. Buttressing may be deficient because of comminution, poor bone quality, or fracture pattern. After applying the plate, the fracture is carefully assessed using an image intensifier. If there is any doubt about the stability of the construct, it is best to proceed with the placement of a medial buttressing plate (some authors prefer a bone strut). Usually an implant with LHS through a separate incision is used. The main difficulty encountered in the medial approach is the femoral artery as it exits Hunter's canal medially before it then runs posteriorly. However, it is not recommended to approach the joint line more proximal than at a distance of 15 cm.

For a very low distal femoral periprosthetic fracture or, in case of a posteriorly stabilized component design just above the central box, screw fixation or blade-plate insertion is unrealistic [13]. The only viable option is revision arthroplasty, even in the presence of well-fixed prosthetic components [14].

An increasing number of patients with knee prosthesis also have an ipsilateral hip prosthesis (chapters 10.6 and 10.17) or a proximal intramedullary-nail device. This combination of implants may produce a critical biomechanical situation by creating stress risers in the interprosthetic diaphyseal segment, which may lead to fractures in the vicinity of one of the prostheses and requiring specific treatment [15].

The basic principle of plate fixation, which is most frequently applied in interprosthetic fractures, is that the plate must be as long as the entire femur in order to overlap with the existing intramedullary implants. This will avoid stress risers and provide the best chance for fracture healing. Published data has not, as yet, precisely determined the exact amount of required overlap. But as a rule of thumb, it seems acceptable that the overlap should be at least half the length of the entire intramedullary implant.

If the fracture is close to the distal femur, one of two situations is encountered: The proximal stem is either short or long. In case of a short stem, the plate used may be solidly fixed with multiple bicortical screws in the diaphysis before it overlaps with the implanted stem. In case of a long stem, monocortical screws, augmented by cerclage wires, cables, or the new locking-attachment plate (LAP) (chapters 5.4.2, 10.16, and 11.5) will be necessary to allow strong fixation proximally. However, multiple cerclages around a diaphysis implanted with an intramedullary stem represent a risk factor for failure due to cortical bone necrosis caused by circulatory disturbances induced by the cerclage wires or cables. On the other hand, short monocortical locked screws may be blamed for damaging the periprosthetic cement mantle, if present. This may, however, be unavoidable in many of these complex situations.

Revision arthroplasty

The prerequisite for successful revision surgery (chapters 5.5 and 11.4) is the availability of the correct information about type and design of the implant, which allows for a minimal amount of bone loss during the explantation or that only one component of the prosthesis has to be replaced. Depending on the extent of the fracture and the quality of the bone, the fracture zone can be bridged using modular revision prostheses with long intramedullary stems that will allow early movement and (partial) weight bearing. If the bone defect is more extensive, it might be necessary to incorporate additional reconstruction techniques using augmentation struts or allografts.

In the presence of an ipsilateral hip prosthesis, caution is advised because a knee arthroplasty with a long stem can lead to stress risers between the two ends of the stems, possibly resulting in a fracture in the unprotected section of the femur. In certain cases in which the amount of healthy bone is considered insufficient to support the implant and provide immediate stability for weight bearing, a so-called "push-through femoral prosthesis"—connecting the stems of both hip and knee implants while retaining the cortical remainder of the femur and the attached muscles—may be used. Total replacement of the femur would be the most extreme option for salvage.

In general, it can be said that the stem of the revision endoprosthesis should bridge the fracture zone by at least two widths of the diaphysis. The stem of the prosthesis should be inserted without cement, thereby preventing the risk of cement leaking into the fracture gaps, which would endanger the healing process. Moreover, a noncemented stem of a knee endoprosthesis can be removed more easily than a cemented one in case further surgery should become necessary. An exception to this rule is the presence of extensive osteolysis or osteoporosis, which make successful healing unlikely. In such a situation, the stem is cemented along its entire length, even bridging the fracture. The prosthetic components in the fragment adjoining the knee joint are usually cemented in place. In case a periprosthetic fracture is associated with a loose prosthesis due to bacterial infection, a one-stage revision procedure—with addition of microbe-specific antibiotics to the cement—represents a promising treatment option for fracture stabilization and simultaneous treatment of the infection.

If the fracture is unstable, it may be useful to explore the fracture during the revision surgery, reducing the fragments and fixing them with a temporary external-fixator frame supplemented by an adequately positioned plate that is held in place by Verbrugge forceps. As soon as the internal instrumentation, ie, the inserted endoprosthesis, has achieved some stabilization of the fracture, the temporary fixation devices can be removed.

Periprosthetic fractures accompanied by loose implants and insufficient bone stock represent the most problematic situation. In circumscribed bone defects, reconstruction can be carried out by applying morselized allograft bone, implant sleeves, or both. If the bone defect is segmental, other concepts have to be applied. Smaller segmental defects (approximately 2 cm on the femoral side and 5 cm on the tibial side) can be substituted by augmentation materials. It is better to replace larger bone defects with augmentation materials on the tibial side than on the femoral side, because on the tibia these can be combined with higher inlays. Extensive preexisting bone defects or those occurring during revision surgery have to be reconstructed with implant-specific components (eg, sleeves), tumor prostheses (mega prosthesis), or structural allografts (chapter 5.6).

Revision surgery is complex and should only be carried out in centers where the appropriate experience and equipment are available. The correct alignment of the limb axis, the reconstruction of leg length and the correct height of the joint spaces are essential for optimal postoperative return of limb function.

Complications and outcome

Outcome after open reduction and internal fixation (ORIF) of periprosthetic fractures has been reported recently by several authors [8, 10, 16–19].

Kolb et al reported on 15 patients with femoral fractures above well-fixed knee arthroplasties seen after a long-term follow-up averaging 9 years and fixed with 95° condylar blade plates [16]. In some cases adjunct bone cement or strut grafts were used. The average range of motion was found to be 101° and the average American Knee Society Score (AKSS) was 77. Only 1 case of implant failure is reported along with 1 case with a developed varus malalignment of 5°.

Ebraheim et al [17] used LCP in 27 patients with a union rate of 89% and a 37% complication rate, which included three cases of delayed and/or nonunion and seven fixation failures.

Hou et al [18] reported 52 patients with above total knee arthroplasty periprosthetic fractures. Of these, 34 were treated with plate fixation and 18 with a retrograde nail. The authors state that at follow-up the results were similar in regard to achieved union and function. In the locking-plate group, six patients sustained nonunion or progressed to malunion, and two had infections. For the retrograde nail group, one patient developed an infected nonunion and two progressed to malunion.

A retrospective study by Kolb et al [10] involved 19 patients treated with the LISS plate after having sustained a periprosthetic fracture above a well-fixed femoral component and followed-up at 46 months All 19 patients healed and they had two cases of delayed union and one patient had a malalignment with 7° varus. The average range of motion was 102° and the average American Knee Society score was 56 points. The advantages of the locked plate, eg, less blood loss, better preservation of the periosteal blood supply, and relative ease of insertion compared with the 95° blade plate [10].

Using single LCPs in 22 consecutive patients with interprosthetic fractures, Sah et al [8] reported that all patients achieved fracture union and recovered satisfactory function at a follow-up of 17.7 months.

In a retrospective study, Hierholzer et al [19] analyzed 115 patients with distal femoral fractures treated either by retrograde IM nailing (59 patients) or by LISS plating (56 patients). In their study, 90% of patients achieved bone union with no statistically significant differences found for the parameters time of osseous healing, rate of nonunion, and postoperative complications between the two techniques.

Some studies reported results of revision arthroplasty with stabilization of the fracture by long, noncemented stems. Chen et al [20] performed eleven prosthesis revisions in a total of 195 supracondylar periprosthetic fractures [20]. Of these, ten patients exhibited satisfactory outcome. McLaren et al [21] searched the literature and found 25 cases of prosthetic revision surgery following supracondylar fractures, of which 24 had satisfactory outcome. Srinivasan et al [22] reported on eight patients who underwent prosthetic revision following complex distal femoral fractures: All fractures had healed and, after an average follow-up of 24 months, the American Knee Society score results were excellent in 1 case, good in 4, satisfactory in 1, and poor in 2 cases [22].

Kraay et al [23] reported seven cases in which large, distal femoral structural allografts were used in combination with unconstrained stem prostheses. Although the outcome for most patients was satisfactory, only two of the allografts exhibited bony incorporation into the host bone, one dislocation occurred, and two patients required an orthotic device at all times because of persistent instability of the knee. Gross [24] reported one case of nonunion and one amputation after an average follow-up of 6 years in a cohort of ten patients with allograft-prosthesis composites following periprosthetic fracture of the knee. Kassab et al [25] followed up twelve patients with such composites for an average of 58.8 months and reported a Hospital for Special Surgery score (HSS-Score) (modified) of 74.7 ± 6.8 (average flexion of 97.7° ± 21.8°) and one patient with an excellent outcome, five good, three satisfactory results, while one had a poor outcome.

Tumor prostheses for distal femoral replacement and/or proximal tibial replacement usually show higher rates of loosening, especially in young, physically active patients, which makes this type of prosthesis more suitable for treating periprosthetic fractures in older patients with lower levels of activity. Keenan et al [26] reported on customized prostheses with very good outcome in all seven cases studied.

References

[1] **Clarius M, Haas D, Aldinger PR, et al.** Periprosthetic tibial fractures in unicompartmental knee arthroplasty as a function of extended sagittal saw cuts: an experimental study. *Knee.* 2010 Jan;17(1):57–60.

[2] **Gujarathi N, Putti AB, Abboud RJ, et al.** Risk of periprosthetic fracture after anterior femoral notching. *Acta Orthop.* 2009 Oct;80(5):553–556.

[3] **Han CD, Han CW, Yang IH.** Femoral component fracture due to osteolysis after cemented mobile–bearing total knee arthroplasty. *J Arthroplasty.* 2009 Feb;24(2):323.e7–12.

[4] **Kumar A, Chambers I, Maistrelli G, et al.** Management of periprosthetic fracture above total knee arthroplasty using intramedullary fibular allograft and plate fixation. *J Arthroplasty.* 2008 Jun;23(4):554–558.

[5] **Beris AE, Lykissas MG, Sioros V, et al.** Femoral periprosthetic fracture in osteoporotic bone after a total knee replacement: treatment with Ilizarov external fixation. *J Arthroplasty.* 2010 Oct;25(7):1168.e9–12.

[6] **Chettiar K, Jackson MP, Brewin J, et al.** Supracondylar periprosthetic femoral fractures following total knee arthroplasty: treatment with a retrograde intramedullary nail. *Int Orthop.* 2009 Aug;33(4):981–985.

[7] **Meyer C, Alt V, Heiss C, et al.** [Intramedullary nailing of periprosthetic femoral fractures after revision for total knee endoprosthesis. Treatment of periprosthetic femoral fractures by inserted knee endoprosthesis with intramedullary shaft by in situ lengthening of the prosthesis with specially prepared slotted hollow nails.] *Unfallchirurg.* 2011 Mar;114(3):241–247. German.

[8] **Sah AP, Marshall A, Virkus WV, et al.** Interprosthetic fractures of the femur: treatment with a single-locked plate. *J Arthroplasty.* 2010 Feb;25(2):280–286.

[9] **AO Foundation.** AO Surgery Reference. Available at: www2.aofoundation.org/wps/portal/surgery. Accessed March 16, 2013.

[10] **Kolb W, Guhlmann H, Windisch C, et al.** Fixation of periprosthetic femur fractures above total knee arthroplasty with the less invasive stabilization system: a midterm follow-up study. *J Trauma.* 2010 Sep;69(3):670–676.

[11] **Large TM, Kellam JF, Bosse MJ, et al.** Locked plating of supracondylar periprosthetic femur fractures. *J Arthroplasty.* 2008 Sep;23(6 Suppl 1):115–120.

[12] **Gautier E, Sommer C.** Guidelines for the clinical application of the LCP. *Injury.* 2003 Nov;34 Suppl 2: B63–76.

[13] **Streubel PN, Gardner MJ, Morshed S, et al.** Are extreme distal periprosthetic supracondylar fractures of the femur too distal to fix using a lateral locked plate? *J Bone Joint Surg Br.* 2010 Apr;92(4):527–534.

[14] **Mortazavi SM, Kurd MF, Bender B, et al.** Distal femoral arthroplasty for the treatment of periprosthetic fractures after total knee arthroplasty. *J Arthroplasty.* 2010 Aug;25(5):775–780.

[15] **Mamczak CN, Gardner MJ, Bolhofner B, et al.** Interprosthetic femoral fractures. *J Orthop Trauma.* 2010 Dec;24(12):740–744.

[16] **Kolb K, Koller H, Lorenz I, et al.** Operative treatment of distal femoral fractures above total knee arthroplasty with the indirect reduction technique: a long-term follow-up study. *Injury.* 2009 Apr;40(4):433–439.

[17] **Ebraheim NA, Liu J, Hashmi SZ, et al.** High complication rate in locking plate fixation of lower periprosthetic distal femur fractures in patients with total knee arthroplasties. *J Arthroplasty.* 2012 May;27(5):809–813.

[18] **Hou Z, Bowen TR, Irgit K, et al.** Locked plating of periprosthetic femur fractures above total knee arthroplasty. *J Orthop Trauma.* 2012 Jul;26(7):427–432.

[19] **Hierholzer C, von Rüden C, Pötzel T, et al.** Outcome analysis of retrograde nailing and less invasive stabilization system in distal femoral fractures: A retrospective analysis. *Indian J Orthop.* 2011 May;45(3):243–250.

[20] **Chen F, Mont MA, Bachner RS.** (1994) Management of ipsilateral supracondylar femur fractures following total knee arthroplasty. *J Arthroplasty.* 1994 Oct;9(5):521–526.

[21] **McLaren AC, Dupont JA, Schroeber DC.** Open reduction internal fixation of supracondylar fractures above total knee arthroplasties using intramedullary supracondylar rod. *Clin Orthop Relat Res.* 1994 May;(302):194–198.

[22] **Srinivasan K, Macdonald DA, Tzioupis CC, et al.** Role of long stem revision knee prosthesis in periprosthetic and complex distal femoral fractures: A review of eight patients. *Injury.* 2005 Sep;36(9):1094–1102.

[23] **Kraay MJ, Goldberg VM, Figgie MP, et al.** Distal femoral replacement with allograft/prosthetic reconstruction for treatment of supracondylar fractures in patients with total knee arthroplasty. *J Arthroplasty.* 1992 Mar;7(1):7–16.

[24] **Gross AE.** Periprosthetic fractures of the knee: puzzle pieces. *J Arthroplasty.* 2004 Jun;19(4 Suppl 1):47–50.

[25] **Kassab M, Zalzal P, Azores GMS, et al.** Management of periprosthetic femoral fractures after total knee arthroplasty using a distal femoral allograft. *J Arthroplasty.* 2004 Apr;19(3):361–368.

[26] **Keenan J, Chakrabarty G, Newman JH.** Treatment of supracondylar femoral fracture above total knee replacement by custom made hinged prosthesis. *Knee.* 2000 Jul;7(3):165–170.

6.5.3 Patella

Authors **Bernd Fink, Marschall B Berkes, Dean G Lorich**

Incidence and risk factors of periprosthetic patellar fractures

Chalidis et al [1] noted a 1.19% rate of periprosthetic patellar fractures in primary cases, with a range of 0.15%–12% for revision procedures. Most (99.1%) occurred in patellae that had had surface replacement (chapter 2). For the patella there are specific risk factors, such as loss of patellar thickness, the presence of surface replacement, thermal necrosis, lateral ligament release, malalignment of the limb, and prosthesis malpositioning (chapter 3.2).

Classification

Up to now, periprosthetic fractures of the patella were classified according to Ortiguea and Berry (chapter 4.2). A new Unified Classification System (UCS) has been proposed (chapter 4.2), which can be applied to the patella (**6.5-7a–b**). The knee joint is numbered "V", the patella "34."

Treatment

A stable retropatellar implant type B1 should only be removed if it would hinder the tension-band fixation as standard treatment. The goal is to reconstruct the extensor mechanism. Periprosthetic fractures of the patella with a loose implant (type B2 or B3) require revision arthroplasty whether the fractured fragments are displaced or not. A patellectomy as another option should be avoided because this type of treatment is expected to lead to a considerable loss of extensor function and strength of approximately 70%.

Tension-band fixation

Simple periprosthetic fractures of the patella type B1 are not common and are best fixed with the typical tension-band wires [2]. If following a fracture with stable implant type V.34-B1 the reconstruction of the extension apparatus fails, a knee revision procedure can be carried out either with replacement or reconstruction of the extension apparatus with allografts or with autogenous soft-tissue reconstruction, eg, the semitendinosus tendon.

Revision arthroplasty

Periprosthetic fractures of the patella are most frequently type B2 or B3 with loose implant components [2]. Usually a two-stage procedure is recommended because the remaining bone stock is often too poor for reimplantation. The loose retropatellar component is first removed and the fracture stabilized using tension bands, screws, or a combination of both.

When combining the tension-band fixation with a cemented implantation of the retropatellar component in a single stage, cement could leak into the fracture site, thereby interfering with safe fracture healing and resulting in nonunion or refracture. Therefore, most authors [2] recommend a resection arthroplasty with smoothing of the contact surfaces of the old retropatellar replacement and fracture fixation. Once the fracture has healed and is stable, a secondary retropatellar replacement can be implanted should the patient report adverse symptoms. The thickness of the remaining patella should be at least 1 cm so that the new retropatellar implant can be securely cemented in position. If this is not the case, retropatellar replacement should not be performed.

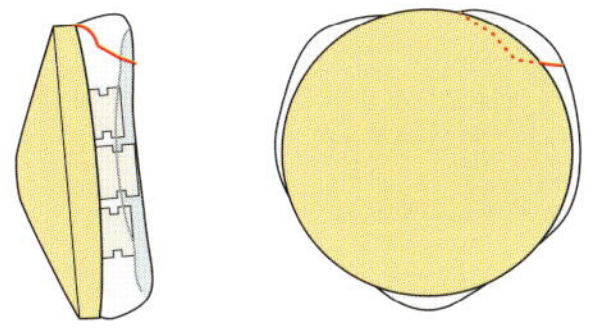
a

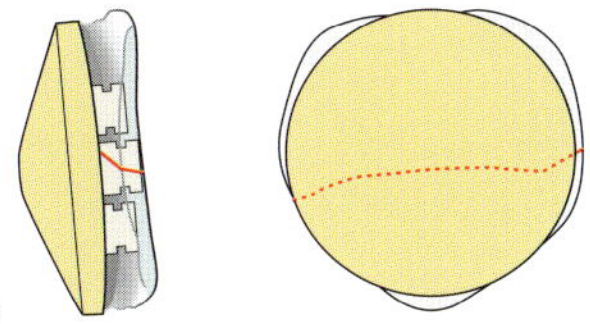
b

6.5-7a–b Examples of periprosthetic fracture types in the proximal femur according to the Unified Classification System (UCS).
a Type V.34-A1.
b Type V.34-B3.

An alternative to the use of cement is the noncemented suturing of a retropatellar replacement with a trabecular-metal backing (**6.5-8a–d**). The high osteointegrative properties of this implant make it highly suitable for noncemented fixation, even if the remaining bone is thin. Using a trabecular-metal patella and a noncemented procedure allows osteosynthesis and reimplantation to be carried out in a one-stage procedure. However, suturing this type of implant into the tendon following patellectomy is not recommended because poor healing is likely to result with a high failure rate.

If the patellar fracture occurred due to considerable malalignment of the femoral or tibial component, causing increased compression onto the contact surfaces, a correction of the malalignment should be performed by partial or total revision arthroplasty in addition to the fixation of the fracture. If left in place, a malaligned femorotibial prosthesis will endanger the healing process due to increased compressive forces [3].

Open fractures

Due to the exposed position and the delicate soft-tissue cover, periprosthetic fractures of the patella are often open fractures. The high infection risk requires special attention because an infected total knee arthroplasty following an open patella fracture represents a major problem. There are two treatment strategies in the clinical scenario of an open-fracture dislocation of a knee arthroplasty. One strategy—presuming that, by definition, the knee joint is infected after an open fracture—involves an aggressive algorithm consisting of explantation of the arthroplasty, debridement, placement of an antibiotic spacer, and osteosynthesis of the patella. In a second stage, and after fracture healing of the patella, a revision arthroplasty is performed. The other strategy uses a more limited approach, consisting only of debridement of the open fracture and thorough irrigation of the knee joint followed by patellar fracture osteosynthesis (chapter 11.1).

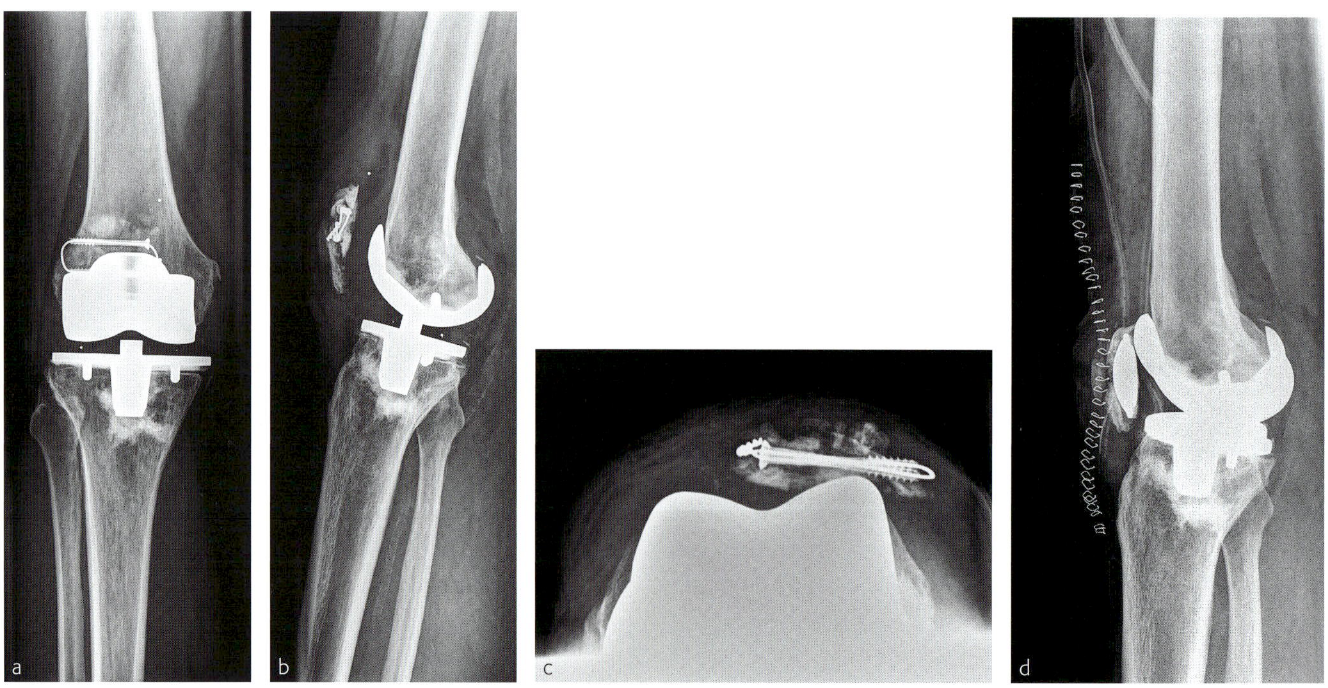

6.5-8a–d X-rays of a 65-year-old man with loosened patellar replacement and nonunion of a patellar fracture with screw fixation.

a AP view of periprosthetic fracture of the patella.
b Lateral view.
c Nonunion after osseosynthesis of the periprosthetic fracture with screws and cerclage, leaving the patellar replacement in place.
d Revision to a trabecular-metal retropatellar replacement resulting in osseointegration and good clinical result, with an average American Knee Society score (AKSS) of 76 and a function score of 75, 12 months postoperatively.

Complications and outcome

Results concerning revision arthroplasty in cases of periprosthetic fractures of the patella are not available in the literature. However, from studies dealing with trabecular metal patellae in revision arthroplasty with bone deficiency it can be presumed that at least 50% of sufficient bone contact is required to achieve good osseointegration of the implant [4]. Ries et al [5] showed that in revision arthroplasties ten of eleven trabecular metal patellae, in which at least 50% of the patellar component surface was covered by host bone, remained stable after a minimum follow-up of 12 months whereas all seven implants failed in cases with no remaining patellar bone stock.

Results of open reduction and internal fixation (ORIF) of periprosthetic fractures reported in the literature are generally poor. High rates of nonunion have been reported and a systematic review on the subject revealed a 90% nonunion rate [1]. This underscores the importance of proper indications for ORIF rather than revision or resection arthroplasty. In addition, a lag of the extensor was present in most reported cases. Despite this, functional range of motion with an arc of at least 80° was usually achieved.

References

[1] **Chalidis BE, Tsiridis E, Tragas AA, et al.** Management of periprosthetic patellar fractures. A systematic review of literature. *Injury*. 2007 Jun;38(6):714–724.

[2] **Sheth NP, Pedowitz DI, Lonner JH.** Periprosthetic patellar fractures. *J Bone Joint Surg Am*. 2007 Oct;89(10):2285–2296.

[3] **Burnett RS, Bourne RB.** Periprosthetic fractures of the tibia and patella in total knee arthroplasty. *Instr Course Lect*. 2004;53:217–235.

[4] **Tigani D, Trentani P, Trentani F, et al.** Trabecular metal patella in total knee arthroplasty with patella bone deficiency. *Knee*. 2009 Jan;16(1):46–49.

[5] **Ries MD, Cabalo A, Bozic KJ, et al.** (2006) Porous tantalum patellar augmentation: the importance of residual bone stock. *Clin Orthop Relat Res*. 2006 Nov;452:166–170.

6.5.4 Proximal tibia

Authors **Michael J Raschke, Bernd Fink**

Introduction

Periprosthetic fractures of the proximal tibia are most challenging and difficult to treat as the proximal fragment is often small and of poor bone quality. Therefore, revision arthroplasties may be indicated in most cases, even if the prosthetic component is still well fixed. Another challenge is the delicate balancing of the ligamentous structures, which is essential for satisfactory knee function.

Since the number of total knee arthroplasties (TKAs) is rising dramatically, the complications of this procedure as well as the number of periprosthetic fractures around the knee are also increasing. As the anatomy and function of the knee is much more complex than that of the hip, the repair of a periprosthetic fracture is much more challenging and technically demanding as well.

Incidence and risk factors

Periprosthetic tibial fractures are the least common periprosthetic fractures around TKA (chapter 2.3.2). General risk factors applying to all periprosthetic fractures are listed and described in chapter 3.2. Local factors that may cause or enhance periprosthetic fractures include:

- Malpositioning of the prosthesis in varus or valgus position
- Noncemented implants
- Poor knee function due to ligamentous imbalance
- Previous revision arthroplasty
- Joint stiffness
- Inflammation or infection.

Classification

Periprosthetic fractures of the tibial component following TKA have been classified by Felix et al [1] according to their location, which takes into consideration the relation of the fracture to the tibial part of the prosthesis, the status of the prosthesis as well as the time of manifestation of the fracture (chapter 4.2). A new Unified Classification System (UCS) has been proposed (chapter 4.2), which can be applied to the proximal tibia (**6.5-9a–c**). The knee joint is number "V", the tibia "4."

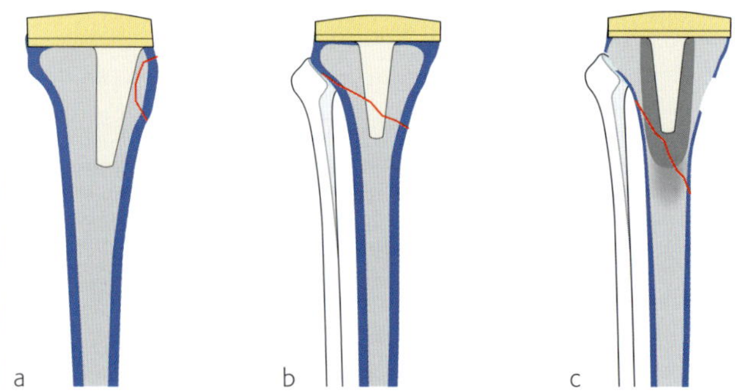

Fig 6.5-9a–c Examples of periprosthetic fracture types in the patella according to the Unified Classification System (UCS).
a Type V.4-A2.
b Type V.4-B1.
c Type V.4-B3.

Treatment

Fractures of the tibial plateau (type V.4) are typically fatigue fractures resulting in an impaction or depression, or a split of the tibial plateau and involve the interface between the tibial tray component and bone. Usually, the patient reports a history of pain and an inadequate trauma that finally leads to the correct diagnosis. This is verified by conventional x-rays and/or computed tomography. If treated conservatively (chapter 5.3), these fractures heal with increasing varus deformity and knee pain. However, since they are often associated with a loosening of the tibial component—corresponding to a type B2 and B3 periprosthetic fracture—revision arthroplasty is typically indicated.

In such cases, metallic or bony augmentation material should be used to supplement the insufficient bone quality of the medial tibial plateau.

A rare complication of unicondylar prostheses is a fracture of the tibial plateau during or after surgery with subsidence of the prosthesis (**6.5-10a–e**). If reduction and a safe operative fixation cannot be guaranteed, revision to bicondylar prosthesis is recommended. If lateral ligaments are stable, an unconstrained surface replacement prosthesis with a lengthened stem of the tibial component can be used. This usually includes augmentation of the tibial defect with appropriate prosthetic spacers. If the stability of the lateral ligaments is compromised by the fracture, then semiconstrained prostheses with an appropriate stem and spacers should be used.

Tibia plateau fractures type V.4 may also be caused by an adequate injury, with the prosthesis acting as an additional stress riser. If the prosthesis is well fixed and stable, corresponding to type B1, and the fragment is large enough, internal fixation is indicated (chapters 11.8–11.10). However, if there are any signs or history of loosening, ie, types B2 and B3 or in case of a short fragment or poor bone quality, revision arthroplasty should be performed. Internal fixation follows the principles of fracture fixation of the proximal tibia, where plates and screws, preferably with angular stability, are used as there is not enough space for intramedullary devices (**6.5-11a–g**).

In case of large segmental bone defects, stem prostheses with sleeves and/or structural allografts should be considered, similar to distal femoral arthroplasties (chapter 5.6). To avoid using larger revision prostheses with metallic or bony augmentation material, or even tumor prostheses, a two-stage procedure is advocated especially in younger patients. As a first step, the distal fracture is fixed by plate and screws and, after fracture healing, in a second step the loose prosthesis is replaced with an adequate implant.

Injuries that involve the extensor mechanism or fractures of the tibial tuberosity (type A2) frequently occur after extensive dissection, during eversion of the patella, or after osteotomy of the tibial tuberosity. The goal is the restoration of the extensor mechanism.

In minimally displaced fractures conservative therapy in a cast may be the first choice. However, in case of dysfunction of the extensor mechanism, operative treatment is indicated. These operations are extremely difficult since the bone stock and the soft-tissue envelope of the tibial tuberosity often are poor. Primary repair of a patellar tendon rupture by suture is usually ineffective. Larger avulsed bony fragments can be fixed with a screw or tension-band fixation; however, immobilization in a cast for 3 months or more is required for healing, which may result in stiffness or impaired function of the knee.

Salvage procedures consisting of an augmentation with autograft or allograft, such as semitendinosus transposition or Achilles tendon with calcaneus allograft, may be indicated, however, with questionable results [2].

Complications and outcome

To our knowledge, no systematic reports in regard to revision arthroplasty for isolated periprosthetic tibial fractures have been published as yet. The available studies concerning periprosthetic tibial fractures provide mixed data, ie, cases of distal femoral fractures and revision arthroplasties are mixed with osteosyntheses. Platzer et al [3] reviewed 41 patients with periprosthetic fractures after TKA. Of these, four patients had periprosthetic fractures of the proximal tibia and 37 of the distal femur. Conservative treatment by long-term cast immobilization was performed in five patients, while 36 underwent operative stabilization by plate fixation (n = 18), intramedullary nailing (n=15), or revision arthroplasty (n = 3). Only 28 patients returned to their preinjury activity level and were satisfied with their clinical results. For ten patients a relevant decrease of knee function and severe limitations in gait and activities of daily living was seen. Successful fracture healing within 6 months was achieved in 33 (87%) of 38 patients. Failures of reduction or fixation occurred in 8 (21%) of 38 patients. Reoperation due to technical failure became necessary in three patients.

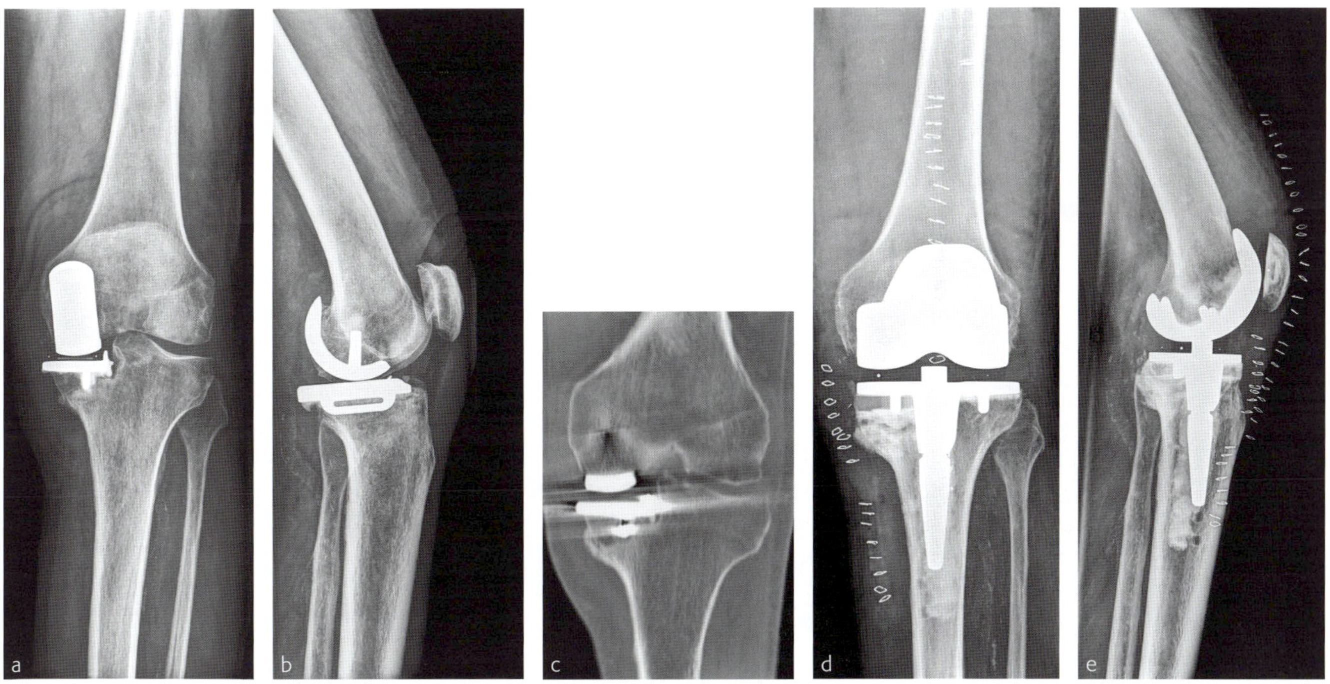

6.5-10a–e X-rays of an 80-year-old man with Parkinson's disease and a spontaneous fracture of the medial tibial plateau 3 months after implantation of a medial unicompartmental knee prosthesis.

- **a** AP view on admission.
- **b** Lateral view on admission.
- **c** CT scan on admission.
- **d–e** Postoperative x-rays after revision to a bicondylar knee prosthesis (rotating platform) with a tibial stem and medial tibial augmentation.
- **d** AP view.
- **e** Lateral view.

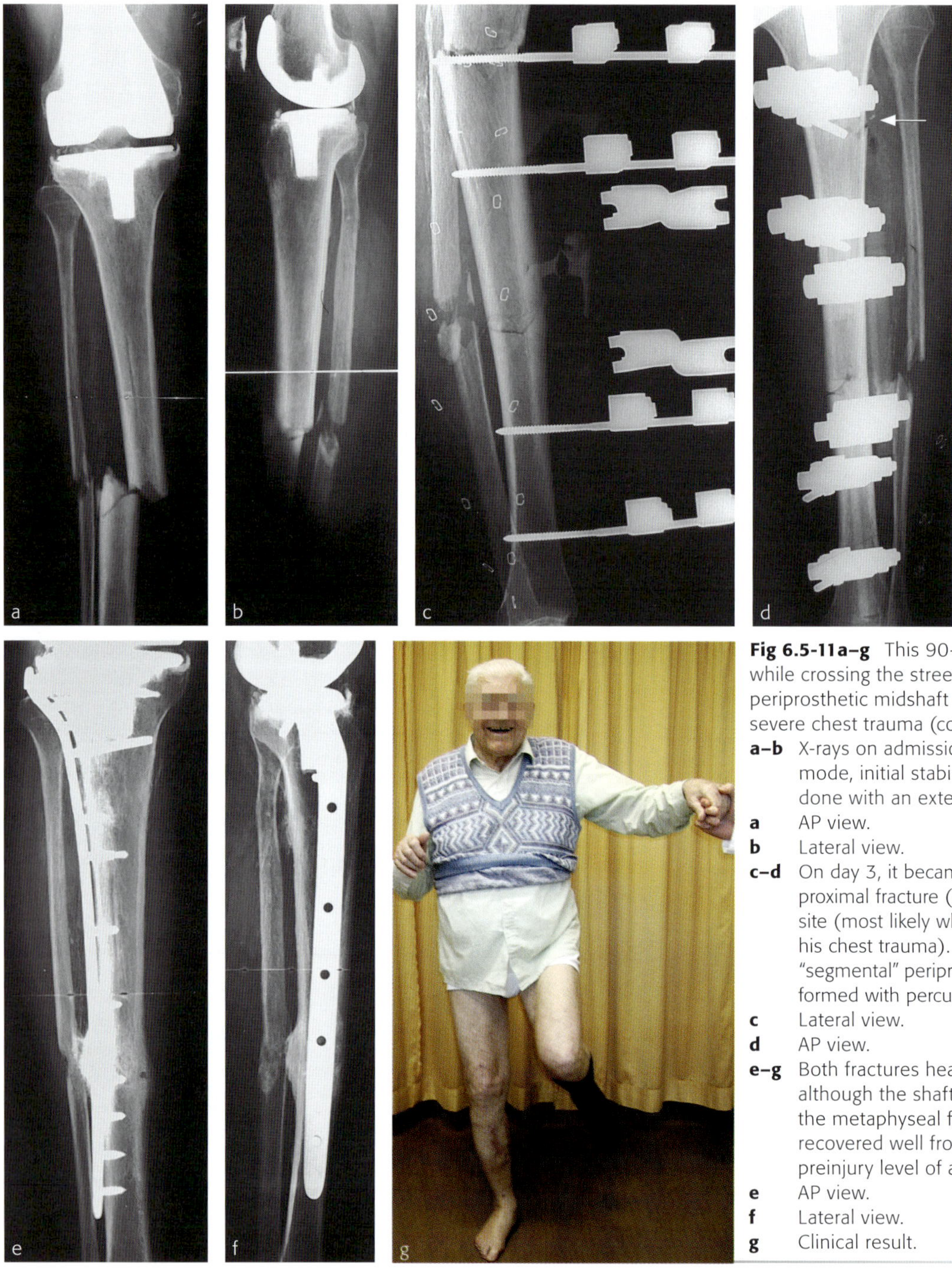

Fig 6.5-11a–g This 90-year-old man was hit by a car while crossing the street and sustained a closed periprosthetic midshaft tibial fracture in addition to severe chest trauma (courtesy of M Schütz).

a–b X-rays on admission. According to damage-control mode, initial stabilization of the tibial shaft was done with an external fixator.

a AP view.

b Lateral view.

c–d On day 3, it became obvious that another more proximal fracture (arrow) had occurred through a pin site (most likely while turning the patient to manage his chest trauma). At this stage, stabilization of the "segmental" periprosthetic tibial fracture was performed with percutaneous locked plating (LISS PLT).

c Lateral view.

d AP view.

e–g Both fractures healed without further intervention, although the shaft fracture took longer to heal than the metaphyseal fracture component. The patient recovered well from all his injuries and regained his preinjury level of activity after 1 year.

e AP view.

f Lateral view.

g Clinical result.

References

[1] **Felix NA, Stuart MJ, Hanssen AD.** Periprosthetic fractures of the tibia associated with total knee arthroplasty. *Clin Orthop Relat Res.* 1997 Dec;(345):113–124.

[2] **Mittlmeier T, Stöckle U, Perka C, et al.** [Periprosthetic fractures after total knee joint arthroplasty.] *Unfallchirurg.* 2005 Jun;108(6):481–496. German.

[3] **Platzer P, Schuster R, Aldrian S, et al.** Management and outcome of periprosthetic fractures after total knee arthroplasty. *J Trauma.* 2010 Jun;68(6):1464–1470.

6.6 Ankle

Authors **Alexej Barg, Beat Hintermann, Sebastian Manegold**

6.6.1 Introduction

There is no doubt that total ankle arthroplasty (TAA) is gaining acceptance as a valuable option for treating patients with end-stage ankle osteoarthritis.

But with increasing numbers of implanted prosthesis, longer survival rates and expanding indications, complications such as periprosthetic fractures occur. These fractures originate either as an intraoperative complication or as a postoperative fracture due to trauma or as a consequence of excessive mechanical overload (stress fracture).

Current reports of TARs show consistently good to excellent midterm results with significant pain relief, good functional outcome, and high-patient satisfaction [1]. Saltzman et al [2] published initial results from a prospective controlled trial of the Scandinavian Total Ankle Replacement System (STAR) versus ankle fusion and reported that TAA led to better function and similar pain relief in comparison with ankles that were fused.

6.6.2 Incidence

While periprosthetic fractures about knee or hip joint replacements as well as their incidence and therapeutic approaches have been widely discussed in an article by Meek et al [3], there are only few reports on this complication in patients with TAA. In most instances, the published literature on patients treated for periprosthetic fractures primarily consists of case reports [4–6] or short annotations within large TAA cohorts (**6.6-1** [5, 7–78]).

Periprosthetic fractures have been described as intraoperative or perioperative complications of TAA [79]. However, the true incidence of this complication is rare and varies significantly according to the study by Yang et al [4]. Nevertheless, these fractures are well-recognized complications in this patient cohort [79, 80].

6.6-1 Literature review addressing periprosthetic fractures in patients with total ankle replacement.

Author	Year	Study	TAR Type (n =)	Periprosthetic Fracture	Treatment	Results
Ali et al [7]	2007	RS, SC	Buechel-Pappas (34)	Intraoperative malleolar Fx (2)	ORIF with partially threaded cancellous screws	Complete healing
Álvarez-Goenaga [8]	2008	RS, SC	Hintegra (25)	Medial malleolar stress Fx (1)	Conservative (1)	Complete healing
Bai et al [9]	2010	RS, SC	Hintegra (67)	Intraoperative malleolar Fx (8)	ORIF (8) with screw	Complete healing
Bardelli and Scoccianti [10]	2006	RS, SC	STAR (7)	Intraoperative lateral malleolar Fx (1)	Conservative (1)	Complete healing
Barg and Hintermann [11] (6)	2010	RS, SC	Hintegra (33)	Intraoperative medial malleolar Fx (3), intraoperative lateral malleolar Fx (1), intraoperative bimalleolar Fx (1)	ORIF (5) with cannulated screw	Complete healing
Besse et al [12]	2009	PS, SC	AES (50)	Intraoperative malleolar Fx (4), tibial Fx (1) during an epileptic seizure 3 weeks postop., nondisplaced talar Fx (1) at 4.5 years postop.	Axial pinning of fibula and screwing for medial malleolus (4), tibial osteosynthesis and graft (1), corticocancellous iliac autograft for talar Fx (1)	Complete healing
Besse et al [13]	2010	RS, MC	Salto TAR (388), AES (173), Hintegra (22), STAR (9)	Intraoperative medial malleolar Fx (35), intraoperative lateral malleolar Fx (18)	NA	NA
Bolton-Maggs et al [14]	1985	RS, SC	ICLH Mark VII TAR (62)	Intraoperative medial malleolar Fx (1), intraoperative lateral malleolar Fx (1)	Conservative	Complete healing

Author	Year	Study	TAR Type (n =)	Periprosthetic Fracture	Treatment	Results
Bonnin et al [15]	2004	RS, SC	Salto TAR (98)	Intraoperative medial malleolar Fx (3), intraoperative lateral malleolar Fx (2), intraoperative pilon Fx (1)	NA	NA
Brunner et al [16]	2010	RS, SC	Hintegra (122)	Medial malleolar Fx (1) at 10 days postop.	ORIF (1) with plate and screw	Complete healing
Buechel et al [17]	1988	PS, MC	New Jersey Low Contact Stress (TAR) (23)	Intraoperative medial malleolar Fx (1)	NA	NA
Buechel et al [18]	2003	PS, SC	Buechel-Pappas (50)	Malleolar Fx (3) at 0.2, 0.8, and 2.7 years postop.	NA	NA
Buechel et al [19]	2004	PS, SC	Buechel-Pappas (115)	Intraoperative malleolar Fx (9)	NA	NA
Claridge and Sagherian [20]	2009	RS, SC	Agility (28)	Intraoperative malleolar Fx (2), medial malleolar stress Fx (1) at 3 weeks postop., medial malleolar stress Fx (1) with tilting of tibial component at 3 weeks postop. lateral malleolar stress Fx at 1 week postop.	All but one case conservative, case with component tilting with ankle fusion	Complete healing
Davies and Saxby [21]	2006	RS, SC	STAR (5)	Intraoperative medial malleolar Fx (1)	Conservative	No symptoms at 4 years, Complete healing
Delagoutte [22]	2002	RS, SC	Buechel-Pappas (36), STAR (8), Ramses (66)	Intraoperative medial malleolar Fx (5), intraoperative lateral malleolar Fx (8)	ORIF (5) with screw, conservative (8)	Complete healing
Dini and Bassett [23]	1980	RS, SC	Smith TAR (21)	Medial malleolar Fx (1)	Ankle fusion	NA
Doets et al [24]	2006	PR, MC	LCS TAR (19), Buechel-Pappas (74)	Intraoperative medial malleolar Fx (15), intraoperative lateral malleolar Fx (5), intraoperative distal tibial Fx (1)	ORIF with screw (9), conservative (12)	Medial malleolus nonunion (2)
Fevang et al [25]	2007	PS, MC	TPR (32), STAR (216), AES (3), Hintegra (6)	(1) in STAR	Revision TAR	NA
Giannini et al [26]	2010	PS, MC	BOX TAR (51)	Intraoperative medial malleolar Fx (1)	ORIF with screw (1)	Complete healing
Giannini et al [27]	2011	PS, MC	BOX TAR (158)	Iintraoperative medial malleolar Fx (2), intraoperative lateral malleolar Fx (1)	ORIF with K-wires (2) and interfragmental compression screw (1)	Complete healing
Harris et al [28]	2009	CR	STAR (1)	Pathological Fx of fibula (1) due to wear debris cyst	Cyst debridement, cast/walker immobilization	No symptoms at 3 months, complete healing
Haskell and Mann [29]	2004	RS, MC	STAR (189)	Iintraoperative medial malleolar Fx (12), intraoperative lateral malleolar Fx (6), medial malleolar stress Fx (3), lateral malleolar stress Fx (3)	ORIF (12), conservative (12)	1 nonunion after conservative treatment of intraop. medial malleolar Fx, complete healing (23)
Hay and Smith [30]	1994	RS, SC	St Georg uniaxial TAR (15)	Intraoperative malleolar Fx (2)	NA	NA
Helm and Stevens [31]	1986	RS, SC	Valdemar Link TAR (1), ICLH (18)	Intraoperative medial malleolar Fx (1), intraoperative lateral malleolar Fx (1)	Conservative (2)	Complete healing
Henricson et al [32]	2010	RS, SC	AES (94)	Intraoperative malleolar Fx (1), medial malleolar stress Fx (1) at 4 years postop.	ORIF (1), ankle fusion (1)	Re-Fx (1)
Hobson et al [33]	2009	RS, SC	STAR (123)	Intraoperative malleolar Fx (4), stress Fx (9)	NA	NA
Karantana et al [34]	2010	RS, SC	STAR (52)	Intraoperative medial malleolar Fx (1), intraoperative lateral malleolar Fx (4), tibial stress Fx (2)	Prolonged immobilization for intraoperative Fx (5), reivision TAR for stress Fx (2)	Complete healing
Karantana et al [35]	2010	RS, SC	STAR (10)	Medial malleolar stress Fx (1) at 10 weeks postop.	Immobilization for 6 weeks	Complete healing
Kim et al [36]	2010	RS, SC	Hintegra (348)	Intraoperative medial malleolar Fx (2)	NA	NA
Kirkup [37]	1985	RS, SC	Richard Smith (24)	Medial malleolar stress Fx (2)	Conservative	Complete healing
Kitaoka and Patzer [38]	1996	PS, SC	Mayo TAR (204)	Intraoperative medial malleolar Fx (4)	ORIF with screws or K-wires (4)	Complete healing

Author	Year	Study	TAR Type (n =)	Periprosthetic Fracture	Treatment	Results
Kopp et al [39] (32)	2006	RS, SC	Agility (43)	Intraoperative medial malleolar Fx (3), intraoperative lateral malleolar Fx (1)	ORIF (4)	Complete healing
Kumar and Dhar [40]	2007	RS, SC	STAR (50)	Intraoperative medial malleolar Fx (3), medial (5) and lateral (1) malleolar stress Fx between 2 and 4 months postop.	Conservative (8), revision TAR (1)	Complete healing
Kurup and Taylor [41]	2006	RS, SC	Buechel-Pappas (34)	Intraoperative medial malleolar Fx (4), intraoperative lateral malleolar Fx (1)	ORIF (1), conservative (4)	Complete healing
Lee et al [42]	2008	RS, SC	Hintegra (50)	Intraoperative malleolar Fx (5)	ORIF with screws (5)	Complete healing
Lee et al [43]	2010	RS, SC	Mobility (30)	Intraoperative medial malleolar Fx (6), intraoperative lateral malleolar Fx (1)	ORIF with screws or K-wires (7)	Complete healing
Mann et al [44]	2011	PS, SC	STAR (84)	Intraoperative medial malleolar Fx (3), intraoperative lateral malleolar Fx (1), medial malleolar stress Fx (3)	ORIF (6), conservative (1)	Complete healing
McGarvey et al [5]	2004	RS, SC	STAR (20), Agility (25)	Intraoperative medial malleolar Fx (Agility 4), intraoperative lateral malleolar Fx (Agility 1, STAR 2), medial malleolar stress Fx (STAR 2) at and 12 months postop.	ORIF with screws or K-wires in intraoperative Fx (7), conservative (2)	Complete healing (7), nonunion (Agility 1, STAR 1)
Mehta et al [45]	2010	RS, SC	Salto (9)	Intraoperative medial malleolar Fx (1), intraoperative distal tibial Fx (1)	ORIF (2)	Complete healing
Mendolia et al [46]	2005	RS, MC	Ramses (73)	Intraoperative malleolar Fx (4)	ORIF (2), conservative (2)	Complete healing
Morgan et al [47] (40)	2010	RS, SC	AES (45)	Talar stress Fx (1)	Tibiocalcaneal fusion	NA
Murnaghan et al [48]	2005	RS, SC	STAR (22)	Intraoperative malleolar Fx (5)	Conservative	1 nonunion
Myerson and Mroczek [49]	2003	RS, SC	Agility (50)	Intraoperative medial malleolar Fx (5), intraoperative lateral malleolar Fx (1), intraoperative bimalleolar Fx (1)	ORIF (3), conservative (4)	Complete healing
Nelissen et al [50]	2006	PS, SC	Buechel-Pappas (15)	Spontaneous distal tibial Fx (2) at the proximal part of the cortical tibial window while in the below-knee plaster	Prolonged immobilization (8 weeks instead of 6)	Complete healing
Nishikawa et al [51]	2004	RS, SC	TNK (32)	Intraoperative medial malleolar Fx (1)	ORIF (1)	Complete healing
Reuver et al [52]	2010	RS, MC	Salto (59)	Intraoperative lateral malleolar Fx (3)	ORIF (3)	Complete healing
Rippstein [53]	2002	RS, SC	Agility (27)	Distal tibial Fx (1)	Conservative	Complete healing
Rippstein et al [54]	2011	RS, SC	Mobility (233)	Intraoperative medial malleolar Fx (4), intraoperative lateral malleolar Fx (5), medial malleolar stress Fx (10)	ORIF (11) with screw or plate, conservative (8)	Complete healing
Rudigier [55]	2005	RS, SC	ESKA (159)	Intraoperative medial malleolar Fx (8)	ORIF (3), conservative (5)	Complete healing
Rzesacz and Gossé [56]	2007	RS, SC	STAR (13)	Intraoperative medial malleolar Fx (1)	ORIF (1) with screw	Complete healing
Saltzman et al [57]	2003	RS, MC	Agility (90)	Intraoperative medial malleolar Fx (8), intraoperative lateral malleolar Fx (4), medial malleolar stress Fx (1), distal tibial insufficiency Fx (1) with stable varus subsidence of tibial component	ORIF (4), conservative (10)	Complete healing
Saltzman et al [58]	2010	RS, MC	STAR (42)	Intraoperative medial or posterior malleolar Fx (5), distal tibial stress Fx (1)	ORIF (5), conservative (1)	Complete healing
San Giovanni et al [59]	2006	RS, SC	Buechel-Pappas (31)	Intraoperative medial malleolar Fx (10), stress Fx (medial malleolus 2, distal tibia 1, distal fibula 1)	All but 2 cases conservative (ORIF medial malleolar stress Fx 1, distal tibial stress Fx 1)	Medial malleolar nonunion (1)
Schenk et al [60]	2011	RS, SC	Salto (413)	Intraoperative malleolar Fx (5)	NA	NA
Schuberth et al [61]	2006	RS, SC	Agility (50)	Intraoperative medial malleolar Fx (13), intraoperative lateral malleolar Fx (5), intraoperative bimalleolar Fx (1)	NA	NA

Author	Year	Study	TAR Type (n =)	Periprosthetic Fracture	Treatment	Results
Schutte and Louwerens [62]	2008	RS, SC	STAR (47)	Intraoperative medial malleolar Fx (6), intraoperative lateral malleolar Fx (2), intraoperative distal tibial Fx (3), medial malleolar stress Fx (1) at 19 months postop.	NA	Complete healing
Shinomiya et al [63]	2003	RS, SC	TNK (20)	Intraoperative medial malleolar Fx (3)	Conservative (3)	Complete healing
Skyttä et al [64]	2010	PS, MC	AES (298), STAR (217), ICLH (32), Hintegra (11), TPR TAR (6), Oregon (4), RCM (3), others (2)	Distal tibial stress Fx (AES 1)	Ankle fusion	NA
Spirt et al [65]	2004	RS, SC	Agility (306)	Intraoperative talus Fx (1)	ORIF	Complete healing
Stauffer [66]	1977	RS, SC	Mayo TAR (76)	Intraoperative medial malleolar Fx (4)	Conservative (4)	Complete healing
Stauffer and Segal [67]	1981	PS, SC	Mayo TAR (102)	Intraoperative medial malleolar Fx (5), intraoperative lateral malleolar Fx (1)	NA	Complete healing
OrthopaedicsOne [68]	1988	RS, SC	TNK (30)	Intraoperative medial malleolar Fx (6)	Conservative	Complete healing
Takakura et al [69]	1990	RS, SC	TNK (69)	Intraoperative medial malleolar Fx (6)	Conservative (6)	Complete healing
Takakura et al [70]	2004	RS, SC	TNK (160)	Intraoperative medial malleolar Fx (4)	Conservative	Complete healing
Thermann et al [71]	2009	CR	Mobility (1)	Iintraoperative medial malleolar Fx (1)	Conservative	Complete healing
van der Heide et al [72]	2009	RS, SC	STAR (37), Buechel-Pappas (21)	Intraoperative medial malleolar Fx (10), intraoperative lateral malleolar Fx (3), intraoperative tibial plafond Fx (3)	ORIF (9), conservative (7)	NA
Vienne and Nothdurft [73]	2005	RS, SC	Agility (10)	Intraoperative medial malleolar Fx (2), intraoperative lateral malleolar Fx (1)	NA	NA
Wood et al [74]	2000	RS, SC	TPR TAR (6), STAR (7)	Intraoperative medial malleolar Fx (STAR 1)	Conservative	Complete healing
Wood and Deakin [75]	2003	PS, SC	STAR (200)	Intraoperative malleolar Fx (9), malleolar stress Fx (10)	ORIF (2), conservative (15), revision TAR or fusion (2)	NA
Wood et al [76]	2008	PS, SC	STAR (200)	Intraoperative malleolar Fx (9), malleolar stress Fx (10) within 12 postop. months	ORIF (2), conservative (15), revision TAR or fusion (2)	NA
Wood et al [77]	2010	PS, SC	Mobility (100)	Intraoperative medial malleolar Fx (2), malleolar medial stress Fx (4), malleolar lateral stress Fx (1)	ORIF (2), conservative (5)	Complete healing
Wynn and Wilde [78]	1992	RS, SC	Conaxial (Beck-Steffee) TAR (36)	Intraoperative malleolar Fx (3), malleolar stress Fx (5) within 2 years postop.	Conservative (8)	Prosthesis loosening (8) at 6–48 months postop.

AES = Ankle Evolutive System (AES)
Fx = Fracture
ICLH = Imperial College London Hospital
NA = Not Available
ORIF = Open Reduction and Internal Fixation
PS = Prospective controlled study (trial)
RS = Randomized study
SC = Study cohort
STAR™ = Scandinavian total ankle replacement
TAR = Total Ankle Replacement
TPR = Thompson-Parkridge-Richards
MC = Mayo Clinic

6.6.3 Classification

As no classification system existed that was based on anatomical features, Glazebrook et al [81] developed an evidence-based classification of complications in patients who underwent TAR using a third-generation ankle prostheses. The following classification system has been proposed based on the rate of failure for a given complication:

- Low grade (very unlikely to cause TAR failure)
- Medium grade (leads to failure < 50% of the time)
- High grade (leads to failure > 50% of the time) [81].

Intraoperative and postoperative bone fractures were classified as low-grade and medium-grade complications respectively.

In the meantime, however, a new Unified Classification System (UCS) has been proposed (chapter 4.2), which can be applied to the ankle (**Fig 6.6-1a–c**). The ankle is joint number "VI," the tibia number "4," and the talus "8."

6.6.4 Treatment

Intraoperative fractures

Total ankle replacement is a demanding surgical procedure with a considerable learning curve. Therefore, intraoperative fractures can occur as an intraoperative complication at every anatomical structure of the ankle, in particular the medial and/or lateral malleolus [42, 49, 57]. Intraoperative malleolar fractures may occur with an incidence of up to 38% of all cases [42, 49, 57]. The overall fracture rate may decrease with increasing surgeon experience [29, 42, 49, 57]. The most common reasons for intraoperative fractures include extensive and inaccurate use of the saw blade in combination with a limited field of vision, insufficient instrumentation, and incorrect sizing of prosthetic components [80, 82]. Furthermore, patients with rheumatoid arthritis and long-term corticosteroid therapy are at higher risk due to reduced bone quality [83].

Anatomical reduction and stable osteosynthetic fixation should be achieved primarily to create a stable bone stock, ensure undisturbed prosthesis osseointegration, and enable an early mobilization of the patient. Therefore, intraoperative medial malleolar fractures should be fixed with screws. Fractures of the distal fibula should be managed with a small fragment plate according to the AO Principles of Fracture Management. Surgeons should be careful when choosing the surgical approaches. When additional medial or lateral incisions are necessary, an adequate skin bridge of at least 4 cm to the anterior approach should be maintained. Some nondisplaced fractures (especially with intact periosteum) can be treated conservatively (chapter 5.3) without any obvious consequences on long-term results [24, 75, 83]. In such cases, prolonged immobilization (8–12 weeks, instead of 6 weeks) in a walking cast or stable walker is proposed. Partial weight bearing (up to 20 kg) is allowed while using a cast or walker. Lack of stabilization is allowed before ambulation. If necessary, union of fractures should be assessed using conventional x-rays or computed tomography (CT).

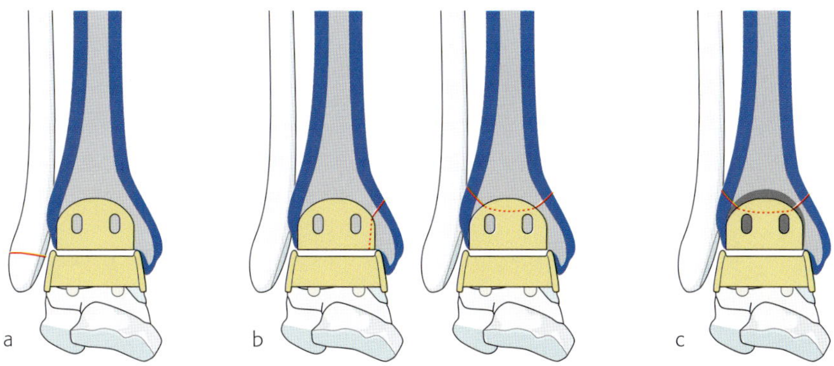

6.6-1a–c Examples of periprosthetic fracture types in the ankle according to the Unified Classification System (UCS).

a Type VI.4-A2.
b Type VI.4-B1.
c Type VI.4-B2.

Some authors reported prophylactic pinning of the malleoli to prevent intraoperative malleolar fractures [5, 41, 59]. However, an intraoperative malleolar fracture may occur despite the prophylactic fixation with K-wires [71]. Furthermore, surgeons should use an image intensifier or other method to assist with the planning of bone cuts and placement of properly sized prosthesis components intraoperatively.

Postoperative fractures

In case of a postoperative periprosthetic fracture, a thorough radiological examination is mandatory to exclude fracture-associated loosening of the prosthesis, regardless of whether it is septic or aseptic. Moreover, the surgeon must differentiate between fracture-independent aseptic and septic loosening (anamnesis, x-ray examination, CT scan, laboratory examination, preexisting periprosthetic osteolysis, joint aspiration, or intraoperative instantaneous section) before therapy.

Stress fractures

Perioperative fractures may occur in the early postoperative course, especially in medial malleolar fractures. Improper bone resection on the medial side may significantly weaken the medial malleolus resulting in a medial malleolus fracture. Incorrect positioning of prosthesis components significantly affects the biomechanics of a replaced ankle including increased joint contact pressures [84], decreased range of motion [85], and pathological restraint in periarticular ligaments [86], resulting in poor clinical outcome [87]. Altered biomechanics due to incorrect prosthesis positioning may also lead to periprosthetic stress fractures.

For nondisplaced stress fractures without any malposition or loosening of the prosthesis, conservative treatment with a prolonged immobilization in a cast or stable walker may be the first-choice treatment (chapter 12.1). In patients with significant dislocation, anatomical reduction and stable osteosynthetic fixation should be achieved. With concomitant malalignment of the biomechanical axis due to prosthesis malposition, corrective osteotomy is recommended to restore leg axis. Patients with aseptic or fracture-associated loosening of the prosthesis should be treated with combined corrective osteotomy or osteosynthesis.

If a stress fracture occurs late after surgery (chapters 12.2 and 12.3), it may be caused by pathologically increased forces across the replaced joint due to hindfoot malalignment. In such cases, careful clinical and radiological analysis of hindfoot alignment should be performed, eg, using the special hindfoot alignment view [88]. In addition, the stability of the prosthesis components should be assessed using CT or single-photon emission CT [89]. In such cases, revision surgery of the prosthesis components and fixation of the fracture alone may not suffice to achieve good long-term results. Therefore, the concomitant hindfoot deformity should be analyzed correctly and treated properly by calcaneal and/or supramalleolar osteotomies [90]. With septic loosening of the prosthesis, removal of TAR and implantation of an antibiotic spacer is recommended. An external fixator will stabilize the fracture and the ankle joint. Once fracture healing is achieved, the revision arthroplasty should be replaced by arthrodesis as second-stage procedure.

Traumatic fractures

Traumatic periprosthetic fractures (chapters 12.1 and 12.4) are rare in patients who have undergone TAA. In these patients, careful diagnostic assessment should be performed clinically and radiologically as the first step to determine the stability of the prosthetic components as it should be done if there is evidence of infection. In patients for whom prosthetic loosening or instability can be excluded, fracture reduction and stable fixation should be performed following the current principles of fracture management.

For evident instability and/or dislocation of prosthetic components, revision TAA can be performed in favorable circumstances, ie, in patients with appropriate bone stock. The affected ankle should be carefully evaluated based on x-rays in three planes as well as CT, which will allow for the assessment of osseous defects, malalignment, and deformities. Based on the authors' experience, prosthetic components with a flat undersurface are the most appropriate for revision TAA due to solid support from the remaining bone stock.

The feasibility of revision TAA has been classified in accordance to the degree of intraoperative osseous defect in the coronal plane after removal of initial prosthesis components and careful debridement:

- Standard components may be used if osseous defect of less than 18 mm and talus is intact
- Revision components should be used if osseous defect is between 18–25 mm and talus is intact
- Custom-made components should be used if osseous defect of more than 25 mm and talus is destroyed [91].

In other cases a salvage procedure by ankle fusion should be performed [92–94]. In the authors' clinic, anterior double plating is used for rigid fixation of isolated tibiotalar arthrodesis with preservation of the subtalar joint as a salvage arthrodesis procedure for failed TAA [95].

6.6.5 Complications and outcome

Periprosthetic ankle fractures are rare events, nevertheless—as an intraoperative complication—they have been described since TAA is in use. However, little is known about their long-term follow-up. Intraoperative periprosthetic fractures should be stabilized by osteosynthesis according to the principles of fracture management irrespective of fracture cause, localization, and extent of dislocation. Thus, a stable bone stock for prosthesis osseointegration is restored, and early mobilization of the patient is possible. From experience, fracture healing is terminated after 6 weeks of immobilization in a walker and long-term follow-up does not differ from patients without fracture complications. The same holds true for postoperative traumatic fractures, as long as prosthesis stability is not affected by the fracture.

Not surprisingly with periprosthetic stress fractures, long-term outcome is determined by prosthesis stability and alignment of the prosthesis. The outcome for patients with nondisplaced periprosthetic stress fractures without any malalignment of the biomechanical leg axis or misalignment of the prosthesis is not restricted. However, long-term follow-up and fracture healing is poor in the presence of prosthesis loosening and hindfoot malalignment, thus, revision surgery is mandatory.

References

[1] **Gougoulias N, Khanna A, Maffulli N.** How successful are current ankle replacements?: a systematic review of the literature. *Clin Orthop Relat Res.* 2010 Jan;468(1):199–208.

[2] **Saltzman CL, Mann RA, Ahrens JE, et al.** Prospective controlled trial of STAR total ankle replacement versus ankle fusion: Initial results. *Foot Ankle Int.* 2009 Jul;30(7):579–596.

[3] **Meek RM, Norwood T, Smith R, et al.** The risk of peri-prosthetic fracture after primary and revision total hip and knee replacement. *J Bone Joint Surg Br.* 2011 Jan;93(1):96–101.

[4] **Yang JH, Kim HJ, Yoon JR, et al.** Minimally invasive plate osteosynthesis (MIPO) for periprosthetic fracture after total ankle arthroplasty: a case report. *Foot Ankle Int.* 2011 Feb;32(2):200–204.

[5] **McGarvey WC, Clanton TO, Lunz D.** Malleolar fracture after total ankle arthroplasty: a comparison of two designs. *Clin Orthop Relat Res.* 2004 Jul;(424):104–110.

[6] **Haendlmayer KT, Fazly FM, Harris NJ.** Periprosthetic fracture after total ankle replacement: surgical technique. *Foot Ankle Int.* 2009 Dec;30(12):1233–1234.

[7] **Ali MS, Higgins GA, Mohamed M.** Intermediate results of Buechel Pappas unconstrained uncemented total ankle replacement for osteoarthritis. *J Foot Ankle Surg.* 2007 Jan-Feb;46(1):16–20.

[8] **Álvarez-Goenaga F.** [Total ankle replacement. First 25 cases]. *Rev Esp Cir Ortop Traumatol.* 2008;52:224–232. Spanish.

[9] **Bai LB, Lee KB, Song EK, et al.** Total ankle arthroplasty outcome comparison for post-traumatic and primary osteoarthritis. *Foot Ankle Int.* 2010 Dec;31(12):1048–1056.

[10] **Bardelli M, Scoccianti G.** Uncemented total ankle arthroplasty in post-traumatic osteoarthritis: 3- to 7-year follow-up. *J Orthopaed Traumatol.* 2006;7:93–96.

[11] **Barg A, Hintermann B.** Takedown of painful ankle fusion and total ankle replacement using a 3-component ankle prosthesis. *Tech Foot & Ankle.* 2010;9(4):190–198.

[12] **Besse JL, Brito N, Lienhart C.** Clinical evaluation and radiographic assessment of bone lysis of the AES total ankle replacement. *Foot Ankle Int.* 2009 Oct;30(10):964–975.

[13] **Besse JL, Colombier JA, Asencio J, et al.** Total ankle arthroplasty in France. *Orthop Traumatol Surg Res.* 2010 May;96(3):291–303.

[14] **Bolton-Maggs BG, Sudlow RA, Freeman MA.** Total ankle arthroplasty. *A long-term review of the London Hospital experience.* J Bone Joint Surg Br. 1985 Nov;67(5):785–790.

[15] **Bonnin M, Judet T, Colombier JA, et al.** Midterm results of the Salto Total Ankle Prosthesis. *Clin Orthop Relat Res.* 2004 Jul;424(424):6–18.

[16] **Brunner S, Knupp M, Hintermann B.** Total ankle replacement for the valgus unstable osteoarthritic ankle. *Tech Foot & Ankle.* 2010;9(4):165–174.

[17] **Buechel FF, Pappas MJ, Iorio LJ.** New Jersey low contact stress total ankle replacement: biomechanical rationale and review of 23 cementless cases. *Foot Ankle.* 1988 Jun;8(6):279–290.

[18] **Buechel FF Sr, Buechel FF Jr, Pappas MJ.** Ten-year evaluation of cementless Buechel-Pappas meniscal bearing total ankle replacement. *Foot Ankle Int.* 2003 Jun;24(6):462–472.

[19] **Buechel FF Sr, Buechel FF Jr, Pappas MJ.** Twenty-year evaluation of cementless mobile-bearing total ankle replacements. *Clin Orthop Relat Res.* 2004 Jul;(424):19–26.

[20] **Claridge RJ, Sagherian BH.** Intermediate term outcome of the agility total ankle arthroplasty. *Foot Ankle Int.* 2009 Sep;30(9):824–835.

[21] **Davies MB, Saxby T.** Ankle arthropathy of hemochromatosis: a case series and review of the literature. *Foot Ankle Int.* 2006 Nov;27(11):902–906.

[22] **Delagoutte JP.** Retrospective analysis of 110 ankle prostheses. *Eur J Orthop Surg Traumatol.* 2002;12:198–205.

[23] **Dini AA, Bassett FH 3rd.** Evaluation of the early result of Smith total ankle replacement. *Clin Orthop Relat Res.* 1980 Jan–Feb;(146):228–230.

[24] **Doets HC, Brand R, Nelissen RG.** Total ankle arthroplasty in inflammatory joint disease with use of two mobile-bearing designs. *J Bone Joint Surg Am.* 2006 Jun;88(6):1272–1284.

[25] **Fevang BT, Lie SA, Havelin LI, et al.** 257 ankle arthroplasties performed in Norway between 1994 and 2005. *Acta Orthop.* 2007 Oct;78(5):575–583.

[26] **Giannini S, Romagnoli M, O'Connor JJ, et al.** Total ankle replacement compatible with ligament function produces mobility, good clinical scores, and low complication rates: an early clinical assessment. *Clin Orthop Relat Res.* 2010 Oct;468(10):2746–2753.

[27] **Giannini S, Romagnoli M, O'Connor JJ, et al.** Early clinical results of the BOX ankle replacement are satisfactory: a multicenter feasibility study of 158 ankles. *J Foot Ankle Surg.* 2011 Nov-Dec;50(6):641–647.

[28] **Harris NJ, Brooke BT, Sturdee S.** A wear debris cyst following S.T.A.R. Total Ankle Replacement—surgical management. *Foot Ankle Surg.* 2009;15(1):43–45.

[29] **Haskell A, Mann RA.** Perioperative complication rate of total ankle replacement is reduced by surgeon experience. *Foot Ankle Int.* 2004 May;25(5):283–289.

[30] **Hay SM, Smith TWD.** Total ankle arthroplasty: a long-term review. *Foot.* 1994;4:1–5.

[31] **Helm R, Stevens J.** Long-term results of total ankle replacement. *J Arthroplasty.* 1986;1(4):271–277.

[32] **Henricson A, Knutson K, Lindahl J, et al.** The AES total ankle replacement: A mid-term analysis of 93 cases. *Foot Ankle Surg.* 2010 Jun;16(2):61–64.

[33] **Hobson SA, Karantana A, Dhar S.** Total ankle replacement in patients with significant pre-operative deformity of the hindfoot. *J Bone Joint Surg Br.* 2009 Apr;91(4):481–486.

[34] **Karantana A, Hobson S, Dhar S.** The Scandinavian total ankle replacement: survivorship at 5 and 8 years comparable to other series. *Clin Orthop Relat Res.* 2010 Apr;468(4):951–957.

[35] **Karantana A, Martin Geoghegan J, Shandil M, et al.** Simultaneous bilateral total ankle replacement using the S.T.A.R.: a case series. *Foot Ankle Int.* 2010 Jan;31(1):86–89.

[36] **Kim BS, Knupp M, Zwicky L, et al.** Total ankle replacement in association with hindfoot fusion: Outcome and complications. *J Bone Joint Surg Br.* 2010 Nov;92(11):1540–1547.

[37] **Kirkup J.** Richard Smith ankle arthroplasty. *J R Soc Med.* 1985 Apr;78(4):301–304.

[38] **Kitaoka HB, Patzer GL.** Clinical results of the Mayo total ankle arthroplasty. *J Bone Joint Surg Am.* 1996 Nov;78(11):1658–1664.

[39] **Kopp FJ, Patel MM, Deland JT, et al.** Total ankle arthroplasty with the Agility prosthesis: clinical and radiographic evaluation. *Foot Ankle Int.* 2006 Feb;27(2):97–103.

[40] **Kumar A, Dhar S.** Total ankle replacement: early results during learning period. *Foot Ankle Surg.* 2007;13:19–23.

[41] **Kurup HV, Taylor GR.** Medial impingement after ankle replacement. *Int Orthop.* 2008 Apr;32(2):243–246.

[42] **Lee KB, Cho SG, Hur CI, et al.** Perioperative complications of HINTEGRA total ankle replacement: our initial 50 cases. *Foot Ankle Int.* 2008 Oct;29(10):978–984.

[43] **Lee KT, Lee YK, Young KW, et al.** Perioperative complications of the MOBILITY total ankle system: comparison with the HINTEGRA total ankle system. *J Orthop Sci.* 2010 May;15(3):317–322.

[44] **Mann JA, Mann RA, Horton E.** STAR™ ankle: long-term results. *Foot Ankle Int.* 2011 May;32(5):S473–484.

[45] **Mehta SK, Donley BG, Jockel JR, et al.** The Salto Talaris total ankle arthroplasty system: a review and report of early results. *Semin Arthroplasty.* 2010 Dec;21(4):282–287.

[46] **Mendolia G, Coillard JY, Cermolacce C, et al.** Long-term (10 to 14 years) results of the Ramses total ankle arthroplasty. *Tech Foot & Ankle.* 2005;4:160–173.

[47] **Morgan SS, Brooke B, Harris NJ.** Total ankle replacement by the Ankle Evolution System: medium-term outcome. *J Bone Joint Surg Br.* 2010 Jan;92(1):61–65.

[48] **Murnaghan JM, Warnock DS, Henderson SA.** Total ankle replacement. Early experiences with STAR prosthesis. *Ulster Med J.* 2005 May;74(1):9–13.

[49] **Myerson MS, Mroczek K.** Perioperative complications of total ankle arthroplasty. *Foot Ankle Int.* 2003 Jan;24(1):17–21.

[50] **Nelissen RG, Doets HC, Valstar ER.** Early migration of the tibial component of the buechel-pappas total ankle prosthesis. *Clin Orthop Relat Res.* 2006 Jul;448:146–151.

[51] **Nishikawa M, Tomita T, Fujii M, et al.** Total ankle replacement in rheumatoid arthritis. *Int Orthop.* 2004 Apr;28(2):123–126.

[52] **Reuver JM, Dayerizadeh N, Burger B, et al.** Total ankle replacement outcome in low volume centers: short-term followup. *Foot Ankle Int.* 2010 Dec;31(12):1064–1068.

[53] **Rippstein PF.** Clinical experiences with three different designs of ankle prostheses. *Foot Ankle Clin.* 2002 Dec;7(4):817–831.

[54] **Rippstein PF, Huber M, Coetzee JC, et al.** Total ankle replacement with use of a new three-component implant. *J Bone Joint Surg Am.* 2011 Aug;93(15):1426–1435.

[55] **Rudigier J.** Ankle replacement by the cementless ESKA endoprosthesis. *Tech Foot & Ankle.* 2005;4:125–136.

[56] **Rzesacz EH, Gossé F.** [Management of posttraumatic osteoarthritis of the upper ankle joint by implantation of the S.T.A.R. ankle prosthesis]. *Oper Orthop Traumatol.* 2007 Dec;19(5-6):527–546. German.

[57] **Saltzman CL, Amendola A, Anderson R, et al.** Surgeon training and complications in total ankle arthroplasty. *Foot Ankle Int.* 2003 Jun;24(6):514–518.

[58] **Saltzman CL.** Ankle osteoarthritis: Five take-home points regarding total ankle arthroplasty in USA. Paper presented at: 26th Annual Summer Meeting of the American Orthopaedic Foot & Ankle Society (AOFAS); July 7–10, 2010; National Habor, MD.

[59] **San Giovanni TP, Keblish DJ, Thomas WH, et al.** Eight-year results of a minimally constrained total ankle arthroplasty. *Foot Ankle Int.* 2006 Jun;27(6):418–426.

[60] **Schenk K, Lieske S, John M, et al.** Prospective study of a cementless, mobile-bearing, third generation total ankle prosthesis. *Foot Ankle Int.* 2011 Aug;32(8):755–763.

[61] **Schuberth JM, Patel S, Zarutsky E.** Perioperative complications of the Agility total ankle replacement in 50 initial, consecutive cases. *J Foot Ankle Surg.* 2006 May–Jun;45(3):139–146.

[62] **Schutte BG, Louwerens JW.** Short-term results of our first 49 Scandanavian total ankle replacements (STAR). *Foot Ankle Int.* 2008 Feb;29(2):124–127.

[63] **Shinomiya F, Okada M, Hamada Y, et al.** Indications of total ankle arthroplasty for rheumatoid arthritis: evaluation at 5 years or more after the operation. *Mod Rheumatol.* 2003;13:153–159.

[64] **Skyttä ET, Koivu H, Eskelinen A, et al.** Total ankle replacement: a population-based study of 515 cases from the Finnish Arthroplasty Register. *Acta Orthop.* 2010 Feb;81(1):114–118.

[65] **Spirt AA, Assal M, Hansen ST Jr.** Complications and failure after total ankle arthroplasty. *J Bone Joint Surg Am.* 2004 Jun;86-A(6):1172–1178.

[66] **Stauffer RN.** Total ankle joint replacement. *Arch Surg.* 1977 Sep;112(9):1105–1109.
[67] **Stauffer RN, Segal NM.** Total ankle arthroplasty: four years' experience. *Clin Orthop Relat Res.* 1981 Oct;160(160):217–221.
[68] **OrthopaedicsOne: The Orthopaedic Knowledge Network.** TNK Total Ankle Replacement. *Available at:* www.orthopaedicsone.com/display/Main/TNK+Total+Ankle+Replacement. Accessed April 21, 2013.
[69] **Takakura Y, Tanaka Y, Sugimoto K, et al.** Ankle arthroplasty. A comparative study of cemented metal and uncemented ceramic prostheses. *Clin Orthop Relat Res.* 1990 Mar;(252):209–216.
[70] **Takakura Y, Tanaka Y, Kumai T, et al.** Ankle arthroplasty using three generations of metal and ceramic prostheses. *Clin Orthop Relat Res.* 2004 Jul;(424):130–136.
[71] **Thermann H, Gavriilidis I, Longo UG, et al.** Total ankle arthroplasty and tibialis posterior tendon transfer for ankle osteoarthritis and drop foot deformity. *Foot Ankle Surg.* 2011 Sep;17(3):203–206.
[72] **van der Heide HJ, Schutte B, Louwerens JW, et al.** Total ankle prostheses in rheumatoid arthropathy: Outcome in 52 patients followed for 1–9 years. *Acta Orthop.* 2009 Aug;80(4):440–444.
[73] **Vienne P, Nothdurft P.** [Total ankle arthroplasty/endoprosthesis Agility: Indications, surgical technique, and results]. *FussSprungg.* 2004;2:17–28. German.
[74] **Wood PLR, Clough TM, Jari S.** Clinical comparison of two total ankle replacements. *Foot Ankle Int.* 2000 Jul;21(7):546–550.
[75] **Wood PL, Deakin S.** Total ankle replacement. The results in 200 ankles. *J Bone Joint Surg Br.* 2003 Apr;85(3):334–341.
[76] **Wood PL, Prem H, Sutton C.** Total ankle replacement: medium-term results in 200 Scandinavian total ankle replacements. *J Bone Joint Surg Br.* 2008 May;90(5):605–609.
[77] **Wood PL, Karski MT, Watmough P.** Total ankle replacement: the results of 100 mobility total ankle replacements. *J Bone Joint Surg Br.* 2010 Jul;92(7):958–962.
[78] **Wynn AH, Wilde AH.** Long-term follow-up of the Conaxial (Beck-Steffee) total ankle arthroplasty. *Foot Ankle.* 1992 Jul-Aug;13(6):303–306.
[79] **Conti SF, Wong YS.** Complications of total ankle replacement. *Clin Orthop Relat Res.* 2001 Oct;(391):105–114.
[80] **Hintermann B, Valderrabano V.** (2003) Total ankle replacement. *Foot Ankle Clin.* 2003 Jun;8(2): 375–405.
[81] **Glazebrook MA, Arsenault K, Dunbar M.** Evidence-based classification of complication in total ankle arthroplasty. *Foot Ankle Int.* 2009 Oct;30(10): 945–949.
[82] **Deorio JK, Easley ME.** Total ankle arthroplasty. *Instr Course Lect.* 2008;57:383–413.
[83] **Wood PL, Crawford LA, Suneja R, et al.** Total ankle replacement for rheumatoid ankle arthritis. *Foot Ankle Clin.* 2007 Sep;12(3):497–508.
[84] **Espinosa N, Walti M, Favre P, et al.** Misalignment of total ankle components can induce high joint contact pressures. *J Bone Joint Surg Am.* 2010 May;92(5):1179–1187.
[85] **Tochigi Y, Rudert MJ, Brown TD, et al.** The effect of accuracy of implantation on range of movement of the Scandinavian Total Ankle Replacement. *J Bone Joint Surg Br.* 2005 May;87(5):736–740.
[86] **Saltzman CL, Tochigi Y, Rudert MJ, et al.** The effect of agility ankle prosthesis misalignment on the peri-ankle ligaments. *Clin Orthop Relat Res.* 2004 Jul;(424):137–142.
[87] **Barg A, Elsner A, Anderson AE, et al.** The effect of three-component total ankle replacement malalignment on clinical outcome: pain relief and functional outcome in 317 consecutive patients. *J Bone Joint Surg Am.* 2011 Nov 2;93(21):1969–1978.
[88] **Saltzman CL, el-Khoury GY.** The hindfoot alignment view. *Foot Ankle Int.* 1995 Sep;16(9):572–576.
[89] **Pagenstert GI, Barg A, Leumann AG, et al.** SPECT-CT imaging in degenerative joint disease of the foot and ankle. *J Bone Joint Surg Br.* 2009 Sep;91(9):1191–1196.
[90] **Knupp M, Stufkens SA, Bolliger L, et al.** Classification and treatment of supramalleolar deformities. *Foot Ankle Int.* 2011 Nov;32(11):1023–1031.
[91] **Hintermann B, Barg A, Knupp M.** [Revision arthroplasty of the ankle joint]. *Orthopade.* 2011 Nov;40(11):1000–1007. German.
[92] **Espinosa N, Wirth SH, Jankauskas L.** Ankle arthrodesis after failed total ankle replacement. Special focus. *Tech Foot Ankle Surg.* 2010;9:199–204.
[93] **Hopgood P, Kumar R, Wood PL.** Ankle arthrodesis for failed total ankle replacement. *J Bone Joint Surg Br.* 2006 Aug;88:1032–1038.
[94] **Kotnis R, Pasapula C, Anwar F, et al.** The management of failed ankle replacement. *J Bone Joint Surg Br.* 2006 Aug;88(8):1039–1047.
[95] **Plaass C, Knupp M, Barg A, et al.** Anterior double plating for rigid fixation of isolated tibiotalar arthrodesis. *Foot Ankle Int.* 2009 Jul;30(7):631–639.

7 Shoulder cases

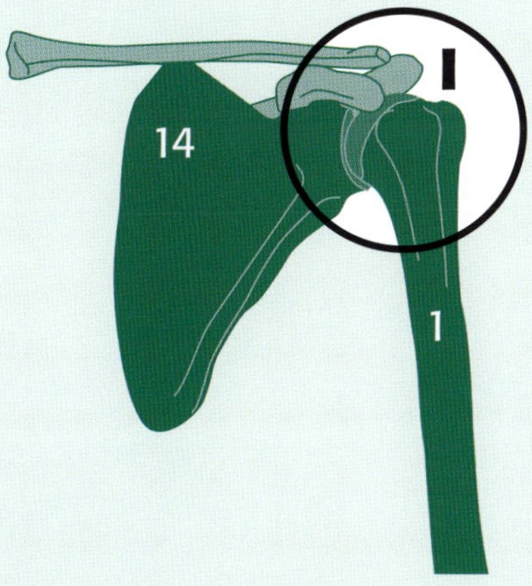

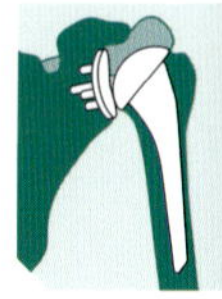

7.1 Proximal humeral fracture, stable prosthesis

Nonoperative treatment: immobilization

Authors **Stephen L Kates, Natasha O'Malley**

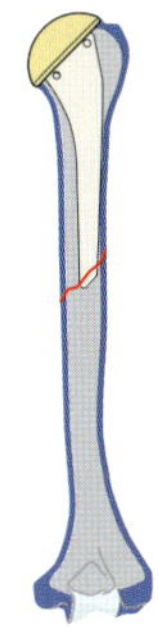

I.1-B1

Case description

A right-handed, 58-year-old woman recently underwent hemiarthroplasty of the right shoulder. Due to extensive comorbidities (including chronic obstructive pulmonary disease and mitral valve replacement with anticoagulation) and surgeon preference, a noncemented prosthesis was used to decrease operative time. X-rays revealed advanced osteoporosis (**7.1-1a–b**).

Two weeks postoperatively, the patient experienced a minor fall forward, with no definite impact, and described feeling a "pop", resulting in new pain in the right shoulder and arm (**7.1-2a–b**).

Classification: Type I.1-B1

Diagnosis: Nondisplaced periprosthetic humeral fracture at the tip of the stem

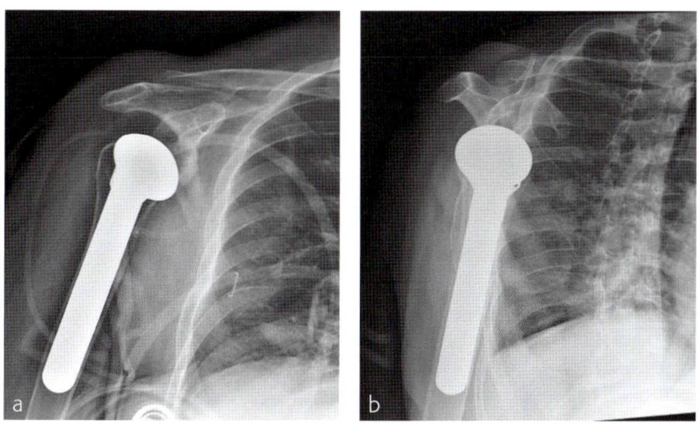

7.1-1a–b Postoperative x-rays of the prosthesis in situ.
a AP view.
b Lateral view.

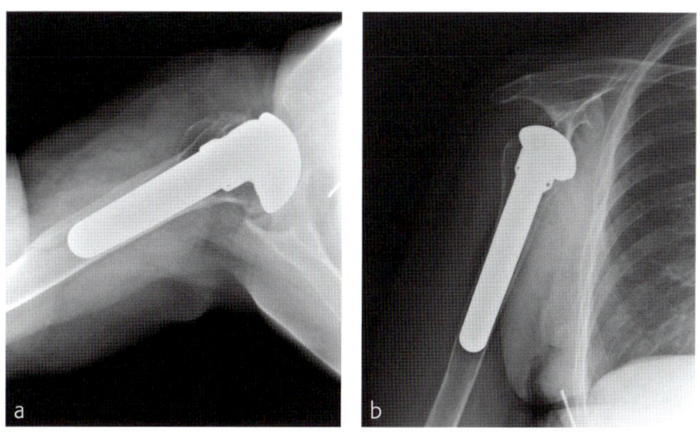

7.1-2a–b X-rays obtained after the patient's fall, 2 weeks postoperatively.
a AP view shows a new periprosthetic fracture at the tip of the stem with distal extension.
a Lateral view shows no apparent fracture.

I.1-B1 Decision making

Treatment options for this type of fracture can be nonoperative or operative. Revision surgery to a longer stem, or a locking plate osteosynthesis, is an option but was not necessary in this patient due to the minimally displaced nature of the fracture, the patient's comfort level, and her extensive comorbidities. Thus, nonoperative treatment with immobilization in a sling was advised (chapter 5.3). Planned, regular clinical and radiological surveillance should be scheduled with the nonoperative treatment to ensure no secondary displacement or extension of the periprosthetic fracture occurs. If either of the latter conditions is present, surgical intervention is indicated. An underlying metabolic bone disorder should be investigated with low-energy mechanisms of injury.

Rehabilitation and follow-up

After 2 weeks of immobilization, passive pendulum range-of-motion exercises were started. Motion was progressed gradually with patient comfort and radiological surveillance.

Fourteen weeks after sustaining the periprosthetic fracture, the patient reported no discomfort. Regular radiological surveillance verified no further displacement, and callus formation was observed (**7.1-3a–b**). At the 1-year follow-up, the patient had 140° of forward elevation and 40° of external rotation, with x-ray evidence of a fracture healing (**7.1-4a–b**).

Points to remember

- Nonoperative treatment of a minimally displaced periprosthetic fracture of the humerus is an option if the implant is securely fixed and the patient complies with treatment.
- Surgical treatment is warranted with secondary extension or displacement of the fracture.
- Patients should be advised about the potential that nonoperative treatment might fail, necessitating extensive revision surgery with the potential for significant loss of function.
- Another fall will worsen the situation.
- Evaluation and optimization of the metabolic bone profile is a priority after any minimally traumatic fracture.

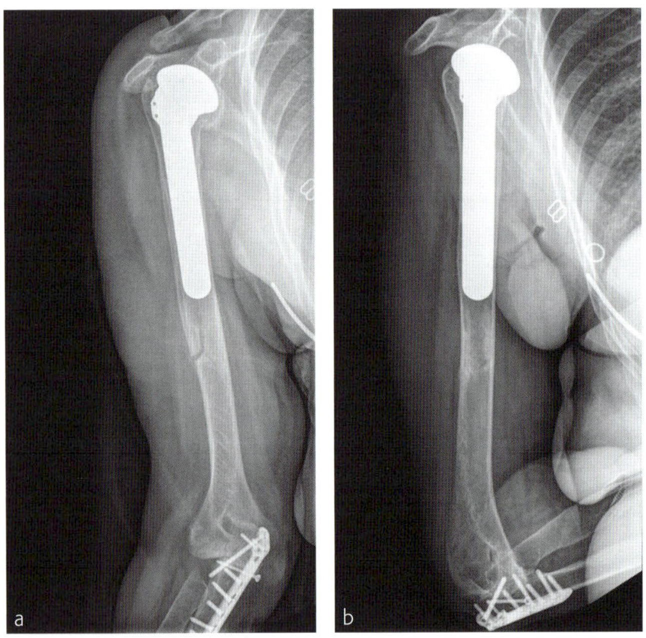

7.1-3a–b Postoperative x-rays obtained 16 weeks after right shoulder hemiarthroplasty and 14 weeks after periprosthetic fracture.

a AP view shows no further displacement. The fracture gap is more visible, and there is some bridging callus.

b Lateral view.

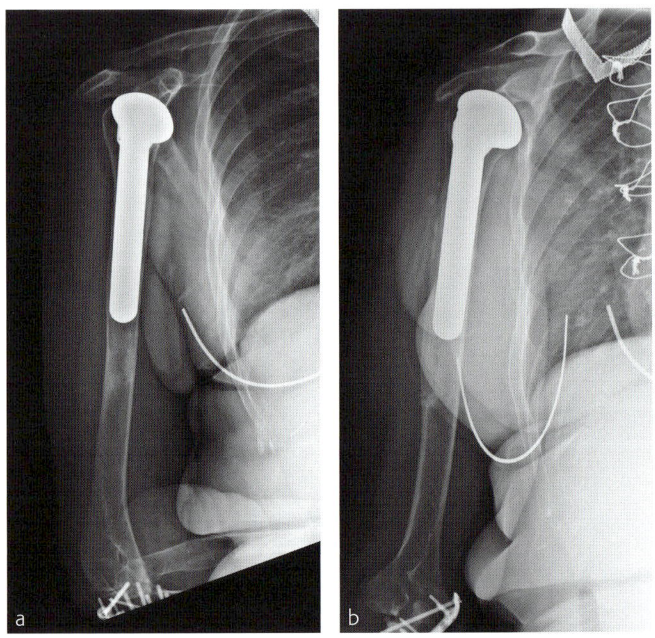

7.1-4a–b X-rays obtained at the 1-year follow-up show the healed fracture.

a AP view.

b Lateral view.

7.2 Humeral shaft fracture, stable prosthesis

ORIF: bridging LCP 4.5/5.0

Author **Simon Lambert**

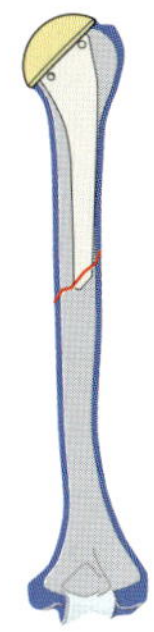

I.1-B1

Case description

A 72-year-old woman underwent arthroplasty for a fracture of the proximal humerus. Initial fracture treatment consisted of midhead resection replacement arthroplasty without glenoid replacement, which was later revised to a long-stem version (**7.2-1**). Comorbidities included Parkinson's disease, cervical spondylosis, and rheumatoid arthritis. Nine months postoperatively, the arthroplasty had failed and was complicated by axillary palsy; therefore, revision surgery with a customized, noncemented total shoulder arthroplasty was required (**7.2-2**). Three weeks after revision surgery, the patient was injured in a fall (**7.2-3a–b**).

Classification: Type I.1-B1

Diagnosis: Humeral shaft fracture distal to the tip of a well-fixed prosthesis

Decision making

Revision of an existing customized cemented implant is not desirable when the implant is well fixed and impacted. The implant can be difficult to remove without causing fragmentation of the humerus. The least invasive technique is application of a long contoured bridging plate (chapter 5.4.1) fixed proximally with cerclage wires.

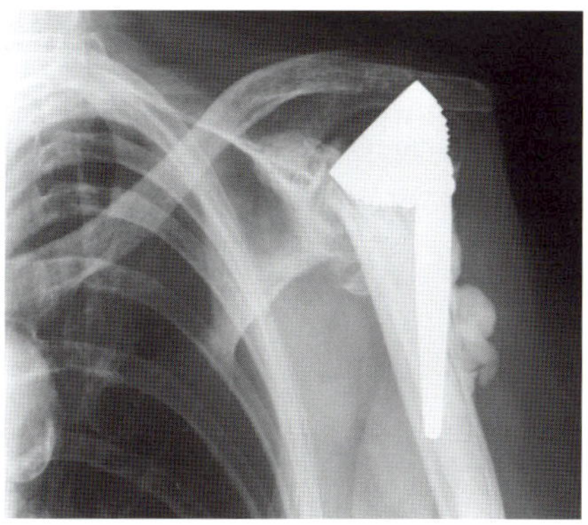

7.2-1 AP x-ray shows osteoporosis of the humeral shaft, lateral diaphyseal insufficiency, a loose cement mantle, and a poor-quality glenoid.

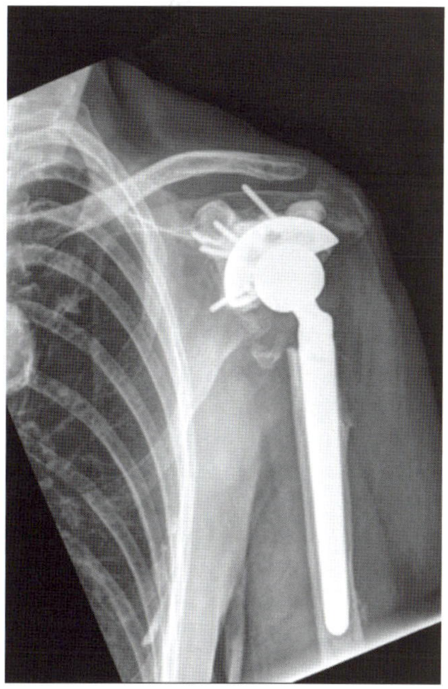

7.2-2 AP x-ray of a customized noncemented revision total shoulder arthroplasty.

1.1-B1

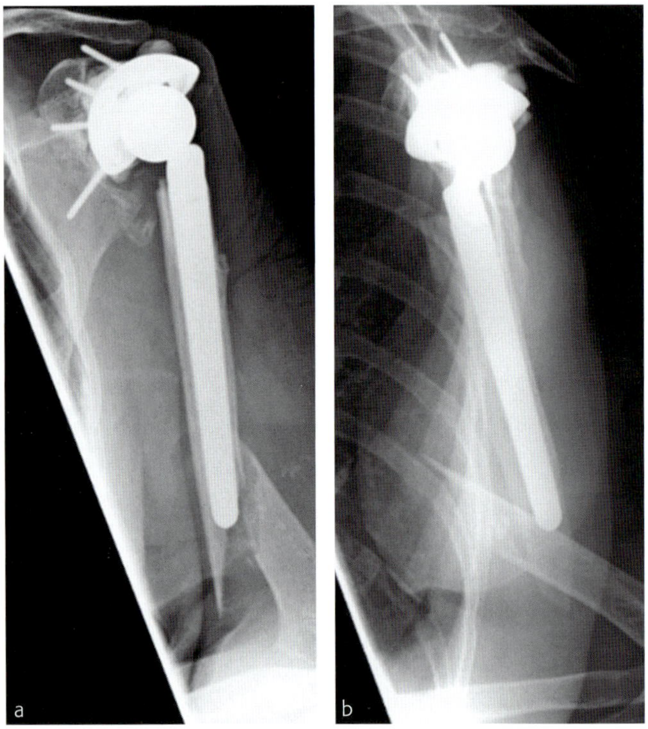

7.2-3a–b X-rays show a periprosthetic humeral fracture 3 weeks after revision arthroplasty.
a AP view.
b Lateral view.

Preoperative planning

Equipment

- 10-hole stainless steel locking compression plate (LCP) 4.5
- 5.0 mm locking-head screws
- 1.2 mm cerclage wiring system

Patient preparation and positioning

- Lateral decubitus position with the arm draped free
- First- or second-generation cephalosporin for antibiotic prophylaxis
- Compression stockings and calf compression for thrombosis prophylaxis
- Patient warming measures
- Neurophysiological monitoring

Reduction and fixation

With the direct posterior (Henry) approach, the incision was made, following the posterior border of the deltoid muscle from the midpoint of the border (to avoid injury to the upper posterolateral cutaneous nerve of the arm) to the midaxial line of the posterior aspect of the arm. It was then extended to a point 4 cm above the tip of the olecranon process, passing slightly to the lateral side of the olecranon process more distally.

The interval between the lateral and medial aspects of the triceps brachii muscle was identified proximally. The seam between the two parts was then split proximodistally, identifying the radial nerve and the arteria profunda brachii proximally. The neurovascular bundle was dissected distally to the lateral intermuscular septum, which was then split to avoid placing adverse traction on the nerve during reduction maneuvers. The remaining seam between the superficial aspects of the triceps brachii muscle was split distally through the triceps aponeurosis to a point 2 cm proximal to the olecranon and then continued slightly laterally to the olecranon. The lateral aspect of the triceps was elevated epiperiosteally from the lateral epicondylar ridge.

The deep part of the triceps brachii muscle was partially dissected by the fracture, with the remaining muscle fibers elevated epiperiosteally at the fracture zone.

Open reduction with manual alignment was used in this patient. Axial alignment is not necessarily required. In this case overlap, adjusting for rotation, was accepted because the interval between the time of the fracture and surgery was longer than 5 weeks, and complete restoration of length could have endangered the associated but distant neurovascular bundles. Proximal cerclage fixation was performed under direct visualization to protect the radial and ulnar neurovascular structures. To achieve "balanced" fixation, a minimum of three cerclage wires should be considered with, distally, four locking-head screws in the relatively good-quality bone of the lateral column of the humerus.

Rehabilitation and follow-up

The patient's arm was placed in a simple sling for 8 weeks. Twice-daily active-assisted elbow full range-of-motion exercises, active-assisted shoulder limited range-of-motion exercises (avoiding external rotation beyond neutral-zero at waist level and limiting flexion elevation to 45°), and postural exercises were encouraged. Simple nonweight-bearing activities of daily living were allowed when union was confirmed by the absence of symptoms and the presence of callus in all four quadrants of the fracture zone at 4.5 months (**7.2-4a–b**).

Points to remember

I.1-B1

- The use of locking-head screws permits optimal plate positioning without devascularization of the compromised bone.
- The radial nerve and its branches are endangered throughout the exposure. Early identification of the nerve proximally (out of the zone of injury) minimizes the risk to the nerve during dissection distally.
- Neurovascular bundles not immediately in the field of surgery (median and ulnar nerves) are at risk during manual realignment of the fracture. Therefore, an anatomical reduction should not be attempted, but an overlap accepted, while still maintaining the correct rotation.
- A fracture reduction instrument could apply too much distraction force and risk traction injury to all nerves "fixed" by scarring near or in the zone of injury. Minimal handling at the fracture zone using manual traction and pointed reduction forceps is recommended.

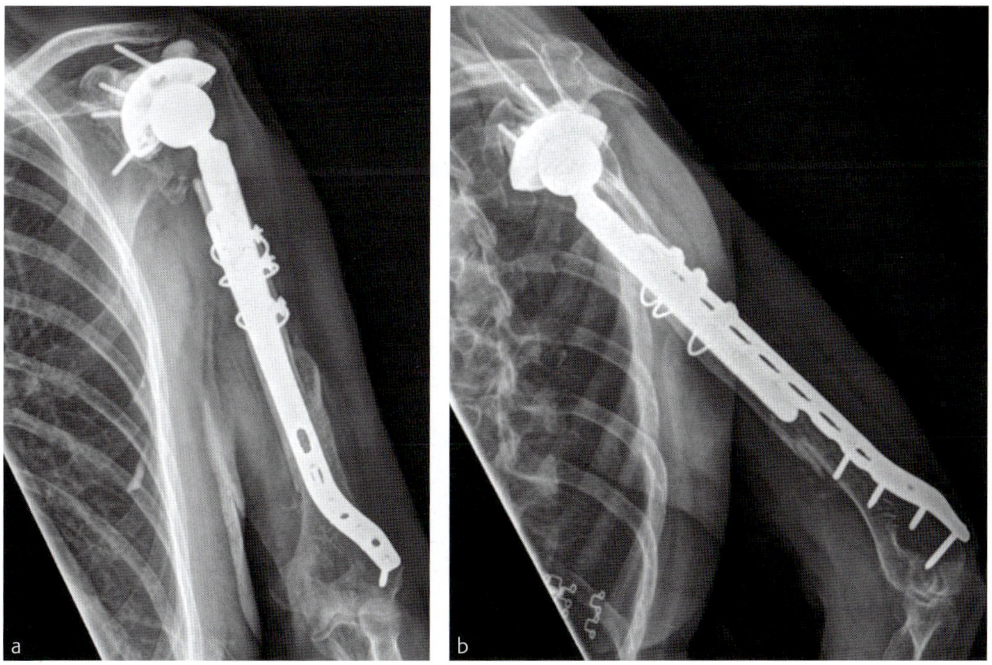

7.2-4a–b Follow-up x-rays obtained at 4.5 months.
a AP view.
b Lateral view.

I.1-B1

7.3 Humeral shaft fracture, stable prosthesis

ORIF: proximal humerus LCP 3.5

Author **David Barei**

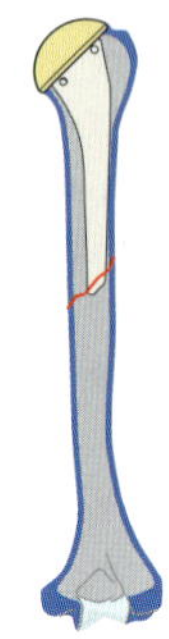

I.1-B1

Case description

An otherwise active, independent 88-year-old woman who sustained a proximal humeral fracture 8 years ago was initially treated with noncemented hemiarthroplasty. She recently fell and sustained a spiral fracture around the tip of the prosthetic stem with complete displacement (**7.3-1a–b**). There were no clinical or radiological signs of loosening of the prosthesis.

Classification: Type I.1-B1

Diagnosis: Periprosthetic fracture of the proximal humerus

Decision making

Different treatment options were discussed with the patient and the family. Because the patient was in good health, independent, and had a well-fixed prosthesis proximally, nonoperative treatment appeared too challenging; therefore, open reduction and internal fixation was recommended. The fracture pattern was simple and thus amenable to an absolute-stability construct. Because of the patient's age-related poor bone quality and the challenges associated with screw placement and purchase around the prosthesis, a long plate with locking-head screws was used to provide a mechanically sound construct (chapter 5.4.1). The goals of treatment were to obtain satisfactory reduction and immediate stability so the patient could quickly return to normal daily activities. Proximal screw fixation was obviously challenging because of the presence of the prosthesis. However, a perimeter around the stem appeared to be available for screw placement. The optimal solution was to use the plate as a long bridging device, spanning almost the entire length of the humerus, to prevent further fractures at either end of the plate. The patient was placed in a coaptation splint and medically cleared for operative treatment within 24 hours of injury.

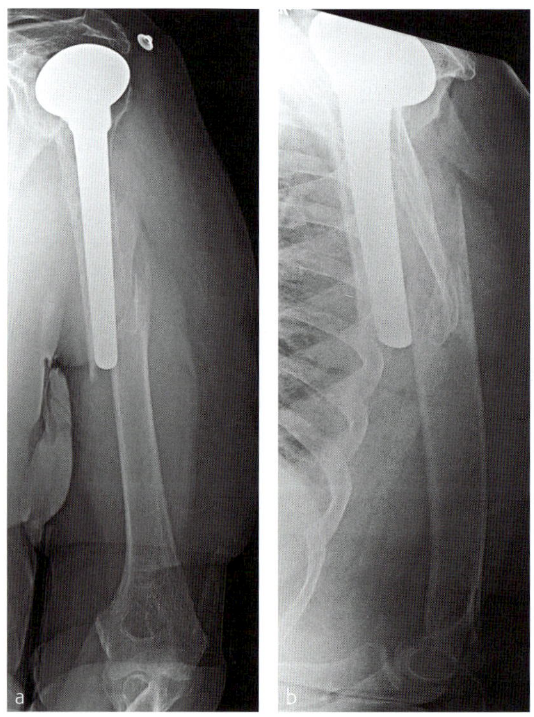

7.3-1a–b X-rays obtained immediately after the injury.
a AP view.
b Lateral view.

Preoperative planning

Equipment

- 14-hole proximal humerus locking plate 3.5
- 3.5 mm locking screws
- 2.4 mm conventional cortex screws
- Large- and small-serrated bone holding forceps
- Radiolucent operating table

Patient preparation and positioning

- Supine position on a radiolucent table
- First-generation cephalosporin for antibiotic prophylaxis
- Entire upper extremity prepared and draped into the surgical field

Reduction and fixation

The previous deltopectoral incision was used and extended distally into the anterior exposure of the humeral shaft. Proximally, the deltopectoral interval was developed and followed distally. The anterolateral third of the deltoid insertion onto the deltoid tuberosity was sharply elevated off the humeral shaft. The biceps musculature was mobilized and retracted medially; the brachialis muscle was divided at its midline and the lateral half elevated. The radial nerve I.1-B1
was identified and protected distally at the brachialis-brachioradialis interval.

The fracture was reduced anatomically around the stem and compressed using large-serrated bone-holding forceps (**7.3-2**). Three 2.4 mm interfragmentary lag screws were then inserted.

Proximal screw fixation is challenging because of the limited areas available for screw insertion and the fixed angle for insertion. However, careful placement of the plate and examination with an image intensifier will frequently identify areas available for screw insertion, either anteriorly or posteriorly. Monocortical locking screws and bicortical conventional screws were placed around the prosthesis. Surprisingly satisfactory purchase can be obtained with conventional screws inserted on a trajectory that prevents them from interfering with the anterior or posterior aspects of the prosthesis. Additionally, a 3.5 mm conventional screw was placed bicortically from the plate across the main fracture line, providing significant additional fixation. The final position of the plate was then confirmed (**7.3-3**). Postoperative x-rays showed a stable construct (**7.3-4a–b**).

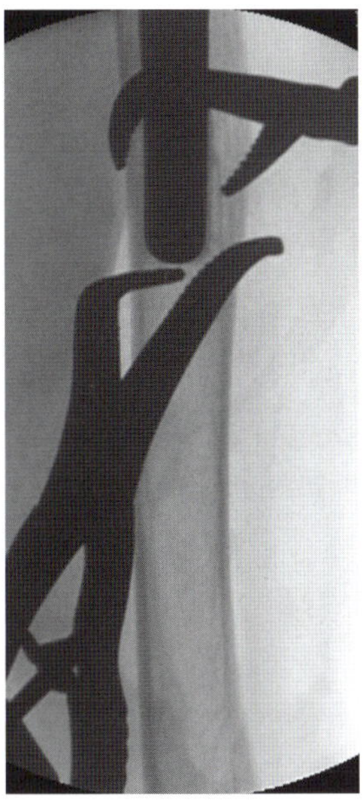

7.3-2 Intraoperative forceps-assisted reduction.

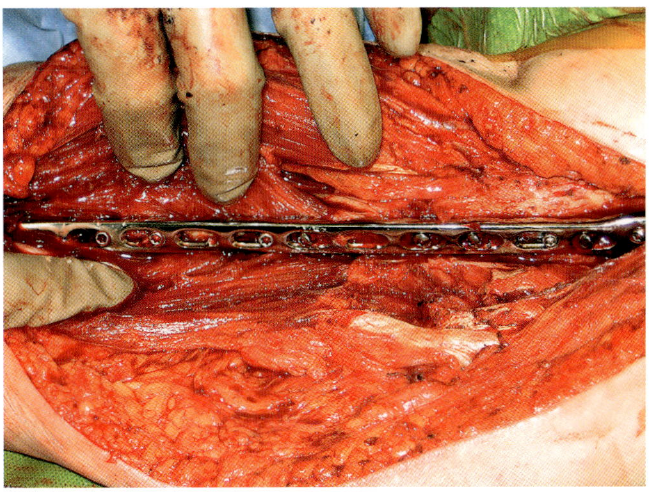

7.3-3 Intraoperative photograph shows final plate position.

I.1-B1

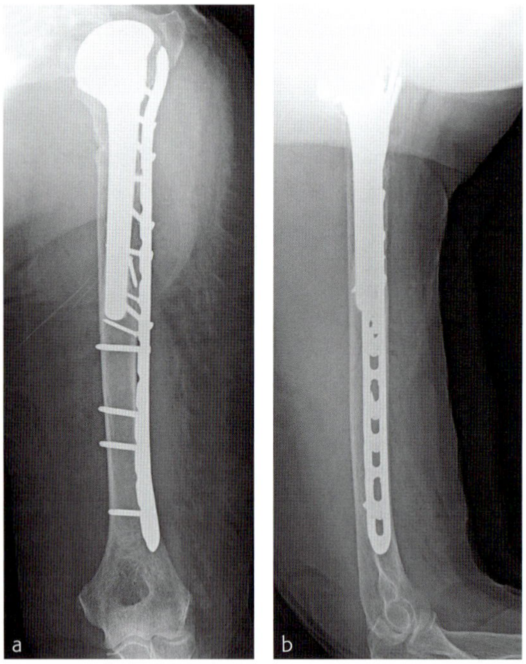

7.3-4a–b X-rays obtained immediately postoperatively.
a AP view.
b Lateral view.

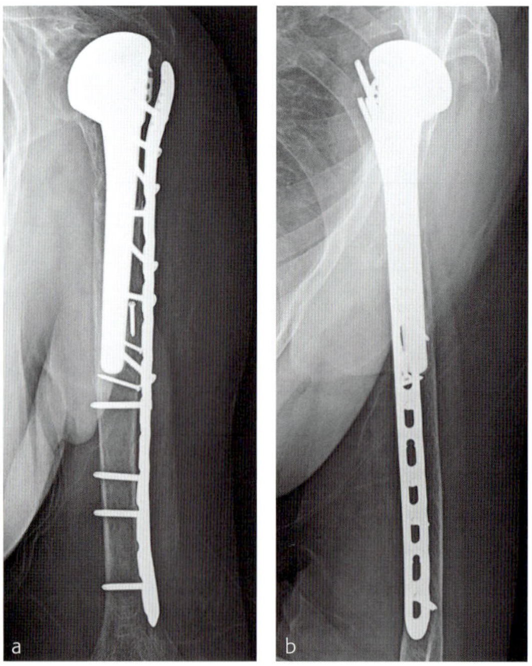

7.3-5a–b X-rays obtained 8 months postoperatively show fracture healing.
a AP view.
b Lateral view.

Rehabilitation and follow-up

The patient was allowed immediate unrestricted range of motion of the shoulder, elbow, forearm, wrist, and hand for activities of daily living. At follow-up 8 months later, x-ray evaluation showed apparent fracture healing (**7.3-5a–b**).

Points to remember

- Care must be taken to preserve as much blood supply to the fracture as possible by minimizing periosteal stripping.
- Proximal fixation has to be secure; there is often adequate bone available for fixation around the surgical neck and the greater and lesser tuberosities.
- Without enough bone around the prosthesis for screw fixation, cables or wires (with or without strut allograft augmentation) should be considered. Bridging the fracture area is another option.
- Long-plate fixation provides several surgical benefits, including offering several options for screw placement in the challenging proximal segment, avoiding future periprosthetic fractures, and maximizing the mechanical stability of the fracture.
- Identification of the radial nerve distally at the brachialis-brachioradialis interval will help to avoid inadvertent traction injury.
- The preoperative plan should ensure that adequate plate lengths are available intraoperatively.
- Care must be taken when applying forceps to osteoporotic bone because of the risk of inadvertent crushing of the cortex.

7.4 Humeral shaft fracture, stable prosthesis

ORIF: double plating with LCPs 3.5 and 2.7

Authors **Marschall B Berkes, Dean G Lorich**

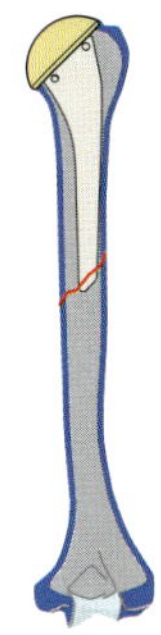

I.1-B1

Case description

A 91-year-old woman who presented with pain and deformity in the right arm after a simple fall from standing position has a history of a right proximal humeral fracture treated with hemiarthroplasty (👁 **7.4-1**).

Classification: Type I.1-B1

Diagnosis: Unstable displaced spiral fracture at the tip of a well-fixed cemented hemiarthroplasty in the distal third of the humeral shaft

Decision making

The best solution for an unstable displaced spiral fracture at the tip of a well-fixed proximal prosthesis is open reduction and internal fixation with one or two plates (chapter 5.4.1). The plates are fixed with screws; proximally, cerclage wires may provide additional fixation.

Preoperative planning

Equipment

- 14-hole extraarticular distal humerus locking compression plate 3.5
- 12-hole reconstruction plate 2.7
- C-arm image intensifier
- Sterile tourniquet

Patient preparation and positioning

- Left lateral decubitus position on a radiolucent table with the right arm placed over a post
- Cefazolin for antibiotic prophylaxis
- Subcutaneous heparin for thrombosis prophylaxis

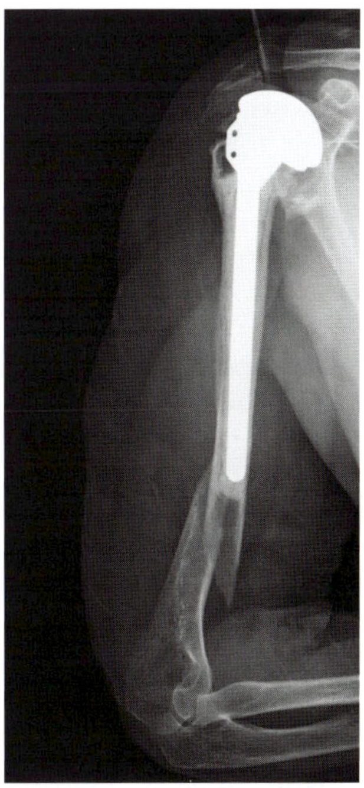

👁 **7.4-1** Lateral x-ray of the injured right humerus.

I.1-B1 Reduction and fixation

With the modified posterior (Gerwin) approach to the humerus (👁 **7.4-2**), a posterior midline incision was made that extended from the proximal aspect of the arm to the tip of the olecranon. The deep fascia was incised in line with the incision. In the lower portion of the wound, the triceps was retracted medially. The lateral brachial cutaneous nerve was identified on the posterior aspect of the lateral intermuscular septum and traced to the main trunk of the radial nerve, proximal to where it pierces the septum. Radial nerve mobilization and neurolysis were performed next by dividing the lateral intermuscular septum in the area where the radial nerve pierces it to allow for intraoperative mobilization. In conjunction with radial nerve mobilization, the triceps musculature was elevated as one subperiosteally and reflected medially to allow direct exposure of the diaphysis up to the level of the axillary nerve proximally. The fracture site was then debrided and irrigated.

One benefit of the modified posterior approach is that it allows for extensile exposure of the humeral shaft in which up to 94% of the humerus can be exposed. This approach also is biologically friendlier. It relies on triceps reflection, rather than splitting, thus reducing the amount of surgical trauma. The risk of injury to the motor branch of the medial head of the triceps also is less when the dissection proceeds from lateral to medial, rather than when the triceps is split directly. Disadvantages of this approach, however, include its technical difficulty and increased operative time compared with more traditional approaches.

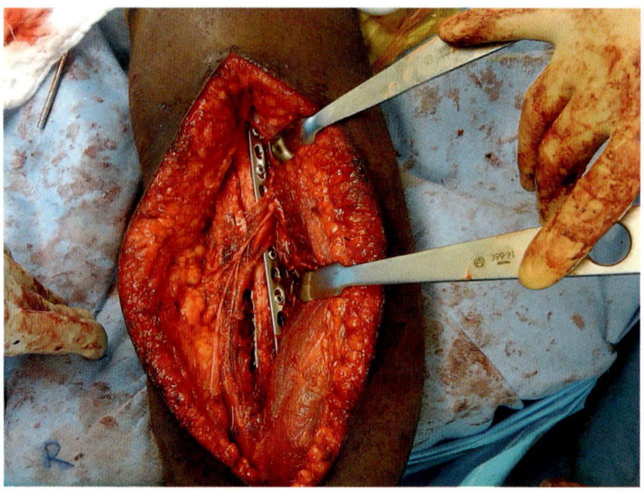

👁 **7.4-2** Modified posterior approach to the humeral shaft.

The spiral fracture was reduced with a Weber forceps. The provisional reduction was secured with a prebent laterally placed reconstruction plate 2.7. Distal fixation was achieved using two conventional screws, proximally with one screw aiming around the stem, followed by two interfragmentary compression screws and an additional screw just distal to the tip of the prosthesis. The extraarticular distal humerus locking compression plate was used in neutralization mode by sliding the plate underneath the well-mobilized radial nerve. Distally, a lag screw and three locking-head screws were placed initially. Just distal to the tip of the stem, a lag screw was inserted into the cement mantle. The most proximal hole was filled with a 2.7 cortex screw and washer and aimed medial to the prosthesis. A single cerclage wire was placed proximally for additional fixation (👁 **7.4-3a–b**).

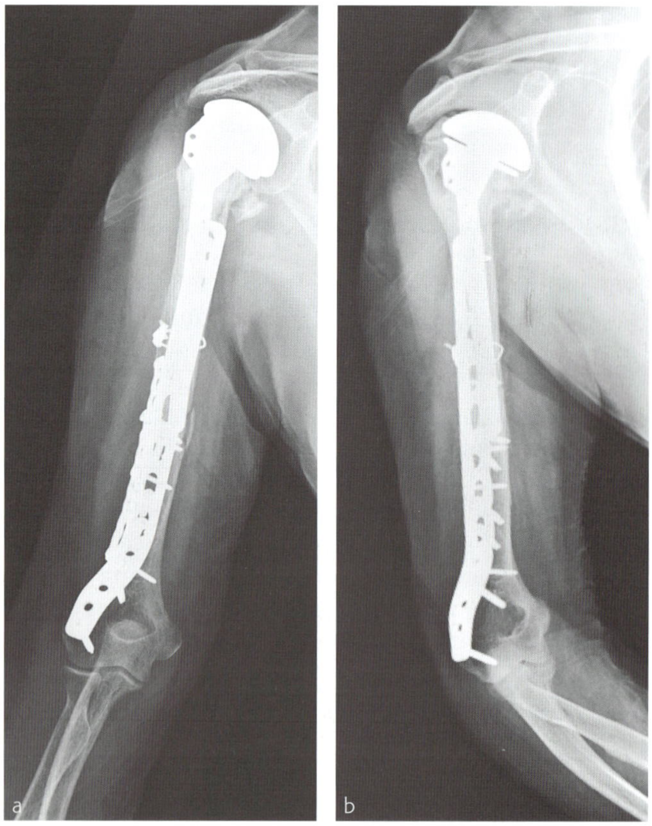

👁 **7.4-3a–b** X-rays of the right humerus obtained immediately after open reduction and internal fixation.

a AP view.

b Lateral view.

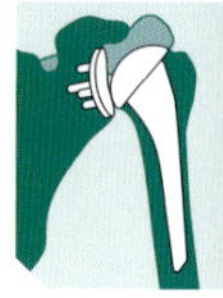

Rehabilitation and follow-up

The patient's arm was placed in an anterior splint in extension immediately postoperatively. An anterior elbow shell was provided for the evenings and a sling for during the day to increase comfort. Occupational therapy included non-weight-bearing and active and passive range of motion of the elbow without limits. Active and gentle passive range of motion of the shoulder was also initiated, with care to avoid torque to the humeral shaft in rotation. Follow-up was scheduled at 2, 4, and 8 weeks postoperatively (**7.4-4a–b**). Progression to full weight bearing and strengthening exercises began 8 weeks postoperatively. At the most recent follow-up, the patient reported no pain and had functional use of the arm. She required no additional surgery.

Points to remember

- The radial nerve must be carefully identified, and the potential for traction injury during reduction and fixation must be avoided.
- Medial soft-tissue dissection and/or stripping must be avoided as it is an unnecessary step and places the ulnar nerve at risk.
- The locking compression plate allows for distal fixation without impinging on the olecranon fossa.
- Orthogonal placement of the plates has two purposes: First, the lateral plate serves as a reduction tool, allowing interfragmentary compression through the plate, thus using it like a large washer. Second, this placement increases the mechanical strength of the construct, which is important in patients with osteoporotic bone.
- Bicortical screw purchase can be achieved proximally by aiming around the implant. This can be assisted through the use of smaller screws (a 2.7 mm screw with a washer in the plate 3.5).

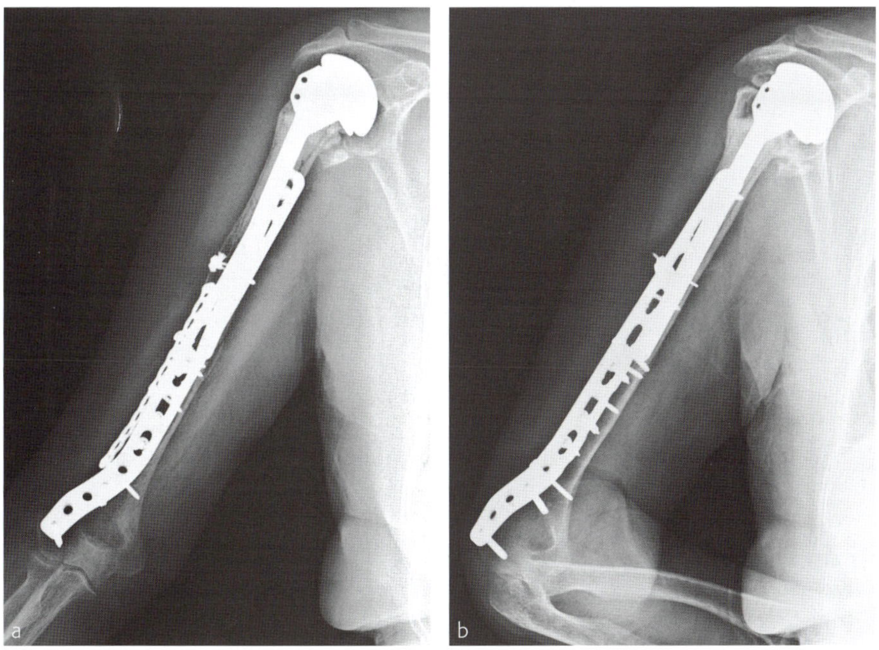

7.4-4a–b X-rays obtained at 8 weeks postoperatively.
a AP view.
b Lateral view.

I.1-B1

7.5 Humeral shaft fracture, stable prosthesis

ORIF: LCP 4.5/5.0 and LAP

Author **Stefaan Nijs**

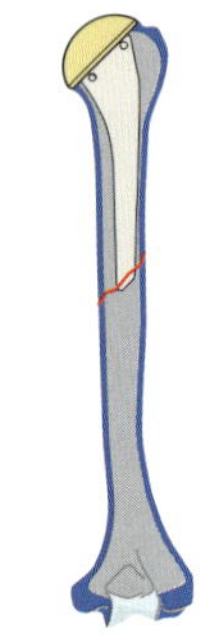

I.1-B1

Case description

A 63-year-old man who is mentally disabled and resides in an assisted living facility underwent hemiarthroplasty 7 years ago due to secondary displacement of a proximal humeral fracture. The functional result was only moderate, but the patient has been quite satisfied.

He presented with a grossly displaced periprosthetic fracture caused by a fall against a parked car (**7.5-1**). There was neither soft-tissue compromise nor any neurovascular deficit. Plaster cast immobilization failed to align the fragments and was poorly tolerated due to the compliance challenges associated with the patient's disability.

Classification: Type I.1-B1

Diagnosis: Humeral shaft fracture with no signs of prosthetic loosening or severe glenoid wear

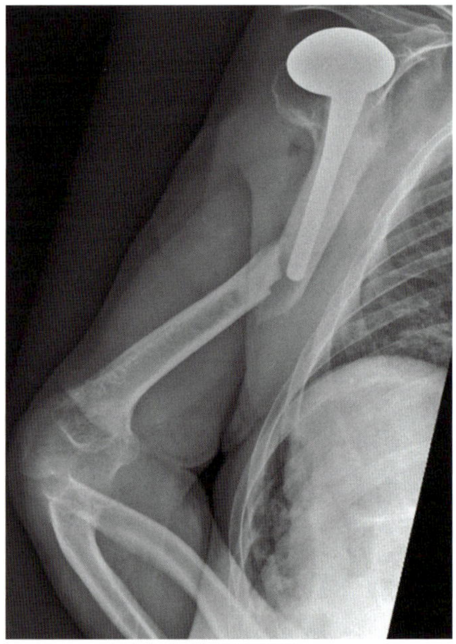

7.5-1 AP x-ray shows a grossly displaced periprosthetic humeral fracture.

Decision making

For an unstable humeral shaft fracture with remaining malalignment in an uncooperative but active patient, the treatment options are revision of the prosthesis or open reduction and internal fixation with a plate (chapter 5.4.1). As the prosthesis appeared to be well fixed on x-rays, the latter technique was selected. The challenge in the proximal humerus is always how to obtain safe fixation of the plate in the thin cortex or osteoporotic tuberosities. Periprosthetic locking-head screws are often difficult to insert as they cannot be angled. Cables or wires may provide only questionable stability while iatrogenic damage to the brittle bone and the vascularity may occur. The locking attachment plate (LAP), while being slightly oversized for the humerus, allows multiplanar angular stable fixation and respects the periosteal blood supply.

Preoperative planning

Equipment

- Broad, straight locking compression plate (LCP) 4.5/5.0
- 4- and 8-hole LAP and fixation screws
- 3.5 and 5 mm locking head screws
- 3.5 and 4.5 mm conventional cortex screws
- Cable system
- Periprosthetic locking screws

Patient preparation and positioning

- Beach chair position with image intensifier allowing AP and pseudoaxial imaging
- Head stabilized in a head holder or helmet
- First- or second-generation cephalosporin for antibiotic prophylaxis

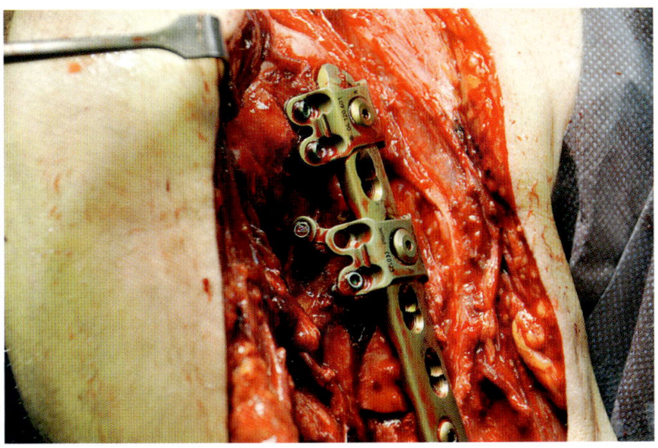

7.5-2 Proximal fixation was obtained using the 4- and 8-hole locking attachment plate (LAP).

Reduction and fixation

I.1-B1

An extended anterolateral approach was used, including the previous incision in the proximal part. The radial nerve must be identified and protected. After careful exposure, anatomical reduction was obtained using reduction forceps and held in position by applying a 3.5 mm lag screw. Next, a broad 10-hole LCP 4.5/5.0 was applied. Proximal fixation was obtained with two LAPs that allow insertion of the screws around the prosthesis (**7.5-2**).

For the fixation distal to the stem, conventional 4.5 mm cortex screws were inserted. In patients with severe osteoporosis, 5.0 mm locking-head screws are recommended (**7.5-3a–b**).

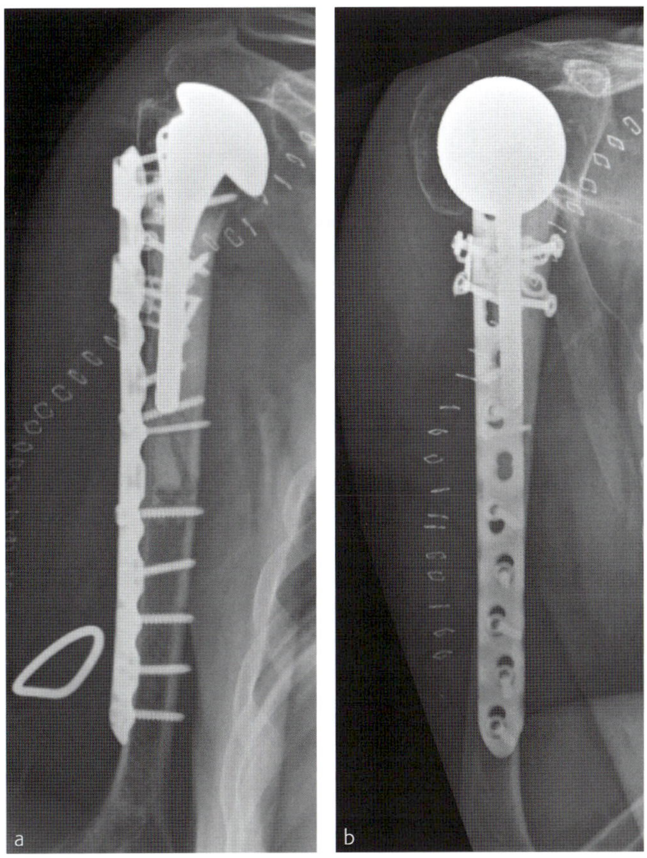

7.5-3a–b X-rays show completed fixation of a periprosthetic fracture of the humerus using LAP.
a AP view.
b Lateral view.

I.1-B1 Depending on the fracture pattern and the quality of local bone, alternative combination osteosyntheses can be performed, including periprosthetic locking-head screws, cables, and/or strut grafts.

Rehabilitation and follow-up

Active mobilization without restrictions was initiated immediately postoperatively. Six weeks postoperatively, the patient began exercises against resistance. The patient had pain-free shoulder motion, and the previous level of function was restored. Follow-up x-rays showed uneventful healing (👁 **7.5-4a–b**).

Points to remember

- Any loose or excessively worn components must be replaced if an osteosynthesis is planned.
- Implants allowing multiplanar angular stable fixation are preferred for this type of fracture.
- Identify and protect the radial nerve.
- Depending on fracture type and bone quality, the combination with strut grafts and cerclage wires or cables is possible.
- Prosthetic exchange may be indicated if there is a loose stem, severe glenoid erosion in case of hemiarthroplasty, or symptomatic secondary rotator-cuff failure necessitating conversion to a reversed polarity shoulder arthroplasty.
- If prosthetic exchange is not indicated, osteosynthesis is the preferred treatment.
- Periprosthetic locking-head screws are often difficult to insert.
- Cables or wires provide only questionable stability, and iatrogenic damage to brittle bone and vascular structures may occur.
- The LAP allows multiplanar angular stable fixation and respects the periosteal blood supply.

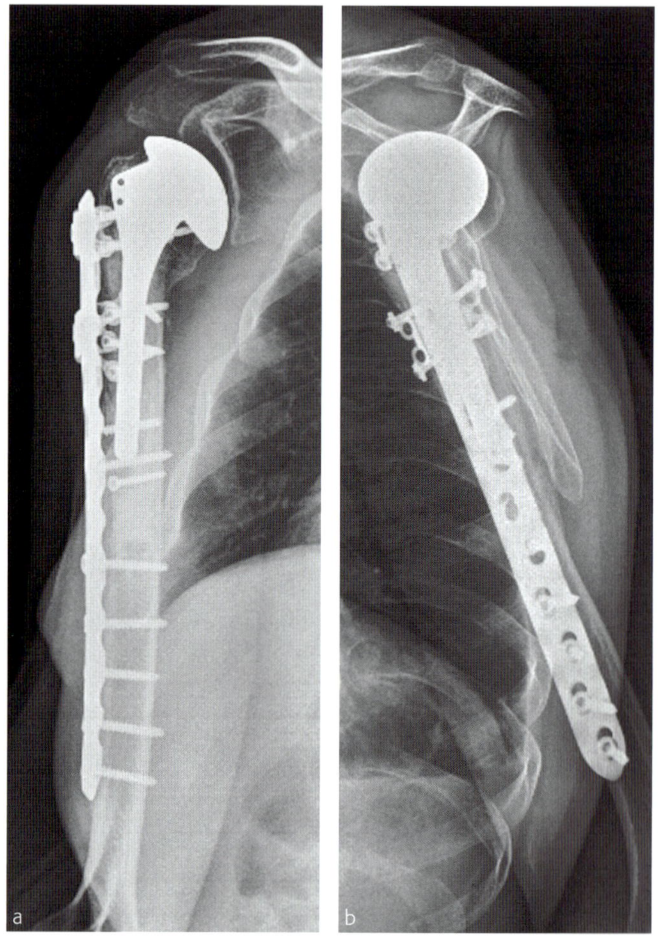

👁 **7.5-4a–b** Follow-up x-rays obtained 6 months postoperatively show fracture healing.
a AP view.
b Lateral view.

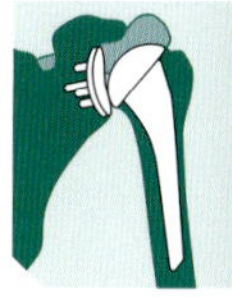

7.6 Humeral shaft fracture, stable prosthesis

ORIF: LCP 4.5/5.0 and LAP

Authors Yves Pascal Acklin, Christoph Sommer

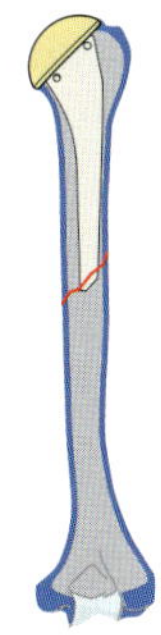

I.1-B1

Case description

An obese 56-year-old woman with an inverse shoulder prosthesis sustained a spiral butterfly periprosthetic humeral fracture after a fall onto her right arm while she was walking. Imaging studies show a large butterfly fragment around a stable-looking stem (7.6-1a–b).

Classification: Type I.1-B1

Diagnosis: Periprosthetic humeral shaft fracture, with a stable prosthesis

Decision making

The long spiral butterfly fracture was characterized by a stable prosthetic stem in the proximal humerus. Although nonoperative treatment consisting of immobilization in an orthosis is possible in slender and compliant patients, it is challenging in obese patients. Surgical fixation allows for immediate mobilization of the injured arm. Although minimally invasive plating in multifragmentary humeral shaft fractures is an attractive alternative, perfect reduction and positioning of the plate is crucial in periprosthetic fractures. An open approach, therefore, seemed more appropriate for this patient. The goal is to achieve anatomical reduction, which helps to increase primary stability by load sharing. Furthermore, the application of a locking attachment plate (LAP) (chapter 5.4.1) required an open approach.

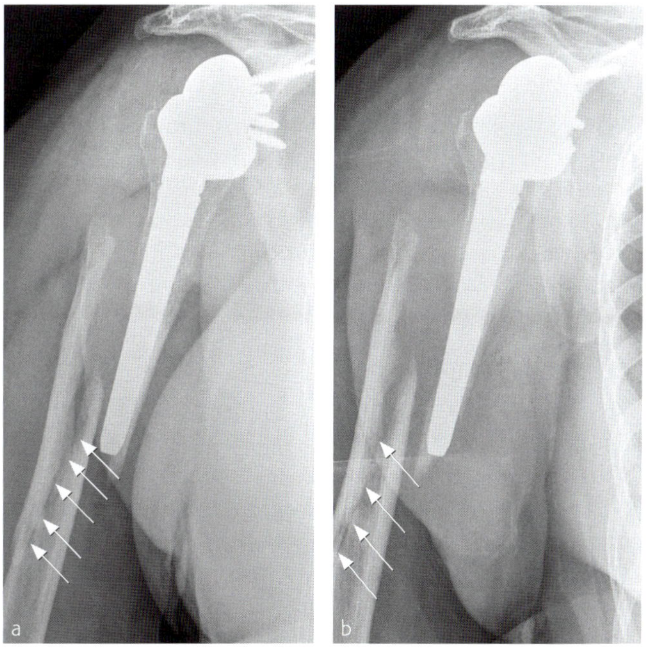

7.6-1a–b Initial x-rays of the periprosthetic fracture of the proximal humerus. The arrows indicate the course of the butterfly fracture distally.
a AP view. The butterfly fragment is difficult to see; however, the prosthesis appears well fixed in the bone.
b Lateral view.

I.1-B1 ## Preoperative planning

Equipment

- Narrow locking compression plate (LCP) 4.5
- 5.0 and 3.5 mm locking-head screws
- 3.5 mm cortex screws
- LAP 3.5
- Cerclage wires

Patient preparation and positioning

- Beach-chair position with the right arm freely draped for intraoperative mobility
- Single shot of first- or second-generation cephalosporin for antibiotic prophylaxis

Reduction and fixation

With the patient in the beach-chair position, a standard anterolateral approach was considered the best choice to obtain good exposure of the proximal humerus and shaft. The humerus must be accessed lateral to the biceps muscle. Identification of the musculocutaneous nerve is mandatory. The brachialis muscle was split in the middle (the medial fibers are supplied by the musculocutaneous nerve, whereas the lateral fibers are controlled by the radial nerve). Elevating the brachialis muscle laterally protects the radial nerve, which lies in the groove between the brachialis and brachioradialis muscles.

After gentle exposure of the fragile fracture fragments, a pointed reduction forceps was used for preliminary fixation, followed by cerclage wires to replace the bone forceps. A narrow LCP 4.5 was first fixed distally using a threaded drill sleeve screwed to the plate and a bicortical drill bit for temporary fixation. The plate was then aligned proximally and an additional cerclage wire applied to secure the plate firmly onto the bone. Due to the thick prosthetic stem in the proximal main fragment, screw fixation with 4.5 mm locking head screws or cortex screws was not possible. This situation was a good indication for applying a locking attachment plate to the proximal end of the plate, which allowed for insertion of four 3.5 mm locking head screws, which do not interfere with the prosthetic stem. One further monocortical periprosthetic locking head screw was inserted through the most proximal plate hole to optimize fracture fixation. Distally, three 4.5 mm locking head screws were inserted and the drill bit was replaced with a conventional screw (**7.6-2a–b**).

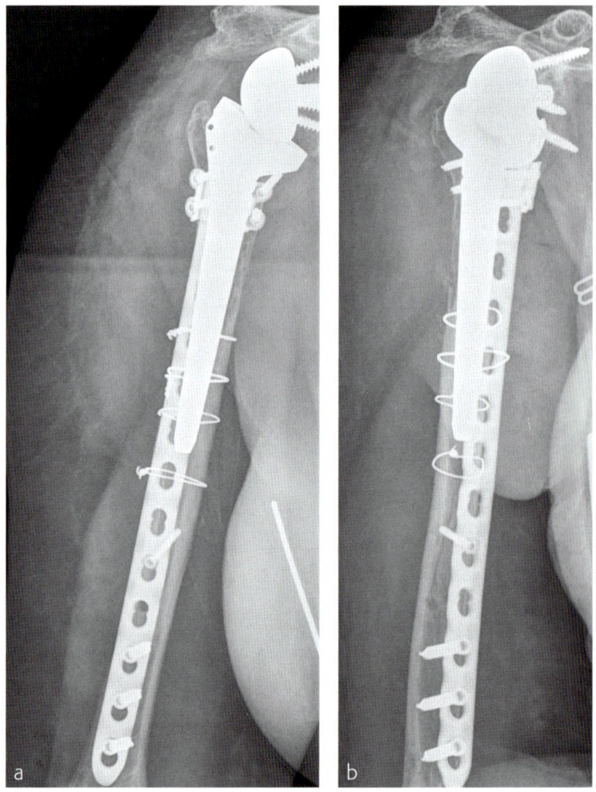

7.6-2a–b Intraoperative x-rays. The fracture is reduced anatomically and fixed with four cerclage wires. Note the locking attachment plate (LAP) at the proximal plate end fixed to the bone with four 3.5 mm locking-head screws without interfering with the stem of the prosthesis.
a AP view.
b Lateral view.

Rehabilitation and follow-up

The patient was allowed immediate active-assisted movement of her right arm. No sling immobilization was necessary. Regular follow-up was recommended after 6 weeks, 3 months, 6 months, and 1 year or at least until definitive fracture healing. In this patient, callus formation was observed at 2 months postoperatively (👁 **7.6-3a–b**) and bone healing after 6 months (👁 **7.6-4a–b**).

Points to remember

- Nonoperative treatment of displaced periprosthetic fractures of the humerus is demanding in obese patients and delays the active mobilization of the arm.
- Locking attachment plates allow 3.5 mm locking-head screws to be inserted that avoid the prosthetic stem or bone cement, thereby providing high postoperative fracture stability (chapter 5.4.1).
- Using the anterolateral approach and splitting the brachialis muscle protects the radial nerve, which is especially important when cerclage wires are applied.

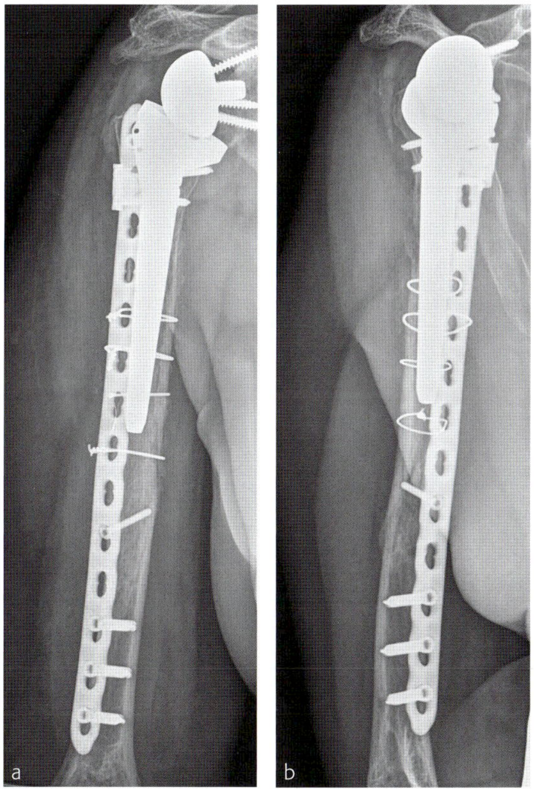

👁 **7.6-3a–b** Follow-up x-rays obtained 2 months postoperatively.
a AP view shows the first signs of callus formation.
b Lateral view shows that all implants appear well fixed.

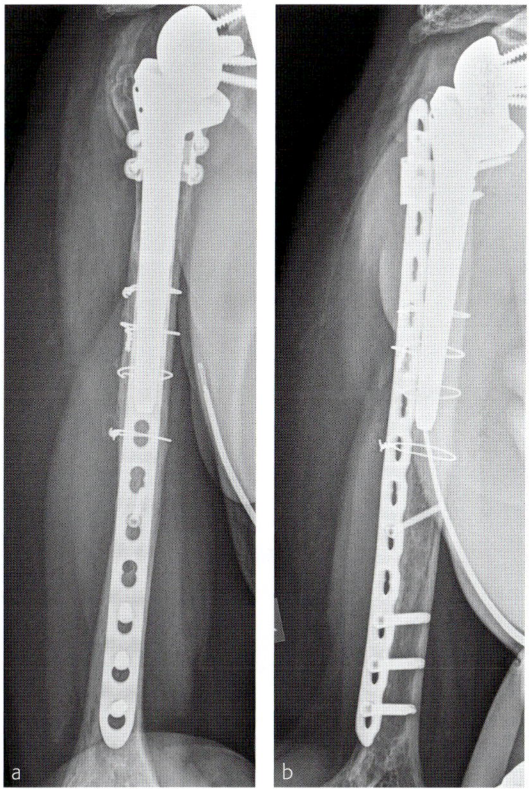

👁 **7.6-4a–b** Follow-up x-rays obtained after 6 months show fracture union and the first signs of remodeling.
a AP view.
b Lateral view.

I.1-B1

7.7 Humeral shaft fracture, stable prosthesis

ORIF: LCP 4.5/5.0 and cerclage wires

Authors Martin Jäger, Norbert P Südkamp

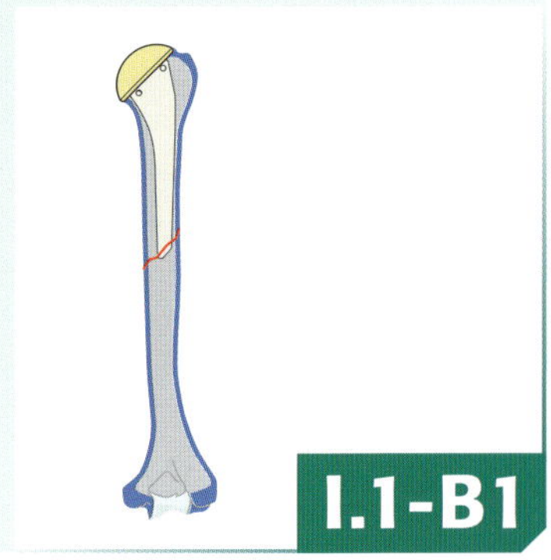

I.1-B1

Case description

An 87-year-old man underwent shoulder hemiarthroplasty for a bilateral displaced four-part fracture of the proximal humerus. Six months postoperatively, he fell on his non-dominant left shoulder, sustaining a periprosthetic fracture of the humeral shaft. Imaging studies revealed a significantly displaced short spiral fracture at the tip of the prosthetic stem with distal fracture extension of approximately 3 cm (**7.7-1a–c**). The stem appeared to be well fixed.

Classification: Type I.1-B1

Diagnosis: Periprosthetic humeral shaft fracture after shoulder hemiarthroplasty

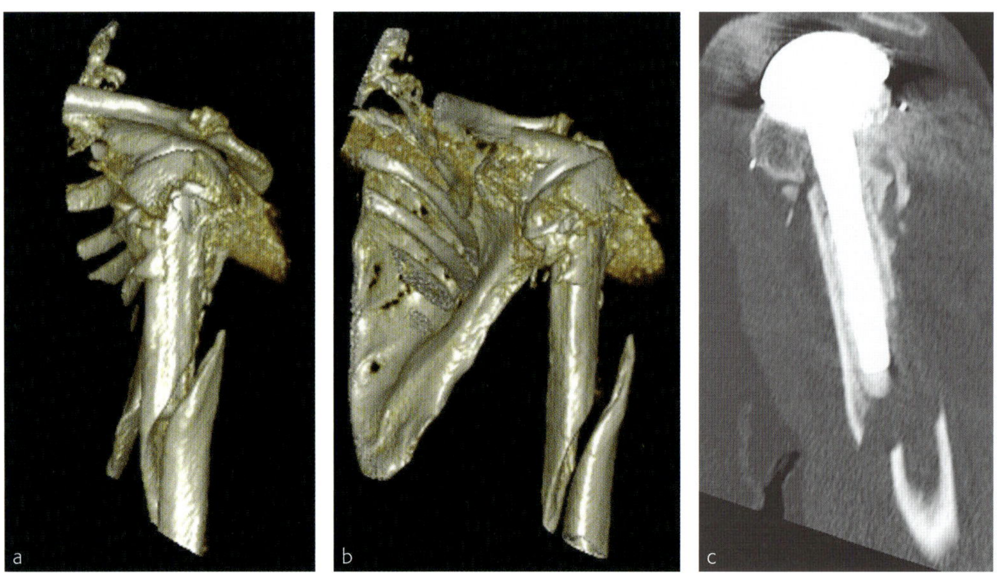

7.7-1a–c Preoperative CT scans show a periprosthetic fracture of the proximal humerus.
a 3D reconstruction, sagittal plane.
b 3D reconstruction, frontal plane.
c CT scan, frontal plane.

I.1-B1

Decision making

With this type of fracture and a well-fixed prosthetic stem, nonoperative treatment could be considered. However, because of the significant degree of fracture displacement and the distal fracture extension in this patient, functional bracing would be difficult, making the success of nonoperative treatment questionable. Therefore, surgical stabilization was selected. Although the tuberosities were fractured initially and fixed with cerclage wires, preoperative CT scans revealed fracture healing without significant displacement. The head of the prosthesis was still centered without signs of proximal migration, and the stem still appeared well fixed. Therefore, replacing the stem for a longer one, with or without conversion to a reverse prosthesis, did not seem to be indicated. Open reduction and internal fixation with a locking compression plate (LCP) was chosen (chapter 5.4.1).

Preoperative planning

Preoperatively, the exact fracture course in respect to the prosthesis must be considered, with the following questions:

- Does it allow for anatomical reduction and interfragmentary compression?
- Is the prosthesis still well fixed?
- Are the tuberosities properly consolidated?
- What is the quality of bone stock at the level and around the stem of the prosthesis?
- Is there room for the insertion of screws?
- Are there any neurological injuries?

Answers to the above questions can be derived from clinical examination of the affected arm, especially in regard to the axillary and radial nerves. Standard imaging studies include plain x-rays of the upper arm in two planes. It is helpful to include the entire humerus on one image to estimate the fracture line in relation to the prosthesis and fragments. Focus should be on any signs of implant loosening. In case of doubt, CT scans can also be beneficial.

The standard implant for the humerus is the narrow plate 4.5. Locking plates such as the LCP are preferred, especially in patients with osteoporotic bone. The cortex around the prosthetic stem appeared very thin in this patient, with little space for proximal screw fixation; therefore, precise positioning of the plate was crucial and verified intraoperatively with the C-arm. If sound screw purchase in the thin cortex cannot be achieved, cerclage wires or cables should be applied to ensure proximal fixation of the plate.

Equipment

- Instruments and implants for plating (LCP recommended)
- Instruments for cerclage application (appropriate cable passers)
- C-arm for intraoperative image intensification

Patient preparation and positioning

- Supine position with the arm placed on the belly
- Lateral position with the arm placed on an arm holder
- Prone position with the arm placed on a radiolucent arm holder (strongly recommended)
- Intraoperative image intensifier
- First- or second-generation cephalosporin for single-shot antibiotic prophylaxis

Reduction and fixation

Both the anterolateral approach and the posterior triceps-splitting approach according to Henry can be used to treat this type of periprosthetic fracture. For the anterolateral approach, the patient is placed in a supine position with a table to support the forearm. Alternatively, the beach chair position can be used for this approach. The anterior deltopectoral approach is typically used in most fracture arthroplasties; the original incision can be used and extended distally. This approach might be helpful, especially if the implanted prosthesis is loose and needs to be replaced by a long-stem prosthesis. Both the musculocutaneous nerve and the radial nerve are at risk during dissection. The latter also is at risk with drilling of the posterior cortex.

The posterior approach offers wide exposure of the distal and middle third of the humerus, although it is limited proximally by the deltoid muscle. In patients with a radial palsy, it is advantageous to explore the nerve via the posterior approach. The radial nerve can be identified as it crosses the humerus approximately 2.5 cm proximal to the apex of the triceps aponeurosis, deep between the muscle bellies of the triceps brachii.

A posterior triceps-splitting approach was used for this patient, and the radial nerve exposed as described above. The fracture was reduced anatomically and temporarily fixed with two pointed reduction forceps. Primary stability was achieved with three lag screws (👁 **7.7-2**). Additionally, a narrow LCP 4.5 was inserted at the posterior aspect of the humerus to neutralize the lag screw fixation. The proximal end of the plate had to be placed under the radial nerve, which was facilitated by release of the lateral intermuscular septum. The

1.1-B1

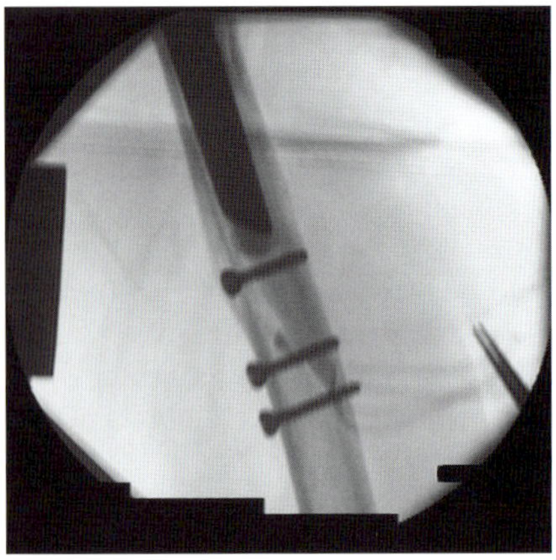

👁 **7.7-2** Intraoperative AP image shows initial lag screw fixation of the fracture.

position of the nerve in relation to the plate must be clearly mentioned in the operative report. Distally, bicortical locking-head screws were used for plate fixation. Proximally, screws could not be inserted without interfering with the cemented stem. Therefore, a cerclage wire was applied using the special threaded cerclage positioning device for the LCP to provide safer fixation (👁 **7.7-3a–b**). Because the radial nerve is identified during the posterior approach, the risk of accidental nerve damage is reduced. If an anterior approach is used, the cable passer must be passed very close to the bone to reduce the risk of nerve and soft-tissue damage.

Rehabilitation and follow-up

Cautious aftercare was recommended for this patient because of osteopenic bone quality and the limited proximal plate fixation. During the first 6 weeks, only active-assisted motion was allowed, supported by lymphatic drainage. X-rays showed no secondary loss of reduction. After 6 weeks, active exercises were encouraged with increased loading. Follow-up at 1 year showed a complete bone healing without secondary loss of reduction (👁 **7.7-4**).

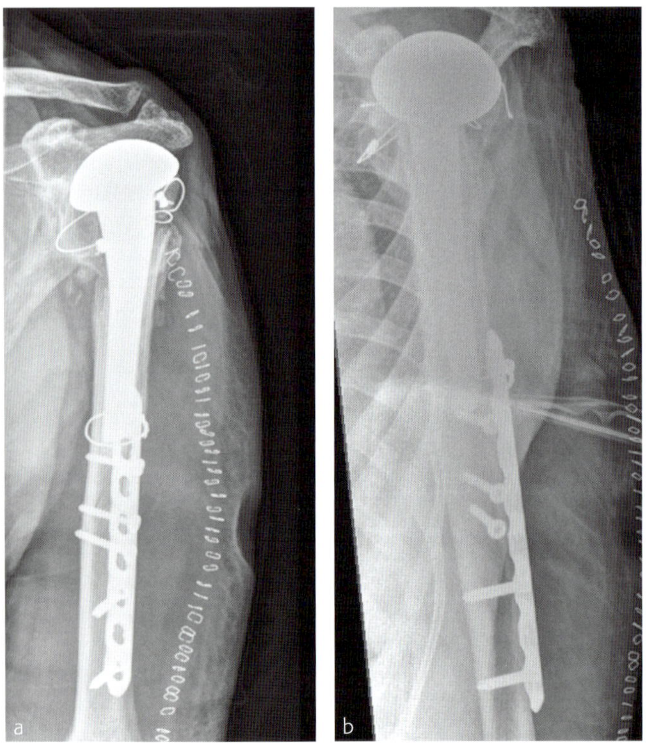

👁 **7.7-3a–b** X-rays obtained immediately postoperatively.

a AP view.

b Lateral view. Note that the small device at the proximal screw hole serves to maintain the cerclage wire in the correct position.

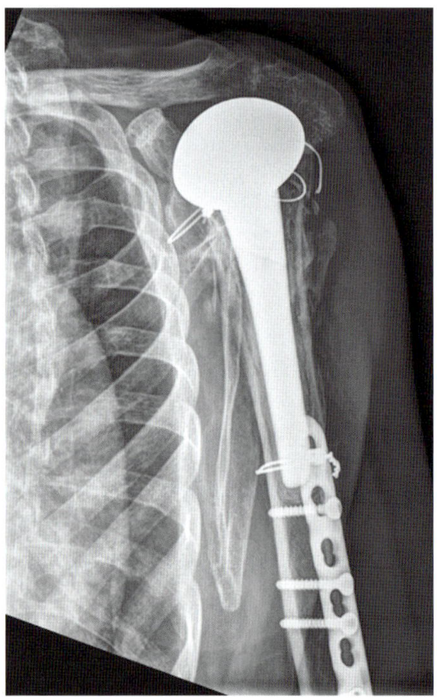

👁 **7.7-4** Lateral view obtained 1 year postoperatively shows complete fracture healing. The use of a longer plate would have improved the fixation.

Points to remember

- The radial nerve is at risk during surgery and thus its course around the humerus must be identified precisely.
- With simple fracture types, anatomical reduction and stable fixation using lag screws and a neutralization plate is recommended.
- If proximal fixation cannot be achieved with screws, a locking attachment plate may be applied knowing that they never provide the same mechanical stability.
- Cerclage wires must be passed around the humerus as close to the bone as possible and perpendicular to the shaft axis. I.1-B1 To secure the position of the cerclage wire to the plate, a special device that is screwed to a plate hole may be used. The course of the radial nerve in relation to the proximal plate holes should be noted in the operative report.
- In this case, the length of the plate was too short proximally. Because it had to be inserted under the radial nerve, a longer plate (two more holes) would have been more appropriate as it would have allowed for insertion of a locking-head screw or a second cerclage wire, thereby improving fixation.

I.1-B1

7.8 Humeral shaft fracture, stable prosthesis

ORIF: LCP 4.5/5.0 and cerclage wires

Authors **Jordanna Forman, Kenneth A Egol**

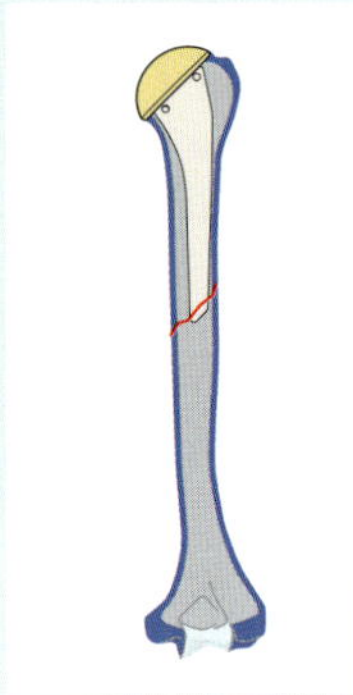

I.1-B1

Case description

A 67-year-old woman underwent several failed arthroplasties on her left shoulder before undergoing a reverse total shoulder arthroplasty as the fourth and most recent procedure 5 months ago. She recently fell off a ladder. X-rays showed a displaced periprosthetic spiral fracture of the proximal humeral shaft with a well-fixed prosthesis (**7.8-1a–b**).

Classification: Type I.1-B1

Diagnosis: Periprosthetic fracture of the humeral shaft, with a well-fixed, cemented prosthesis

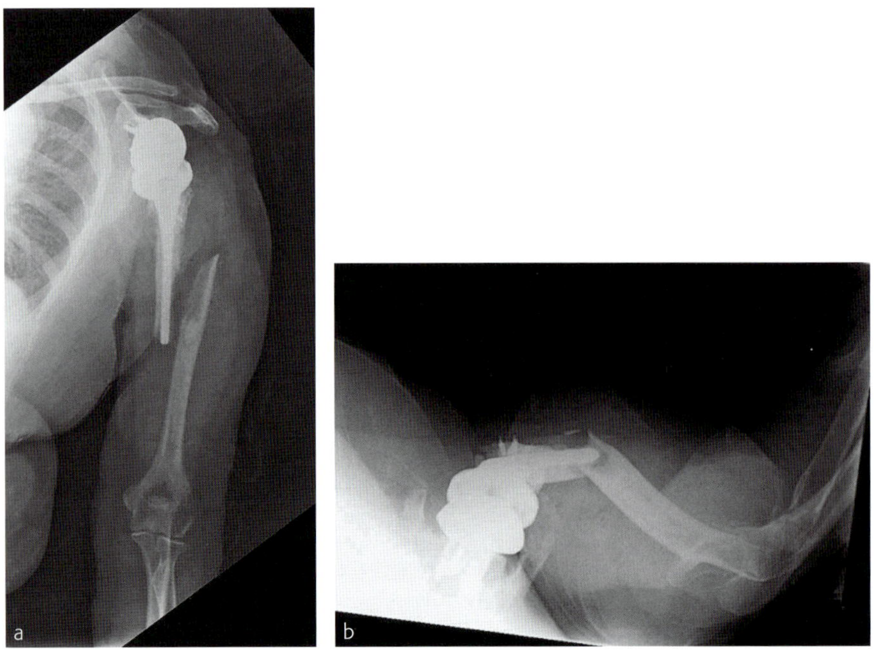

7.8-1a–b X-rays obtained shortly after the injury.
a AP view.
b Axillary view.

Decision making

The primary objectives in treating these fractures are to obtain bony union, ensure prosthesis stability, and maintain range of motion about the shoulder and elbow. Major concerns associated with operative treatment of this type of fracture are the quality of proximal bone stock and the ability to obtain adequate purchase in the proximal fragment with the intramedullary implant in place. Due to the significant displacement and the unstable nature of the patient's fracture, nonoperative treatment was not considered. No gross loosening of the cement mantle of the humeral prosthesis was identified preoperatively. Therefore, open reduction and internal fixation was selected using a narrow locking compression plate (LCP) 4.5/5.0 with locking-head screws distally and cerclage wires proximally (chapter 5.4.1). Alternatively, revision surgery for replacement with a long-stem prosthesis could be used with loosening of the humeral prosthetic component.

Preoperative planning

Equipment

- Narrow LCPs 4.5/5.0
- 1.7 mm cerclage wire
- Wire-tension device
- Wire cutters

Patient preparation and positioning

- Either regional block or general anesthesia
- Supine position on a flat table with a radiolucent arm board or hand table
- Beach-chair position with the patient in a half-sitting position (alternative positioning)
- Preparation and sterile draping from the acromioclavicular joint to the hand
- Prophylactic antibiotics

Reduction and fixation

Proximally a deltopectoral approach was made. The incision was extended distally full thickness down to the biceps muscle. The biceps was retracted medially, exposing the brachialis muscle belly. Due to its dual innervation, the brachialis muscle was split down to the humerus. The deltoid muscle was partially elevated from its humeral insertion, fully exposing both the anterior and lateral aspects of the humerus. The radial nerve was identified distally in the wound in the interval between the brachialis and brachioradialis muscle where it pierces the lateral intermuscular septum. The soft tissue about the proximal fragment was elevated to protect the radial nerve at the spiral groove during wire passage. I.1-B1

The stem of the humeral component was reduced within the distal medullary canal, and anatomical alignment could be obtained by manual reduction and confirmed by an image intensifier. Usually, the stemmed component precludes use of a lag screw in these fractures. A narrow LCP 4.5/5.0 was placed on the lateral aspect of the humerus. First, a conventional one was placed distally to the fracture to pull the plate to the bone. Because of the intramedullary implant, three cerclage wires were placed and tensioned about the proximal fragment to obtain fixation. In some patients, conventional screws may be placed obliquely in the plate holes to catch the far cortex and avoid the stem. This technique is easier in large-diameter bones such as the femur. Distally, several bicortical locking-head screws were inserted. X-rays confirmed anatomical reduction and correct implant placement, as well as reduction of the prosthesis (👁 **7.8-2a–b**). Bone grafting or osteobiological enhancement of the fracture site may be considered at this point due to impaired bone healing potential of the host and the fracture site milieu following open reduction.

Rehabilitation and follow-up

Postoperative immobilization in a sling and early exercises, primarily for the elbow, wrist, and hand were initiated, followed by passive range of motion of the shoulder after 2 weeks. Patients can progress to active motion as healing permits. A structured, supervised physiotherapy program should be initiated and followed throughout the healing phase. At the 1-year follow-up, x-rays confirmed fracture healing (👁 **7.8-3a–c**). The patient had an excellent recovery, with full active range of elbow motion. Shoulder range of motion also returned to prefracture levels.

Points to remember

- The deltopectoral approach is considered the standard approach for shoulder arthroplasty and most types of fracture fixation of the humerus. Therefore, periprosthetic fractures of the shoulder often require reuse of the deltopectoral incision in which the cephalic vein is at risk. Extension of the deltopectoral approach to the anterolateral approach of the humerus is easily performed. However, distal extension of the incision can endanger

I.1-B1 the radial nerve, which must be identified and protected to avoid further intraoperative disruption.

- Patients who have had multiple procedures require evaluation for indolent infection, and deep-tissue cultures should be obtained at the time of any revision or fracture surgery.
- Factors associated with delayed or malunion include the presence of a transverse or short oblique fracture, as well as fractures of the humeral shaft that extend past the stem of the prosthesis and have more than 2 mm of residual gap at the fracture site after rigid fixation.

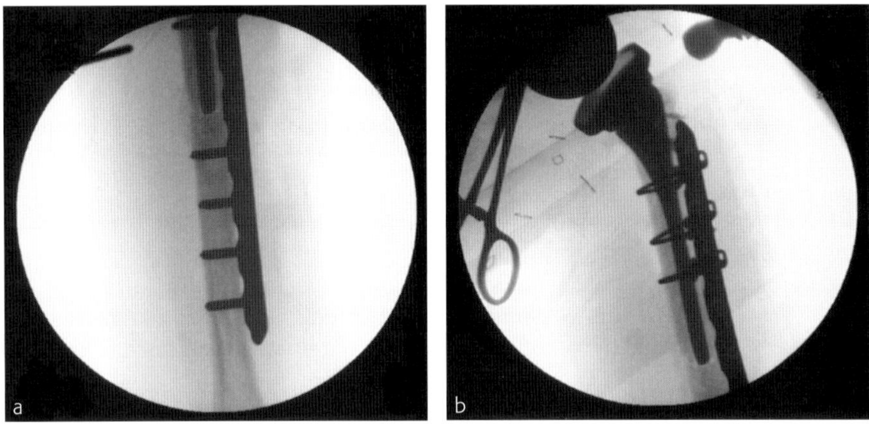

7.8-2a–b X-rays confirm anatomical reduction and correct positioning of the prosthesis.
a Axillary view.
b Lateral view.

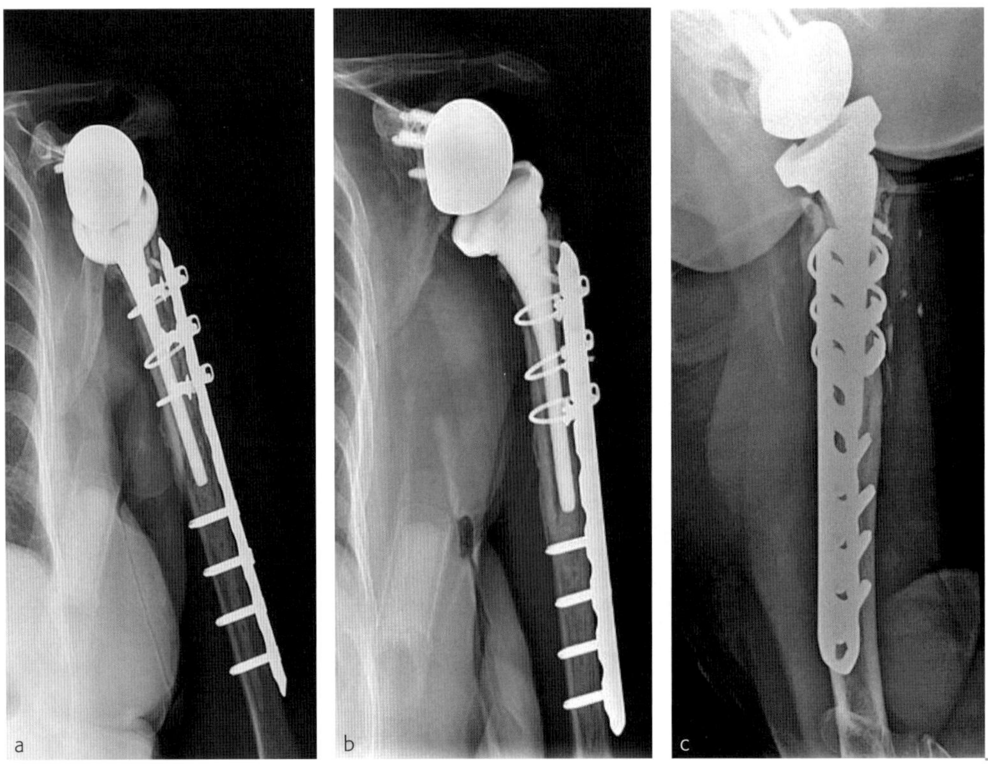

7.8-3a–c Follow-up x-rays obtained 1 year postoperatively.
a Internal rotation AP view.
b External rotation AP view.
c Axillary view.

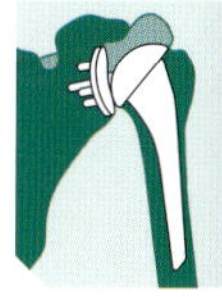

7.9 Surgical neck fracture after humeral surface replacement
ORIF: PHILOS

Authors **Martin Jäger, Norbert P Südkamp**

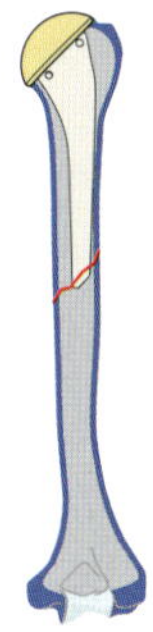

I.1-B1

Case description

An 81-year-old woman sustained a periprosthetic surgical neck fracture of the left nondominant arm as a result of a fall at home. Ten months earlier she underwent humeral surface replacement using a shoulder-resurfacing head (👁 **7.9-1**). Plain x-ray and 3-D CT reconstruction revealed a varus displaced surgical neck fracture (👁 **7.9-2a–b**), but the prosthesis was still well fixed. There were no additional injuries.

Classification: Type I.1-B1

Diagnosis: Periprosthetic fracture of the surgical humeral neck after surface replacement

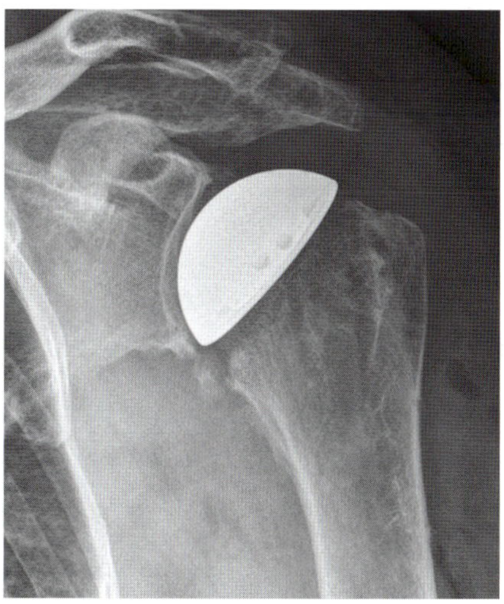

👁 **7.9-1** X-ray obtained after surface replacement of the humeral head.

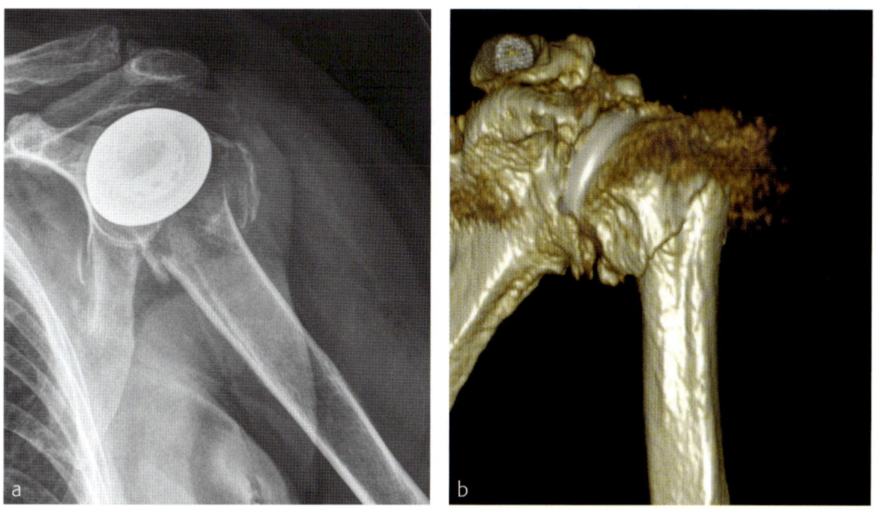

👁 **7.9-2a–b** Periprosthetic fracture of the proximal metaphysis.
a Axial view.
b 3-D CT reconstruction in the frontal plane.

I.1-B1 Decision making

The resurfacing prosthesis just covers the subchondral bone of the former humeral head; therefore, this type of periprosthetic fracture often appears similar to other proximal humeral fractures, with a still remaining humeral bone stock. The head resurfacing implant rarely becomes loose before or as a result of trauma. A loose resurfaced humeral head is best replaced by a long-stem implant, either anatomical or reverse, depending on the condition of the rotator cuff and tuberosities. In this patient, the implant appeared well fixed and the humeral head well centered, indicating that the rotator cuff was still sufficient. This situation corresponds to a 2-part fracture of the surgical neck without involvement of the tuberosities, which can be fixed surgically or treated nonoperatively. If internal fixation with a plate is planned (chapter 5.4.1), an implant design (eg, central peg or crown) must be selected that does not interfere with the screws.

Preoperative planning

Equipment

- Radiolucent shoulder support with patient in supine position
- Instruments and implants for proximal humerus internal locking system (PHILOS) plates
- C-arm for intraoperative image intensification

Patient preparation and positioning

- Preoperative CT scans (mandatory)
- Beach-chair position (or supine position alternatively)
- Perioperative image intensification to obtain two perpendicular planes
- First- or second-generation cephalosporin for single-shot antibiotic prophylaxis

Reduction and fixation

A standard anterior deltopectoral approach was used for the index procedure. The same approach was used for the osteosynthesis because it provides good exposure of the proximal humerus with minimal risk to the axillary nerve. The cephalic vein was retracted laterally.

Open anatomical reduction was performed and checked with an image intensifier. After temporary fixation with two 1.8 mm K-wires (**7.9-3**), a three-hole PHILOS plate was placed on the lateral side of the proximal humerus just dorsal to the bicipital sulcus and fixed with a lag screw in the oval plate hole. After second confirmation of the correct plate position, five locking-head screws were inserted into the head using the guiding block (**7.9-4**). Two locking-head screws fixed the plate to the shaft.

Rehabilitation and follow-up

A Gilchrist bandage was applied for the first 2 days postoperatively. Physiotherapy including active pain-adapted motion was started immediately. The last follow-up was approximately 1.5 years after surgery at which time x-rays showed complete bone healing without secondary loss of reduction (**7.9-5a–b**). Range of motion was 90° for abduction and adduction. The patient was able to reach her neck with the hand.

Points to remember

- Periprosthetic fractures of the humeral head with surface replacement can be treated like any proximal humeral fracture, provided that the prosthetic component is well fixed.
- Anatomical reduction is crucial; therefore, special care must be taken to reduce any varus deformity and restore the calcar of the humeral neck.
- The PHILOS plate must be positioned correctly to prevent the locking-head screws from interfering with the prosthesis.
- Placing the patient in a supine position on radiolucent shoulder supports helps achieve a true axial image intensifier view without rotation of the arm. This step might be valuable in patients with unstable fracture patterns.

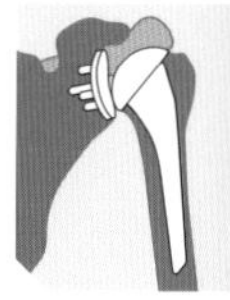

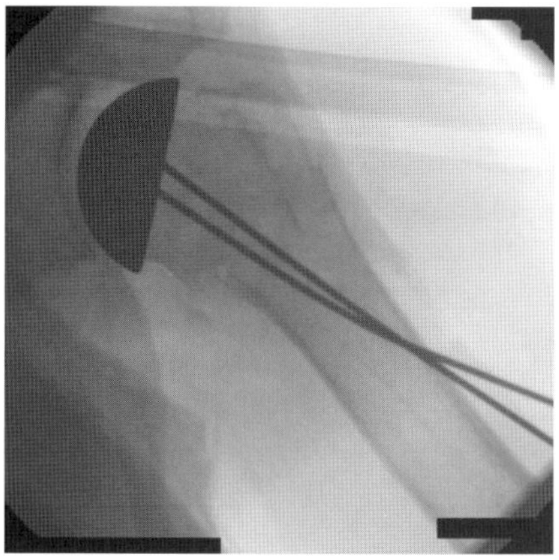

7.9-3 Intraoperative image shows temporary fixation of the humeral head with two K-wires.

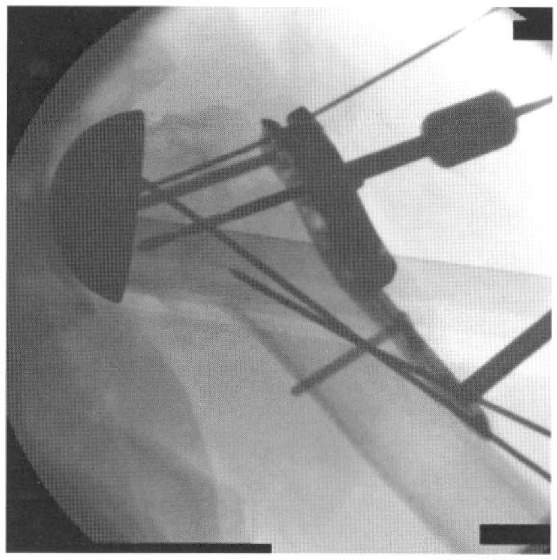

7.9-4 Intraoperative image shows screw fixation after confirmation of correct position of PHILOS plate.

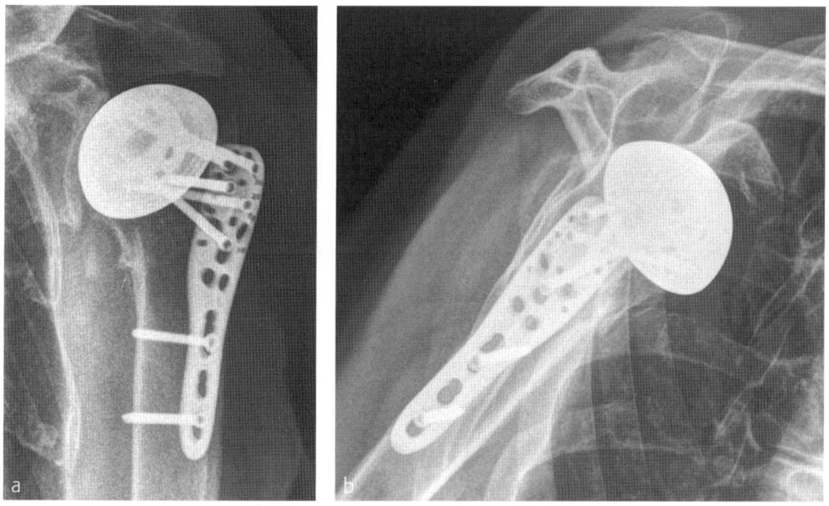

7.9-5a–b Follow-up x-rays obtained 1.5 years postoperatively.
a AP view.
b Lateral view.

I.1-B1(C)

7.10 Segmental humeral shaft fracture, stable prosthesis

ORIF: metaphyseal LCP 3.5/4.5 and two reconstruction plates

Authors **Marschall B Berkes, Dean G Lorich**

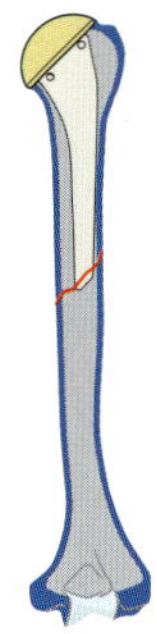

I.1-B1(C)

Case description

A 78-year-old woman with a history of avascular necrosis of the right proximal humerus treated by hemiarthroplasty, sustained a mechanical fall from standing height (**7.10-1a–b**). She presented with pain and deformity in the right arm, as well as signs and symptoms consistent with radial nerve palsy.

Classification: Type I.1-B1(C)

Diagnosis: Segmental humeral shaft fracture, consisting of a distal third displaced spiral fracture at the tip of a well-fixed, noncemented hemiarthroplasty

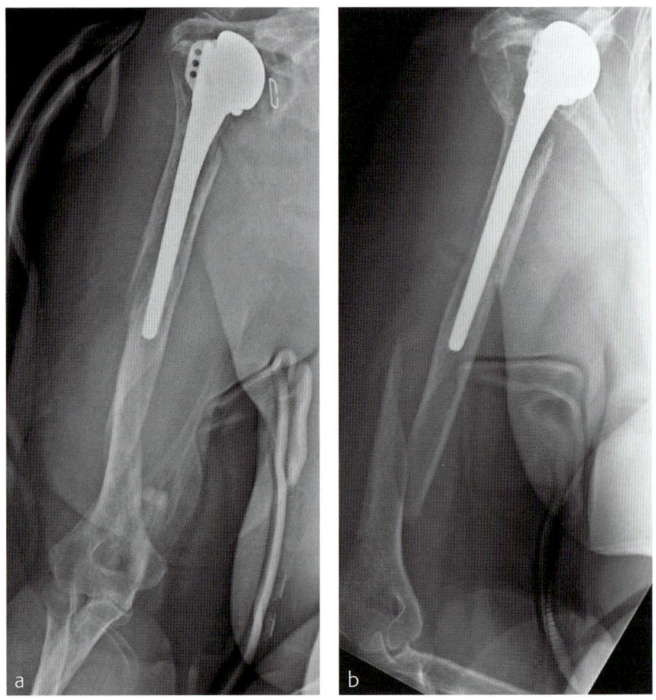

7.10-1a–b X-rays of the injured right humerus. The radial nerve was incarcerated in the fracture.
a AP view.
b Lateral view.

Decision making

Assessing implant stability requires critical analysis of radiographic, clinical, and intraoperative information. Patients should be asked about any previous arm pain, which might indicate loosening prior to the injury. X-rays should be examined for any obvious gross displacement of the stem from the proximal bone stock. Previous x-rays also should be examined for implant subsidence, osteolysis, or any other signs of loosening. The prosthetic stem should be stressed in the operating room to assess its stability.

Based on the patient's preoperative x-rays, in particular the additional fracture fragment that extended proximally, it was difficult to definitively determine if the prosthesis was well fixed. Stressing the stem through the proximal fracture plane was necessary to confirm implant stability.

The best solution to fix a displaced segmental humeral shaft fracture with a well-fixed proximal prosthesis and concomitant radial nerve palsy appears to be open reduction and internal fixation with one or more plates and screws supplemented with cerclage wires (chapter 5.4.1). The radial nerve must be explored carefully and neurolysis performed, if required.

Preoperative planning

Equipment

- 14-hole metaphyseal locking compression plate (LCP) 3.5/4.5
- 7-hole reconstruction plate 2.7
- 7-hole reconstruction plate 3.5
- Cerclage wiring
- C-arm image intensifier
- Sterile tourniquet

Patient preparation and positioning

- Relaxed lateral position on a radiolucent table with a bean bag
- Preparation and draping of the entire right shoulder and upper extremity
- Cefazolin for antibiotic prophylaxis
- Subcutaneous heparin for thrombosis prophylaxis

Reduction and fixation

An extended anterolateral approach was used in which the previous deltopectoral incision was incorporated proximally, and distally, the incision oriented laterally, passing the lateral epicondyle. Proximally, deep dissection proceeded between the anterior and middle raphe of the deltoid muscle. The axillary nerve was identified and protected, as were the circumflex vessels. Distally, deep dissection continued between the brachialis and the posterior compartment. The radial nerve was identified as it pierces the intermuscular septum and from there it was traced proximally and distally. The radial nerve was found to be incarcerated in the distal spiral fracture and was thus dissected free and protected during the remainder of the procedure. The fracture sites were then debrided and irrigated. The prosthesis was assessed with manual stress and found to be stable.

The distal spiral fracture was reduced anatomically with Weber forceps. I.1-B1(C)
The provisional reduction was secured with an anterior 7-hole reconstruction plate 2.7 fixed with lag screws. The proximal fracture fragments also were reduced with Weber forceps and stabilized with an anterolaterally placed 7-hole reconstruction plate 3.5. Finally, a 14-hole metaphyseal LCP 3.5/4.5 was applied to bridge the entire construct. The plate was inserted under the radial nerve distally and the axillary nerve proximally. Distally, the fixation was secured with one conventional and two locking-head screws. Proximally, locking-head screws were inserted bypassing the prosthesis. For additional fixation, two cerclage wires were placed around the obliquity of the proximal fracture. The final result was verified radiologically (◉ **7.10-2a–b**).

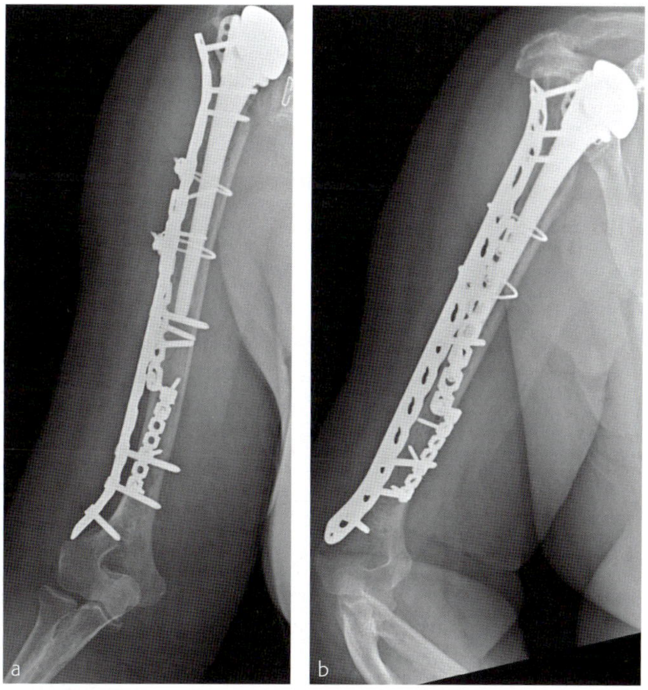

◉ **7.10-2a–b** Postoperative x-rays of the right humerus.
a AP view.
b Lateral view.

I.1-B1(C) Rehabilitation and follow-up

The patient's arm was placed in a sling for comfort, and a cock-up wrist splint was used because of the radial nerve palsy. Occupational therapy included active and passive range of motion of the elbow without limits, active and gentle passive range of motion of the shoulder, and passive range of motion of the fingers and wrist distally. The patient was seen at 2, 8, 12, and 18 weeks postoperatively. At the 8-week follow-up, the patient reported no pain at the surgical site, but radial nerve function had not yet been restored. X-rays obtained at this time showed that the reduction was maintained and interval healing had been achieved (**7.10-3a–b**). Unrestricted active and passive motion of the shoulder and elbow and passive motion of the wrist and fingers were continued. Progression to full weight bearing and strengthening exercises began at 12 weeks postoperatively. X-rays obtained at 18 weeks postoperatively showed bony union (**7.10-4a–b**). Because radial nerve function still was not restored, the patient was referred first to a neurologist and then to a hand surgeon for tendon transfers. At the 7-year follow-up, the patient was pain free and had full function of both the shoulder and elbow. Her activity was limited only by the sequelae of the radial nerve palsy and subsequent tendon transfers.

Points to remember

- Stem loosening is a possible pitfall in this situation. Implant stability is of paramount importance. Fracture fixation with a residual loose stem will result in an unsuccessful clinical outcome, necessitating revision arthroplasty. In this situation, implant stability was confirmed, obviating the need for revision arthroplasty.
- Both the radial and axillary nerves must be identified and traction injury avoided during reduction and fixation.
- Medial soft-tissue dissection and stripping should be avoided, as it places the ulnar nerve at risk.
- The extended anterolateral approach allows for an extensile approach to the entire humerus, providing access to the anterior and lateral aspects of the humerus.
- Small reconstruction plates allow for provisional fixation while assisting with reduction of each individual fracture line.
- Bicortical screw purchase can be achieved proximally by aiming around the implant. This can be assisted by using smaller screws (2.7 mm screw with a washer in the plate 3.5).

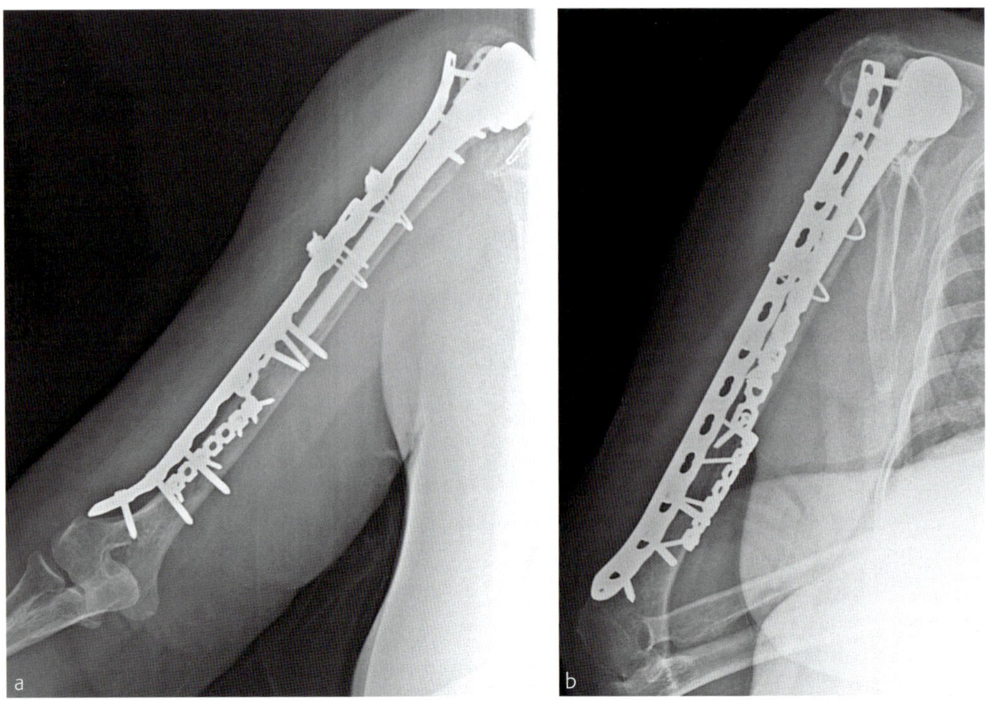

Fig 7.10-3a–b Follow-up x-rays obtained 8 weeks postoperatively.
a AP view
b Lateral view.

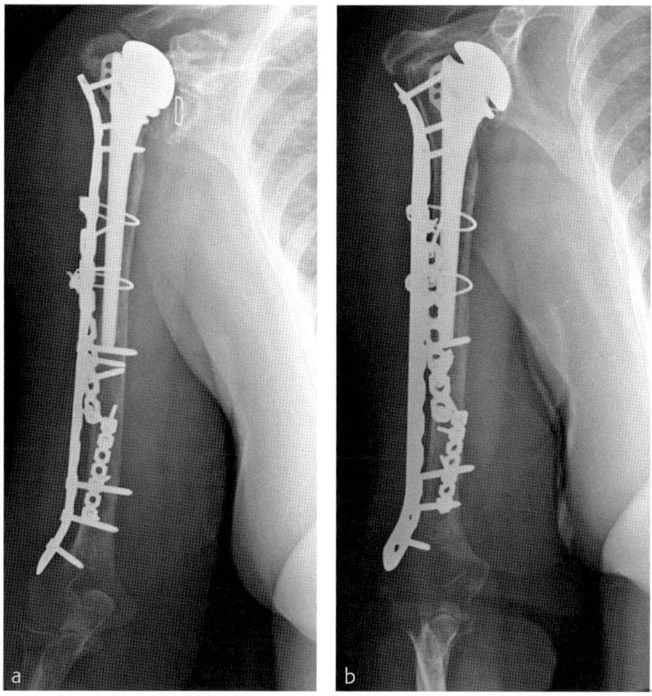

Fig 7.10-4a–b Follow-up x-rays of the humerus obtained 18 weeks postoperatively show bony union. The radial palsy had not recovered and required tendon transfer.
a AP view.
b Lateral view.

I.1-B2

7.11 Proximal humeral fracture, loose reverse prosthesis

Revision: replacement of prosthesis stem

Authors **Martin Jäger, Norbert P Südkamp**

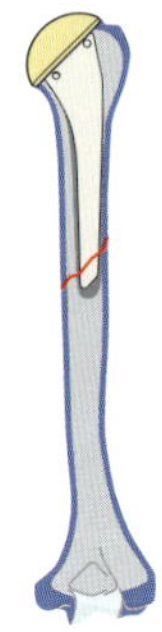

I.1-B2

Case description

An 86-year-old woman with cuff-tear arthropathy of the right dominant shoulder underwent a procedure using a stemless total evolutive shoulder system (TESS) reverse shoulder system. She subsequently fell on the right arm, resulting in a periprosthetic fracture of the proximal humerus (**7.11-1a–b**). X-rays and CT scans showed loosening of the humeral component, while the metaglene (36 mm) appeared well fixed.

Classification: Type I.1-B2

Diagnosis: Periprosthetic fracture of the proximal humerus after implantation of TESS reverse

Decision making

Despite the patient's advanced age, surgical revision appeared indicated because nonoperative treatment was not an option. Because the corolla component was clearly loose and the metaglene appeared well fixed, partial replacement of the prosthesis was considered appropriate (chapter 5.5). There were no options for osteosynthesis due to the very short proximal fragment and poor-quality bone stock. The challenge in this case was identifying the most appropriate prosthesis. A long-stem version of the TESS reverse shoulder system is available, but its humeral component is not recommended in patients with fractures and its use has not been approved for this indication because a disconnection between the corolla and the stem might occur. Alternatively,

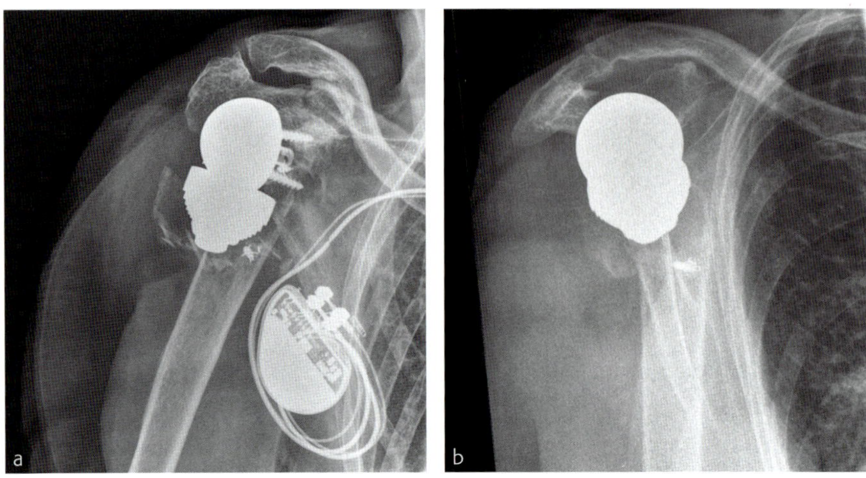

7.11-1a–b Preoperative x-rays show a grossly displaced periprosthetic fracture of the Total Evolutive Shoulder System® (TESS). The corolla component is loose.
a AP view.
b Lateral view.

a comprehensive shoulder system with a reverse option using a 36 mm glenosphere is also available. This system is a stack-on system that leads to a marked extension and lateralization of the humerus, which was not favored. Currently, few products provide a 36 mm glenosphere with an equivalent geometry and a built-in design that minimizes lateralization and extension. The stem of the trabecular metal reverse shoulder system seemed to meet this patient's requirements.

Preoperative planning

Equipment

- Instruments and implants of the trabecular metal reverse shoulder system that minimize lateralization and extension
- Instruments for cementing, including a humeral stem plug
- Bone cement
- Special shoulder retractors
- C-arm for intraoperative image intensification

Patient preparation and positioning

- Preoperative CT scans (mandatory)
- Beach-chair position
- Free draping of the injured extremity
- Adduction and external rotation should be possible and checked perioperatively
- Intraoperative image intensifier
- First- or second-generation cephalosporin for single-shot antibiotic prophylaxis

Reduction and fixation

I.1-B2

A standard anterior deltopectoral approach was used, which is strongly recommended in any revision surgery to explore and expose the axillary nerve. This approach is easier and safer than either the lateral or anterolateral approach.

The metaphyseal area of the proximal humerus was fractured. Remnants of the infraspinatus and teres minor tendons still existed and were attached to stay (permanent) sutures. The same was done with what was left of the subscapularis tendon. The metaphyseal component of the TESS was loose so its removal was not a problem (**7.11-2**). Exploration of the glenosphere revealed that it was stable and thus remained untouched and in situ. The stem of the trabecular metal reverse shoulder system was implanted in 10° retrotorsion after cementing. The height of the prosthesis was adjusted to the glenosphere by adding a 9 mm spacer to achieve a proper soft-tissue tension (**7.11-3a–b**). The remaining rotator-cuff structures were then attached to the stem using nonresorbable fiber wires.

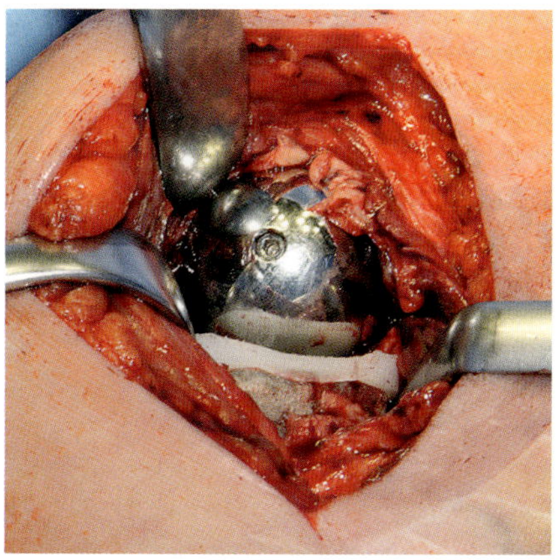

7.11-2 Intraoperative image of the TESS. Note marked polyethylene wear at the medial side of the inlay.

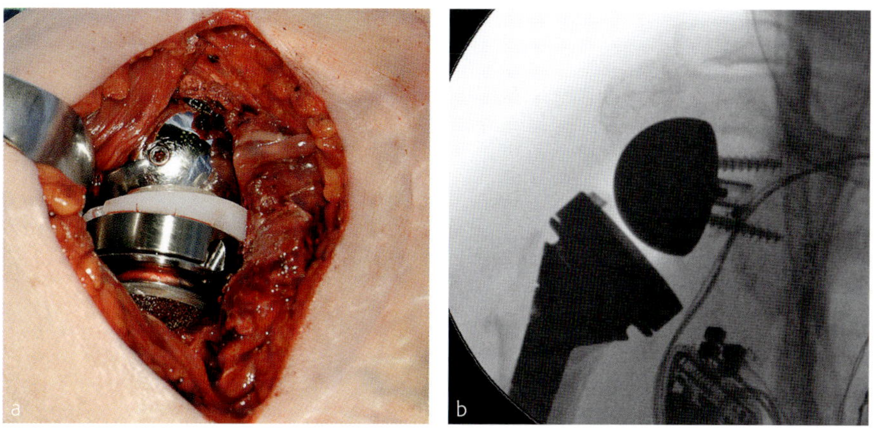

7.11-3a–b Intraoperative images obtained after implantation of the new long-stem humeral component.
a Intraoperative photograph.
b AP view.

I.1-B2 Rehabilitation and follow-up

The right arm was immobilized for 3 weeks using a 15° abduction pillow to decrease tension on the deltoid muscle. During this period, active-assisted exercises and lymphatic drainage were performed. A chair for continuous passive motion was also used. This initial program was followed by an active pain-adapted therapy. Follow-up x-rays obtained 3 months postoperatively showed correct positioning of the reverse prosthesis (👁 **7.11-4**).

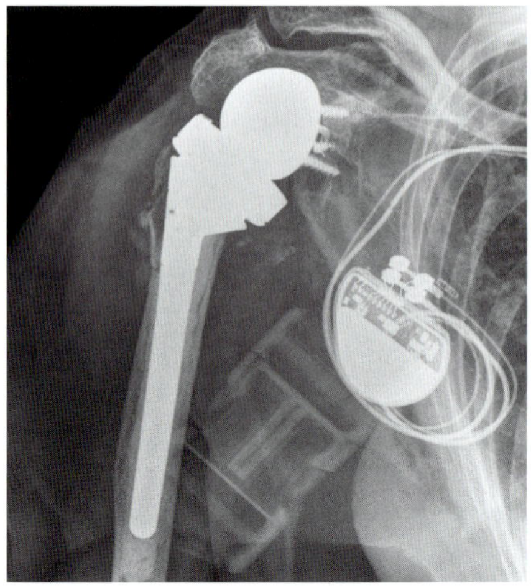

👁 **7.11-4** Follow-up AP view obtained 3 months postoperatively shows correct positioning of the reverse prosthesis.

Points to remember

- Adequate exposure of the site is crucial; use of special shoulder retractors is helpful.
- Special care is needed to ensure adequate soft-tissue release.
- The prosthesis must be implanted in the correct position according to the producers guidelines.
- The remaining rotator cuff must be fixed to preserve rotational function.
- Adequate soft-tissue tension is crucial.
- Any overtensioning of the soft tissues should be avoided.

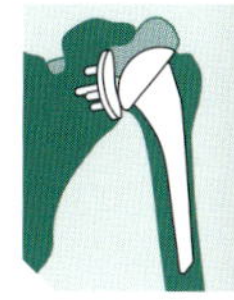

7.12 Humeral shaft malunion, loose prosthesis

Revision: long-stem reverse arthroplasty

Author Simon Lambert

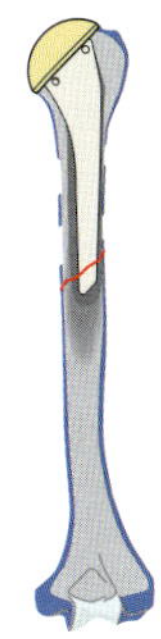

I.1-B3

Case description

A 68-year-old patient underwent hemiarthroplasty for painful shoulder dysfunction caused by glenohumeral degeneration. One year postoperatively, the patient presented with pain, no useful motion in the dominant right shoulder, and fixed internal rotation of 45°. Nonoperative treatment was attempted, but imaging studies showed a severe malunion of a periprosthetic humeral midshaft fracture (**7.12-1a–b**). Both axillary and radial nerves were functioning normally. Preoperative MRI revealed deficiency of the supraequatorial rotator cuff.

Classification: Type I.1-B3

Diagnosis: Malunion of a periprosthetic fracture of the humerus, with a loose prosthesis

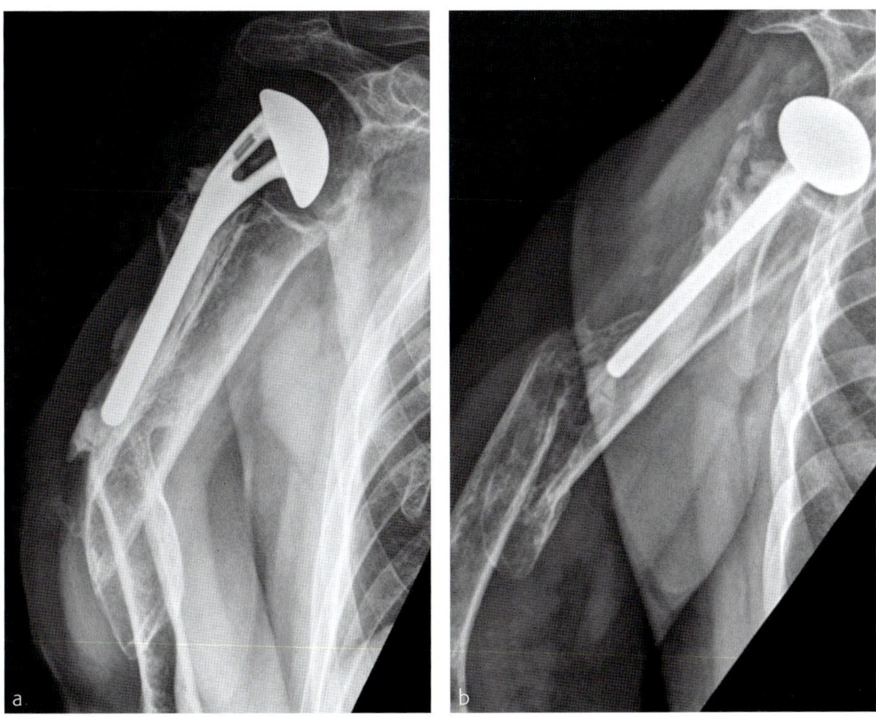

7.12-1a–b X-rays of a failed hemiarthroplasty and malunion of a periprosthetic humeral fracture that had been treated nonoperatively in a sling.
a AP view.
b Lateral view.

I.1-B3 Decision making

Revision of the existing implant was required due to a combination of painful rotator-cuff failure and poor arm position. The fact that the implant was not completely in the bone precluded a simple humeral osteotomy and plate osteosynthesis. Furthermore, the rotator-cuff deficiency required a form of reverse-polarity prosthesis, but the specific form and site of the osteotomy (ie, a lateral closing wedge close to or at the deltoid tuberosity) suggested that deltoid function might be compromised (shortening of the humerus at the site of insertion of the muscle). This would risk instability of a standard reverse-polarity prosthesis. Therefore, a fixed-fulcrum type of prosthesis was extended as a custom-built humeral component with a long stem. The custom stem provided rotational stability of the proximal humeral segment and a smooth tip cemented into the distal humerus. Rotational stability was required in the proximal humerus to provide for muscle attachment and activity and was obtained by use of extrinsic flutes in the proximal segment. The isthmic region was not cemented to encourage bone formation at the osteotomy site. The need for healing of the osteotomy meant that the cement needed to be removed and avoided at the osteotomy site.

Preoperative planning

Equipment

- Fixed-fulcrum total shoulder replacement device
- Fixed-fulcrum glenoid component (hydroxyapatite-coated large-pitch titanium screw with a 22 mm bearing head)
- Custom-built humeral component with extra-long stem (Cobalt-chrome standard receiving proximal end with an ultra-high-molecular-weight polyethylene captive liner, and custom-made stem with hydroxyapatite-coated flutes 1 mm high proximal to the isthmic zone)

Patient preparation and positioning

- Reclining position with the arm draped free
- Neurosurgical head support with neck protection
- First- or second-generation cephalosporin for antibiotic prophylaxis
- Compression stockings and calf compression for thrombosis prophylaxis
- Patient warming measures
- Neurophysiological monitoring

Reduction and fixation

An extensile anterolateral (Henry) approach was used in which the incision follows the deltopectoral interval proximally and cephalic vein distally, lateral to the lateral border of the biceps brachii at least as far as the level of the emergence of the radial nerve through the lateral intermuscular septum.

The interval between the biceps brachii and brachialis was identified proximally, and the seam between the two muscles split proximodistally, identifying the musculocutaneous nerve and the lateral cutaneous nerve of the forearm proximally. The remaining seam between the muscles was split distally, protecting the lateral cutaneous nerve of the forearm, to a point about 5 cm proximal to the anterior flexor crease of the elbow. The brachialis was split, cauterizing the distal transverse intramuscular vessels. Strong medial or lateral retraction should be avoided at this level to avoid injury to the radial and ulnar nerves.

The loose prosthesis and cement mantle were easily removed in this patient. In a more typical presentation, in which the prosthesis is contained within the medulla, standard techniques for removal of the prosthesis and cement mantle (eg, the limited longitudinal humeral split [Gohlke technique] and/or ultrasound cement removal equipment) are used. The revision implant is designed to be at least 5 cm longer than the planned length of the limited longitudinal osteotomy to allow sufficient intramedullary length for stable distal cement fixation.

The malunion was exposed, with elevation of the periosteum sufficient to identify the malunion zone and prepare the osteotomy. The periosteum commonly adheres to the fibrous tissue of the malunion and requires sharp dissection to free the bone circumferentially. This step is necessary to protect the radial nerve passing behind during the osteotomy. The osteotomy was planned as a simple closing wedge laterally and was made by first perforating the diaphysis with a cooled drill and then connecting the perforations using a sharp osteotome. Excess bone was not removed from outside the osteotomy zone, as removal risks damage to the radial nerve; this bone will usually remodel (as in this case). The ends of the bone at the osteotomy site were petaled in the Judet manner (intracortical corticotomy) to promote vascular diversion and thus bone healing. Local bone, which can be safely harvested from the exophytes, was morcelized and used to graft the osteotomy site.

To obtain axial and rotational alignment, the custom implant was introduced through the proximal part of the humerus until the tip of the stem was visible at the osteotomy site. The rotational alignment of the proximal segment was gauged by reference to the bicipital sulcus, the attachment zone of the pectoralis major, and the deltoid tuberosity.

The distal humeral preparation was then completed, and antibiotic-loaded cement was introduced into the distal humerus only. The implant was finally advanced into the distal segment and compression carried out manually, clearing excess cement as it presented at the osteotomy site.

Rehabilitation and follow-up

The construct seemed stable at 6 weeks postoperatively (**7.12-2a–b**). The arm rested in a simple sling for 6 weeks. Twice-daily active-assisted elbow full range-of-motion exercises, active-assisted shoulder limited range-of-motion exercises (avoiding external rotation beyond neutral zero at waist level and limiting flexion-elevation to 45°) and postural exercises were encouraged. Simple nonweight-bearing activities of daily living were allowed when union was confirmed by the absence of symptoms and the presence of callus in all four quadrants of the fracture zone on x-rays at 6 months. The final result after 1 year was good (**7.12-3a–b**). I.1-B3

Points to remember

- The musculocutaneous nerve and its terminal branch are at risk throughout the exposure; dissection lateral to the nerve provides protection.
- The radial nerve and its branches are at risk throughout the distal exposure; avoiding strong lateral retraction minimizes this risk during dissection distally.
- Neurovascular bundles not immediately in the field of surgery are at risk during the osteotomy and manual realignment of the bone.
- Rotational malalignment is avoided by specific reference to the bicipital sulcus proximally and to the anterior crest

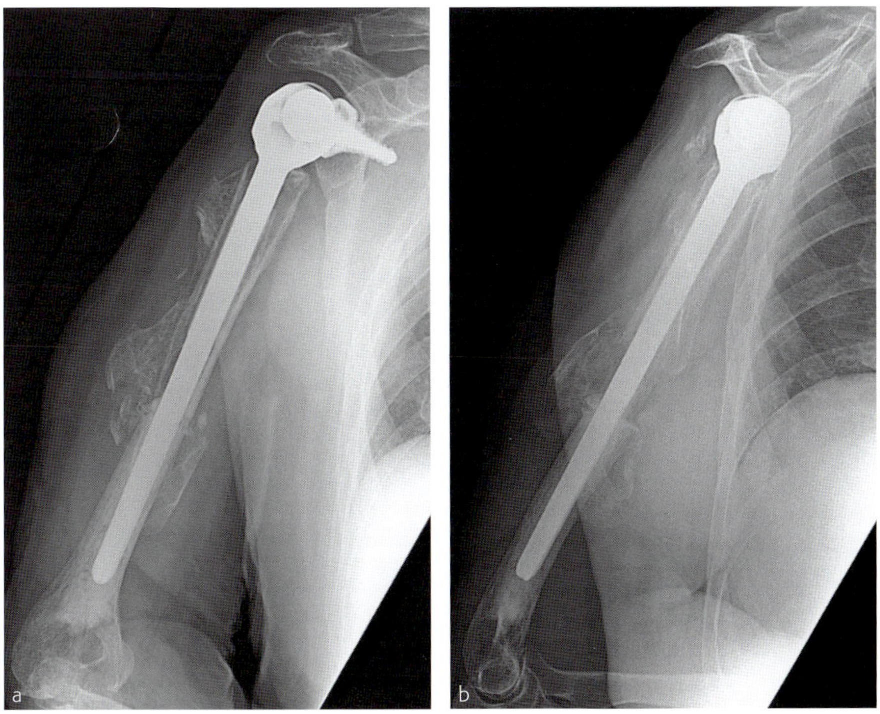

7.12-2a–b X-rays obtained 6 weeks after reconstruction with revision total shoulder arthroplasty and simple corrective diaphyseal osteotomy. Autogenous bone from the residual exophytes was used as a morcelized graft.
a AP view.
b Lateral view shows close apposition of the osteotomy surfaces.

I.1-B3 of the humerus distally. The line of the crest should lie just medial to the line of the bicipital sulcus.

- Although gentamicin-enriched cement may have an inhibiting effect on bone healing, the risk of infection was considered to be potentially greater.
- Intramedullary fixation of a transverse osteotomy, as in a transverse fracture, carries the risk of nonunion due to high strain within the fracture/osteotomy zone. Both the proximal and distal segments of the diaphysis must be rotationally stable with respect to each other. Although cementing the entire construct is possible, bone healing would almost certainly be delayed or prevented. Therefore, a customized implant with distal primary stability through cementation, and primary proximal stability through derotation fins, which also permits/enhances bone on growth for secondary stability, is a useful alternative to standard long-stemmed revision components.

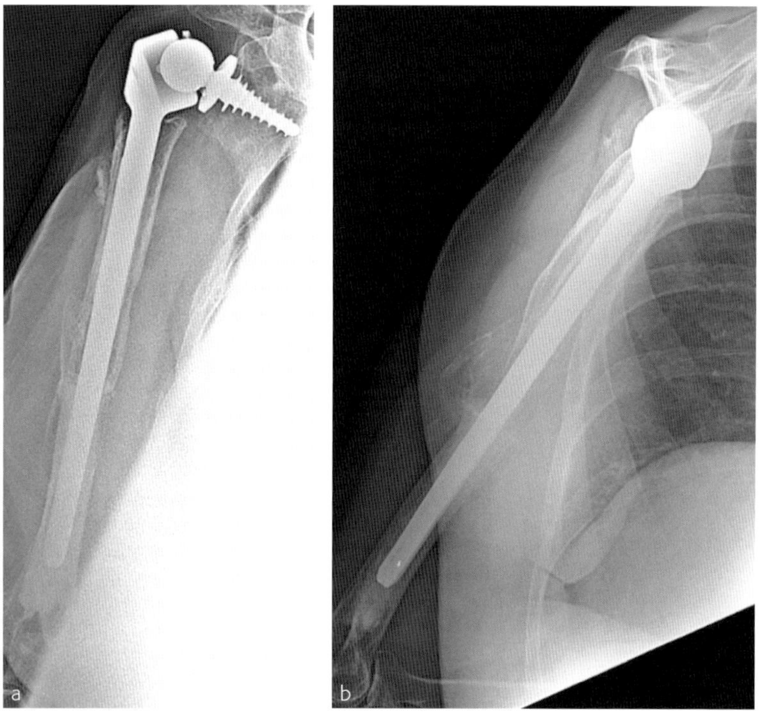

7.12-3a–b Follow-up x-rays obtained 1 year after reconstruction with revision total shoulder arthroplasty and simple corrective diaphyseal osteotomy. Union at the osteotomy and remodeling occurred with no prosthetic complications. The glenoid screw was secure, even in the presence of a long lever arm and load bearing, suggesting excellent incorporation into the glenoid vault.

a AP view.
b Lateral view.

7.13 Humeral shaft fracture, stable prosthesis
ORIF: LCP 4.5/5.0

Authors **Martin Jäger, Norbert P Südkamp**

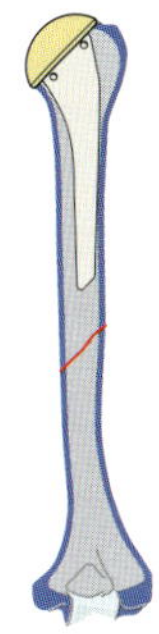

I.1-C

Case description

A 64-year-old man underwent anatomical total shoulder arthroplasty of his left nondominant shoulder because of secondary omarthrosis due to polyarthritis 9 years ago. Four months postoperatively, he sustained a humeral shaft fracture with concomitant palsy of the radial nerve as a result of a fall at home.

Classification: Type I.1-C

Diagnosis: Periprosthetic fracture of the humeral shaft, distal to a well-fixed stem

Decision making

X-rays showed a spiral fracture of the humeral shaft well distal to the tip of a well-fixed prosthetic stem. Nonoperative treatment was considered, which with functional bracing works in displaced fractures. In this patient, however, the preoperative neurological examination showed a concomitant palsy of the radial nerve, which led to exploration of the radial nerve via a posterior approach combined with plate fixation. This approach seemed appropriate because bone quality was still good and the fracture was approximately 4 cm distal to the tip of the stem allowing for safe screw purchase (**7.13-1a–c**). The stability of the prosthetic stem must be checked; in case of any doubt, CT is strongly recommended. The following questions also should be answered:

- Is the quality of the bone stock adequate for safe implant purchase?
- What is the distance between the fracture line and the tip of the stem?
- Is there enough room beside the stem to allow safe insertion of screws or are cerclage wires required?
- Does the spiral or oblique fracture allow for placement of a lag screw to obtain interfragmentary compression?

In this case, anatomical reduction with a stable plate osteosynthesis seemed possible without use of cerclage wires (chapter 5.4.1).

Preoperative planning

Equipment

- Instruments and implants for plating (locking compression plate [LCP] recommended)
- Instruments and wire for cerclage osteosynthesis (appropriate cable passers)
- C-arm for intraoperative image intensification

Patient preparation and positioning

- Preoperative CT (mandatory)
- Supine position with the arm placed on the abdomen
- Prone position with the arm placed on a radiolucent arm holder (strongly recommended for best intraoperative image intensification)
- Lateral position with the arm placed on an arm holder (alternative)
- First- or second-generation cephalosporin for single-shot antibiotic prophylaxis

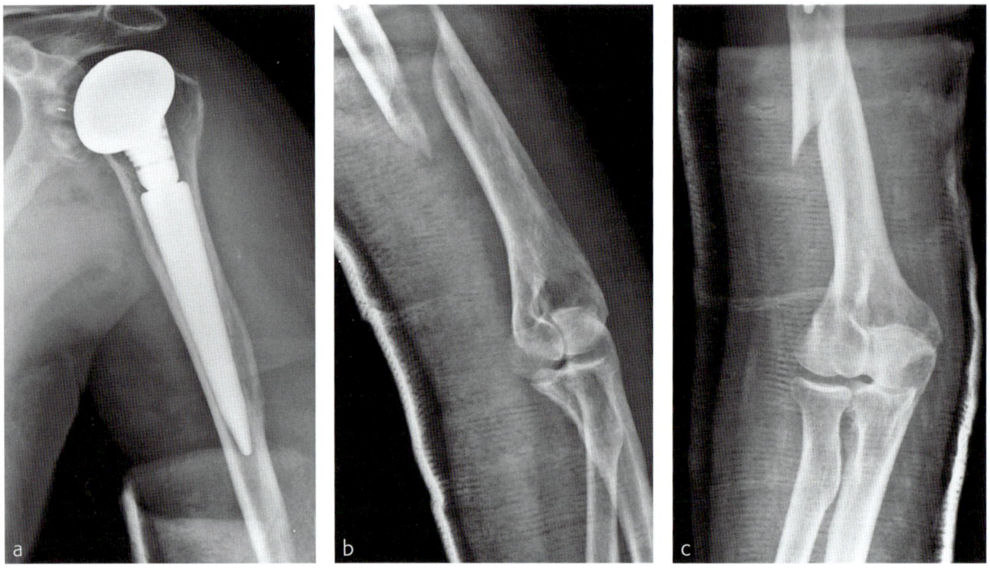

7.13-1a–c Preoperative x-rays show a periprosthetic fracture of the humeral shaft well distal to the tip of the stem.
a AP view of the shoulder.
b AP view of the elbow.
c Lateral view of the elbow.

Reduction and fixation

A standard posterior Henry approach was used with exploration of the radial nerve. There is a close relationship between the apex of the triceps aponeurosis and the course of the radial nerve, which can be identified approximately 2.5 cm proximal to this apex after splitting the muscle bellies of the triceps brachii muscle. In this case, the radial nerve appeared macroscopically intact. An additional neurolysis was performed (**7.13-2**). Release of the intermuscular septum is recommended.

After anatomical fracture reduction, two lag screws were inserted and a 12-hole LCP 3.5 was placed on the posterior aspect of the humerus, slipping the proximal end underneath the radial nerve. Two bicortical and one monocortical locking-head screws were placed into the proximal fragment without interfering with the stem. Additional cerclage wires were not needed. Intraoperative x-rays confirmed the anatomical reduction and correct positioning of the implant.

Rehabilitation and follow-up

A Gilchrist bandage was used for pain relief for the first 2 days postoperatively. Immediate physiotherapy was started with active pain-adapted exercises without restrictions. The patient also received lymphatic drainage. A dynamic forearm orthosis served to counterbalance the temporary radial nerve palsy. Clinical and radiological follow up after 1 year showed bony healing of the humerus without secondary loss of reduction (**7.13-3a–b**).

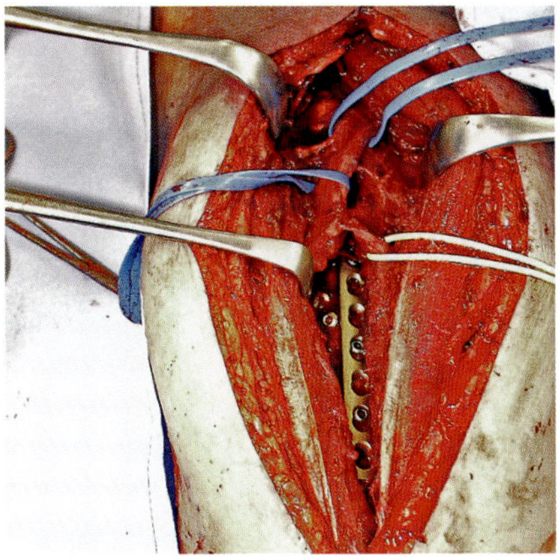

7.13-2 Intraoperative image after plating the humerus via a posterior approach. Note the course of the macroscopically intact radial nerve over the plate (blue slings).

Points to remember

I.1-C

- In simple fracture types, anatomical reduction and stable fixation is a reliable treatment option.
- Slightly lateral placement of the plate might allow screw placement beside the stem.
- Intraoperative x-rays are helpful to verify correct plate and screw positioning.
- The radial nerve is at risk and should be explored in every patient. When using the standard Henry posterior approach, the mean distance of the crossing of the radial nerve from the apex of the triceps aponeurosis is approximately 2.5 cm. This distance correlates with the patient's height and arm length.
- The course of the radial nerve in relation to the proximal plate holes must be noted in the operative report, which helps to spare it in the event that plate removal or revision surgery is needed.

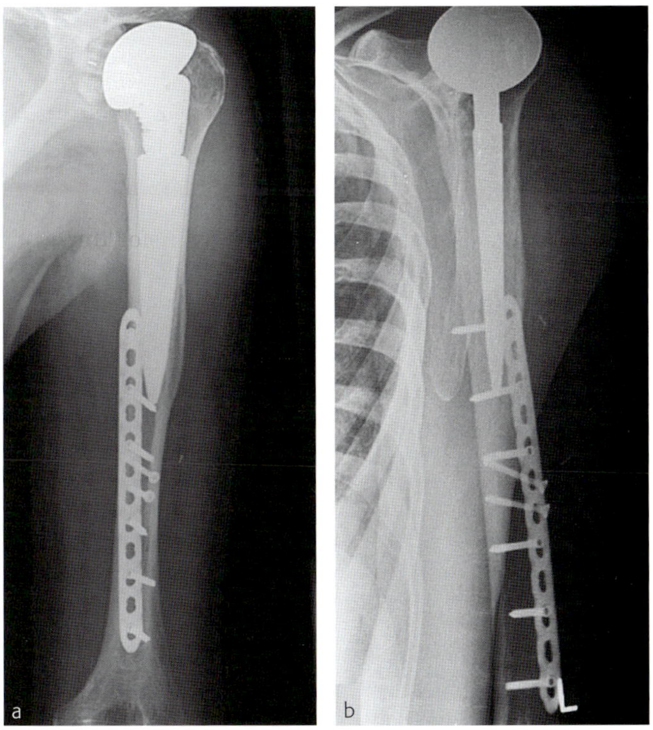

7.13-3a–b X-rays obtained 1 year postoperatively show complete healing of the fracture.
a AP view.
b Lateral view.

I.1-C

7.14 Humeral shaft fracture, stable prosthesis

ORIF: LCP 4.5/5.0 and cerclage wires

Authors **Martin Jäger, Norbert P Südkamp**

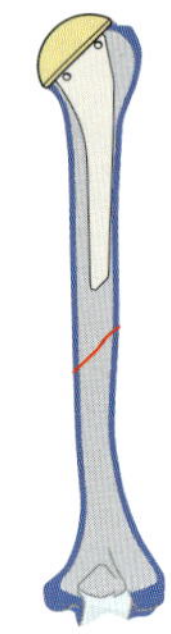

I.1-C

Case description

An 82-year-old woman underwent bilateral shoulder hemiarthroplasties for displaced four-part fractures on both sides 5 years ago. Three months postoperatively, she fell on her dominant right shoulder, resulting in a periprosthetic fracture of the right arm. X-rays showed a significantly displaced, short spiral fracture, approximately 3 cm distal to the stem and approximately 1 cm distal to the cement plug combined with a marked shortening of the humerus (**7.14-1**). The prosthetic stem appeared well fixed.

Classification: Type I.1-C

Diagnosis: Periprosthetic fracture of the humerus distal to a well-fixed hemiarthroplasty

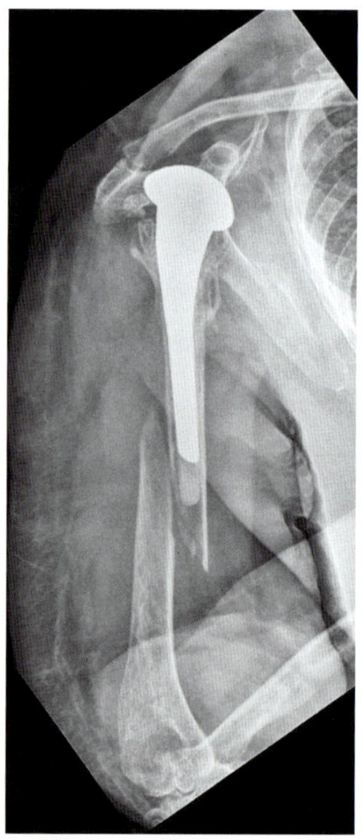

7.14-1 X-ray shows a periprosthetic fracture of the humeral shaft distal to the well-fixed cemented hemiprosthesis.

Decision making

This type of humeral shaft fracture can be treated nonoperatively, but open reduction and internal fixation was selected for this patient due to the marked shortening and displacement of the fracture, as well as the age of the patient. Although the tuberosities seemed healed with only minor displacement, slight proximal migration of the prosthesis head was evident, indicating a rotator-cuff insufficiency. Because the stem was well fixed and the patient was satisfied with shoulder function before the most recent fall, replacing the hemiprosthesis or converting to a reverse system was not indicated.

The challenge preoperatively was to estimate the options for internal fixation. Even though the type of fracture and the remaining bone stock distal to the stem seemed to allow for anatomical reduction and stable plate fixation, the question was if proximally the integrity of the remaining cortical bone thickness around the prosthetic stem would permit screw placement. The thin cortex indicated that cerclage wires would most likely be required for proximal plate fixation (chapter 5.4.1).

Preoperative planning

Equipment

- Instruments and implants for plating (locking compression plates [LCP] recommended)
- Instruments and wire for cerclage osteosynthesis (appropriate cable passers)
- C-arm for intraoperative fluoroscopy

Patient preparation and positioning

- Preoperative CT scans (mandatory)
- Supine or beach-chair position with the arm placed on the abdomen
- First- or second-generation cephalosporin for single-shot antibiotic prophylaxis

Reduction and fixation

Both the anterolateral and posterior approach are appropriate to treat this periprosthetic fracture. The posterior approach has a limited extension proximally due to the deltoid muscle but allows direct visualization of the radial nerve. In contrast, the anterolateral approach allows exposure of the entire humerus, especially the proximal part. In this case it was anticipated that screw fixation at the level of the stem might fail and cerclage wires might become necessary. Therefore, an anterolateral approach was chosen even though it may render the identification of the radial nerve in its entire course more difficult.

The patient was placed in a beach-chair position. A standard anterolateral approach to the humerus according to Henry was performed, using the distal part of the preexisting deltopectoral approach. Deep dissection was carried out in the interval just posterior to the biceps brachii muscle and distally anterior to the brachioradialis muscle. With this approach, the biceps brachii and brachialis muscles should be carefully retracted medially because of the musculocutaneous nerve. The radial nerve comes around the posterior aspect of the humerus, penetrating the lateral intermuscular septum entering the anterior compartment of the arm between the brachioradialis and brachialis muscles. The radial nerve must be identified and protected by retracting it to the ulnar side of the arm. It is helpful to release the lateral intermuscular septum to reduce its tension on the radial nerve.

The challenge in this patient was the diameter of the stem, filling the humeral shaft on one hand and the thin cortex on the other. Both make the use of screws for proximal plate fixation uncertain and risky. Because the bone appeared to be quite fragile, temporary fixation with reduction forceps was not possible. Therefore, the LCP was first inserted extraperiosteally and fixed distally with locking-head screws, followed by reduction of the distal humerus and plate application to the proximal fragment. Once approximate reduction was obtained, cable cerclage wires were used to fix the plate proximally at the level of the stem to prevent migration of the cerclage wires. Threaded cerclage positioning screws were used to achieve additional stability for the LCP. Slightly distal to the stem, a bicortical screw was inserted through the cement plug to provide additional fixation.

Rehabilitation and follow-up

Postoperative x-rays showed a stable osteosynthesis (👁 **7.14-2a–b**). However, due to the osteopenic bone and the cerclage wires used proximally, physiotherapy was limited to active-assisted motion for the first 6 weeks after which time active motion was initiated. Follow-up 1 year later showed complete bony healing without secondary loss of reduction (👁 **7.14-3a–b**).

Points to remember

- The lateral cutaneous branch of the musculocutaneous nerve is at risk at the distal end of the incision as it exits the biceps muscle laterally.
- The radial nerve must be identified before any incision is made into the brachialis muscle or before periosteal elevation of the brachialis.
- The course of the radial nerve in relation to the proximal plate holes should be noted in the operative report.
- Instruments to place cerclage wires must be introduced gently around the humerus to ensure they stay directly on the bone to avoid damaging the radial nerve.
- To improve fixation the plate should be 2–3 holes longer proximally (comment by the editors).

I.1-C

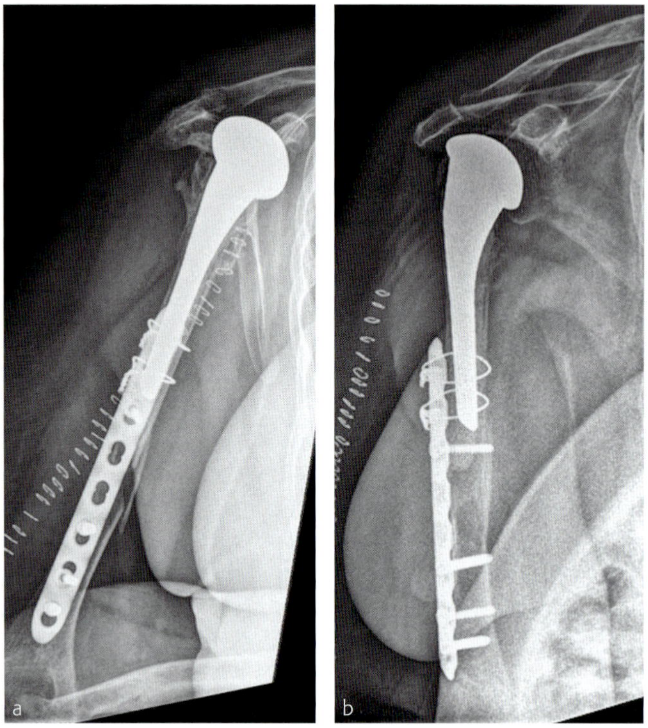

7.14-2a–b X-rays of the humerus obtained immediately postoperatively. A longer plate proximally would have been preferable.
a AP view.
b Lateral view.

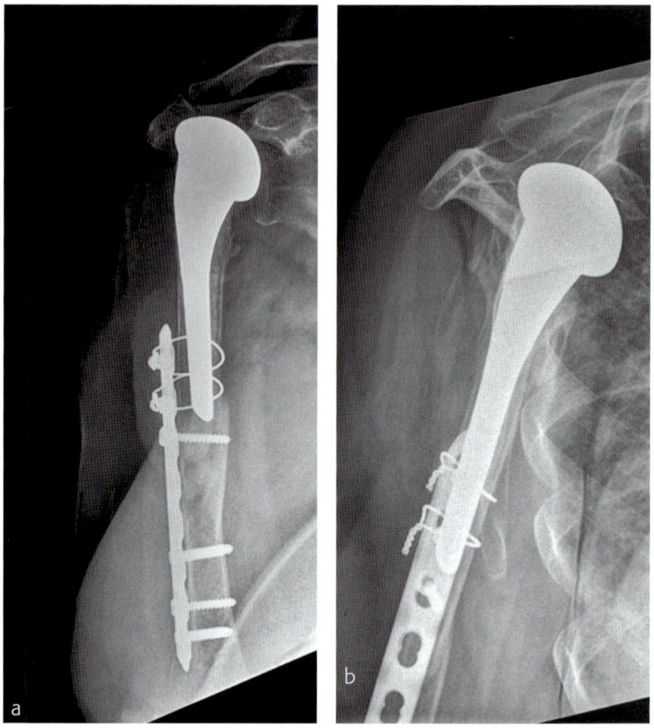

7.14-3a–b Follow-up x-rays obtained 1 year postoperatively.
a AP view of the humerus shows complete fracture healing.
b Axial view of the shoulder.

8 Elbow cases

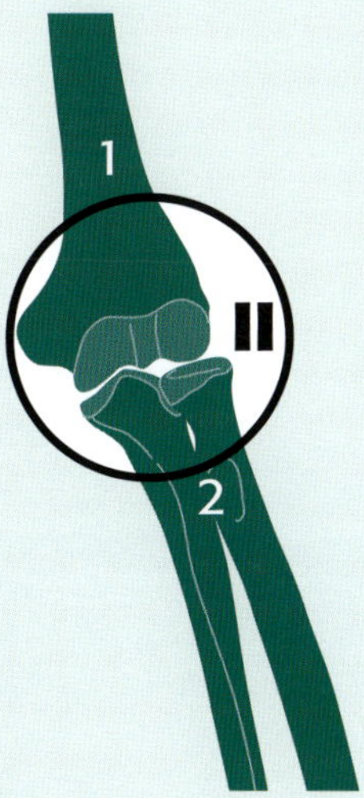

8.1 Distal humeral fracture, loose elbow prosthesis

Reconstruction: allograft prosthetic composite and plate fixation

Authors **Stephen L Kates, Natasha O'Malley**

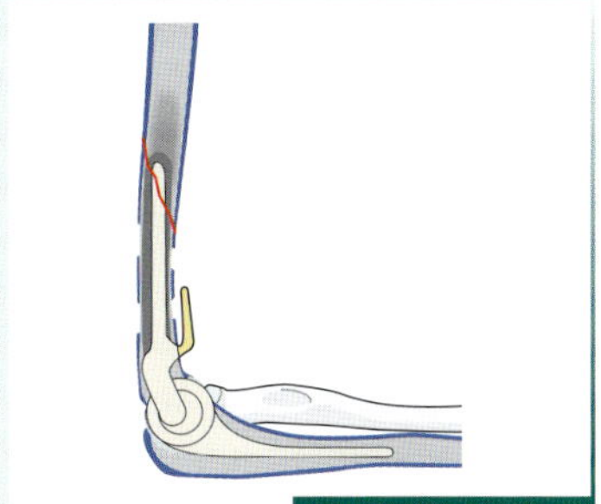

II.1-B3

Case description

An 80-year-old woman presented with increasing pain in her dominant right arm after a fall (👁 **8.1-1a–c**). She underwent total elbow arthroplasty and radial head resection of that arm 6 years ago.

Classification: Type II.1-B3

Diagnosis: Periprosthetic distal humeral fracture, with a loose prosthesis

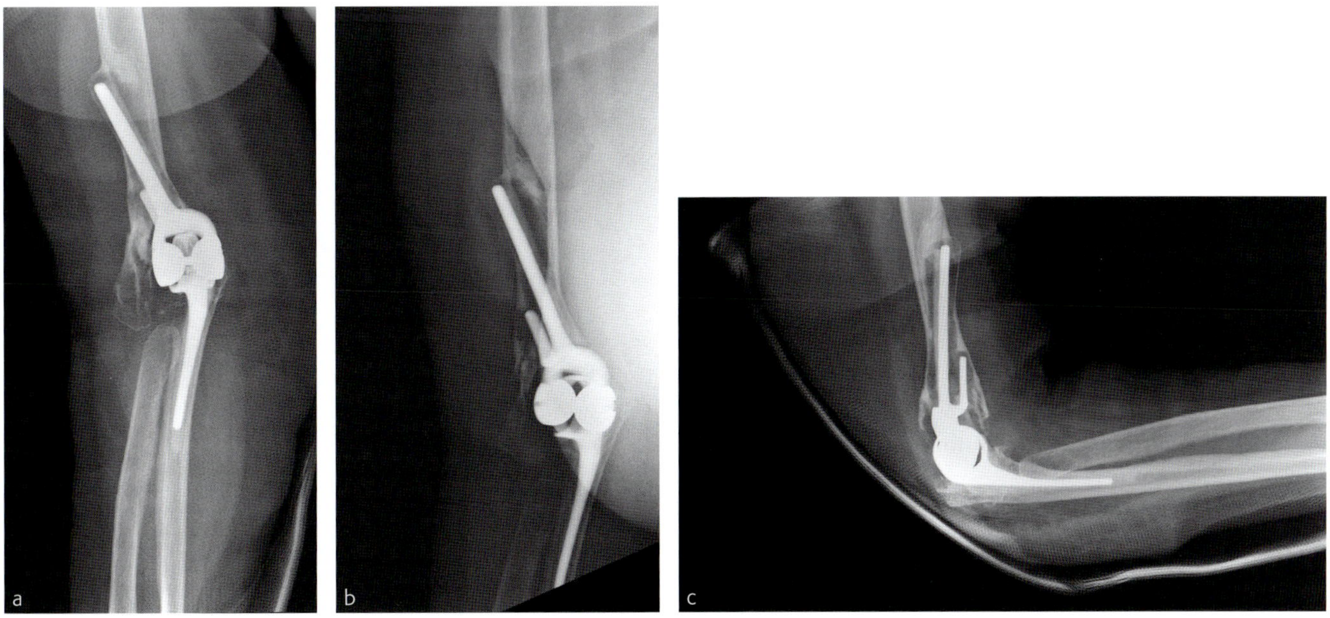

👁 **8.1-1a–c** X-rays show radial head resection and total elbow arthroplasty in situ with extensive osteolysis and cortical perforation of the humerus.
a AP view.
b AP view.
c Lateral view.

II.1-B3 Decision making

Due to extensive osteolysis and destruction of the distal humerus, fracture reduction was not possible. Therefore, the surgical solution was to replace the distal humerus with an allograft (chapter 5.6) to accommodate a long-stem revision prosthesis, allowing implantation in native healthy bone to restore maximum function.

The presence of infection must be excluded. The brand of prosthesis already in situ must be available, and the long-stem revision humeral component should be technically compatible with the current ulnar component, which appeared solidly fixed.

Complete revision and exchange of the ulnar component is necessary if the component is loose at the time of surgery or if there is any hardware mismatch.

An appropriate and screened humeral allograft must be ordered. Patient consent for the procedure is needed, including the possibility of a two-staged procedure if infection is a concern at time of surgery or if amputation is needed as a consequence of bone destruction.

Preoperative planning

Equipment

- Humeral allograft
- Cement removal device
- 10-hole locking compression plate (LCP)
- Locking-head screws (range of sizes 10–20 mm)
- Cable system
- Humeral-sized reamers
- Burr for cement removal
- Cement
- Matching revision prostheses (humeral and ulnar)

Patient preparation and positioning

- Lateral decubitus position
- Antibiotics after cultures from prosthesis

Reduction and fixation

The surgical approach was through the previous posterior midline incision. The ulnar nerve was identified and protected throughout the procedure. To rule out concomitant infection, a sample of synovial fluid and tissue was obtained for urgent culture and frozen section. Results of both studies were negative. Intraoperative findings included a grossly loose humeral prosthesis with complete resorption of the humeral condyles. The ulnar component appeared stable. After further dissection, the radial nerve was identified and protected throughout the procedure. The midline of the proximal humerus was marked with diathermy to orient with a flare remnant of the humeral condyle in anticipation of aligning the final prosthesis before decoupling the humeral and ulnar components of the prosthesis.

The distal humerus was resected from the perforation point and the proximal cement removed. The humeral allograft was then prepared and sized, sequentially reamed, and the prosthesis trial component was tested (**8.1-2**). A trial with the actual prosthesis was then carried out, with orientation in line with the healthy premarked proximal humerus, with 60 mm of the humeral prosthesis in native bone and coupled to the originally implanted ulnar component. A cement restrictor was inserted in native bone 75 mm from the distal edge, and the prosthesis was cemented in situ with the humeral allograft aligned and oriented with the initial diathermy markings. Thus, a total of 100 mm of the distal humerus had been excised. A 160 mm humeral prosthesis was used, and the cement restrictor placed at 75 mm of the native proximal humeral mantle.

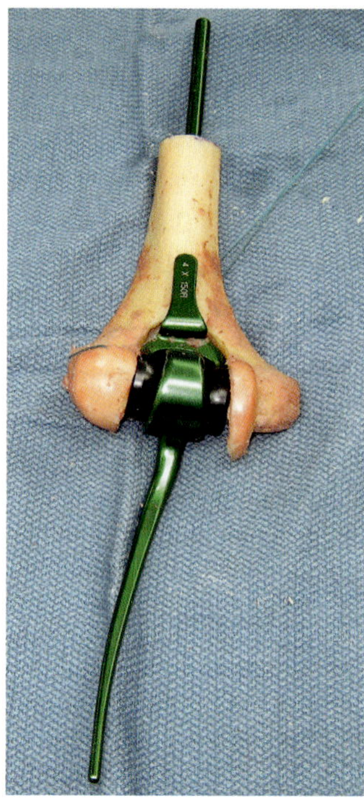

8.1-2 Prepared humeral allograft (100 mm) with trial prostheses in situ (image courtesy of John Elfar, Rochester, USA).

A 10-hole LCP was then applied with proximal and distal screw fixation and with cable augmentation (**8.1-3a–b**).

Rehabilitation and follow-up

Range-of-motion exercises were initiated at 2 weeks postoperatively. A 1 kg limit to weights was imposed on the side of surgery and was gradually increased with a supervised rehabilitation program. At the 6-month follow-up, elbow range of motion was from 10° to 130°, and x-rays showed that the prosthesis was well fixed. Follow-up x-rays obtained 10 months postoperatively showed that the allograft was well incorporated (**8.1-4a–b**).

Points to remember

- Loose displaced prosthetic components must be revised; they cannot be reconstructed with plating.
- In patients with a bone defect or severe osteolysis, an allograft must be considered, which when combined with a long-stem prosthesis can be used to reconstruct the distal humerus.
- The ulnar and medial nerves are at risk due to multiple previous surgeries and use of an extensile approach.
- Malalignment of allograft and prosthesis will compromise eventual function.
- Orientation of humeral condyles should be premarked proximally in native bone before excision.
- Multiple practice trials of the implants with allograft and the in situ ulnar component are necessary to correct and ensure correct positioning with optimal range of motion before cementing in situ.

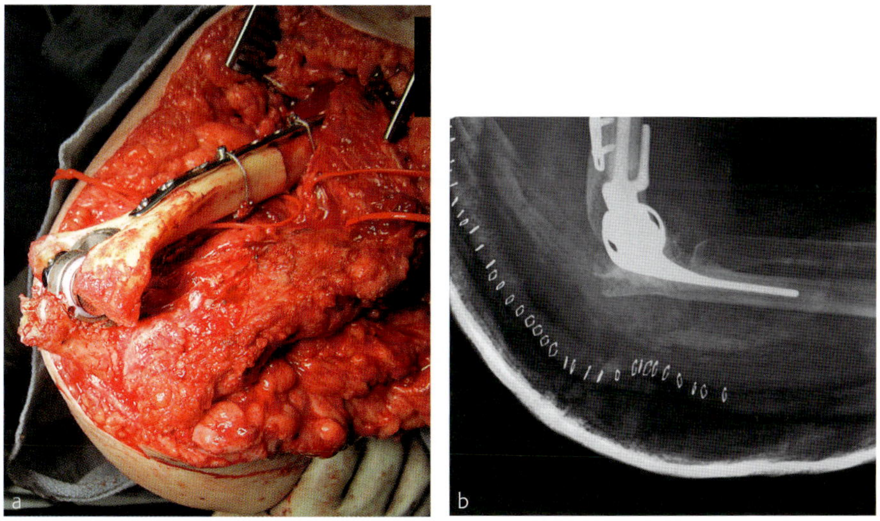

8.1-3a–b Locking compression plate (LCP) is applied with proximal and distal screw fixation and with cable augmentation.

a Intraoperative photograph shows humeral allograft and native humerus interface, the coupled prosthesis, and LCP with screw and cable fixation.

b X-ray confirms the coupled prosthesis and position of the plate.

II.1-B3

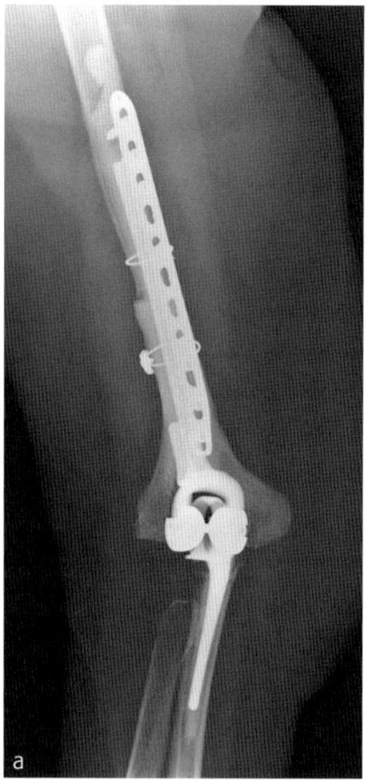

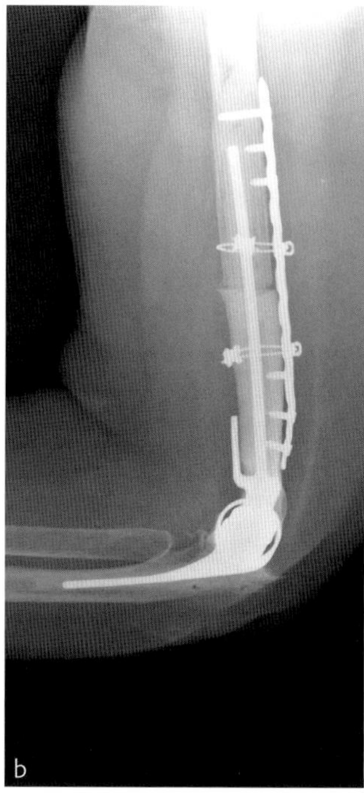

8.1-4a–b X-rays obtained 10 months postoperatively after revision of the right total elbow arthroplasty using humeral bone prosthetic allograft with a 160 mm prosthesis. The cement restrictor is visible 75 mm proximal to the native humeral mantle with augmentation of the fixation by a 10-hole LCP with locking-head screws and cable fixation.

a AP view.
b Lateral view.

8.2 Lateral humeral condyle fracture with impeding humeral fracture, loose prosthesis

Reconstruction: allograft struts and impaction grafting, cerclage fixation

Authors **Antonio M Foruria de Diego, Joaquín Sanchez-Sotelo**

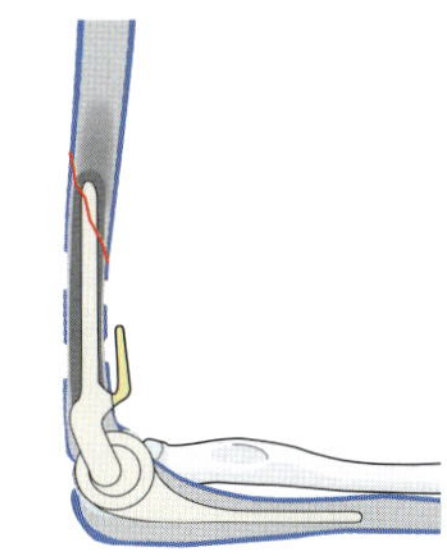

II.1-B3

Case description

A 72-year-old woman with posttraumatic osteoarthritis underwent total elbow arthroplasty 2 years ago. She had progressive pain, a sensation of instability, and experienced a cracking sound when bending the elbow. X-rays showed proximal radiolucency around an otherwise well-fixed long ulnar component (**8.2-1a–b**). The patient had a completely loose 10 cm long humeral component with dramatic cortical thinning of the humeral diaphysis around the prosthetic stem due to osteolysis.

Classification: Type II.1-B3

Diagnosis: Periprosthetic fracture of the lateral humeral condyle with displacement, with a loose prosthesis

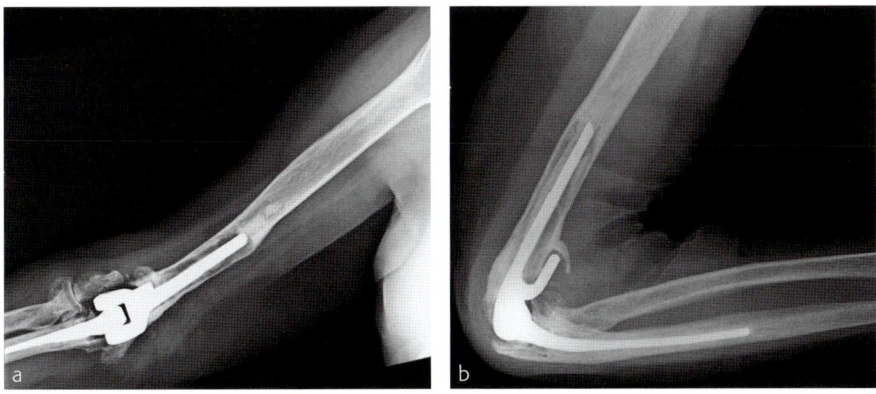

8.2-1a–b X-rays of the elbow arthroplasty show a loose humeral component, extensive osteolysis, and a displaced fracture of the lateral humeral condyle.
a AP view.
b Lateral view.

II.1-B3

Decision making

Such extensive bone resorption and prosthetic loosening after only 2 years could be the result of an infection or mechanical failure. A two-staged procedure was planned, although results of blood studies were negative, and no fluid was obtained by aspiration.

In patients with an osteolysis with such extreme cortical thinning, the possibility of salvage is limited to the use of struts and impaction grafting techniques or allograft prosthetic composite or customized tumor prosthesis of the distal humerus (chapter 5.6.2).

The humeral component and all cement were first removed, and tissue samples were obtained for bacteriological culture. The implant was sent for sonication and cultures. The ulnar component appeared well fixed and was left in place. A handmade cement spacer loaded with gentamicin and vancomycin was placed inside the medullary canal of the humerus and used to maintain elbow alignment (👁 **8.2-2a–b**). After 2 weeks, results of all cultures came back negative, which facilitated final surgical planning.

The thinned, weakened humeral shaft was reinforced on the outside with two allograft cortical bone struts fixed with cerclage wires and inside with morcelized allograft cancellous bone before insertion of the new cemented 15 cm long humeral component (chapter 5.6).

Preoperative planning

Equipment

- Fresh-frozen allograft of proximal half of humerus
- Fresh-frozen allograft of a femoral head
- Cerclage wires and wire passers
- Complete set for elbow arthroplasty with instrumentation
- Acetabular reamers to harvest bone graft from femoral and humeral head
- Antibiotic-loaded, low-viscosity bone cement

Patient preparation and positioning

- Supine position with the forearm placed across the chest
- Cefazolin for antibiotic prophylaxis

Reduction and fixation

The previous direct posterior midline incision was used, with extension proximally to the level of the deltoid insertion. After the ulnar and radial nerves were identified and protected, the triceps brachii muscle was isolated, allowing displacement of the extensor mechanism and the forearm medially, thereby delivering the humeral shaft through the space left open after resection of the lateral condyle. The fractured lateral condyle was resected, morcelized, and mixed to the allograft. The cement spacer was removed and the medullary canal cleaned and irrigated.

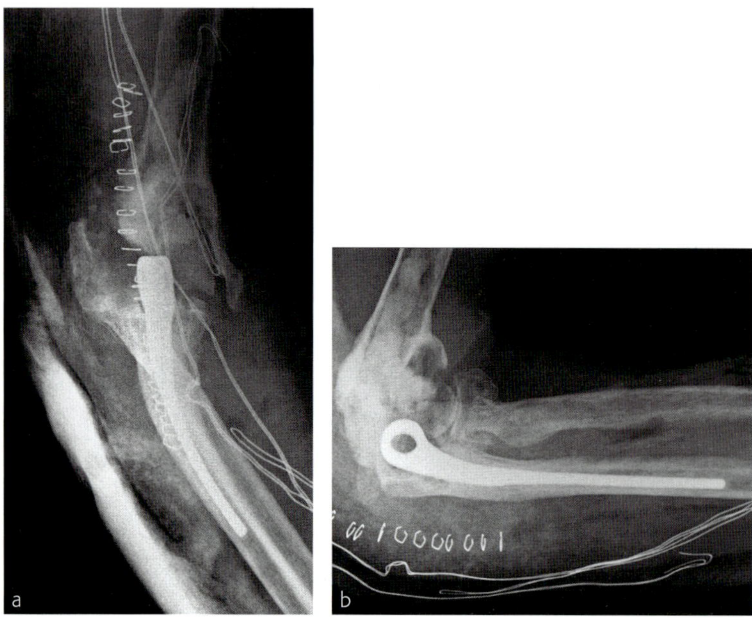

👁 **8.2-2a–b** X-rays obtained after removal of the humeral component and placement of a cement spacer as a first step. The ulnar prosthetic component appears firmly fixed and held between the humeral condyles.

a AP view.

b Lateral view shows a reduced radial head.

II.1-B3

The humeral allograft head then was cut at the anatomical neck, and the cancellous bone extracted with an acetabular reamer. An additional femoral head allograft was reamed and mixed with the humeral allograft. The condylar autograft was morcelized and mixed with the allograft. Two cortical struts of the humeral allograft were obtained long enough to reach across and reinforce the weakened cortex of the humeral shaft.

The two allograft cortical bone struts were then placed anteriorly and posteriorly flush with the olecranon fossa distally and well past the weak area in the proximal humerus. Three cerclage wires were applied for fixation.

The medullary canal was broached to accept the new 15 cm long humeral component (**8.2-3**). The trial component was placed to test soft-tissue tension and to verify correct positioning of the stem and the prosthetic flange engaging the anterior strut. The impactor sleeve was cut to the length of the deficient canal, and the cement nozzle was cut accordingly to the length of the selected humeral component (approximately 18 cm). A cement stopper was placed inside the medullary canal. The impactor sleeve with the cement nozzle was centered in the humeral canal, and the morcelized allograft was impacted circumferentially around it into the humeral shaft.

Cement was deployed early, in a still fairly liquid state, through the cement nozzle and the impactor sleeve, which were then slowly retrieved in a retrograde fashion. The selected humeral component with a long flange was then inserted into the medullary canal (**8.2-4**). Once the cement cured, the prosthesis was linked to the ulnar component and the extensor-pronator structures sutured to the lateral edge of the triceps brachii tendon.

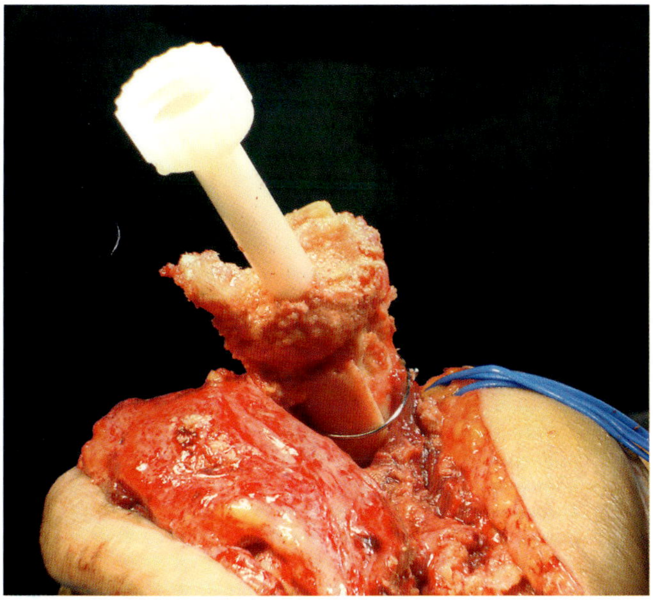

8.2-3 Second step: Two cortical allograft struts are fixed anteriorly and posteriorly to the humerus shaft with three cerclage wires. An impaction sleeve is inserted into the medullary canal of the humerus, with the morcelized allograft bone inserted and impacted around it.

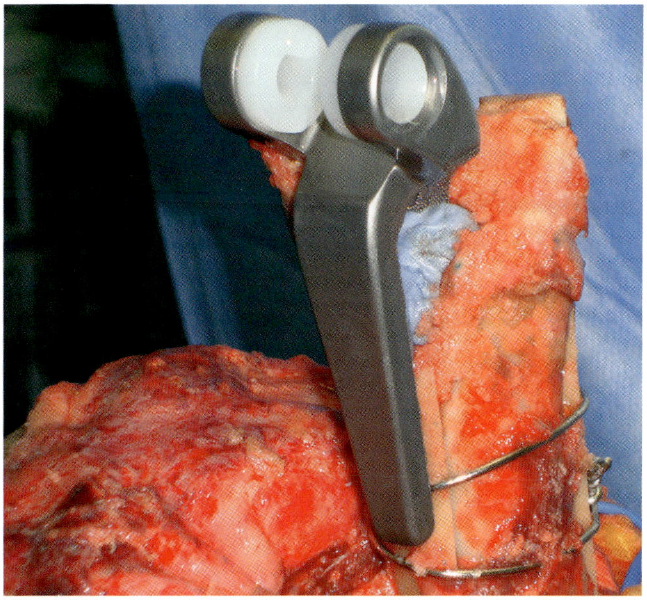

8.2-4 The final reconstruction shows the humeral prosthetic component cemented into the reinforced humeral shaft.

II.1-B3 Rehabilitation and follow-up

An extension splint was used for 3 days (👁 **8.2-5a–b**). Active and active-assisted elbow flexion and extension exercises were started from postoperative day 4. Weight lifting was restricted to no more than a glass of water for 3 months. No formal physiotherapy was required.

X-rays obtained 1 year postoperatively showed incorporation of the impaction grafts and struts with no signs of loosening. The clinical result was satisfactory with 15–145° of extension and flexion and 75–85° of pronation and supination (👁 **8.2-6a–b**).

Points to remember

- In patients with pain and severe osteolysis around the prosthetic stem, the presence of infection must be excluded before undertaking complex reconstruction with allograft augmentation.
- A 2-step procedure may be advisable to exclude the presence of a low-grade infection.
- Ulnar and radial nerve identification and protection are paramount during revision elbow arthroplasty, especially with fractures of the humeral epicondyles and shaft.
- Exposing the humerus without damaging the extensor apparatus is important when working on both sides of the triceps brachii muscle and using the spaces left by resected or deficient condyles.
- The nerves must be protected from extruding cement or motorized instruments used to remove cement.
- Complex reconstruction requires careful attention to multiple steps, including implant and cement removal, preparation of the medullary canal of the humerus, strut fixation with cerclage wires avoiding radial nerve damage, allograft preparation and impaction grafting, cement technique, and soft-tissue tension.

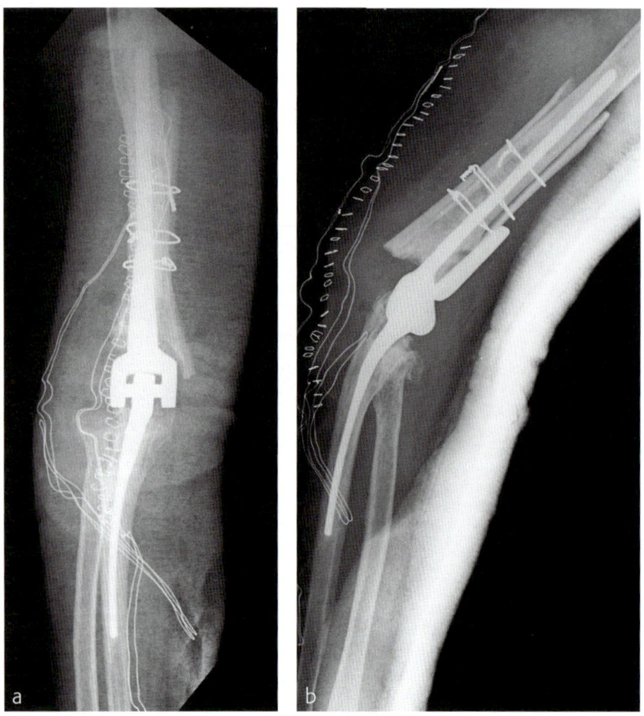

👁 **8.2-5a–b** X-rays obtained immediately postoperatively show the arm fixed in an extension splint.
a AP view.
b Lateral view.

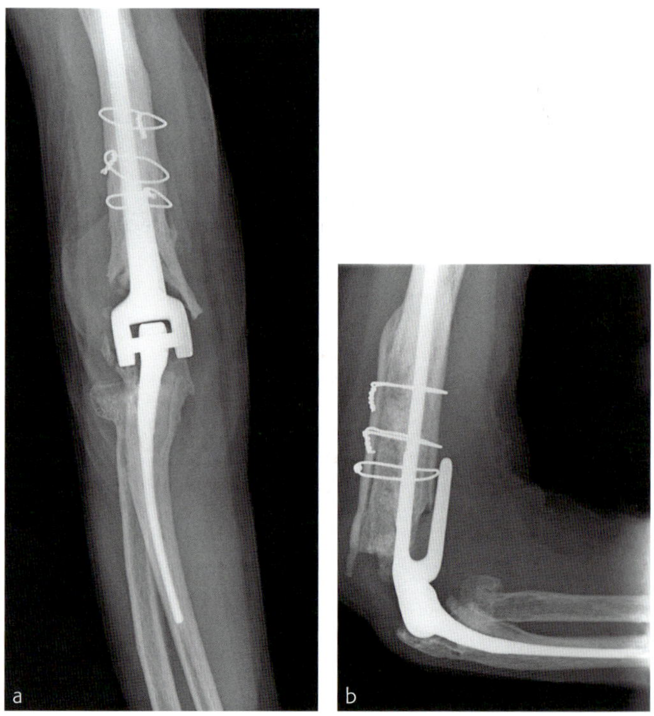

👁 **8.2-6a–b** Follow-up x-rays obtained 1 year postoperatively.
a AP view.
b Lateral view.

8.3 Proximal ulnar fracture, stable prosthesis

ORIF: LCP 3.5

Authors **Antonio M Foruria de Diego, Joaquín Sanchez-Sotelo**

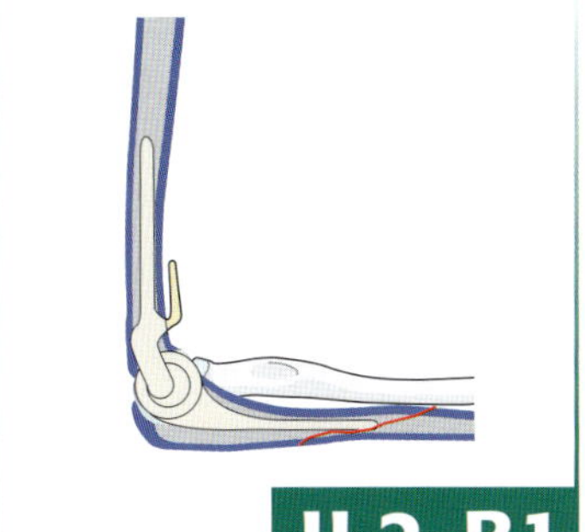

II.2-B1

Case description

A 68-year-old patient sustained a displaced fracture with ulnar angulation, which impaired pronation and supination, as a result of a fall from standing height. Five years ago, the patient underwent total elbow arthroplasty for posttraumatic osteoarthritis. X-rays showed a periprosthetic fracture at the tip of the ulnar stem, which appeared still well fixed (**8.3-1a–b**). Surgery was recommended based on persistent pain and functional limitations.

Classification: Type II.2-B1

Diagnosis: Displaced proximal ulnar fracture with a well-fixed component

Decision making

If the ulnar prosthetic component proves to be well fixed, internal fixation of the fracture with a plate is the simplest and best solution (chapter 5.4.1). If the components are loose, revision arthroplasty must be considered with at least an exchange of the ulnar component (chapter 5.5).

Preoperative planning

Equipment

- Locking compression plates (LCP) of different sizes
- Locking-head and conventional screws
- Prosthesis and instrumentation for exchange (available in the operating room)

Patient preparation and positioning

- Supine position with the forearm placed across the chest
- Cefazolin for antibiotic prophylaxis

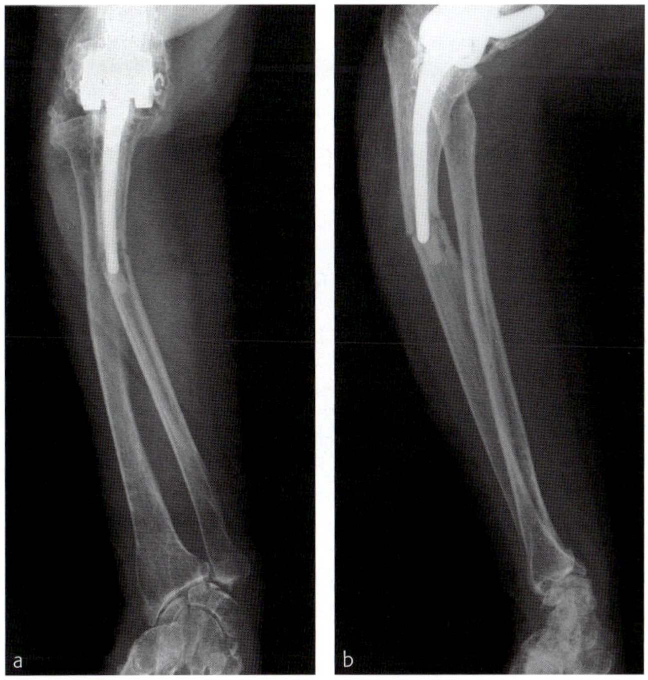

8.3-1a–b X-rays show a periprosthetic fracture of the ulna at the tip of the well-fixed implant.
a AP view.
b Lateral view.

II.2-B1 ## Reduction and fixation

The previous posterior midline incision was used. The ulnar nerve had already been transposed and was identified and protected throughout the procedure. The posterior and lateral aspects of the proximal ulna and ulnar shaft were exposed subperiosteally.

Since the ulnar component was well fixed in the bone, the fracture was reduced, and the LCP 3.5 was contoured to match the lateral side of the ulna. Fixation was started with compression of the fracture site and subsequent placement of two locking-head screws in each main fragment. Bicortical locking-head screws were used proximally as well, since the lateral placement of the plate allows insertion of such long screws posterior to the ulnar component (**8.3-2a–d**).

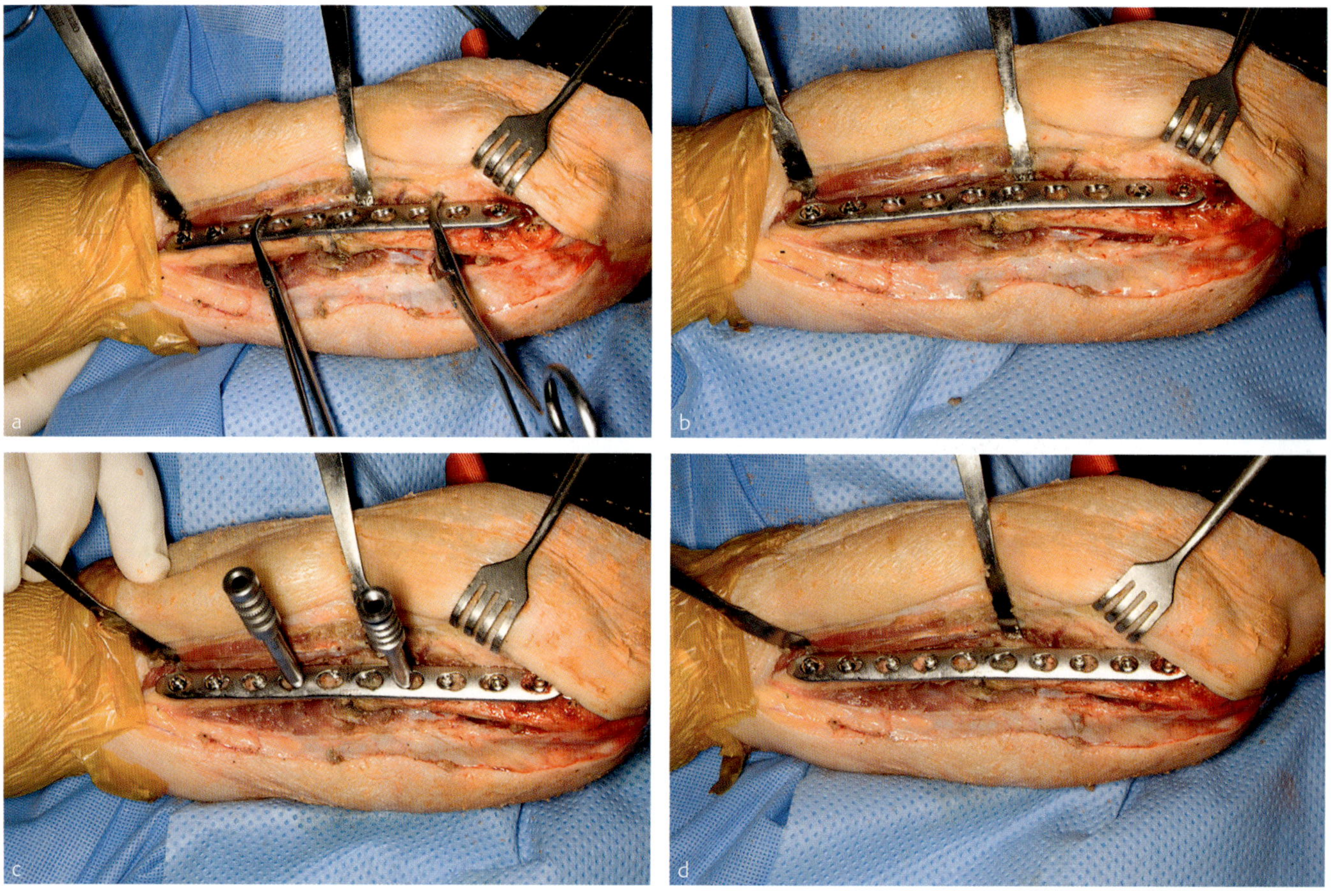

8.3-2a–d Reduction and fracture fixation.
a Fracture reduction.
b Fracture compression with eccentrically placed conventional cortex screws at either end of the pate.
c Insertion of bicortical locking-head screws.
d Definitive fixation.

Rehabilitation and follow-up

The elbow was immobilized and splinted in extension for 48 hours to prevent swelling. Active and active-assisted range-of-motion exercises were initiated the day after surgery. Weight lifting was avoided until fracture consolidation was achieved, which is typically 8 weeks postoperatively. No formal physiotherapy usually is required.

Six weeks postoperatively, the patient reported no pain and had active motion ranging from 10° of lack of extension to 135° of flexion and full pronosupination. Follow-up x-rays showed excellent fragment alignment and a well-fixed implant (**8.3-3a–b**).

Points to remember

- Lateral placement of the plate allows bicortical screw placement proximally and better soft-tissue coverage of the plate.
- Lateral placement of the plate can decrease the possibility of implant-related pain requiring implant removal.
- Long plates should be used for bridging of the fracture.

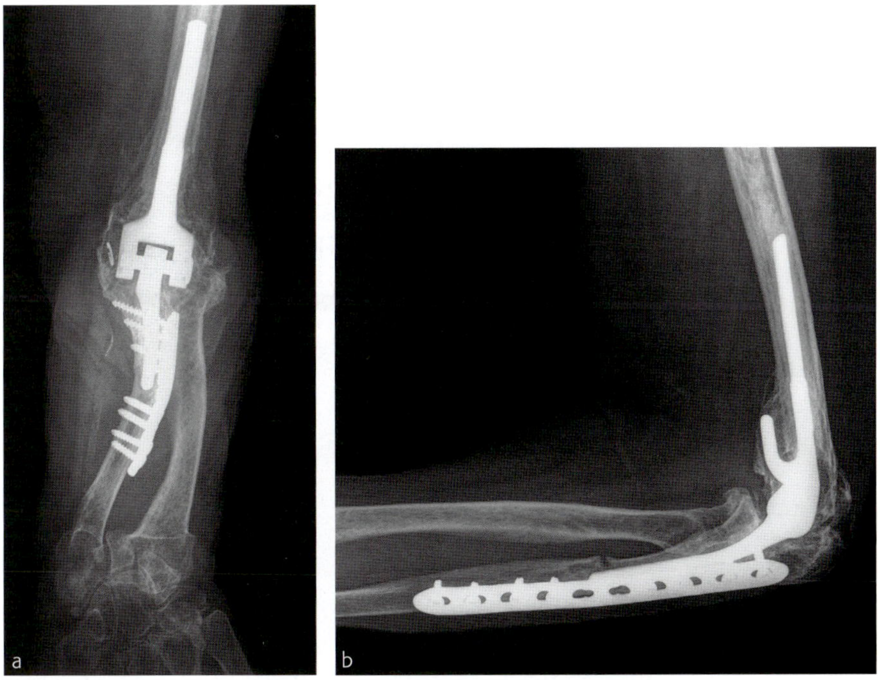

8.3-3a–b Follow-up x-rays obtained 6 weeks postoperatively.
a AP view.
b Lateral view.

II.2-B3

8.4 Proximal ulnar fracture, loose prosthesis

Reconstruction: allograft prosthetic composite and reconstruction plate 3.5

Authors **Antonio M Foruria de Diego, Joaquín Sanchez-Sotelo**

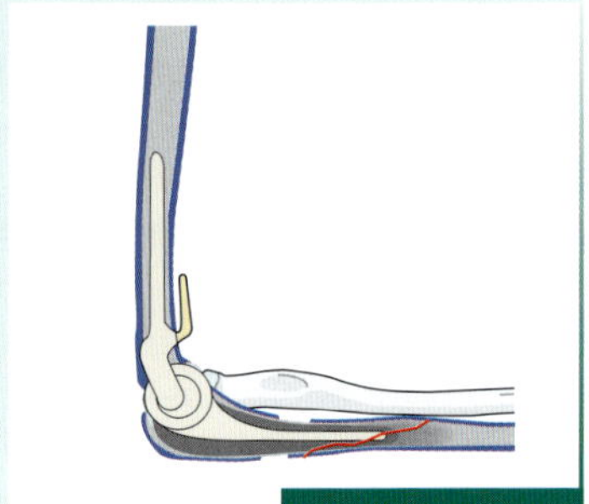

II.2-B3

Case description

A 72-year-old patient with rheumatoid arthritis and a total elbow arthroplasty (TEA) felt a cracking sensation while getting up from a chair. X-rays confirmed a fracture of the ulna (**8.4-1a–b**), with malalignment of the forearm and dislocation of the radial head. An olecranon nonunion was also present as well as considerable resorption around the prosthesis.

Classification: Type II.2-B3

Diagnosis: Displaced periprosthetic fracture of the ulna around a loose implant

Decision making

The periprosthetic fracture was located around the ulnar stem, with implant loosening and poor bone stock at the proximal ulna. Isolated implant revision was considered inadequate to obtain implant stability (chapter 5.5). Bone augmentation was required to restore bone stock and improve implant fixation. The extensor mechanism required reconstruction in an effort to restore extension strength and improve function. An allograft prosthetic composite (APC) with a proximal ulnar allograft was considered the best option (chapter 5.6).

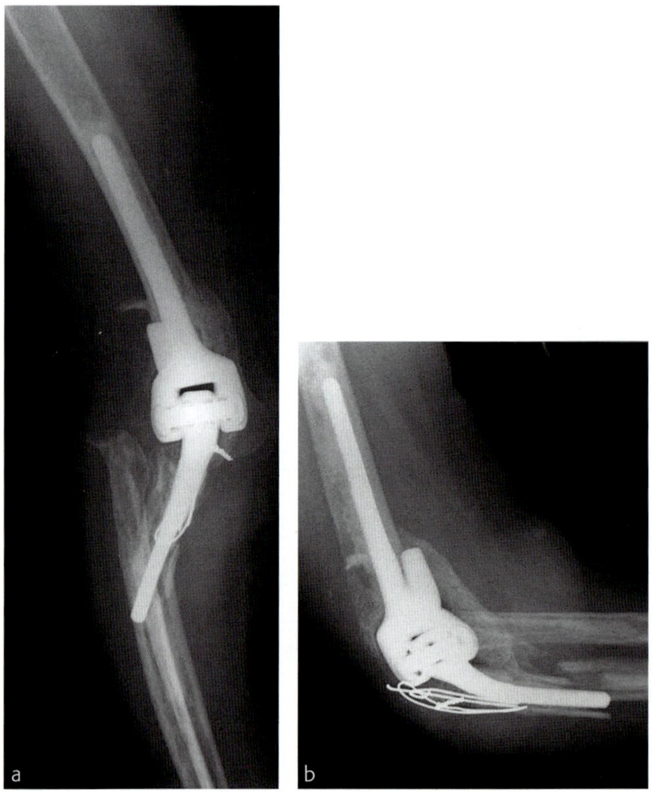

8.4-1a–b X-rays of a periprosthetic ulnar fracture.
a AP view.
b Lateral view.

Preoperative planning

Equipment

- Same-side fresh-frozen ulnar allograft with the triceps brachii tendon attached
- Elbow arthroplasty components and instrumentation matching the humeral component
- Antibiotic-loaded, low-viscosity bone cement
- Small-fragment locking compression and reconstruction plates 3.5

Patient preparation and positioning

- Supine position with the forearm across the chest
- Cefazolin for antibiotic prophylaxis

Reduction and fixation

The previous posterior midline incision was used to access the fracture. The ulnar nerve had already been transposed and was protected throughout the case. The posterior and lateral aspects of proximal ulna and ulnar shaft were exposed. The prosthesis was disengaged, and the ulnar component with the surrounding fractured osteolytic bone was resected circumferentially (**8.4-2a–b**). The distal ulnar bone cement was partially removed. An anterior step cut was made distally on the native ulna to match a complementary posterior step cut that was then made on the allograft. The length of the step cut was approximately two ulnar bone diameters. II.2-B3

The canal of the ulnar allograft was opened and reamed to accommodate the ulnar component. The bone defect was long enough to use a standard ulnar component without bypassing the junction (**8.4-3a**). The ulnar allograft was marked and cut circumferentially to maintain the length of the resected ulna and create a posterior step cut to match the one created in the native ulna. The ulnar component was cemented into the allograft on the back table (**8.4-3b**).

The APC was tried on the patient, and fine contouring of the allograft step cut was performed with a small burr to match that of the native bone. The APC was linked to the humeral component and the native bone aligned with the allograft (**8.4-4a**). The reconstruction plate was bent to match the shape of the bone and placed laterally on the ulna. Hybrid fixation was performed with compression at the host bone-allograft junction and subsequent fixation with locking-head screws. Bicortical screws were used proximally because lateral placement of the plate allows screw positioning posterior to the ulnar component (**8.4-4b**). The allograft triceps brachii tendon was sutured to the native triceps brachii tendon using nonresorbable sutures in a running, locking, Krackow-like fashion.

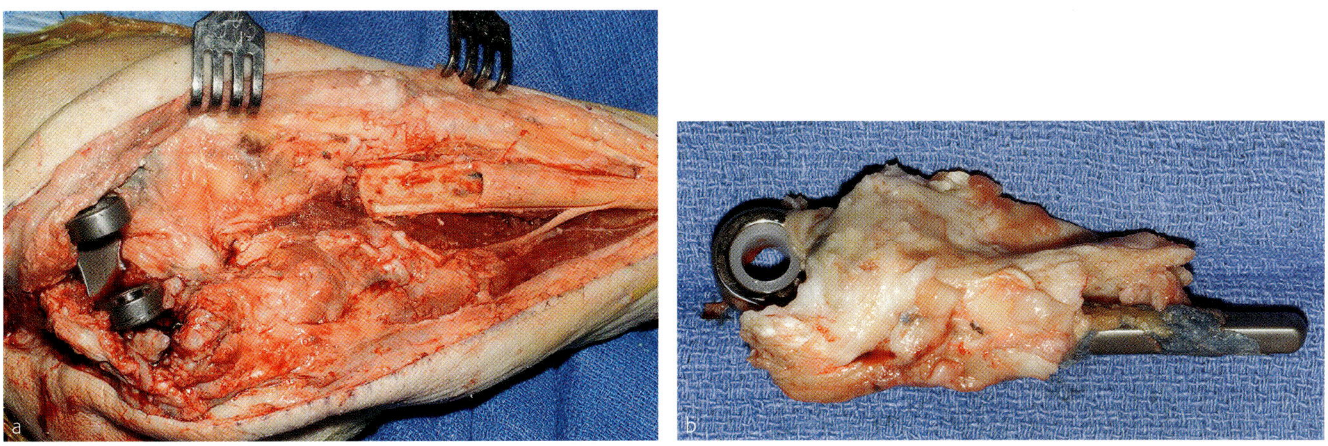

8.4-2a–b Intraoperative photographs show resection of the ulnar component with the surrounding fractured osteolytic bone.
a Aspect of the surgical field after proximal ulna resection and step-cut osteotomy.
b Removed specimen with ulnar component resected along with deficient proximal ulna.

II.2-B3

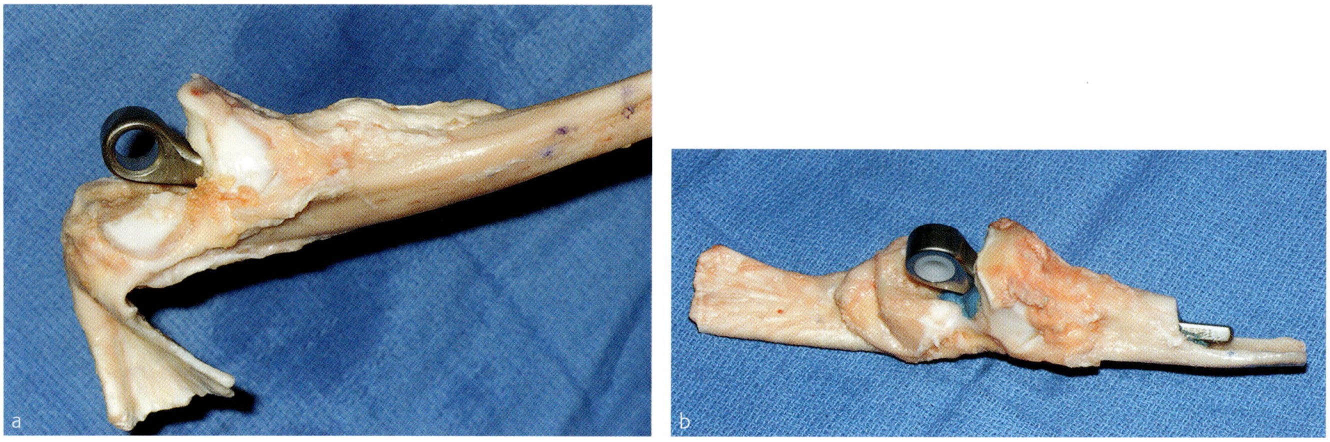

8.4-3a–b Intraoperative photographs show insertion of the ulnar component.
a Prosthetic trial component inside the ulnar allograft with triceps brachii tendon.
b Definitive prosthetic component cemented into the prepared ulnar allograft to form the allograft prosthetic composite (APC).

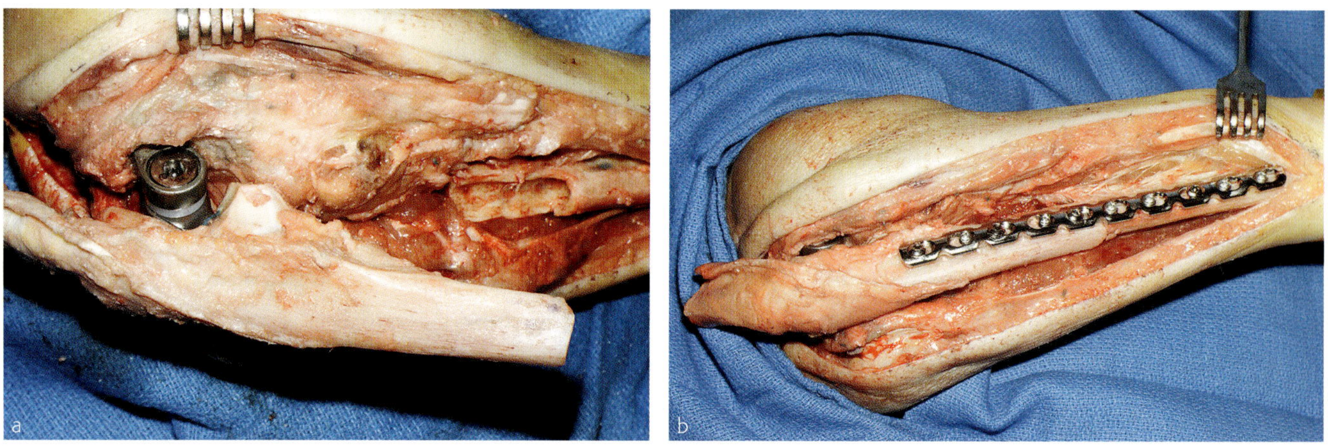

8.4-4a–b Intraoperative photographs show completed insertion of the ulnar component.
a APC linked to the humeral component.
b Completed internal fixation using the reconstruction plate before triceps brachii tendon reconstruction.

Rehabilitation and follow-up

The elbow was maintained in extension and elevated for the first 48 hours postoperatively. Active and active-assisted elbow flexion and pronation and supination exercises were started on postoperative day 3. Gravity-assisted passive elbow extension exercises were started on that day as well. Active elbow-extension exercises began at 6 weeks, and active against resistance exercises at 3 months.

Four years postoperatively, the osteotomy was well healed and the graft was incorporated (**8.4-5a–b**). The patient reported no pain and had excellent range of motion.

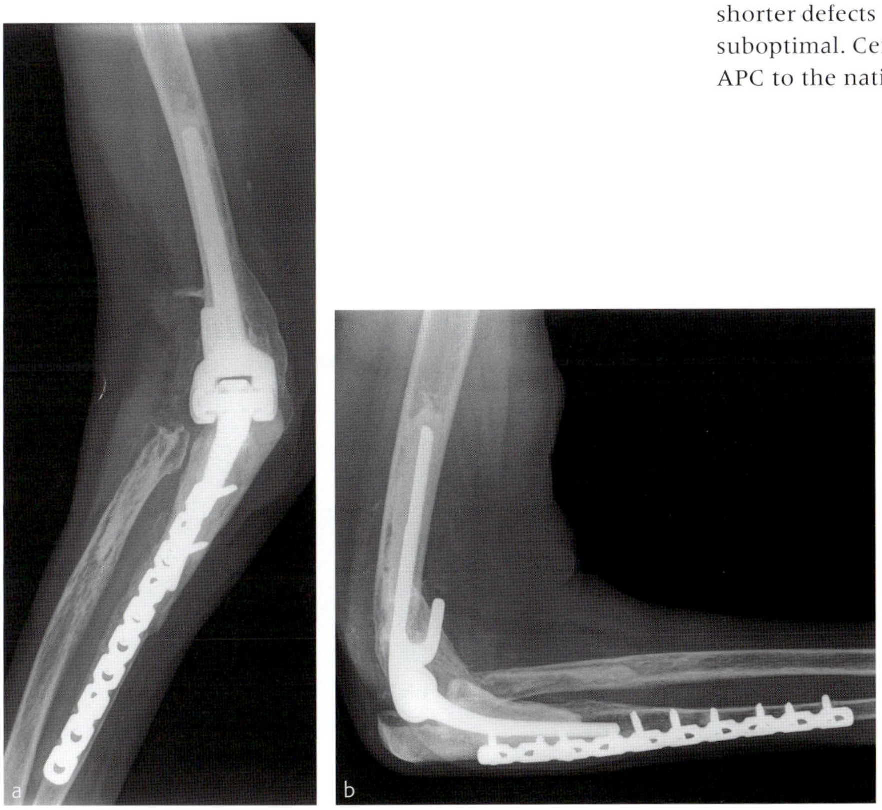

8.4-5a–b X-rays obtained 4 years postoperatively show allograft incorporation.
a AP view.
b Lateral view.

Points to remember

II.2-B3

- Identify and protect the ulnar nerve at all times to avoid iatrogenic injury.
- Preserve as much healthy tissue as possible when resecting a fractured osteolytic poor-quality bone.
- Obtain perfect matching of the osteotomized bone ends and interfragmentary compression at the host bone-allograft junction.
- Use a long enough plate and solid screw fixation both proximally and distally, preferably with locking-head screws.
- Restore adequate overall ulnar length, as determined by the patient's size and the condition of the soft tissues.
- Consider bypassing the junction with a longer stem for shorter defects or when plate fixation is anticipated to be suboptimal. Cerclage wires can then be helpful to fix the APC to the native bone.

II.2-B3

8.5 Proximal ulnar fracture, loose prosthesis

Reconstruction: allograft prosthetic composite and cerclage wires

Authors **Angus Keogh, Gregory Bain**

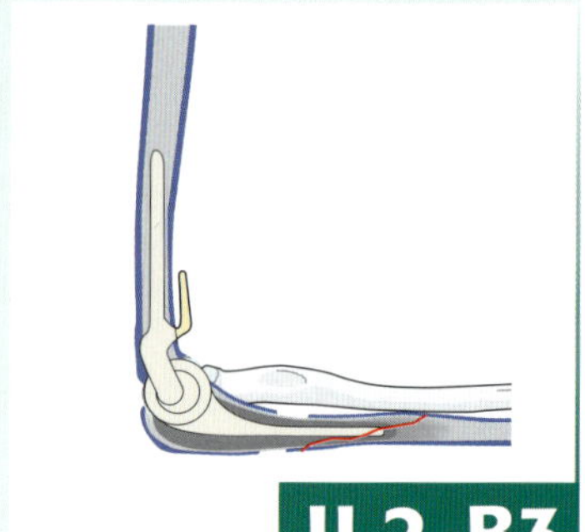

II.2-B3

Case description

A 65-year-old woman with rheumatoid arthritis sustained a supracondylar fracture of the left humerus and was treated with open reduction and internal fixation. Four years after the original injury and treatment, she presented with pain and restricted movement, particularly supination, in the left elbow. At that time, she underwent primary total elbow arthroplasty. A modified Bryan-Morrey approach, was inserted without complication. Range of motion postoperatively was limited only in extension to 40°.

Eight years later, when the patient was 77 years old, she presented with a 3-month history of clicking with movement into full extension. Plain x-rays at that time suggested loosening of the ulnar component (**8.5-1a–b**), which was confirmed by image intensification. The patient was asked to consider revision surgery on the elbow at that time which she refused.

The patient is now 80 years old and presented with a 2-month history of increasing mechanical pain and swelling of the proximal ulna. X-rays confirmed a fracture of the proximal ulna (**8.5-2a–b**) with associated osteolysis and loss of proximal ulnar bone stock. The patient agreed to revision surgery.

Classification: Type II.2-B3

Diagnosis: Proximal ulnar fracture with associated osteolysis and loss of proximal ulnar bone stock

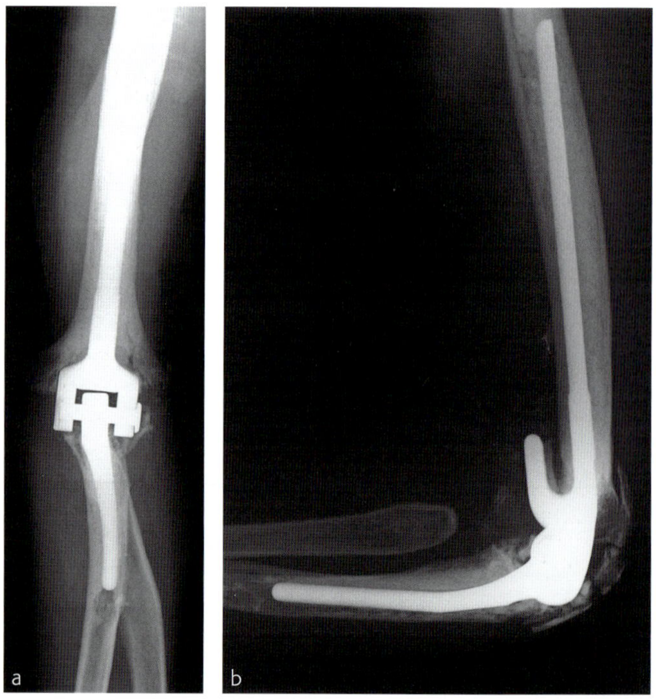

8.5-1a–b X-rays obtained 8 years after total elbow arthroplasty. Osteolysis can be seen at the ulnar stem tip and a cement/prosthesis lucent line is present proximally. The patient refused revision surgery at this time.
a AP view.
b Lateral view.

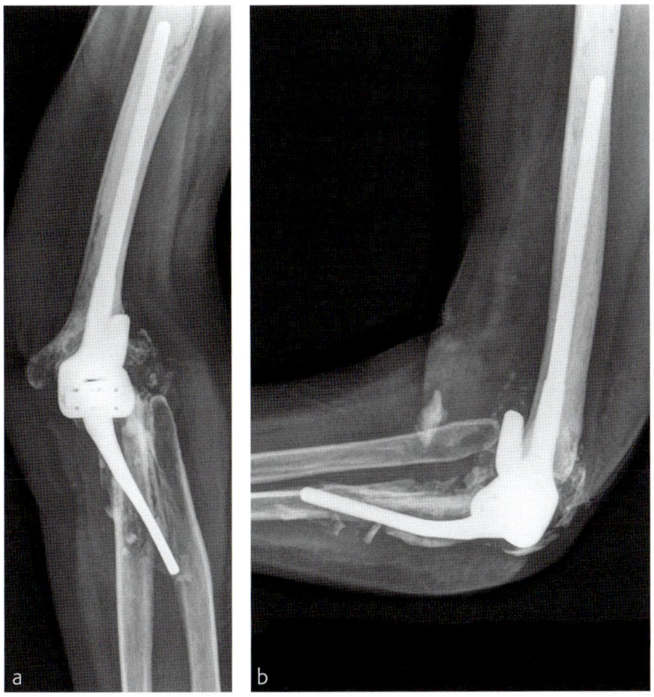

8.5-2a–b X-rays obtained 3 years after fracture of the proximal ulna. The fracture is at the level of the prosthesis with inadequate proximal ulnar bone stock. The humeral component remained well fixed.

a AP view.
b Lateral view.

Decision making

The combination of a fracture around a loose implant in the ulna can be salvaged only by a combination of revision prosthesis with an allograft prosthetic composite (APC) of the proximal ulna. A reinforcement with struts and impaction grafting could be considered as an alternative, if the soft-tissue envelope allows for covering a larger portion of the ulna.

In this patient, 3 years elapsed between the initial deterioration in symptoms and the revision procedure. The proximal ulnar fracture and the subsequent need to use APC could have been avoided if the patient had agreed to revision surgery soon after the component loosening was first identified. Revision at that time would have consisted of either bypassing the critical zone of the proximal ulna with a long stem or impaction grafting. Regular radiological monitoring is recommended with aseptic loosening, and if there is steady progression, then elective revision of the loose components is advised. The advantage of early revision is that the procedure can be performed with an intact bony envelope rather than when there is the inevitable periprosthetic fracture and consequent uncontained bony defect.

The use of APC (chapter 5.6) has some theoretical advantages compared to endoprosthetic replacement. Allograft provides a biological attachment for soft tissues such as the triceps in the case of elbow arthroplasty or for the abductors in revision total hip arthroplasty. There is the additional advantage of load sharing between the biological allograft and the prosthesis. An endoprosthesis, meanwhile, bears the entire load and is therefore at risk for failure. Conventional prostheses can be used with allograft and hence may be more affordable than a custom endoprosthesis. Bone stock is restored with allograft, making future revisions less technically difficult.

Preoperative planning

Equipment

- Custom proximal ulnar prosthesis
- Proximal ulnar allograft of appropriate size
- Saws and burrs
- Cerclage wire
- Cement removal tools

Patient preparation and positioning

- Prophylactic antibiotics
- Lateral position with the arm over a bolster

Reduction and fixation

A posterior midline approach was used, and a modified Bryan-Morrey incision was made. Intraoperatively, a piece of proximal ulna with the insertion of the triceps brachii tendon attached was identified and maintained intact to reattach the triceps at the end of the procedure. Multiple swabs and deep-tissue samples were obtained for analysis during the revision surgery; all results were negative on delayed bacterial culture. The ulnar part of the prosthesis was removed. The allograft of the proximal ulna was fashioned with a step cut and predrilled for suture placement (**8.5-3**). The custom ulnar prosthesis was first cemented into the proximal ulnar allograft. The APC was then inserted and cemented into the ulnar shaft with two cerclage wires applied to maintain stability. Bone graft from the iliac crest was placed around the junction of the composite and native bone. Bone graft was also placed between the reattached

II.2-B3 piece of bone with the triceps insertion and the proximal ulnar allograft. The triceps brachii with its bony attachment was secured with two transosseous fiber wire sutures (**8.5-4a–b**).

Rehabilitation and follow-up

The patient's arm was placed in a cast until the wound healed. Gentle passive range-of-motion exercises were performed for 6 weeks. Thereafter, active range-of-motion exercises were performed.

Six months postoperatively, the patient reported arm weakness and lack of ability to push away. Neurological examination was normal other than reduced power of elbow extension (MRC grade 1). The patient requested a physiotherapy referral.

Follow-up after 18 months confirmed that the prosthesis was functioning well, with range of motion from 30° to 130° of flexion (**8.5-5a–b**). Plain x-rays suggested incorporation of the APC with the ulnar shaft and the presence of bridging callus, particularly on the radial side. The triceps mechanism, however, had not incorporated either clinically or radiologically. X-rays showed that the sleeve of ulnar bone with the triceps attachment had migrated proximally. Thus, the patient experienced persistent weakness of elbow extension (MRC grade 1). The allograft incorporated at the ulnar shaft (**8.5-6a–b**). Both components remained well fixed.

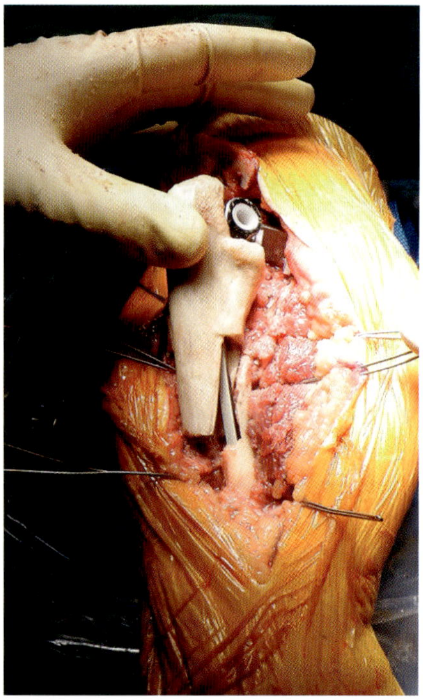

8.5-3 Insertion of the allograft prosthesis composite (APC). Note the cerclage wires and the step cut of the allograft and native ulna.

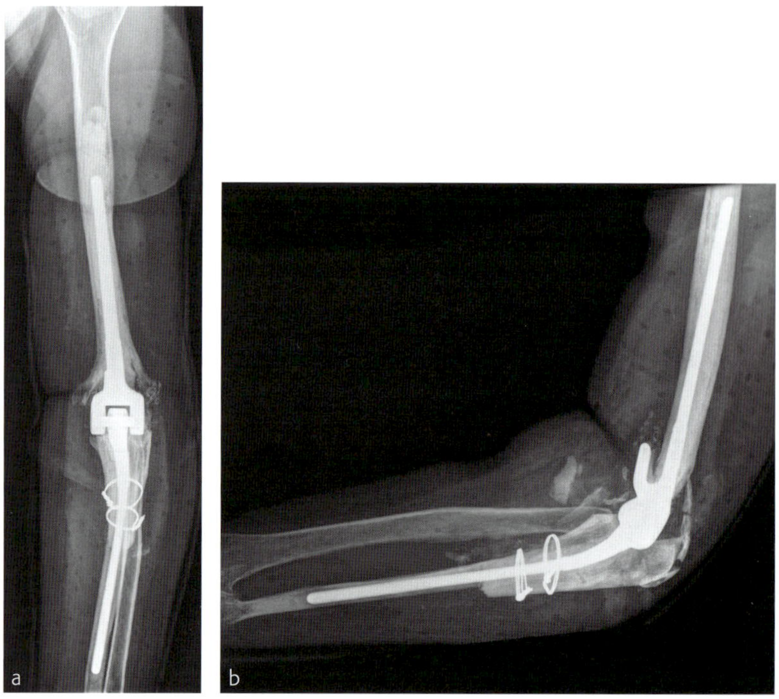

8.5-4a–b X-rays show the revision component and proximal ulnar allograft 1 month postoperatively. Note the proximal migration of the triceps attachment and proximal ulnar bone. Cerclage wires secure the allograft to the shaft.

a Lateral view.

b AP view.

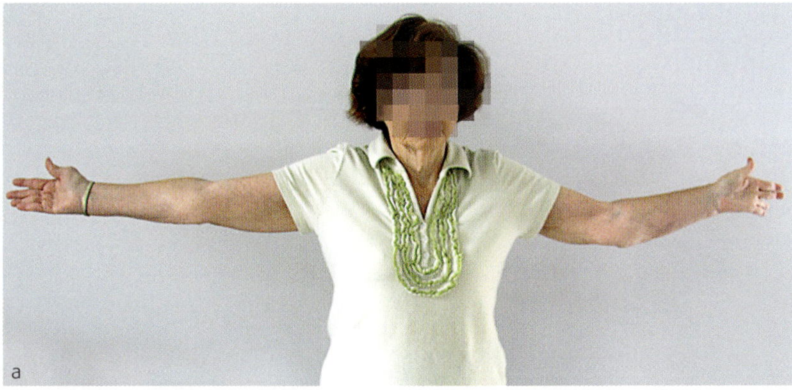

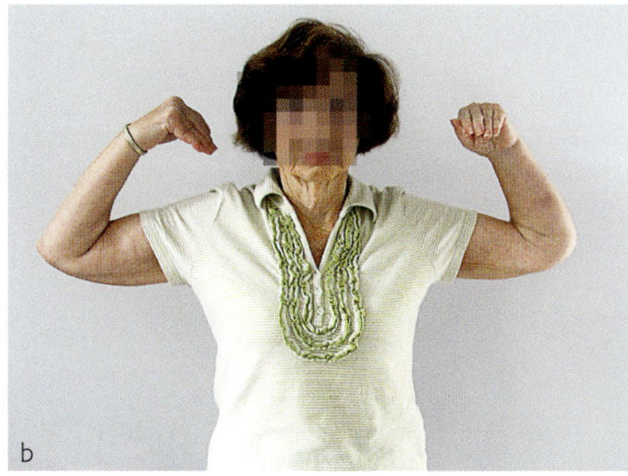

8.5-5a–b Range of motion following revision surgery.
a Extension to 30°.
b Flexion to 130°.

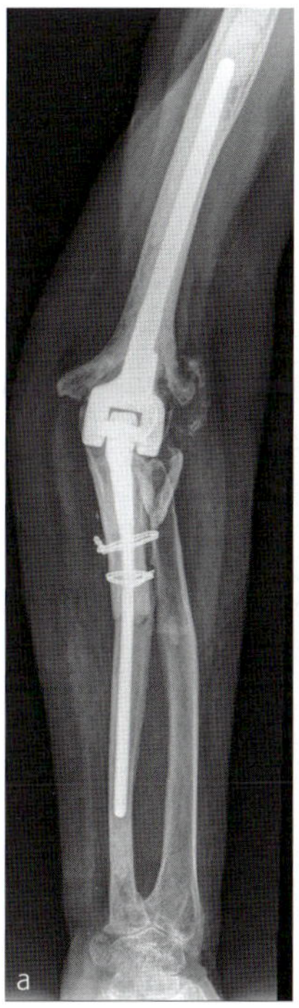

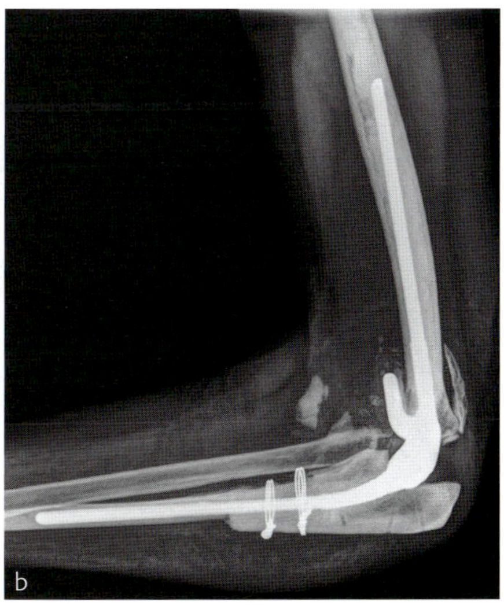

8.5-6a–b X-rays obtained 18 months following revision surgery show incorporation of the allograft with native bone, a stable cement mantle, and proximal migration of the triceps attachment (bone posterior to humeral shaft at the joint level). The humeral component remained well fixed.
a AP view.
b Lateral view.

Points to remember

- Optimal timing of revision total elbow arthroplasty for aseptic loosening probably is at the first radiological signs of loosening. Surgery should not be delayed until symptoms develop, which indicates that the construct has already begun to fail.
- Loose components with imminent risk of fracture, even in the absence of pain, might also be an indication for revision.
- One of the challenges of allograft surgery is incorporation of host and allograft bone.
- Incorporation requires the gradual replacement of bony trabeculae at the host bone-allograft junction by creeping substitution, either by intramembranous or endochondral ossification. In this situation, two surfaces are needed to incorporate: the ulnar shaft and the triceps mechanism with the native ulnar attachment.
- Bone loss can be accommodated with the use of an APC, with the aim of allograft incorporation at the ulnar shaft.
- Reattachment of the triceps mechanism is problematic but may not constitute a significant functional problem, even if the reattachment fails.

9 Wrist cases

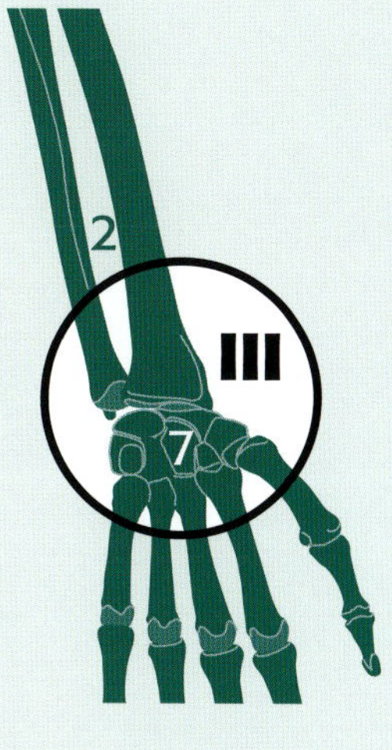

9.1 Loose prosthesis, imminent metacarpal fracture

Fusion: total wrist fusion with plates

Authors **Shian-Chao Tay, Alexander Y Shin**

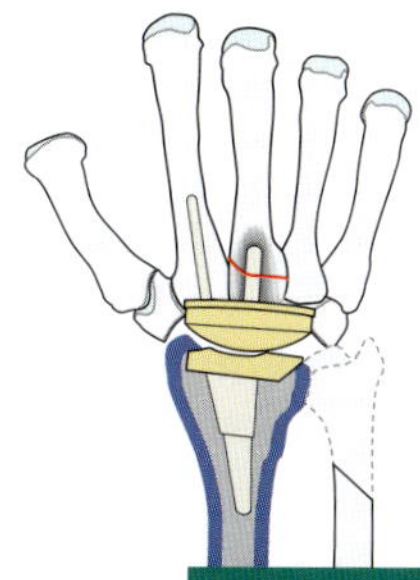

III.7-B3

Case description

A 75-year-old woman with Kienböck's disease of the right wrist underwent proximal row carpectomy 13 years ago. Eight years after the initial surgery, she underwent hemiarthroplasty of the right capitate in which a pyrolytic metacarpophalangeal implant was used as an unconventional method of salvage to address her painful radiocapitate arthritis. This was revised to a total wrist arthroplasty 1 year later because of dorsal impingement. She was well for about 1 year after the last surgery but reported increasing pain, and x-rays showed loosening of the distal component screws (**9.1-1a–b**).

Classification: Type III.7-B3

Diagnosis: Distal component loosening of total wrist arthroplasty with pain

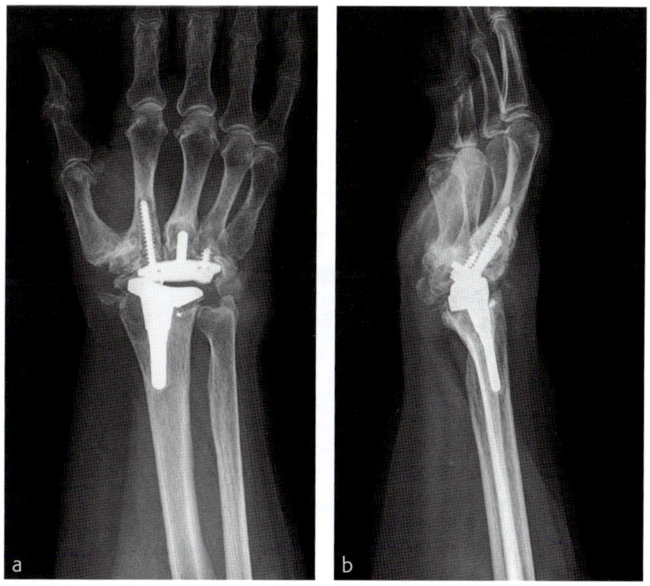

9.1-1a–b Preoperative x-rays show the halo around the distal component screws.
a AP view.
b Lateral view.

Decision making

The concern here was progressive erosion of the distal component, resulting in eventual fracture at the metacarpals. Implant removal was needed, followed by total wrist fusion with autogenous iliac crest bone graft supplemented with fresh-frozen femoral head allograft.

III.7-B3 ## Preoperative planning

Equipment

- Straight 10-hole wrist fusion locking compression plate (LCP)
- Straight small-fragment LCP
- Iliac crest autograft
- Fresh-frozen allograft of the femoral head

Patient preparation and positioning

- Supine position
- Upper arm tourniquet set to 250 mm Hg during the procedure

Reduction and fixation

A longitudinal dorsal midline approach was used with laterally based extensor retinacular flaps created through the third extensor compartment and release of the extensor pollicis longus tendon, followed by capsulotomy for exposure of the wrist. In this patient, a longitudinal capsulotomy was used (**9.1-2**).

Tissue and fluid specimens were obtained intraoperatively for analysis to exclude infection. Removal of the distal component was easier and performed before removal of the proximal component. Because of significant bony ingrowth, dorsal osteotomies were required to facilitate removal of the components (**9.1-3**). A rongeur and burr were used to ensure that all bony surfaces were debrided to healthy bleeding surfaces in preparation for bone grafting.

A significant defect was noted after removal of the components and debridement of the bone (**9.1-4a**). Pulsed irrigation lavage with at least 3 L of fluid was performed to ensure any potential contaminants and necrotic tissue were flushed out. The femoral head allograft was fashioned into a disc or a shape appropriate for the defect and supplemented with autogenous corticocancellous bone graft from the iliac crest (**9.1-4b–c**). Final fixation was achieved using a 10-hole wrist-fusion LCP between the radius and third metacarpal. In addition, a straight small-fragment LCP was added between the radius and index metacarpal (**9.1-4d**).

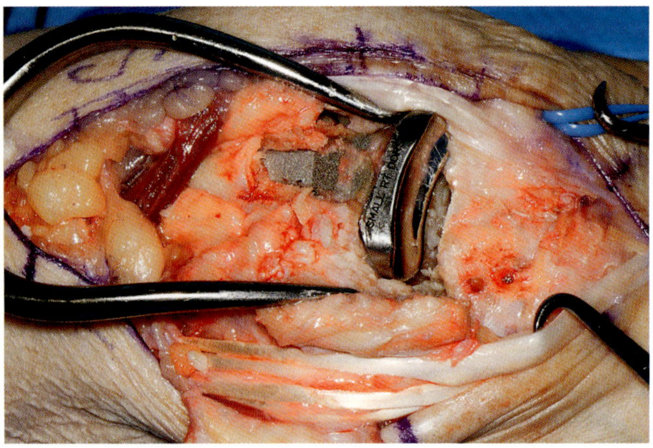

9.1-2 Dorsal radial osteotomy performed to facilitate removal of proximal component.

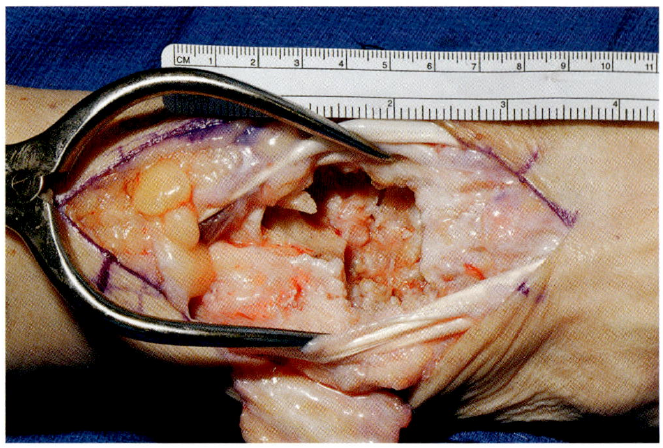

9.1-3 Large defect after complete removal of implants and surface debridement.

III.7-B3

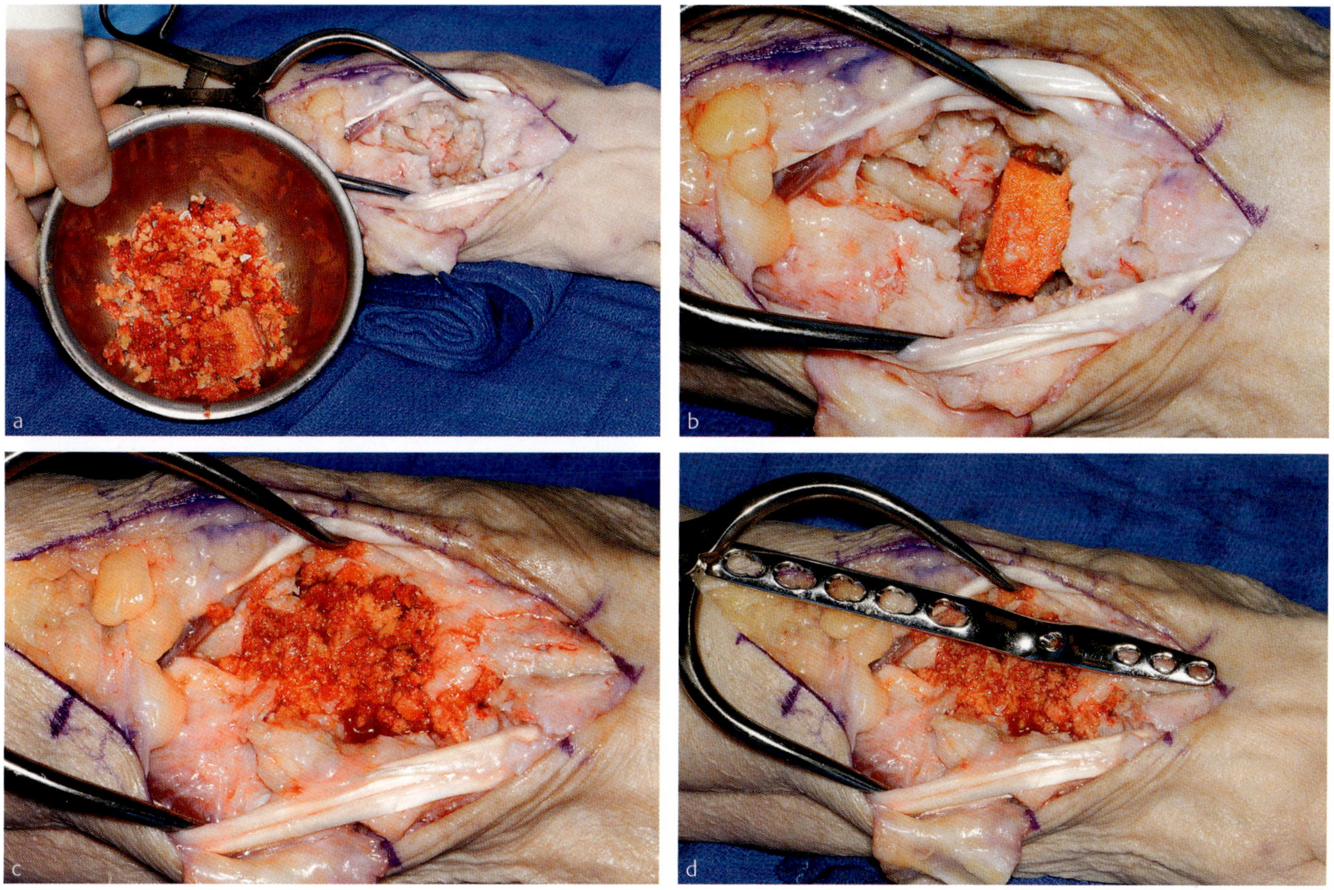

9.1-4a–d Filling of the considerable defect before final wrist fusion with a fresh-frozen femoral head allograft augmented by an autogenous bone graft.

- **a** Bone graft after harvesting.
- **b** Fresh-frozen femoral head allograft shaped to fit into the defect.
- **c** Autogenous iliac crest bone graft filled in the defect around the femoral head allograft.
- **d** Plates were used to stabilize the index metacarpal to the radius and achieve complete fusion of the wrist.

III.7-B3

Rehabilitation and follow-up

The patient's wrist was placed in a cast for 8 weeks, followed by 4 weeks in a removable splint. X-rays obtained 3 months postoperatively showed complete fusion of the wrist (**9.1-5a–b**).

At the 1-year follow-up, the wrist fusion was solid. The patient maintained excellent pronation, supination, and digital function. The pain was eliminated, and she was able to perform activities of daily living without pain or problems.

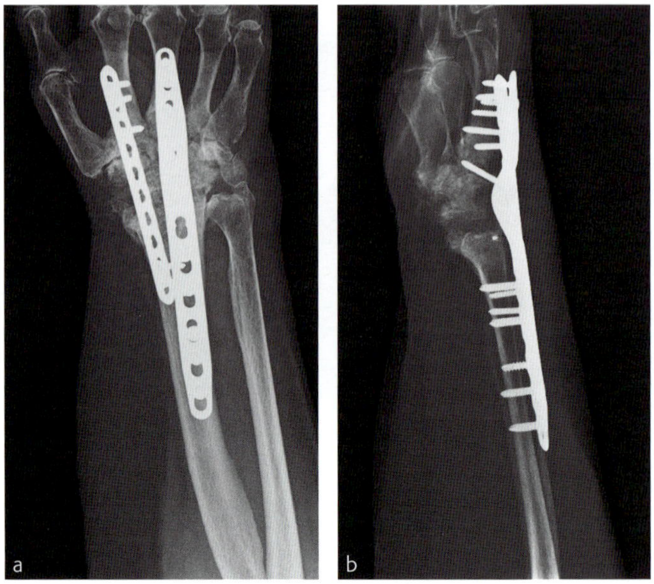

9.1-5a–b X-rays obtained 3 months postoperatively showed complete fusion of the wrist.
a AP view.
b Lateral view.

Points to remember

- Complications of total wrist arthroplasty include subluxation and dislocation. These should be corrected as soon as possible before soft-tissue contractures develop. Once soft-tissue contracture has occurred, revision arthroplasty is difficult to perform. In such circumstances, revision to a total wrist fusion is recommended.
- Loosening will eventually result in component protrusion and fracture. This can occur in the proximal or distal component, although protrusion of the distal component is at least two to five times more common. With significant loosening or risk of protrusion, the wrist should be protected with splinting and/or restricted activities.
- Surgery is indicated before significant protrusion occurs to avoid a more complicated surgical procedure. Options for revision include a revision hemiarthroplasty with cement and/or bone graft or a total wrist fusion.
- Total wrist arthroplasty that is revised to a total wrist fusion requires significant amounts of corticocancellous bone graft as a result of the large bony defect, following component removal, debridement, and possibly osteotomies. As such, supplementary sources of bone graft such as allograft will have to be used.

10 Hip cases

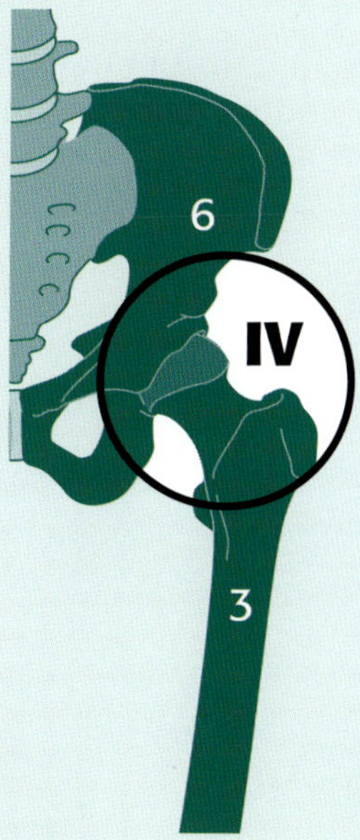

10.1 Transverse acetabular fracture, stable hemiarthroplasty

ORIF: reconstruction plate and total hip arthroplasty

Authors **Gregory G Polkowski, John C Clohisy, Jay R Lieberman**

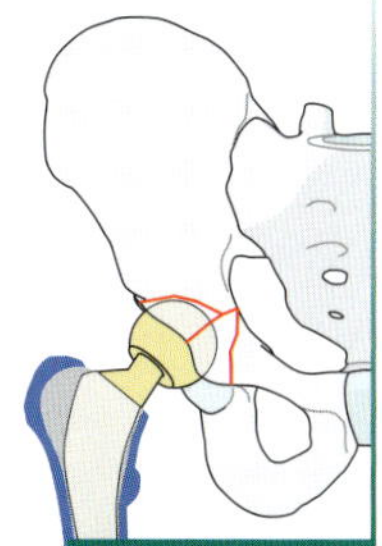

IV.6-F

Case description

A 66-year-old woman presented to the emergency department with pain in the left hip and the inability to bear weight after falling at home. Approximately 1 year ago she underwent a cemented left hip hemiarthroplasty for a displaced femoral neck fracture. She had no history of antecedent hip pain and was functioning well until her fall. X-rays revealed a transverse acetabular fracture (**10.1-1a–b**).

Classification: Type IV.6-F

Diagnosis: Periprosthetic fracture of the acetabulum after hemiarthroplasty

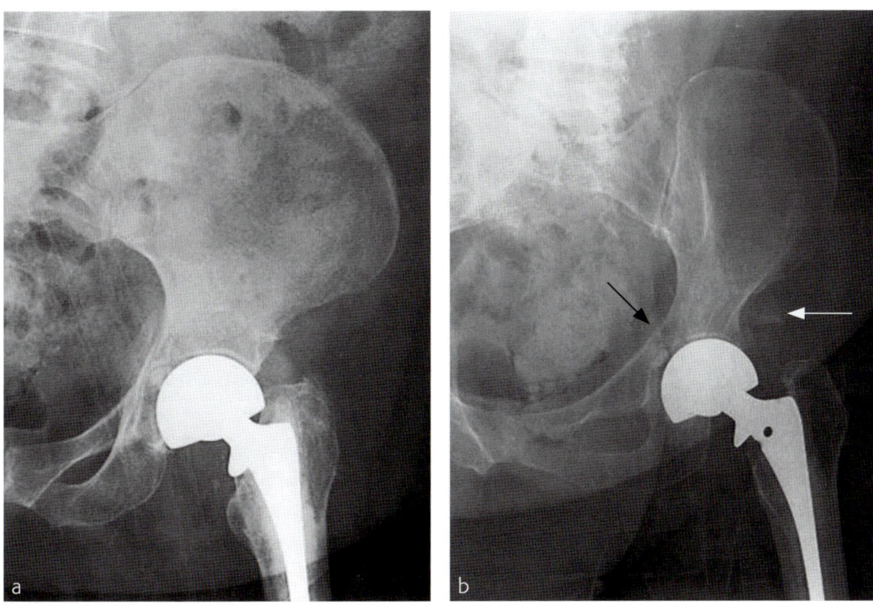

10.1-1a–b X-rays obtained shortly after the injury show a cemented left hip hemiarthroplasty with transverse acetabular fracture.

- **a** AP view. The femoral stem shows no radiographic signs of loosening.
- **b** Oblique view. The transverse fracture line is seen exiting anteriorly (black arrow) and there is a large posterior-wall fragment that is displaced posterior-superiorly (white arrow).

IV.6-F

Decision making

The patient was functioning well until her fall, and given her young age and complex intraarticular fracture, conversion to total hip arthroplasty with open reduction and internal fixation (chapter 5.5) of her transverse/posterior wall acetabular fracture was recommended. Plating of the posterior column and posterior wall were planned through a posterior approach (chapter 5.4.1). The well-fixed cemented stem would be left in place and not revised.

Preoperative planning

Equipment

- Pelvic reconstruction plates
- Porous revision acetabular sockets
- Structural allograft (distal femur or femoral head)
- Porous wedge augmentation
- Revision acetabular cage

Patient preparation and positioning

- Lateral decubitus position
- Wide surgical draping for extensile exposure

Reduction and fixation

A posterior lateral approach was used through the previous surgical incision, and the gluteus maximus tendon was released at its distal insertion to facilitate wide exposure. The scarred posterior capsule and short external rotators were reflected posteriorly after release as one large sleeve off the proximal femur. Care was taken to identify the posterior border of the gluteus medius muscle to minimize trauma to the hip abductor musculature. The modular hemiarthroplasty head was removed, and the stem and proximal femur were retracted anteriorly to expose the acetabulum and fracture. The amount of fracture displacement and bone quality were assessed.

The fractures were then identified and exposed. There was a large posterior wall fragment with extensive comminution and impaction. Any attempts to mobilize and reduce this fragment resulted in further fragmentation of the posterior wall piece. A structural femoral head allograft was necessary to reconstruct the posterior wall and provide support for a new acetabular component. The posterior wall defect was reamed with a hemispherical reamer to accept a comparably sized femoral head allograft, and the bone graft was secured with a small fragment screw. A 10-hole pelvic reconstruction plate was contoured and applied to the posterior column after reduction of the transverse acetabular fracture. The acetabulum was then reamed to accept a porous tantalum acetabular component, which was carefully impacted into place and secured with screws.

Rehabilitation and follow-up

An abduction brace was used for 2 months postoperatively to minimize hip motion and reduce the risk of dislocation. Prophylaxis for deep vein thrombosis was initiated with warfarin, and the patient was instructed to maintain toe-touch weight bearing restrictions on the operative side for 3 months until the acetabular fracture healed and her acetabular component demonstrated good ingrowth.

At the 13-month follow-up, the patient was free of pain and ambulating with minimal limp (👁 **10.1-2a–b**).

Points to remember

- Care must be taken during exposure to minimize trauma to the abductor muscles.
- The sciatic nerve also is at risk and care must be taken to avoid undue retraction, especially during exposure and plating of the ischium.
- Options to increase hip offset will often be limited when converting a hemiarthroplasty to a total hip arthroplasty if the surgeon intends to leave a well-fixed stem. This problem can be magnified in the setting of the displaced acetabular fracture, as the acetabular component may be placed more medial than normal. In situations like this, it is helpful to have extended-offset head and high-offset liner options available to help restore appropriate soft-tissue tension to the joint. This improves the biomechanics of the prosthetic joint and helps to ensure hip stability. Revision femoral components should be available in the event that the appropriate offset cannot be attained through neck, cup, and liner options.

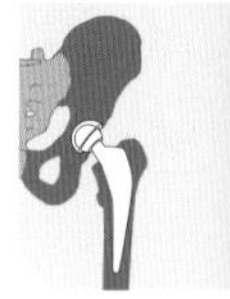

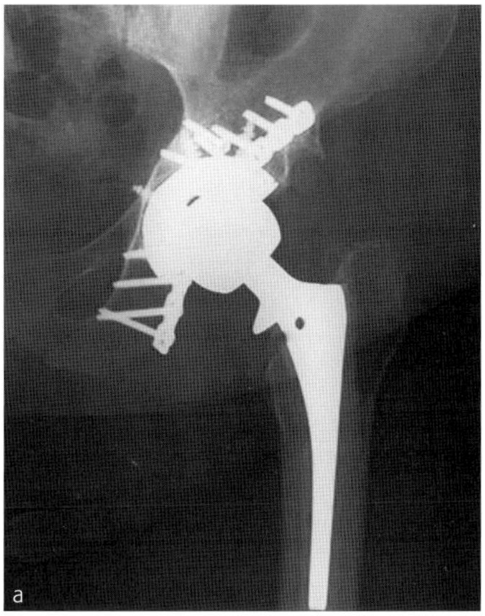

a

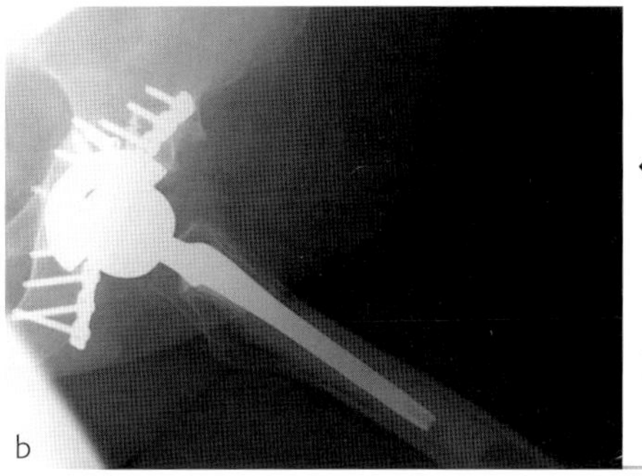

b

10.1-2a–b X-rays obtained 13 months postoperatively. The transverse fracture has healed. The acetabular component is well fixed and continues to be supported by the femoral head allograft. The femoral stem is also well fixed.

a AP view.
b Cross-table lateral view.

IV.6-B2

10.2 Transverse acetabular fracture, loose acetabular cup

Reconstruction: two plates and revision arthroplasty, Burch-Schneider antiprotrusio cage, hook plate

Author Emanuel Gautier

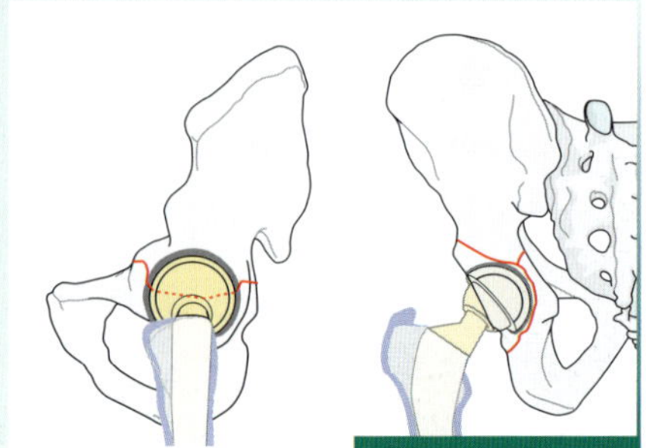

IV.6-B2

Case description

An 81-year-old woman who underwent left total hip arthroplasty 13 years ago presented to the emergency department after a fall at home. She could ambulate with crutches but reported mechanical pain around the left hip. Plain x-rays and CT scans (**10.2-1a–g**) showed no fracture around the hip prosthesis; however, excessive wear of the polyethylene liner with eccentricity of the prosthetic head and considerable osteolysis in the supraacetabular bone were observed. The patient refused revision arthroplasty and was discharged home some days later.

Four months later, she presented with persistent mechanical pain around the left hip. Follow-up AP pelvic and iliac oblique views showed no fracture lines, but the obturator oblique view now showed a clear periprosthetic fracture of the anterior column (**10.2-2a–c**). The patient agreed to revision arthroplasty. CT scans obtained for preoperative planning and to confirm the diagnosis of a periprosthetic acetabular fracture showed a somewhat displaced periprosthetic transverse acetabular fracture on the left side (**10.2-3a–f**).

Classification: Type IV.6-B2

Diagnosis: Transverse periprosthetic acetabular fracture due to osteolysis of the cup

10.2 **Transverse acetabular fracture, loose acetabular cup**

Reconstruction: two plates and revision arthroplasty, Burch-Schneider antiprotrusio cage, hook plate

IV.6-B2

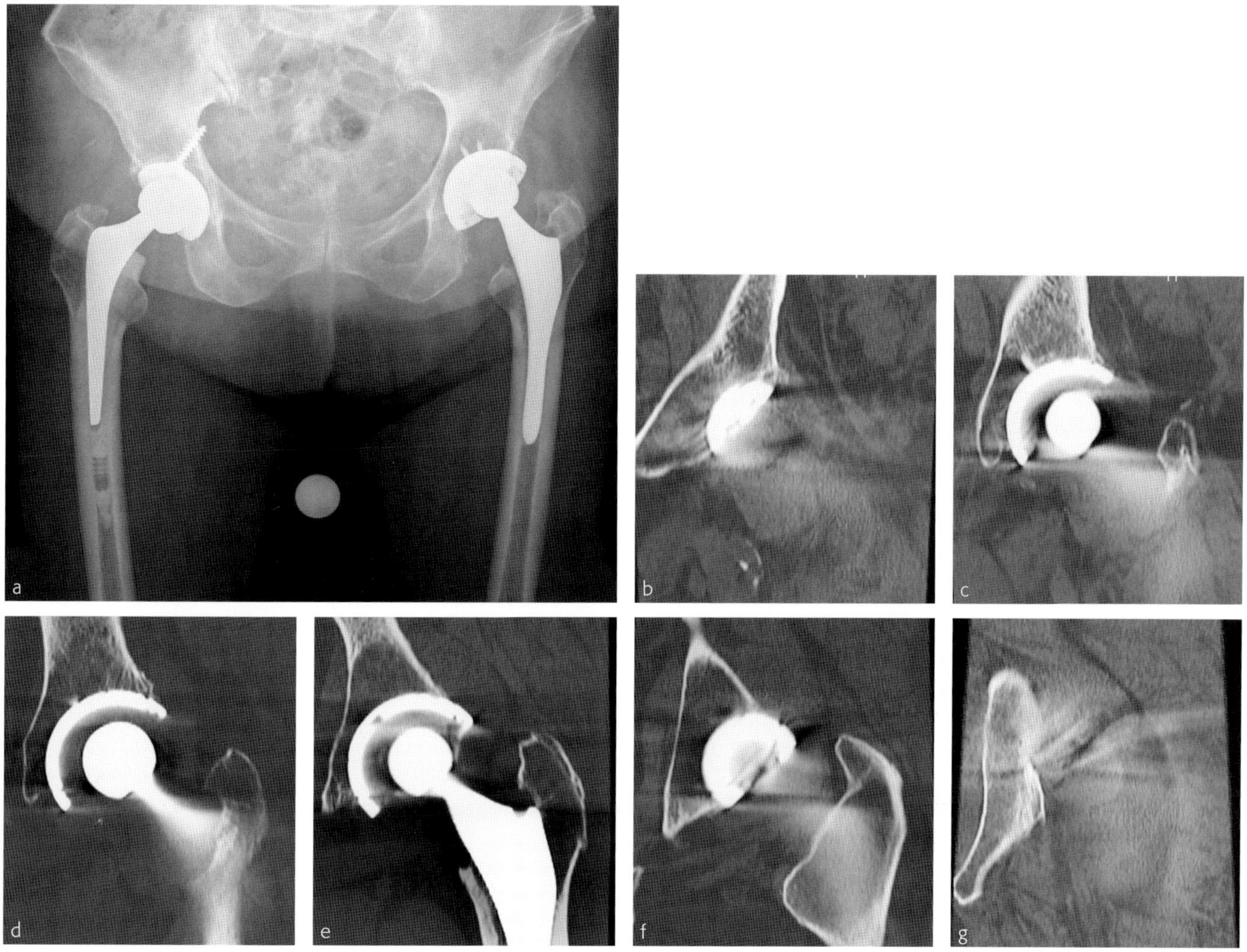

10.2-1a–g Imaging studies obtained at initial presentation.

a AP view shows bilateral total hip arthroplasty; the left side is painful, no clear evidence of a fracture.

b–g CT scans with frontal reconstruction. Note eccentricity of prosthetic head as a sign of polyethylene wear.

IV.6-B2

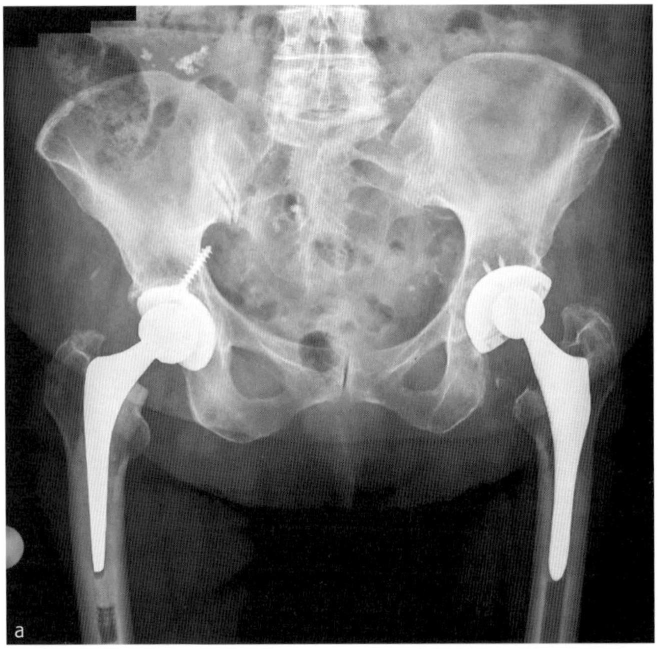

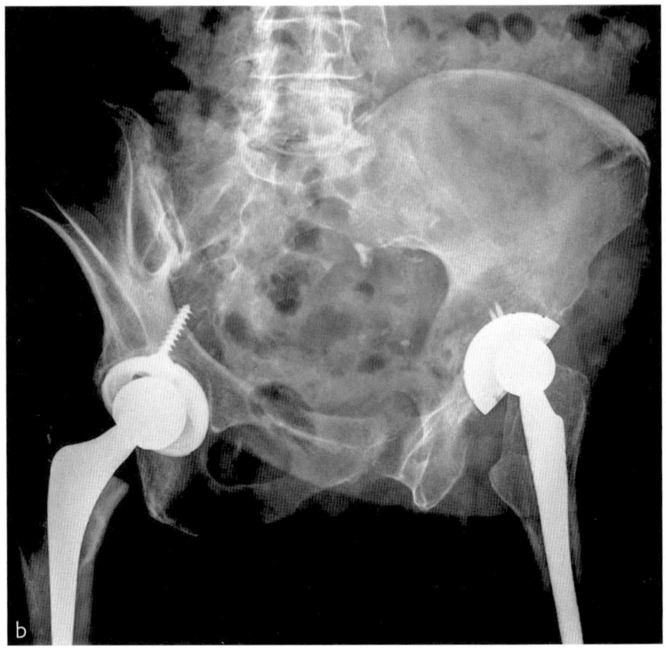

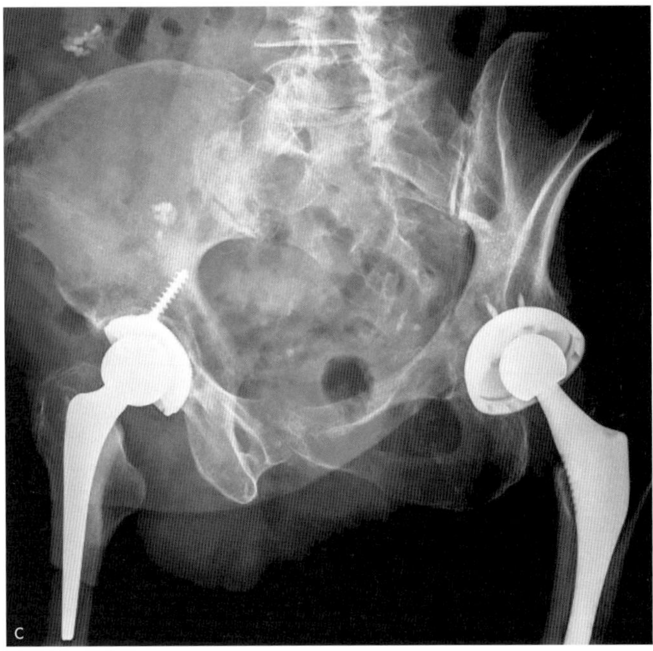

10.2-2a–c X-rays obtained 4 months after initial presentation.
- **a** AP view.
- **b** Iliac oblique view.
- **c** Obturator oblique view shows a fracture line in the anterior column.

10.2 Transverse acetabular fracture, loose acetabular cup

Reconstruction: two plates and revision arthroplasty, Burch-Schneider antiprotrusio cage, hook plate

IV.6-B2

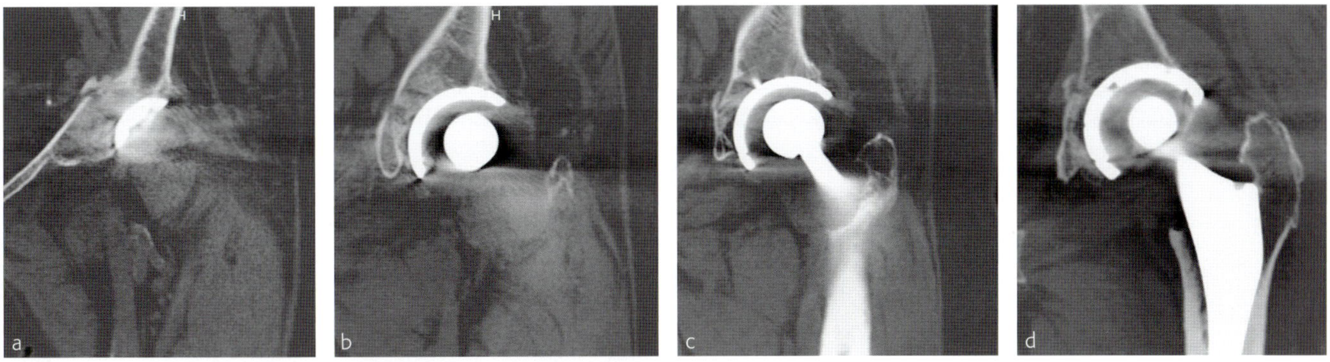

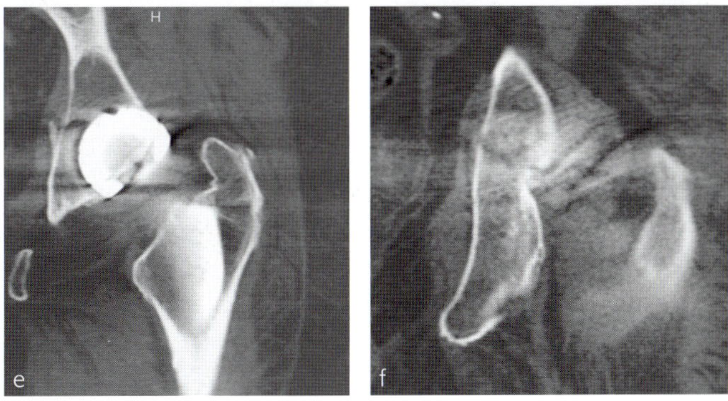

10.2-3a–f Preoperative CT scans with frontal reconstruction show the little displaced infratectal transverse acetabular fracture.

Decision making

Careful workup, including plain x-rays (AP and oblique views according to Letournel) and CT scans (multiplanar and 3-D reconstructions), are mandatory. The classification for acetabular deficiencies proposed by the American Academy of Orthopaedic Surgeons does not give clear guidelines for the need of internal fixation for safe cup anchorage. It is therefore proposed to use the new unified classification system, or the one according to Letournel.

The patient has a somewhat displaced periprosthetic transverse fracture of the left acetabulum. Because there is no osseous continuity between the stable dome fragment and the ischium, internal fixation of the posterior column of the acetabulum is mandatory to safely anchor the cup (chapter 5.4.1). For legal reasons, the mix of prosthetic components from different manufacturers is not permitted in some countries. Therefore, the exchange of the cup must be combined with an appropriate new femoral component (chapter 5.5), even though the original stem was solidly anchored.

Preoperative planning

Equipment

- Complete set of pelvic instruments
- Pelvic reconstruction plates 3.5, curved and straight
- 3.5 mm cortex screws
- 3.5 mm locking-head screws
- Complete set of total hip arthroplasty instruments
- Complete set of revision total hip arthroplasty instruments
- Noncemented hip prosthesis cups (press-fit system)
- Acetabular reinforcement rings or Burch-Schneider antiprotrusio cages
- Cemented flat profile standard or highly cross-linked polyethylene cups
- Cemented or noncemented hip prosthesis stems
- Revision total hip femoral system (preferably modular system)
- Cable system
- Trochanter grip plates of different lengths
- Instrument set for cable system

IV.6-B2

Patient preparation and positioning

- First- or second-generation cephalosporin for antibiotic prophylaxis
- Low-molecular-weight heparin for thrombosis prophylaxis
- Lateral position with a pelvic support on the sacrum and the pubic symphysis
- The posterosuperior iliac spine is marked with a pen and must remain palpable during the entire procedure to guarantee correct orientation of the cup
- Free draping of the involved lower leg

Reduction and fixation

Depending on the specific needs of the surgical plan and whether additional revision of the stem is needed, one of three approaches can be used: a standard Kocher-Langenbeck approach, a Kocher-Langenbeck-like approach with digastric trochanteric slide osteotomy, or a transfemoral approach. The latter two approaches offer partial visualization of the anterior column (from inside the acetabulum) and complete visualization of the posterior column.

In this case, the transfemoral approach was used with the hemitransverse femoral osteotomy at a distance of 12–13 cm distally to the tip of the greater trochanter.

Careful preparation of the external rotators and identification of the sciatic nerve was done to avoid injury to the nerve.

In most patients with periprosthetic transverse or T-shaped acetabular fractures, stability is only required between the stable dome fragment and the ischium. After removal of the loose cup, the entire acetabulum is usually accessible from posterior as well as from the inside. Fracture fragments are then cleared of any existing hematoma, interposed early callus, and granulation tissue. Rotational alignment can be achieved with a Schanz screw placed into the ischium. The posterior column is reduced with a large or small Jungbluth forceps applied to screws in the proximal and distal posterior column fragments. The posterior column is then fixed with one or two straight or curved pelvic reconstruction plates 3.5, spanning from the ischium to the supraacetabular area. A 4- to 5-hole straight reconstruction plate 3.5 is placed along the greater sciatic notch with the Jungbluth forceps remaining in position. The forceps can then be removed, and fixation is completed with a second curved 6- to 8-hole pelvic reconstruction plate 3.5. The first screw is inserted at the infracotyloid fossa just proximally to the ischial tuberosity, followed by at least two additional screws in the proximal fragment and into the ischial tuberosity.

The acetabular cavity is prepared using standard acetabular reamers. Depending on the situation, reconstruction of the bone stock of the medial wall and the dome segment with autogenous bone chips is required.

Proper inclination of the cup (45° ± 2.5) as well as antiversion (20° ± 2.5) are ensured when the seating instrument of the cup is aligned in the direction of the posterosuperior iliac spine.

With a highly stable fixation of the posterior column that tolerates radial prestress around the acetabular cup, insertion of a press-fit cup system with additional screw fixation is a possible technical solution. In case of any doubt, insertion of an acetabular antiprotrusio cage (Burch-Schneider) with a cemented polyethylene liner is a safe option. The insertion of the wing of the Burch-Schneider antiprotrusio cage can be demanding because at least the two most distal plate screws need space in the ischial bone. These screws should be retightened after wing insertion. If a transfemoral approach is used, internal fixation of the proximal femur is performed using a cable system with or without a trochanter grip plate.

Rehabilitation and follow-up

Intravenous antibiotics were administrated for 24 hours according to hospital prophylaxis protocol. Prophylaxis for deep vein thrombosis with low-molecular-weight heparin was maintained for 6 weeks.

Partial weight bearing (15 kg) was initiated within the first 48 hours postoperatively. This patient remained on crutches for 3 months, but progressive loading can be allowed after 6 weeks depending on the situation and progress of bone healing. X-rays should be obtained immediately and at 6 and 12 weeks after surgery. At the 1-year follow-up, the patient was pain free and walking without crutches and without a limp (**10.2-4a–b**). Hip joint mobility was satisfactory, and the patient could put her shoes on without any help.

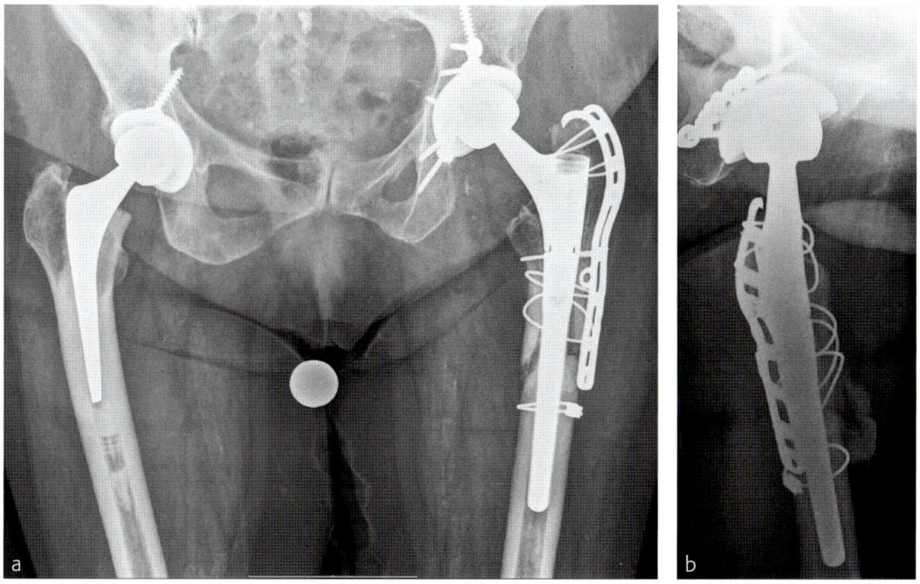

10.2-4a–b X-rays obtained 1 year postoperatively.
a AP view shows that the acetabular fracture has healed. The transverse part of the femoral osteotomy is still visible but does not show secondary displacement. The medial fragment shows bone healing.
b Axial view.

Points to remember

- Use of the transfemoral or trochanteric slide approach allows easy visualization of the entire acetabulum from inside and direct access to the entire posterior column.
- One-stage internal fixation, bone-stock reconstruction, and revision total hip arthroplasty are possible.
- Careful preparation is required to avoid injury to the sciatic nerve.
- If there is a posterior column fracture or a transverse or T-shaped fracture with or without posterior-wall component, exposure of the entire posterior column will allow for correct reduction and positioning of the plates on the posterior column.
- Safe anchoring of an acetabular antiprotrusio cage or a press-fit cup system is possible.
- Correct orientation of the prosthetic components is possible, reducing the risk of hip dislocation due to prosthetic component impingement.
- Stable fixation of the bony flap in case of a transfemoral approach using cerclage wiring or a cable system is mandatory to reduce the risk of nonunion or secondary displacement of the femoral fragment.
- Nonunion of the periprosthetic acetabular fracture component can occur.
- If in doubt about healing of the transfemoral approach, the integration of homogenous bone-stock reconstruction, or fracture healing of the acetabulum, CT scans may be obtained, if necessary.

IV.6-B3

10.3 Acetabular fracture, osteolysis, and loose cup

Reconstruction: cage, morcelized allograft, cemented new cup

Authors Gregory G Polkowski, John C Clohisy, Jay R Lieberman

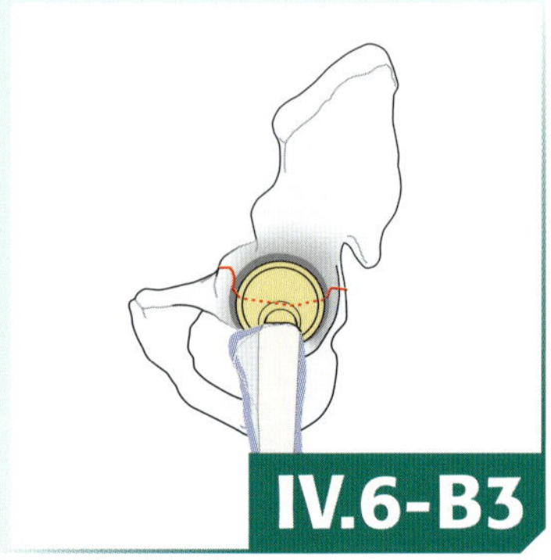

IV.6-B3

Case description

A 73-year-old woman who presented with increasing pain in the right hip after a fall, had undergone a noncemented total hip arthroplasty 8 years ago. She had antecedent pain in the right hip region for several months before she fell but no complications associated with the initial arthroplasty procedure. She is a community ambulator with mild dementia, but otherwise healthy. X-rays revealed a fracture with a transverse pattern, involving both anterior and posterior columns of the acetabulum (**10.3-1a–b**). There is loosening of the acetabular component.

Classification: Type IV.6-B3

Diagnosis: Periprosthetic acetabular fracture with osteolysis and pelvic discontinuity on the right side

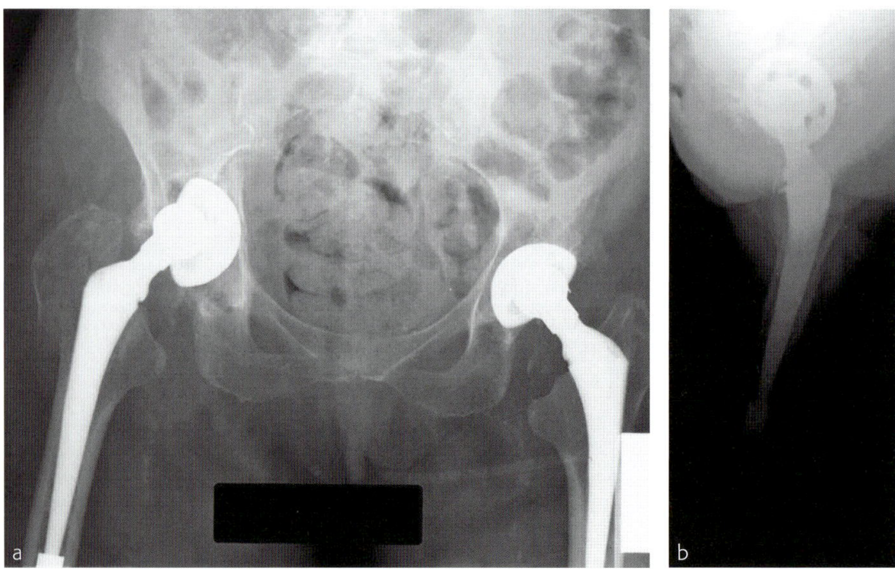

10.3-1a–b X-rays obtained shortly after injury.

- **a** AP view shows bilateral noncemented total hip arthroplasties with periprosthetic fracture of the right acetabulum. The femoral stem is well fixed. Osteolysis is seen at the right acetabulum.
- **b** Cross-table lateral view. Soft-tissue shadows obscure much of the pelvis, but loosening of the acetabular component is apparent from the radiolucent area between the os ischium and the acetabular component.

Decision making

Given the history of antecedent pain in the months before her fall, periacetabular osteolysis was suspected. Revision of the acetabular component, combined with fixation of the acetabular fracture and bone grafting of osteolytic lesions, was required to reconstruct the acetabulum. The transverse fracture through the pelvic osteolysis represents a pelvic discontinuity, which complicates the reconstruction. A variety of techniques would be needed to fix the discontinuity, including posterior column plating to provide stable fixation of a new acetabular component (chapter 5.6). In the case of a larger osteolytic defect, porous wedge augmentation or structural femoral allograft may be necessary to enhance acetabular component support. A revision acetabular cage with bone grafting may be required in more extreme cases of pelvic osteolysis in which initial revision component stability cannot be achieved.

Preoperative planning

Equipment

- Pelvic reconstruction plates
- Porous revision acetabular sockets
- Structural allograft (distal femur or femoral head)
- Porous wedge augmentation
- Revision acetabular cage

Patient preparation and positioning

- Lateral decubitus position
- Wide surgical draping for extensile exposure

Reduction and fixation

A posterolateral approach was used through the previous surgical incision, and the gluteus maximus tendon was released at its distal insertion to facilitate wide exposure. The scarred posterior capsule and short external rotators were reflected posteriorly after release as one large sleeve off the proximal femur. Care was taken to identify the posterior border of the gluteus medius muscle to minimize trauma to the hip abductor musculature. The modular head was removed, and the stem and proximal femur were retracted anteriorly to expose the socket and fracture. The bone quality, fracture displacement, and extent of osteolysis were assessed after meticulous debridement following removal of the loose acetabular component.

Careful assessment of the bone stock of the anterior and posterior columns revealed extensive superior, medial, and anterior osteolysis. The transverse fracture was identified superior to the acetabulum, exiting the acetabulum anteriorly in the form of two separate fracture lines, one anterior, and one inferior. Given the poor bone quality and osteolysis, plate and screw fixation of the transverse fracture and discontinuity would not be adequate; therefore, a cage reconstruction was necessary. The pelvic reconstruction cage was fixed to the acetabulum with screws after performing extensive morcelized bone grafting to the osteolytic defects and fracture. An acetabular liner was cemented into the cage, and a new modular head was applied. IV.6-B3

Rehabilitation and follow-up

An abduction brace was used for 2 months postoperatively to minimize hip motion and reduce the risk of dislocation. Prophylaxis for deep vein thrombosis was initiated with warfarin, and the patient was instructed to maintain toe-touch weight bearing restrictions on the operative side for 3 months until the acetabular bone graft had an opportunity to heal and incorporate.

At the 3-year follow-up, the patient walked with a limp but remained pain free without complications. X-rays showed incorporation of the acetabular bone graft (**10.3-2**).

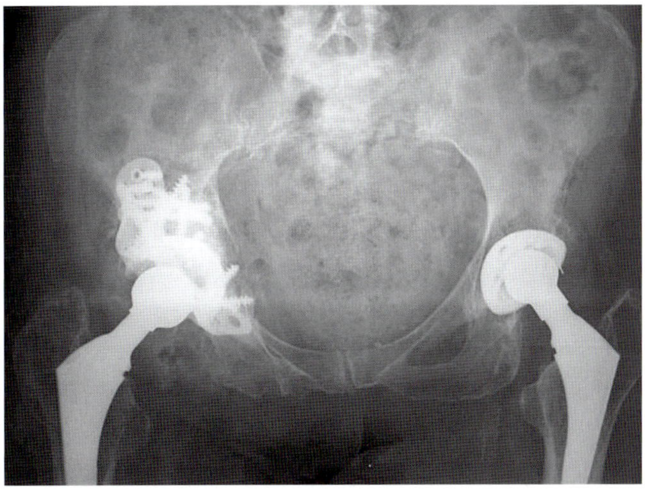

10.3-2 AP x-ray obtained 3 years postoperatively shows stable fixation of the acetabular cage and bone-graft construct. The cancellous bone graft in the osteolytic defects medial to the cage has been incorporated.

IV.6-B3 Points to remember

- Care must be taken to preserve the insertion of the abductor muscles on the greater trochanter, as these play an important role for long-term hip function and maintaining adequate soft-tissue tension that affords greater hip stability.
- Though not used in this case, preoperative CT is helpful to assess the extent of pelvic osteolysis, better characterize the fracture, and assess pelvic bone stock to aid with operative planning.
- The sciatic nerve is at risk with the posterior approach to the hip, and in revision situations it can be extensively encased in scar tissue from previous surgical procedures. This structure should be isolated and protected, especially when additional exposure is required for cage reconstructions or posterior column plating.

10.4 Proximal femoral fracture, stable prosthesis

MIPO: LCP hook plate 4.5/5.0

Author Rodrigo Pesantez

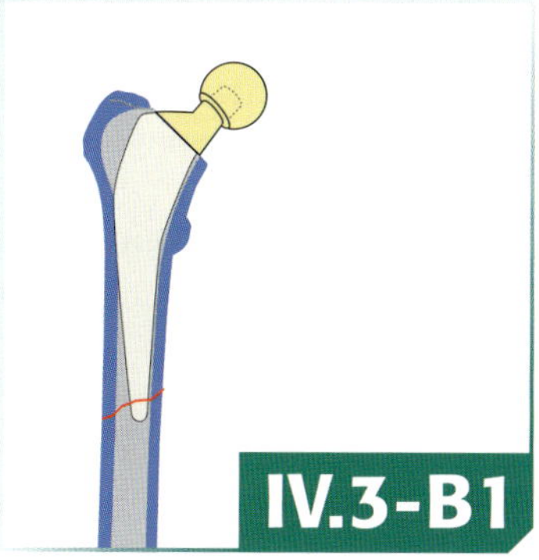

IV.3-B1

Case description

An 87-year-old woman sustained a fall from standing height while on vacation. She underwent total hip arthroplasty 1 year ago, with no postoperative complaints or symptoms. X-rays showed a stable prosthesis and a long spiral fracture around a noncemented stem (**10.4-1a–c**). She was cleared for surgery and then operated on 24 hours after the accident.

Classification: Type IV.3-B1

Diagnosis: Long spiral periprosthetic fracture of the proximal femur with a stable well-fixed, noncemented stem

Decision making

Because the patient had a simple fracture, direct reduction and absolute stability with lag screws and a locking compression hook plate using a minimally invasive plate osteosynthesis (MIPO) technique and cables for proximal fixation was considered the best solution (chapter 5.4.1).

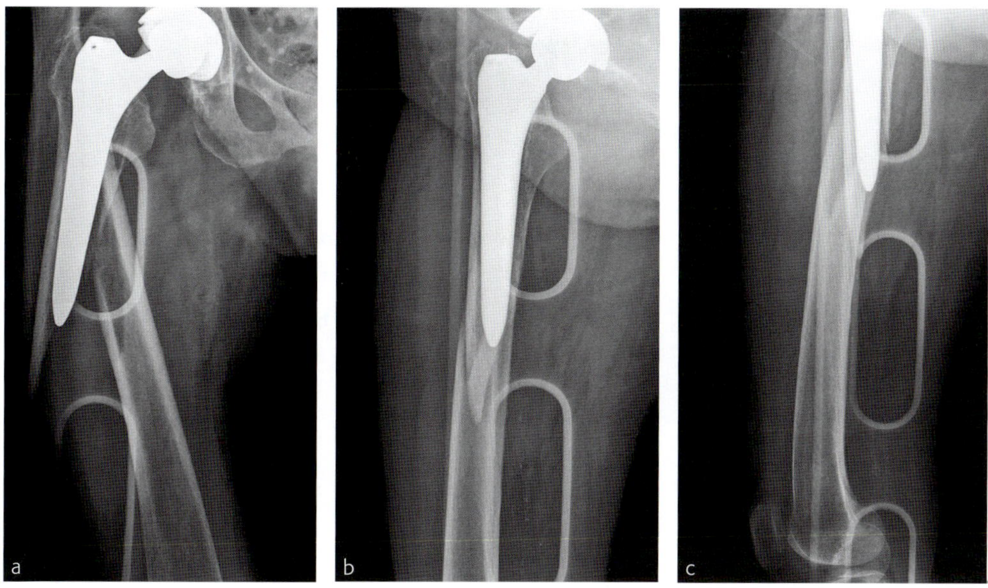

10.4-1a–c X-rays show a spiral fracture of the femur around a well-fixed noncemented stem.
- **a** AP view of the proximal femur.
- **b** Lateral view of the proximal femur.
- **c** Lateral view including the distal femur.

IV.3-B1 ## Preoperative planning

Equipment

- Proximal femur locking compression hook plate 4.5/5.0
- 5 mm locking-head screws
- Cables and attachments for locking plate
- 3.5 mm cortex screws

Preparation and patient positioning

- Supine position on a radiolucent table with a bolster under the ipsilateral buttock
- First- or second-generation cephalosporin for antibiotic prophylaxis
- Low-molecular-weight heparin for thrombosis prophylaxis

Reduction and fixation

The fracture site was identified with an image intensifier, and a short ventral incision was made to expose the fracture. Reduction was done under manual traction with a reduction forceps and more proximally a temporary cerclage wire (👁 **10.4-2a–b**).

For percutaneous submuscular insertion of the locking compression hook plate, lateral incisions were made over the greater trochanter and distal femur. The fracture was fixed by percutaneous insertion of two plate-independent 3.5 mm lag screws just distal to the stem. The 17-hole locking compression hook plate was inserted from proximal to distal after preparing a submuscular tunnel. The position of the plate was confirmed with the image intensifier. Proximal fixation of the plate was secured with two cerclage cables and distally with two locking-head screws and one conventional screw. Immediate postoperative x-rays were obtained (👁 **10.4-3a–c**).

Rehabilitation and follow-up

Physiotherapy was initiated immediately to restore hip and knee motion. Partial weight bearing was advised for 6 weeks, with progression to full weight bearing at 12 weeks. Prophylaxis for deep vein thrombosis included low-molecular-weight heparin for 35 days and use of compression stockings. Follow-up was recommended at 3, 6, and 12 weeks when she returned home. X-rays obtained 3 months postoperatively showed fracture consolidation (👁 **10.4-4a–b**).

Two years postoperatively, the patient was doing fine and living independently. She did not require more surgery and was walking without supporting aids.

Points to remember

- Use a radiolucent table. Place a bump under the ipsilateral buttock to obtain an AP view (left) and a lateral (right) view of the femur.
- Position the C-arm on the opposite side of the fracture with the screens distal (at the patient's feet).
- Use the image intensifier to identify the skin incisions for plate and clamp placement.

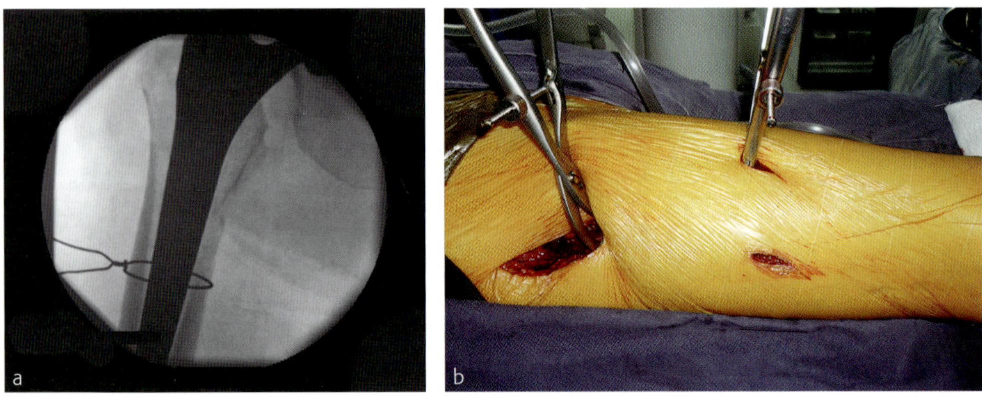

👁 **10.4-2a–b** Surgical reduction.
a Minimally invasive cerclage wiring to reduce the fracture.
b Lateral and anterior incisions made with two Verbrugge forceps to reduce and hold the fracture in place.

10.4 **Proximal femoral fracture, stable prosthesis**

MIPO: LCP hook plate 4.5/5.0

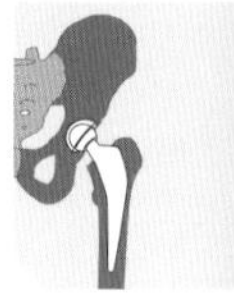

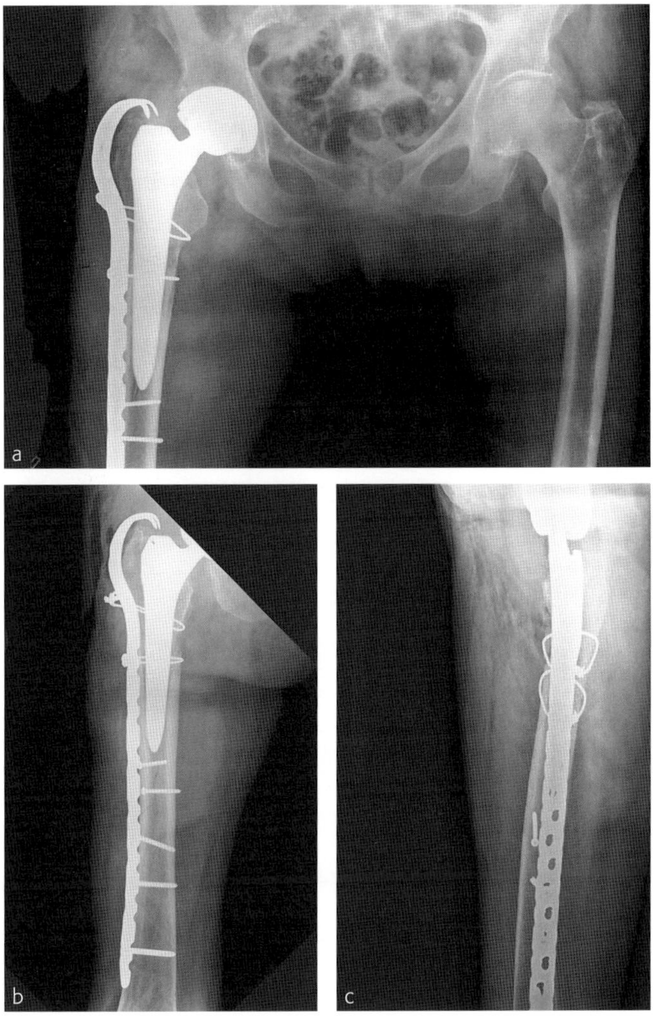

10.4-3a–c X-rays obtained immediately postoperatively.

a AP view of the pelvis.
b AP view of the femur.
c Lateral view.

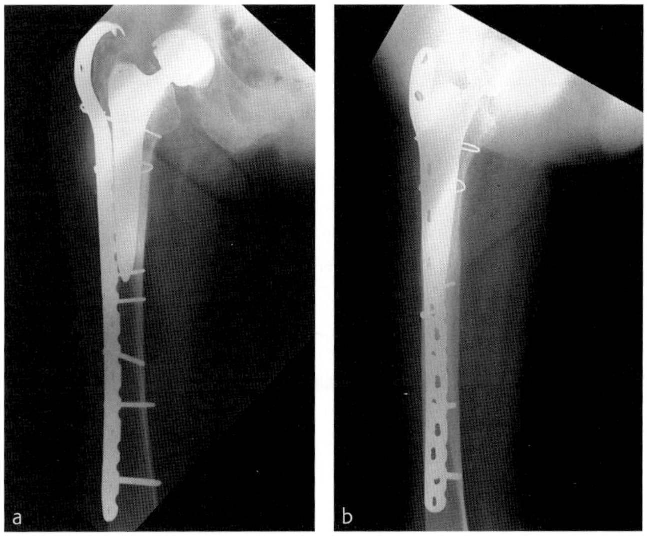

10.4-4a–b X-rays obtained 3 months postoperatively showed good progress of fracture healing.

a AP view.
b Lateral view.

IV.3-B1

10.5 Proximal femoral fracture, stable prosthesis

ORIF: LCP hook plate 4.5/5.0

Author **Rodrigo Pesantez**

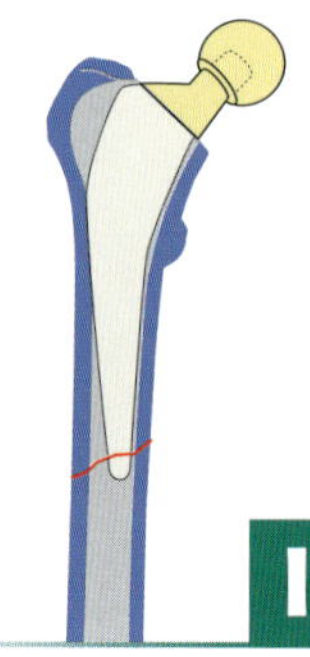

IV.3-B1

Case description

An 82-year-old woman fell from a standing height while intoxicated. She had undergone bilateral total hip arthroplasties more than 12 years ago and had been asymptomatic. X-rays showed a spiral fracture with a possible butterfly fragment and a well-fixed cemented prosthesis (👁 **10.5-1a–c**).

Classification: Type IV.3-B1

Diagnosis: Spiral butterfly periprosthetic fracture of the proximal femur, with a well-fixed cemented stem

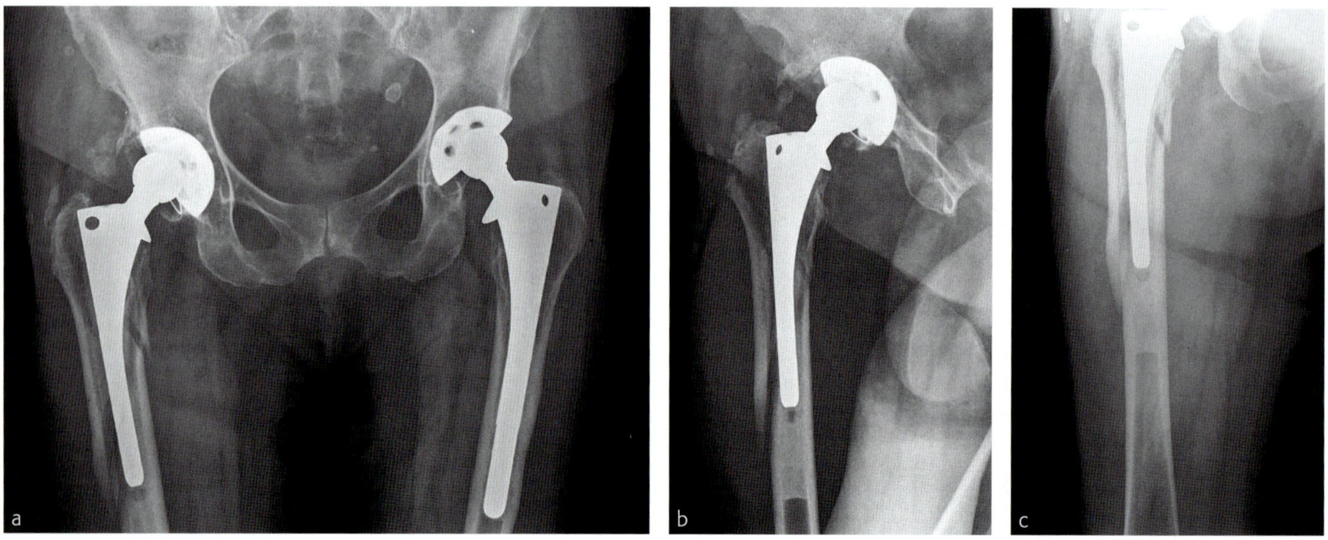

👁 **10.5-1a–c** Preoperative x-rays.

a AP view of the pelvis shows previous bilateral total hip arthroplasties. On the right side, the hybrid total hip arthroplasty shows a spiral fracture with a butterfly around the cemented stem.
b AP view of the femur.
c Lateral view of the femur.

Decision making

The patient has a simple fracture, which is best approached by direct reduction and fixation to provide absolute stability. Lag screws and a neutralization plate are indicated (chapter 5.4.1).

Preoperative planning

Equipment

- 17-hole proximal femur locking compression hook plate 4.5/5.0
- 3.5 and 4.5 mm cortex screws
- Wires and cables, if needed

Patient preparation and positioning

- Supine position on a radiolucent table with a bolster placed under the ipsilateral buttock
- First- or second-generation cephalosporin for antibiotic prophylaxis
- Low-molecular-weight heparin for thrombosis prophylaxis

Reduction and fixation IV.3-B1

Short lateral incisions were made over the greater trochanter and distal femur. Once the fracture was exposed, it was reduced under manual traction with the use of two bone forceps. Two 3.5 mm lag screws were inserted to secure the reduction. A 17-hole locking compression hook plate was then applied from proximal to distal following preparation of a submuscular tunnel. Correct positioning of the plate was then verified. Conventional 4.5 mm cortex screws were inserted percutaneously at different angles to resist pull-out. Postoperative x-rays were obtained immediately (👁 **10.5-2a–c**).

Rehabilitation and follow-up

Physiotherapy was initiated immediately to restore hip and knee motion. Partial weight bearing was recommended for 6 weeks, with progression to full weight bearing at 12 weeks. Prophylaxis for deep vein thrombosis included low-molecular-weight heparin for 35 days and compression stockings. The patient returned for follow-up at 3, 6, and 12 weeks, 6 months, and 1 year. Follow-up x-rays were obtained after 2 years (👁 **10.5-3a–b**). The patient was well, independent, and able to walk without assistance.

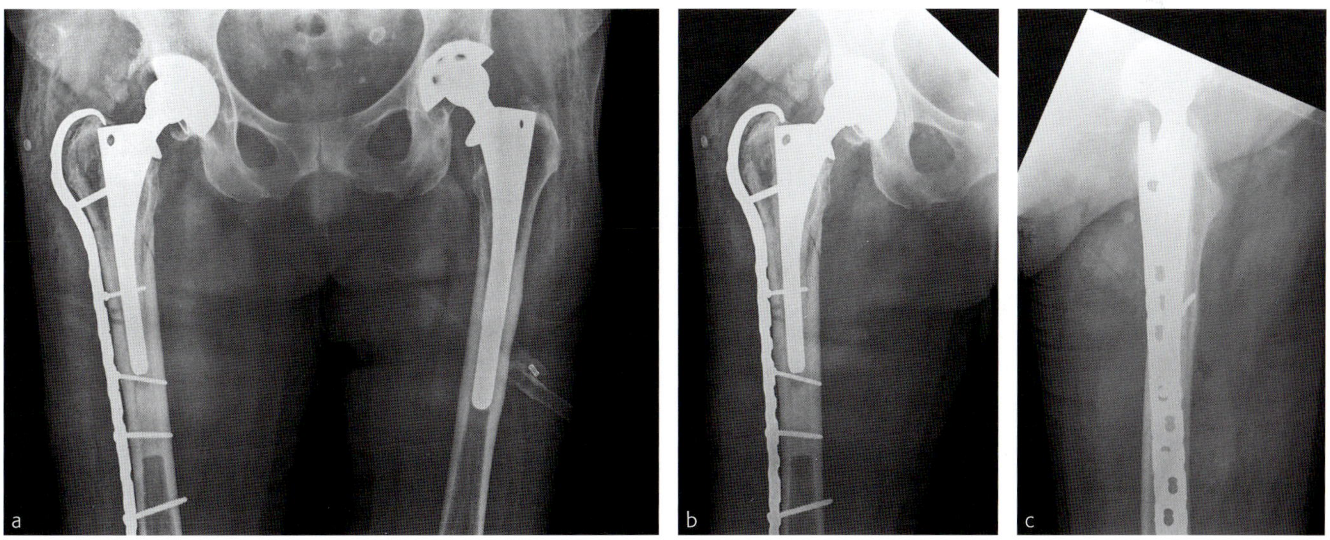

👁 **10.5-2a–c** Immediate postoperative x-rays.
a AP view of the pelvis.
b AP view of the femur.
c Lateral view of the femur.

IV.3-B1

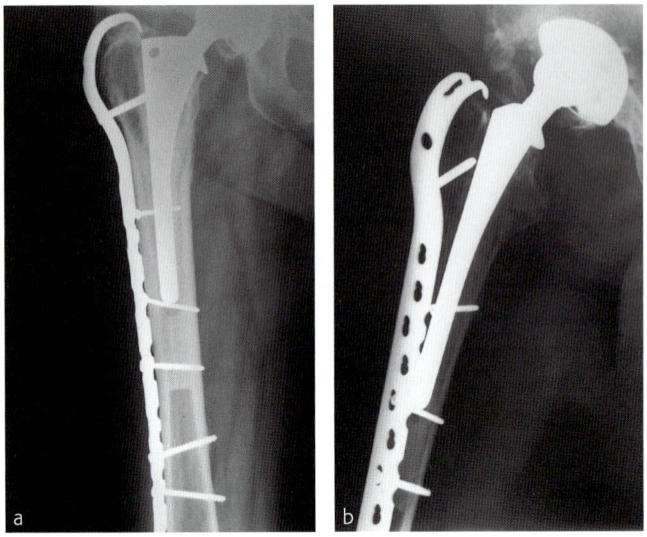

10.5-3a–b X-rays of the femur obtained 2 year postoperatively show a well-healed fracture and no signs of prosthetic loosening.
a AP view.
b Lateral view.

Points to remember

- Use a radiolucent table. Place a bolster under the ipsilateral buttock to obtain AP and laterals view of the femur.
- Position the C-arm on the opposite side of the fracture with the screens at the patient's feet.
- Use the image intensifier to identify the skin incisions for plate and clamp placement.
- Have available the cables and attachments for the cables. Another option is the locking attachment plate 3.5.
- In case there are no locking-head screws available, conventional 4.5 mm cortex screws may be used. If they are inserted at different angles, they have a higher resistance to pull-out.

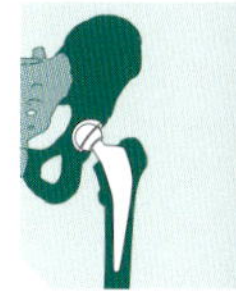

10.6 Spiral femoral fracture, stable prosthesis

MIPO: lag screw and LCP 4.5/5.0

Author **Takeshi Sawaguchi**

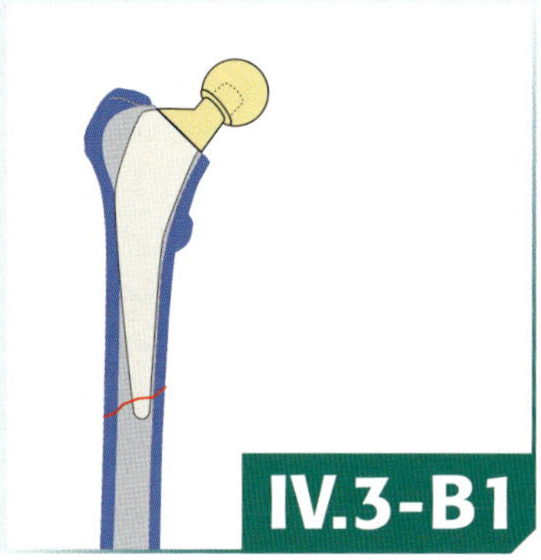

IV.3-B1

Case description

An 86-year-old woman, who underwent a cemented endoprosthesis 10 years ago for a right femoral neck fracture, fell while walking inside her house. X-rays obtained immediately after the injury showed a simple spiral fracture extending from the lesser trochanter to the midshaft of the femur (**10.6-1a–b**). The cemented stem appeared well fixed despite the proximal extension of the fracture.

Classification: Type IV.3-B1

Diagnosis: Periprosthetic fracture of the proximal femur/femoral shaft, with a stable prosthesis

Decision making

Exchange of the prosthesis would require an osteosynthesis; therefore, the best solution for this patient was anatomical reduction and bridging of the fracture with a locking internal fixator plate with a minimally invasive plate osteosynthesis technique (chapter 5.4.1).

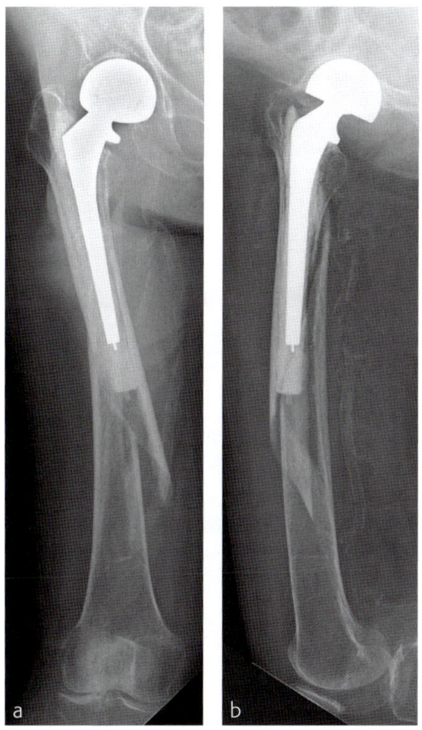

10.6-1a–b X-rays obtained immediately after the injury.
a AP view.
b Lateral view.

IV.3-B1 ## Preoperative planning

Equipment

- 16-hole narrow locking compression plate (LCP) 4.5/5.0
- 5.0 mm locking-head screws
- 4.5 mm cortex screws
- 2.0 mm K-wires
- Pointed reduction forceps

Patient preparation and positioning

- First- or second-generation cephalosporin for antibiotic prophylaxis
- Low-molecular-weight heparin for thrombosis prophylaxis

Reduction and fixation

A minimally invasive surgical approach was used through three short incisions: on the lateral side of the femur over the lateral condyle, the trochanteric area, and over the fracture site to reduce the fracture anatomically. Care was used to minimize soft-tissue damage.

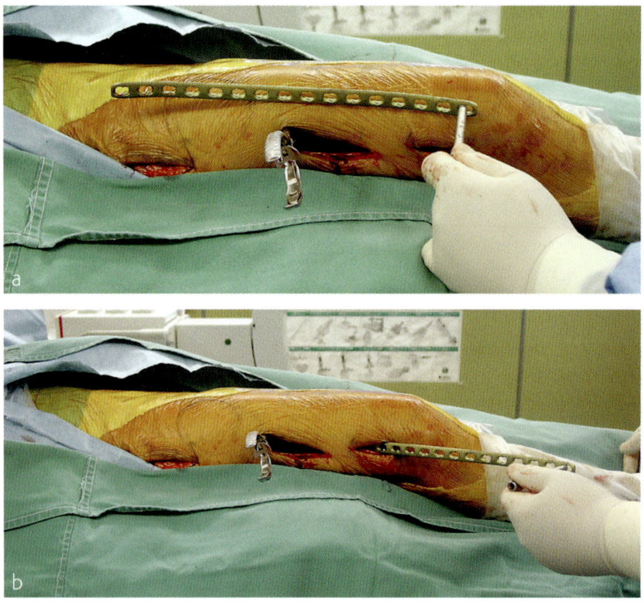

10.6-2a–b Surgical reduction.
a Verification of plate length; contouring is required.
b Plate insertion from distal to proximal.

A short incision was made using two pointed reduction forceps with manual traction; control of the reduction was facilitated with an image intensifier. Plate length was verified (**10.6-2a**); the plate was inserted from distal to proximal (**10.6-2b**); and then K-wires were used for temporary fixation at the distal and proximal fragments. The fracture was first fixed with a lag screw through the plate, followed by insertion of four locking-head screws in the distal fragment and five monocortical locking-head screws in the proximal fragment. The monocortical screws were placed anteriorly to the prosthesis because there was more room for better purchase. One bicortical screw was inserted distal to the stem of the prosthesis. The result was verified radiologically (**10.6-3a–b**).

Rehabilitation and follow-up

Partial weight bearing was recommended for 8 weeks. The patient returned for follow-up at 4, 12, and 16 weeks and one year postoperatively (**10.6-4a–c**). At 16 weeks, the patient needed only a cane for walking. One year postoperatively, the patient had no major problems, despite slight subsidence of the prosthesis as a sign of possible loosening (**10.6-5a–b**). She continued to walk with a cane until her death 3 years later.

Points to remember

- Minimal fracture exposure is necessary to obtain anatomical reduction in simple long spiral fractures.
- Locking-head screws simplify minimally invasive procedures because the plate does not have to be precisely contoured. However, when using very long implants, as in this situation, the plate ends must be slightly bent.
- Narrow LCPs 4.5/5.0 are useful for women of small stature. Broad plates are required in men.
- Monocortical screws are inserted into the long overlapping portion of the proximal segment anterior to the prosthesis and into the bone cement for improved stability.

10.6 **Spiral femoral fracture, stable prosthesis**

MIPO: lag screw and LCP 4.5/5.0

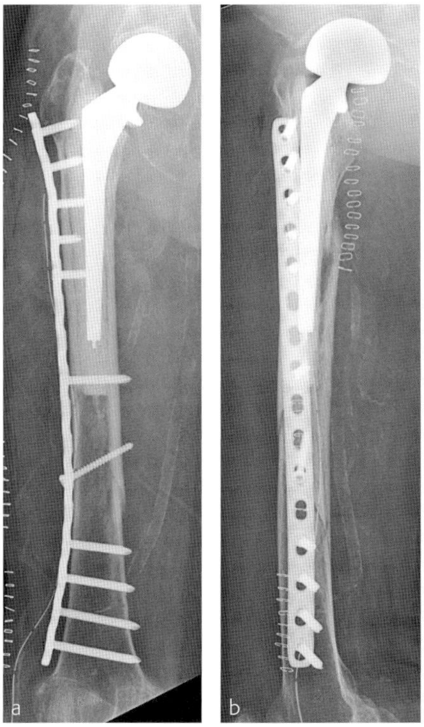

10.6-3a–b X-rays obtained immediately postoperatively.

a AP view.

b Lateral view.

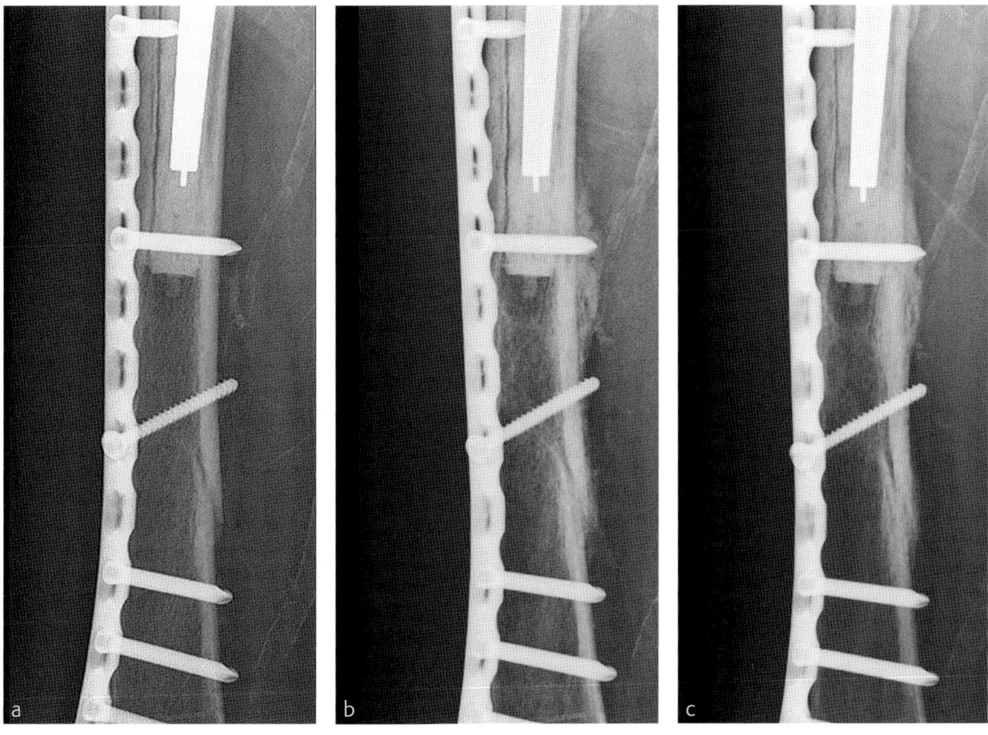

10.6-4a–c X-rays obtained at 4, 12, and 16 weeks postoperatively document the progress to bony union.

a AP view 4 weeks postoperatively.

b AP view 12 weeks postoperatively.

c AP view 16 weeks postoperatively.

IV.3-B1

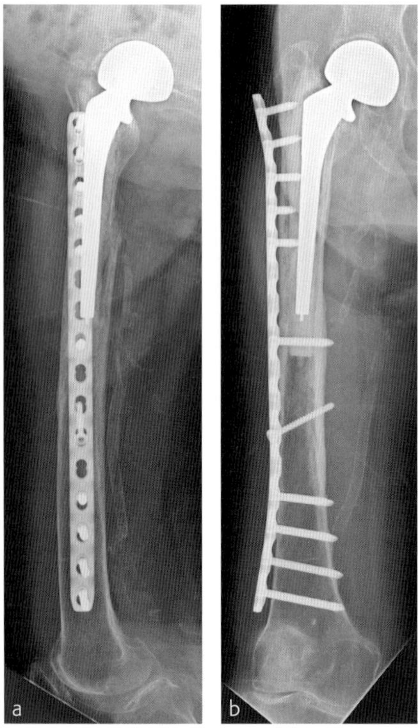

10.6-5a–b X-rays obtained 1 year postoperatively show slight subsidence of the prosthesis.
a AP view.
b Lateral view.

10.7 **Spiral femoral fracture at the tip of a stable prosthesis**

MIPO: long LCP distal femur, secondary revision with long-stem prosthesis

IV.3-B1

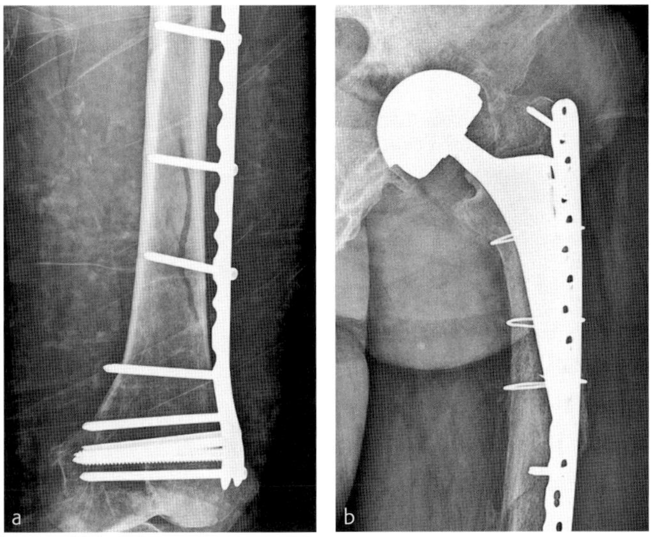

10.7-2a–b X-rays of the femur after fixation with a long locking compression plate distal femur and additional cerclage wires proximally.

a AP view.
b Lateral view.

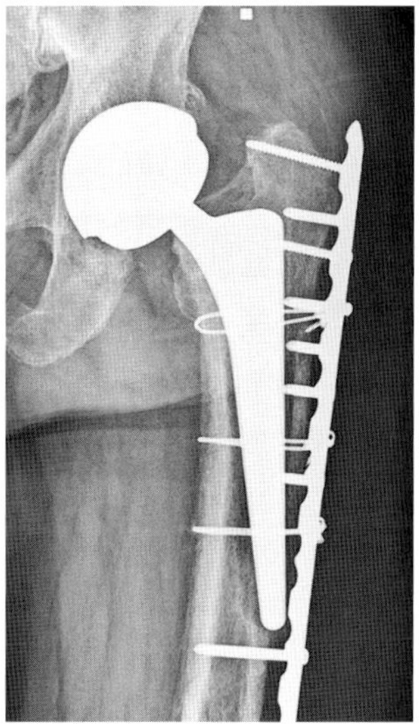

10.7-3 Progressive loosening and cut out of the prosthetic stem through the fracture, necessitating revision surgery.

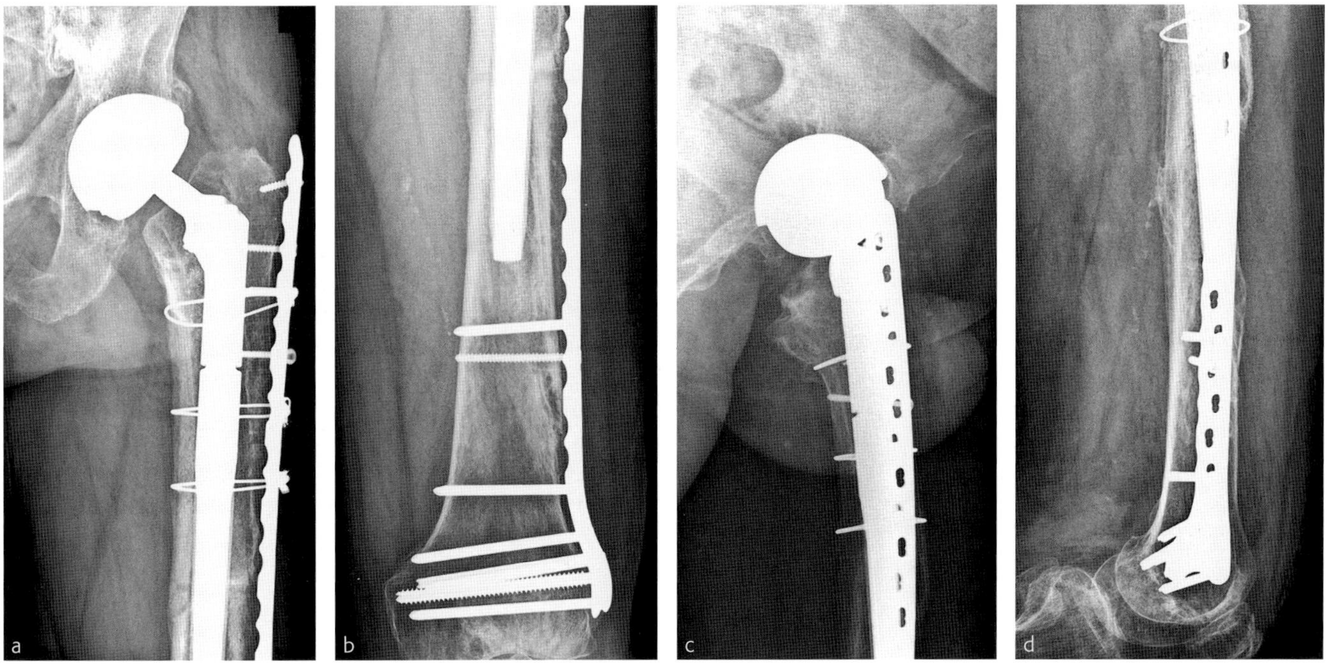

10.7-4a–d One year postoperatively the distal fractures appeared healed. Exchange for a long-stemmed femoral component after removal of several screws.

a AP view of the proximal femur after revision.
b AP view of the distal femur.
c Lateral view of the proximal femur.
d Lateral view of the distal femur.

IV.3-B1

10.8 Femoral shaft fracture, stable long-stem prosthesis

ORIF: locked retrograde intramedullary nail

Author **Aart D Verburg**

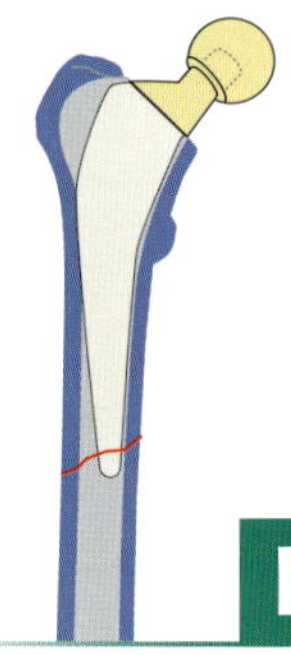

Case description

A 70-year-old woman with a femoral canal-filling Wagner revision prosthesis fell at home sustaining a long spiral fracture (**10.8-1a–c**).

Classification: Type IV.3-B1

Diagnosis: Periprosthetic fracture around a stable long-stem prosthesis

Decision making

The rather distal spiral fracture around a slender prosthetic stem lends itself to the use of an appropriate slotted or tubular retrograde intramedullary nail. Plate osteosynthesis seems less suitable due to the short distal fragment and the marked osteoporosis. The intramedullary nail should provide a solid construction that permits immediate partial weight bearing (chapter 5.4.2).

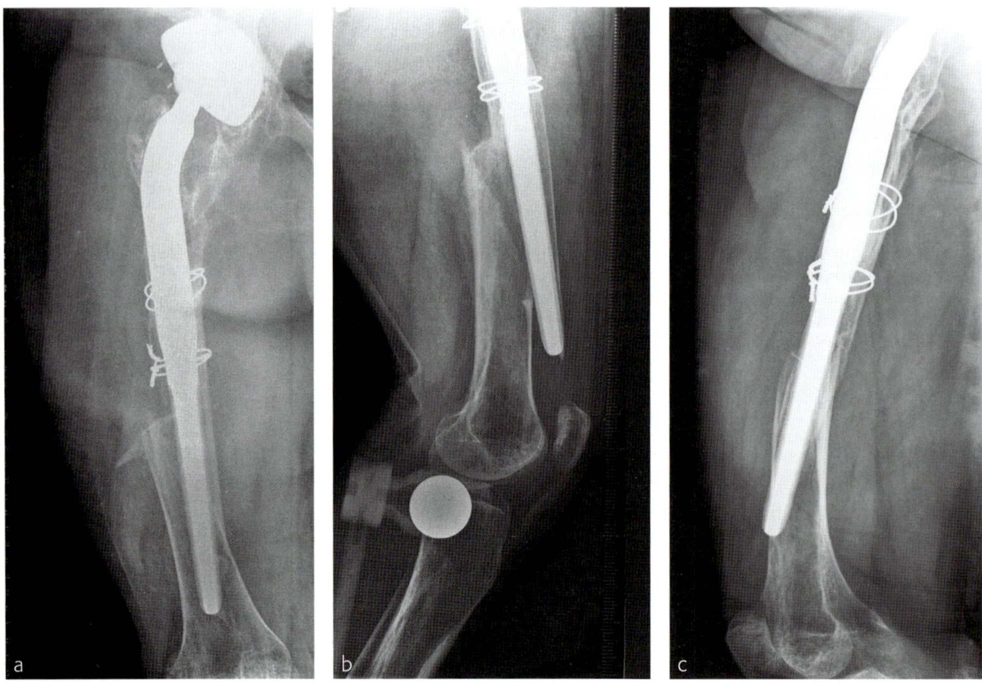

10.8-1a–c X-rays show marked osteoporosis and a fracture around the tip of the prosthetic stem that reaches far distally.
a AP view.
b–c Lateral views.

IV.3-B1

Preoperative planning

It is advisable to obtain leg-length x-rays before the operation.

Equipment

- Custom-made, semi-slotted intramedullary nail of proper length and diameter for retrograde insertion
- Locking bolts

Patient preparation and positioning

- First- or second-generation cephalosporin for antibiotic prophylaxis
- Low-molecular-weight heparin for thrombosis prophylaxis
- Supine position with the affected knee flexed to 70° over a bolster or post for the lower leg, mounted on the traction table. The elevated leg facilitates the use of the image intensifier in two planes.

Reduction and fixation

A miniarthrotomy (2–3 cm) was performed medial to the patellar tendon followed by retrograde introduction of a Steinmann pin at the femoral notch with correct axial alignment. The fracture was reduced with traction and bypassed with a guide wire. The medullary canal was reamed up to the diameter of the nail, with the correct length and rotation under image intensifier control. The custom-made retrograde nail was inserted 3–4 cm over the tip of the prosthesis. Distal locking was achieved with three bolts.

Rehabilitation and follow-up

Progressive weight bearing was initiated 6 weeks postoperatively, just as with standard locking intramedullary nailing of the femur. X-rays obtained 6 weeks postoperatively show the first signs of callus formation (**10.8-2a–c**). Follow-up after 4 years showed fracture healing and a stable prosthesis (**10.8-3a–c**).

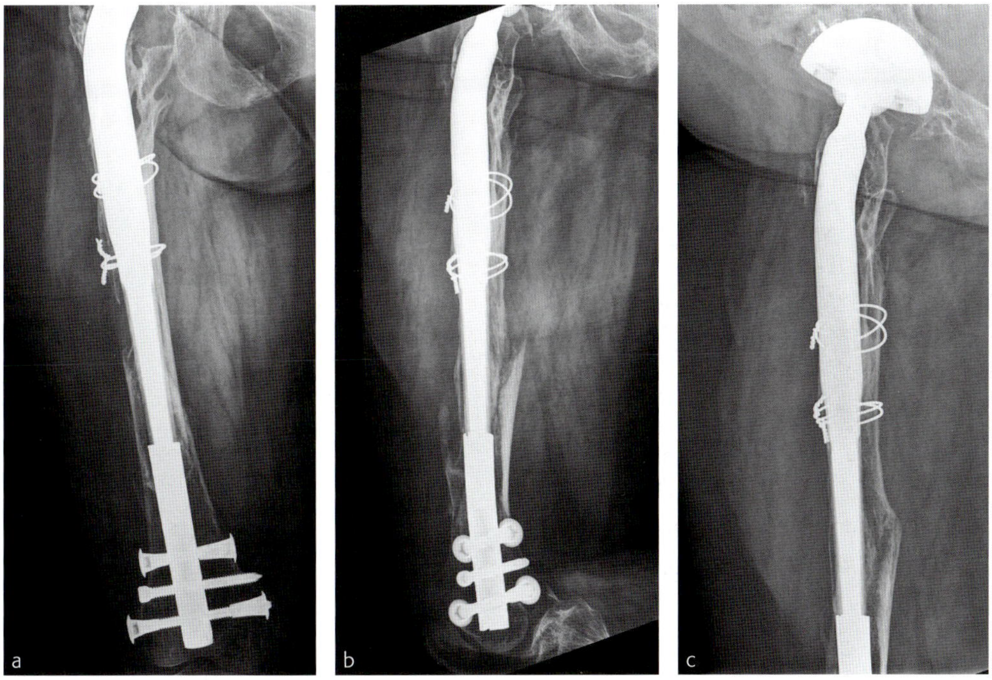

10.8-2a–c X-rays obtained 6 weeks postoperatively.
a AP view.
b–c Lateral views.

IV.3-B1

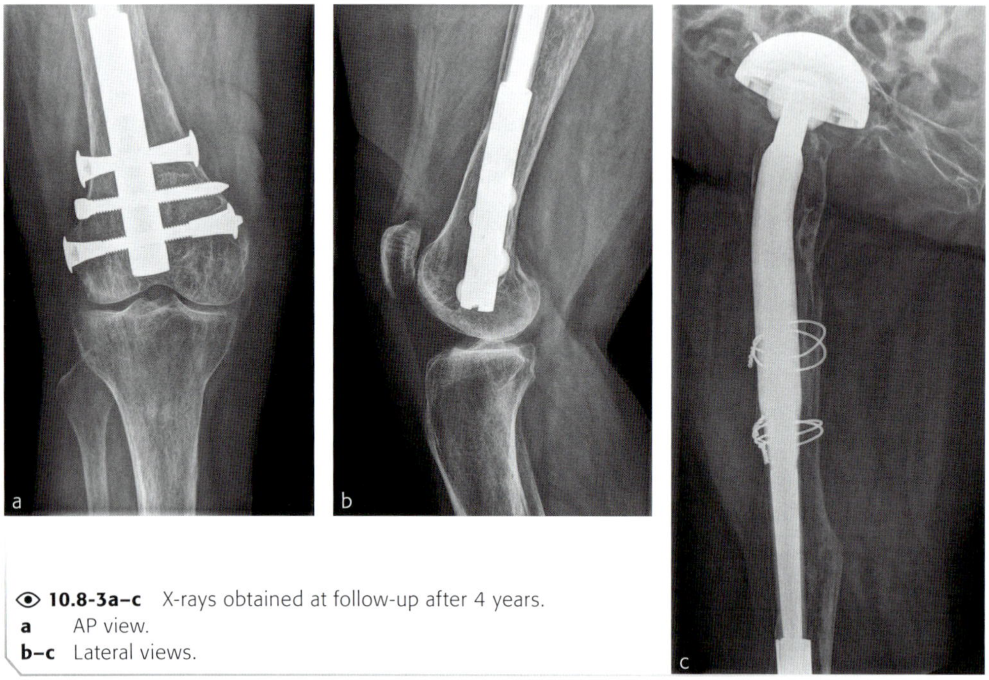

10.8-3a–c X-rays obtained at follow-up after 4 years.
a AP view.
b–c Lateral views.

Points to remember

- A retrograde nail that engages to the tip of a slender stem of a well-fixed prosthesis is the most stable internal fixation, especially in patients with osteoporosis.
- A careful, exact preoperative plan and a custom-made tubular nail that allows safe locking in the supracondylar region are required.
- The intramedullary nail and other implants used in this patient were custom-made by a local company and therefore not widely available.

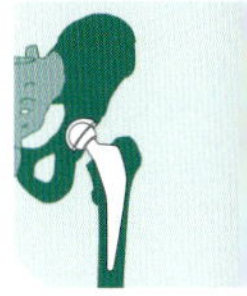

10.9 Proximal femoral fracture, stable prosthesis
ORIF: locked retrograde intramedullary nail

Author **Rutger G Zuurmond**

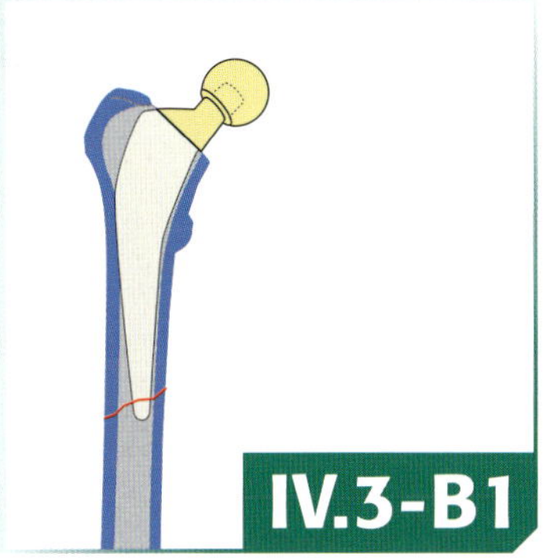

Case description

An 86-year-old woman with a cemented total hip arthroplasty for the past 12 years and comorbidities sustained a periprosthetic fracture after falling at home on her right hip (**10.9-1a–b**).

Classification: Type IV.3-B1

Diagnosis: Periprosthetic spiral fracture of the right proximal femur, with a stable prosthesis

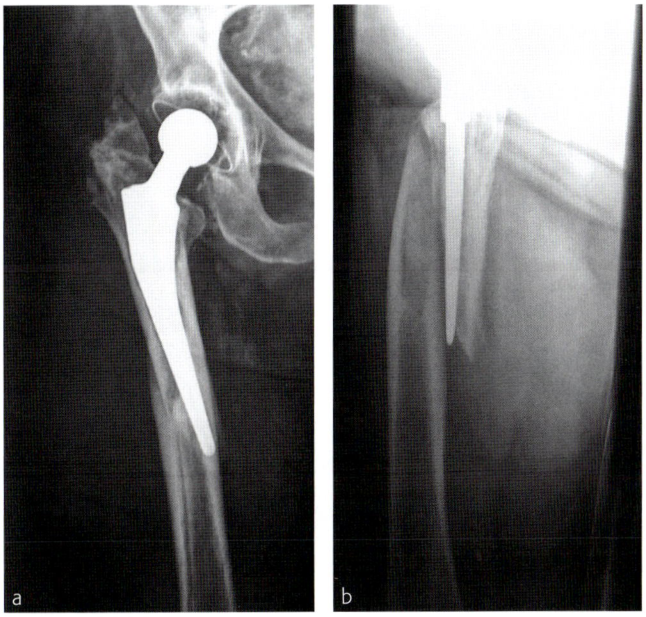

10.9-1a–b X-rays obtained shortly after the injury.
a AP view of the proximal femur shows that the prosthesis appears well fixed.
b Lateral view.

Decision making

Considering the general medical condition of the patient, the goal was to minimize the risks associated with surgery and create acceptable conditions for early mobilization. Open reduction and internal fixation with a plate was considered more problematic than a closed procedure with an intramedullary nail. To bridge the long spiral fracture and to obtain a stable junction with the stem of the prosthesis, a retrograde tubular intramedullary nail to be slipped over the tip of nail was preferred, despite considerable knee osteoarthritis (chapter 5.4.2).

IV.3-B1

Preoperative planning

Equipment

- 12 mm universal intramedullary nail (tubular and slotted), according to preoperative plan with exact measurements of the diameters of tip of the stem and nail. The nail is preoperatively prepared regarding the desired length, which is measured on the contralateral femur.
- Two 5 mm locking bolts

Patient preparation and positioning

- First- or second-generation cephalosporin for antibiotic prophylaxis
- Low-molecular-weight heparin for thrombosis prophylaxis
- Supine position with a bolster under the knee for appropriate flexion, allowing use of an image intensifier

Reduction and fixation

Closed reduction was not successful; therefore, an incision was made to reduce the fracture with a bone forceps under image intensifier control. A short incision medial to be parapatellar tendon was appropriate to expose the intercondylar notch of the distal femur (**10.9-2**). A speculum was used to protect the soft tissues and patellar tendon during insertion of the guide wire and reamers.

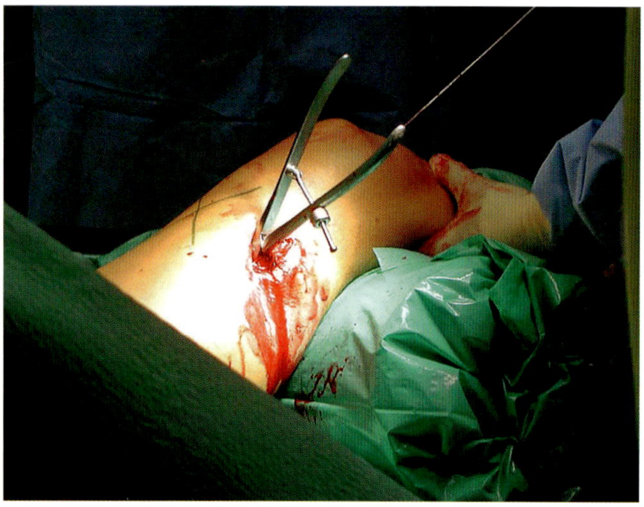

10.9-2 A small open medial approach was used to reduce the fracture and guide the intramedullary nail properly.

The medullary canal was reamed in a retrograde fashion, as far as the tip of the prosthetic stem. Any bone cement or debris was removed with a long curette. The tubular slotted intramedullary nail was inserted and engaged the prosthetic tip by gentle hammering.

Rehabilitation and follow-up

Weight bearing was allowed as tolerated after surgery. The patient was able to walk with a walking aid after 3 weeks, although remained housebound. Follow-up occurred at 3, 6, and 9 months postoperatively, with slow progress in mobility but no complications. At the 9-month follow-up, full range of motion was restored to both the hip and knee and the fracture had healed (**10.9-3a–c**).

Points to remember

- The entry point for the intramedullary nail must be in the longitudinal axis of the medullary canal. A position that is too far anterior will inhibit introduction of the intramedullary nail.
- The diameter and length of the intramedullary nail, as well as the size of the tip of the prosthetic stem, must be measured carefully.
- Any cement or debris must be removed with the drill or long curette. If the cement cannot be removed, a small lateral approach may be used to remove it.
- The nail must engage well around the tip of the stem. However, care must be taken to avoid creating a false route.
- Rigid intramedullary fixation is achieved when the nail is driven at least 3 cm over the tip of the prosthetic stem. The implant can serve as a definitive implant.
- This construction allows for early weight bearing as tolerated.
- Using only a small medial approach, blood loss and trauma will be limited.

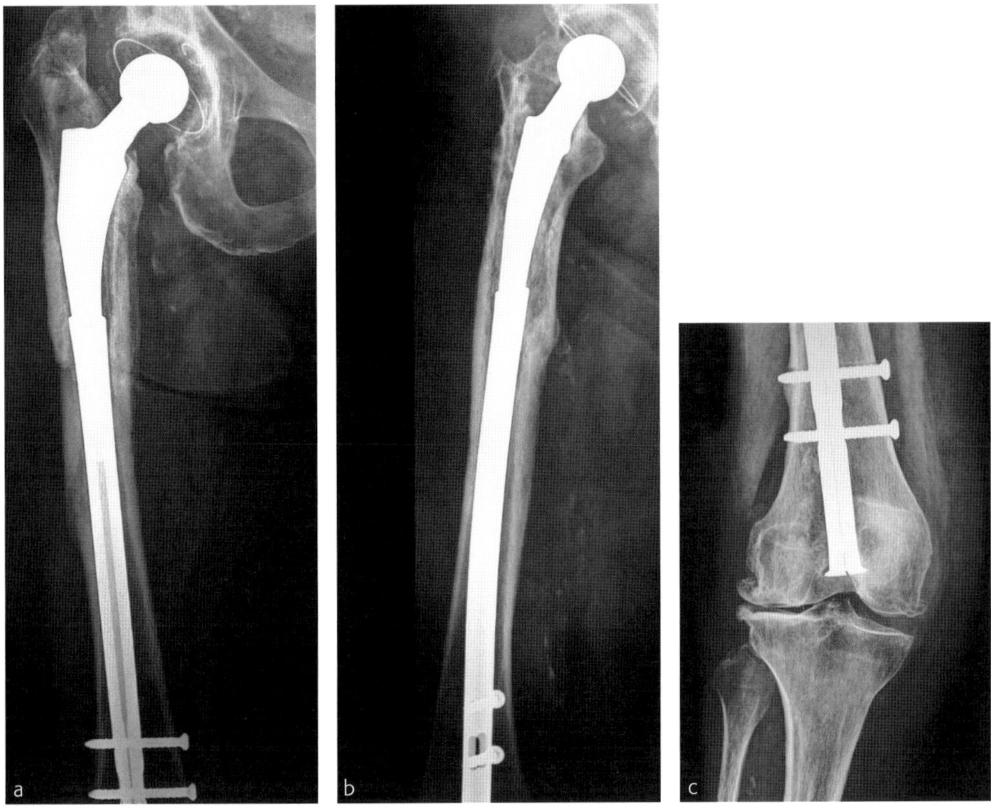

10.9-3a–c X-rays obtained 9 months postoperatively show complete union of the fracture.
- **a** AP view of the proximal femur.
- **b** Lateral view of the proximal femur.
- **c** AP view of the distal femur.

IV.3-B2

10.10 Refracture/nonunion of the proximal femur, stable prosthesis

ORIF: distal femoral locking plate

Author **William M Ricci**

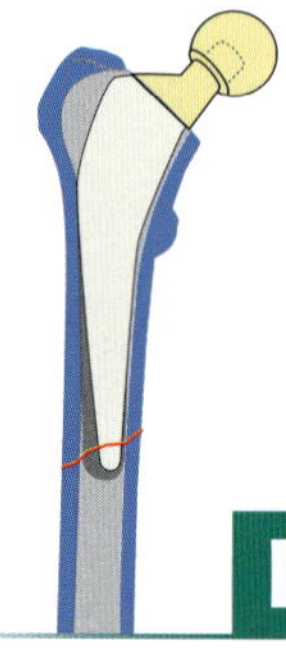

IV.3-B2

Case description

An 84-year-old woman with a previous Vancouver type B1 fracture at the tip of a hip arthroplasty stem approximately 2 years ago fell again while walking. The index open reduction and internal fixation was complicated by a nonunion and subsequent multiple revision procedures. Before her recent fall, she was ambulating with a cane with mild thigh pain. Presently, she reported increased pain, especially with weight bearing. Current x-rays showed slight angulation of the femur and evidence of multiple previous attempts at fracture fixation (👁 **10.10-1a–b**). Without comparable pre-injury x-rays, it remains unclear whether the acute fall resulted in a new fracture or, more probably, in displacement of an existing nonunion.

The patient refused further imaging studies (such as CT scan) or treatment and returned to full weight bearing. Three weeks later she returned unable to bear weight. X-rays obtained at that time confirmed a nonunion (👁 **10.10-2**) with failure of proximal fixation and varus angulation.

Classification: Type IV.3-B2

Diagnosis: Periprosthetic refracture/nonunion of the proximal femur, with a stable prosthesis

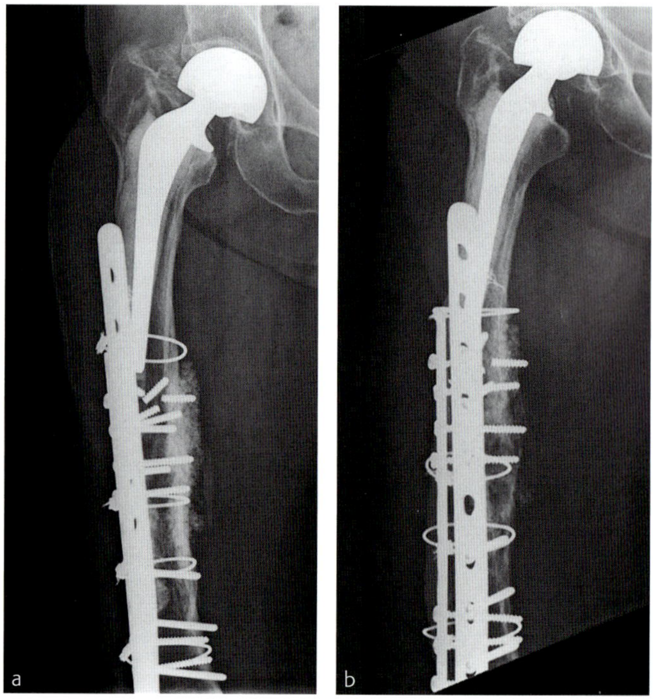

👁 **10.10-1a–b** X-rays obtained after a recent fall show evidence of multiple previous attempts at open reduction and internal fixation.
a AP view.
b Lateral view.

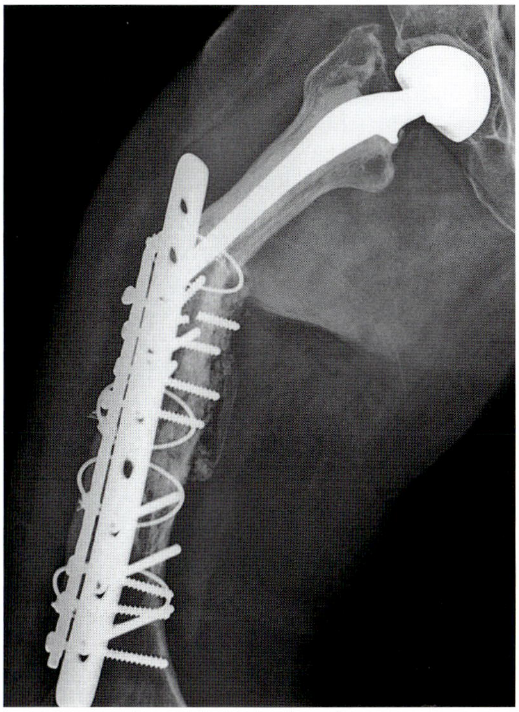

10.10-2 Oblique view x-ray showing progressive varus displacement of the fracture and nonunion. The prosthesis appears well fixed.

Decision making

This patient underwent ill-conceived prior attempts at open reduction and internal fixation of a Vancouver type B1 fracture with a well-fixed prosthesis. The basic principles of biological fracture treatment were ignored. The fixation construct provided inadequate mechanical stability proximally, despite the presence of both lateral and anterior plates. Neither plate was long enough to adequately stabilize the proximal femur that carries the prosthesis, which was clearly demonstrated by the loss of proximal fixation. As revision of the femoral component with a long-stem prosthesis and removal of all broken screws and other implants would be quite invasive, this option was not selected. An extra-long locking compression plate (LCP) was used to bridge almost the entire femur with support from a strut allograft (chapter 5.4.1).

Preoperative planning

IV.3-B2

Equipment

- 16- and 19-hole distal femur locking plate
- 4.5 mm locking-head and conventional screws
- 1.7 mm cables
- Allogenic strut graft of one third of the femur
- Acetabular reamers (for harvesting of iliac crest autograft)
- Broken-screw removal set
- Revision hip arthroplasty implants and instruments

Patient preparation and positioning

- Antibiotics (held in reserve until accurate cultures from the nonunion site are obtained)
- Low-molecular-weight heparin for thrombosis prophylaxis
- Lateral position on a radiolucent table with the entire leg and pelvis disinfected and draped

Reduction and fixation

A lateral exposure to the entire femur was used. The iliotibial band was incised longitudinally and the vastus lateralis muscle elevated off the intermuscular septum. The lateral and anterior plates were then exposed and removed. The dissection performed in this patient was more extensive than in a patient with an acute fracture because additional exposure was required to remove both plates and cerclage wires. A separate oblique incision over the iliac crest or proximal extension of the lateral thigh incision can be used to harvest iliac crest autograft.

The general principles for the treatment of nonunion were applied initially. The nonunion was taken down by removing interfering fibrous tissue without healing capacity. The stability of the hip stem was evaluated through the nonunion and found to be stable, indicating no requirement for revision arthroplasty. The bone defect at the nonunion site was then assessed and considered to be substantial enough to warrant an allogenic strut graft. An extra-long lateral LCP was used to provide the required mechanical stability, and an anterior femoral strut allograft to support the biology together with a cancellous autograft were used to fill any remaining defects in the area of the nonunion. Proximally in the zone of the hip stem, the plate was secured with multiple cables, while distally both locking-head and conventional screws were used. The strut graft also was secured with cables. The final construct was checked and appeared stable (**10.10-3**).

IV.3-B2

Rehabilitation and follow-up

Toe-touch weight bearing was recommended for 8 weeks, followed by increasing load, based on radiological and clinical signs of healing. At 6 months postoperatively, the patient ambulated at full weight bearing, and x-rays confirmed healing of the nonunion and progressive incorporation of the allograft (**10.10-4a–b**). At the final follow-up at 1 year, the reduction was maintained and the allograft completely incorporated (**10.10-5**).

Points to remember

- If a periprosthetic B1 fracture is fixed with a plate, the plate must reach at least 4–5 cm above the tip of the prosthetic stem to prevent refracture or nonunion.
- Fixation around the stem can be done with short locking-head screws, cerclage wires, cables, or the locking attachment plate (chapter 5.4.1).
- Care must be taken when applying cables to avoid stripping the periosteum circumferentially. Exclusive use of monocortical locking-head screws in the zone of the hip implant may be insufficient. When monocortical screws are used, the fixation should be supplemented with either cables or bicortical screws placed around the hip stem.
- A distal femoral LCP, long enough to span the entire length of the femur to protect against future fractures at or near the end of the plate, could be used. In this patient, a 19-hole distal femoral locking plate provided an anatomical preshape for the curved shaft and distal femur that makes the plate especially useful as a reduction aid. A tabletop bending press was used to further contour the plate to fit the trochanteric anatomy.
- Whenever a plate and a strut graft are used in concert, separate cables that independently secure each are preferred. This way, a loose cable will affect only one aspect of the fixation construct.
- A careful examination of the hip stem is warranted. Synovial fluid emanating from the fracture or nonunion site from around the stem is evidence of stem loosening with or without infection.

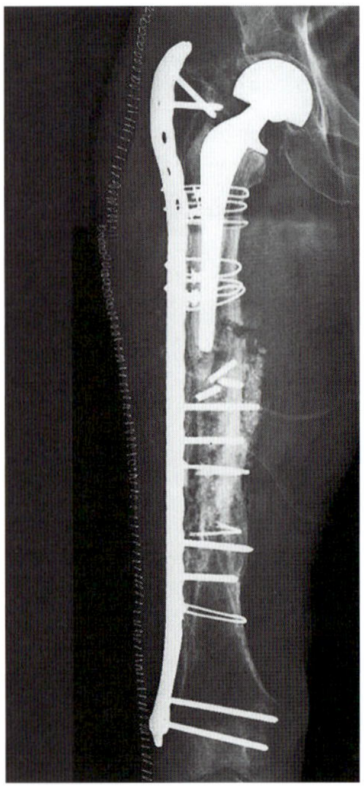

10.10-3 AP x-ray obtained immediately after reconstruction and fixation of the nonunion with a long locking plate and strut grafts.

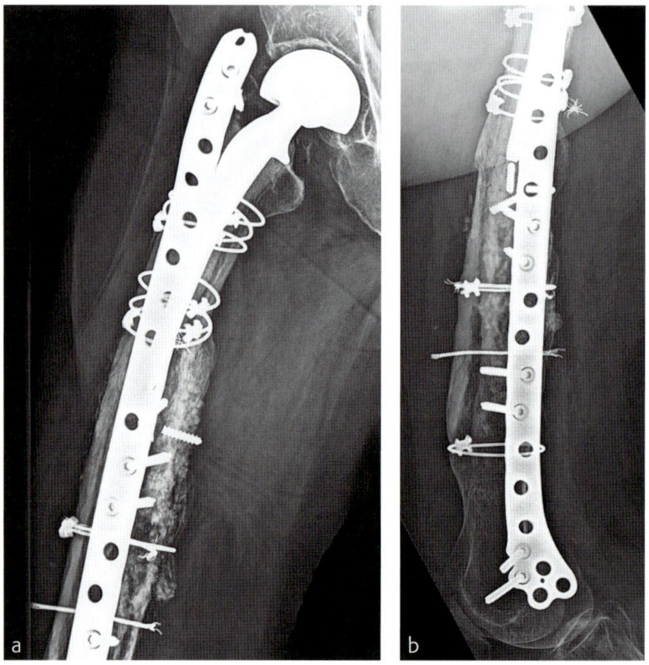

10.10-4a–b X-rays obtained 6 months postoperatively show a healed nonunion and progressive incorporation of the allograft strut.
a AP view.
b Lateral view.

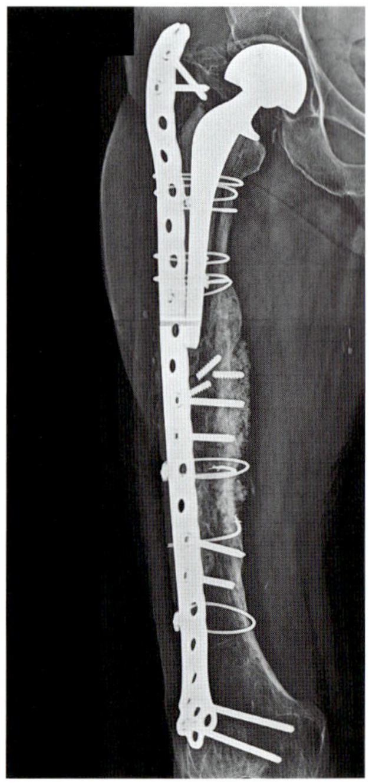

10.10-5 AP x-ray obtained at final follow-up 1 year postoperatively shows a healed nonunion, maintained alignment, and complete incorporation of the allograft.

10.11 Multifragmentary segmental femoral fracture, apparently stable prosthesis

ORIF: locked retrograde intramedullary nail with cerclage bands

Authors **Christof Meyer, Reinhard Schnettler**

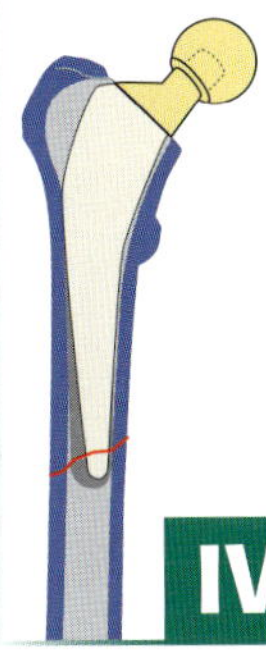

IV.3-B2(C)

Case description

A 77-year-old man sustained a comminuted segmental periprosthetic fracture of the left femur (**10.11-1a–c**) and an ipsilateral open fracture of the lower leg with severe soft-tissue damage as a result of a scooter accident. The patient also had a history of diabetes mellitus, arteriosclerosis, coronary heart disease, and cardiac insufficiency.

Classification: Type IV.3- B2(C)

Diagnosis: Comminuted, segmental periprosthetic femoral fracture after total hip arthroplasty, with an apparently well-fixed femoral component

Decision making

A variety of treatment options were considered for fixation of this patient's segmental comminuted femoral fracture: plate osteosynthesis, retrograde intramedullary nailing, and external fixation. This decision was complicated by the fact that the salvage of the lower leg was questionable. Revision arthroplasty with a custom-made long-stem prosthesis and transfemoral amputation were alternative treatment options.

Primary amputation without fixation was not appropriate because the resulting amputation stump would be extremely short, making prosthetic care difficult. Revision arthroplasty was not considered because of the open fracture and serious soft-tissue damage in the lower leg.

External fixation was not favored because of insufficient stability, as well as the expected time required for bony consolidation (discomfort and soft-tissue problems).

Thus, internal fixation with retrograde intramedullary nailing was preferred to plating because of its increased stability and its less invasive technique, which would prevent additional soft-tissue damage (chapter 5.4.2). Furthermore, there was a high risk that the concomitant open fracture of the lower leg could result in a secondary amputation. Therefore, the aim was to achieve a situation that would still allow early prosthetic care.

CT scans were used to ascertain the stability of the prosthetic component and the length of the femur and diameter of the medullar canal in the contralateral leg. Based on this data, a custom-made intramedullary nail was manufactured.

Preoperative planning

Equipment

- Hollow slotted, retrograde, custom-made femoral nail, and two transverse distal locking holes
- Corresponding locking nail system

Patient preparation and positioning

- Supine position without use of a traction table
- Knee positioned in 60° of flexion

IV.3-B2(C)

Reduction and fixation

By a classical approach through the knee, the medullary canal was opened and the distal fragments were drilled up to 15 mm. The proximal fracture was exposed and any remaining cement removed. The tip of the prosthesis was then cleared of adherent cement and bone fragments for a length of approximately 4 cm. Finally, the custom-made intramedullary nail was inserted in a retrograde manner and coupled to the tip of the prosthesis under visual control; the bony sleeve was reconstructed with two metal bands (**10.11-2**). Distally, the fixation was completed with two locking bolts.

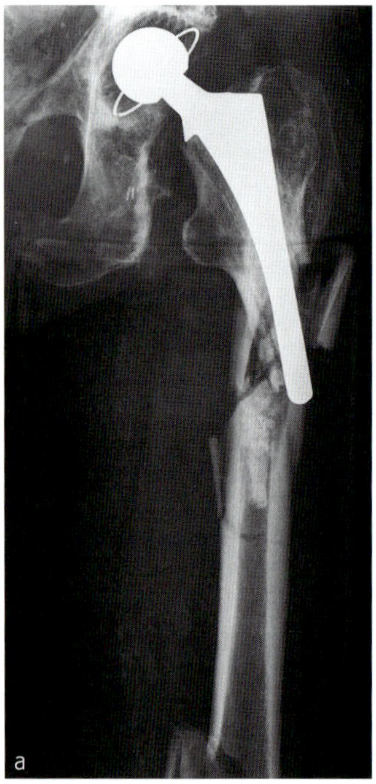

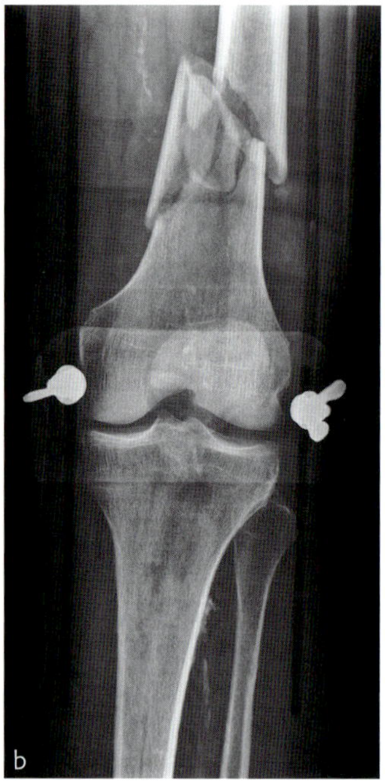

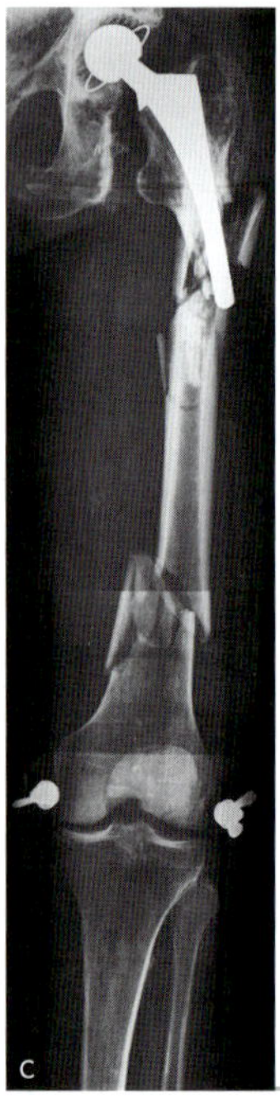

10.11-1a–c X-rays show a comminuted segmental periprosthetic fracture of the proximal femur.

- **a** AP view shows that the proximal femoral prosthetic component appears radiologically well fixed despite comminution.
- **b** AP view of the distal femur shows a second comminuted fracture.
- **c** View of the entire femur shows the segmental fracture.

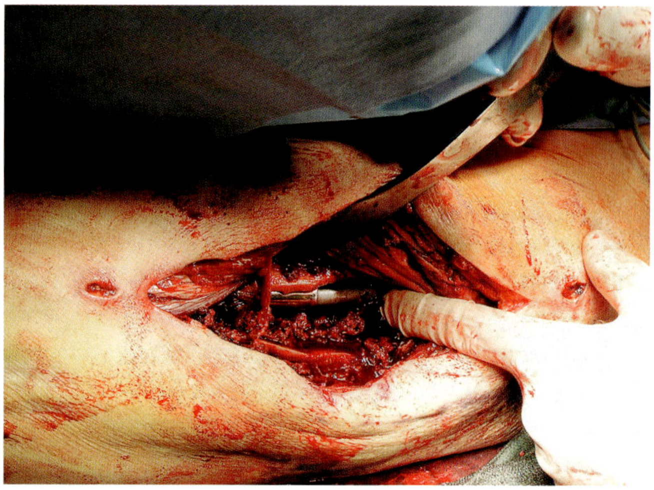

10.11-2 Intraoperative coupling of the custom-made intramedullary nail to the tip of the prosthesis before the fractured bony sleeve is closed and fixed with metal bands.

Rehabilitation and follow-up

Wound healing was uneventful; however, 6 weeks postoperatively the severe open fracture of the lower leg required amputation due to uncontrollable soft-tissue problems and infection. After 3 months, the patient could walk independently with a limb prosthesis using a walker. At the 9-month follow-up, x-rays showed complete consolidation of the distal femur, while proximally some callus formation was visible (**10.11-3a–d**).

Points to remember

- In this patient who, ultimately, required a through-knee amputation, intramedullary stabilization allowed for early fitting of an artificial limb.
- As an alternative to a long-stem revision prosthesis, an extension of the prosthesis with a retrograde nail is possible in severely comminuted periprosthetic fractures.
- Such in-situ extension of the prosthesis allows mobilization under full weight bearing earlier than after plate osteosynthesis.
- In patients with comminuted fractures, length and diameter of the bone can be measured with CT of the contralateral leg.
- In cases of nonunion, infection, or severe soft-tissue complications, primary amputation must be carefully considered.

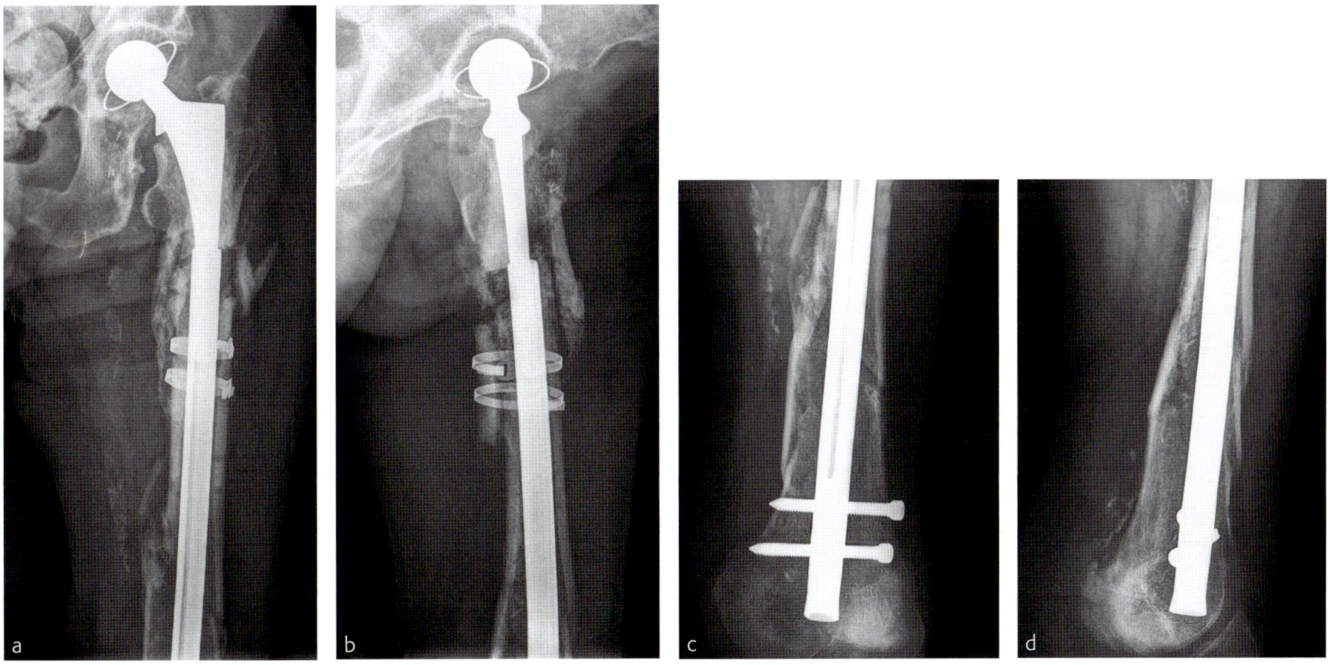

10.11-3a–d X-rays show the extended prosthesis with the distally locked retrograde intramedullary nail. Fracture consolidation occurred at 9 months. At 6 weeks the lower leg had to be amputated.

a AP view of the proximal femur shows some callus formation.
b Lateral view of the proximal femur.
c AP view of the distal femur shows a well-consolidated fracture.
d Lateral view of the distal femur.

IV.3-B2

10.12 Proximal femoral fracture, loose prosthesis

Revision: arthroplasty with allograft and cable plate

Author **Christopher Morrey**

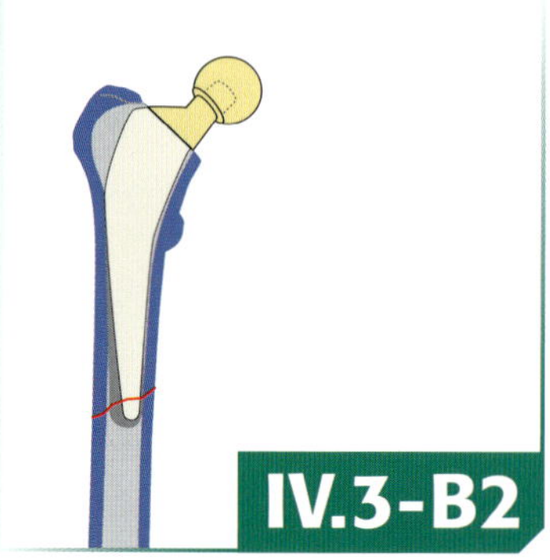

Case description

A 76-year-old woman with previous revision total hip arthroplasty of the right hip fell in the bathroom (**10.12-1a–b**).

Classification: Type IV.3-B2

Diagnosis: Periprosthetic fracture of the right proximal femur with a loose and protruding stem

Decision making

Simple fixation of the femoral shaft was not considered adequate because the femoral prosthesis was loose and protruding distally. The best solution to this problem was a revision arthroplasty of both components as the cup also seemed loose (chapter 5.5). Because the patient also had poor bone stock, this construct was combined with an allograft strut and a cable plate. The acetabulum was planned to be revised to a noncemented component.

Preoperative planning

A preoperative drawing was made depicting the prosthesis and fracture line extending to approximately 260 mm distal to the tip of the trochanter. This required a prosthesis of at least 290 mm in length to obtain two cortical diameters below the fracture line. The cable plate needed to be at least 160 mm long to span the fracture site.

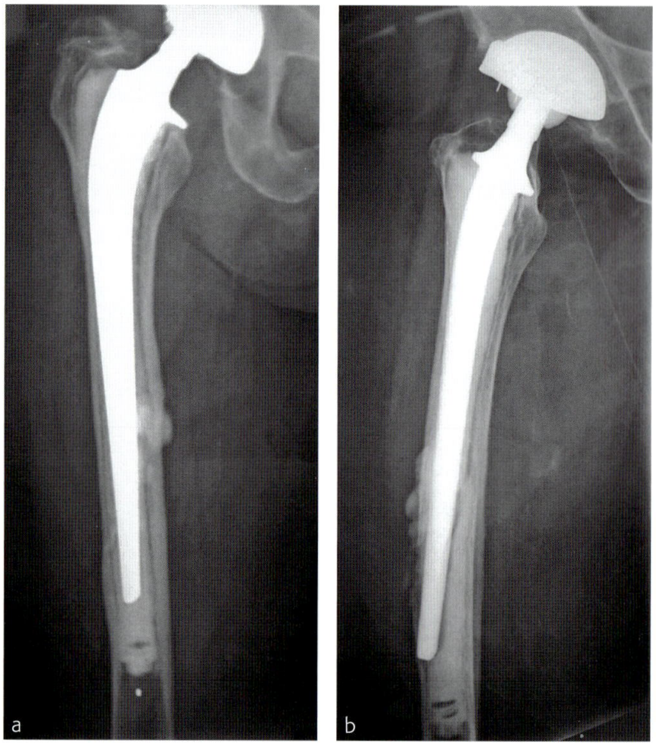

10.12-1a–b X-rays obtained shortly after the injury, displaying the protrusion of the tip of the loose prosthesis.
a AP view.
b Lateral view.

Equipment

- 8-hole cable plate
- Cables and tensioner
- Whole-tibia allograft to cut the strut
- Noncemented 16 × 290 mm prosthetic stem
- 56–58 mm noncemented R3 Acetabular Cup® with 36 mm liner

Patient preparation and positioning

- 2 g intravenous cephalothin for antibiotic prophylaxis
- Compression stockings and sequential compression devices for deep vein thrombosis prophylaxis
- 1,000 IU intravenous heparin (upon reaming of the femoral canal)
- Right lateral decubitus position

Reduction and fixation

A curved lateral incision was made through the previous scar and extended distally along the line of the femur. The posterior approach to the hip joint was used, staying on the bone to protect the sciatic nerve. A lateral approach to the midshaft and distal femur was used to access the femur.

The femoral prosthesis was easily removed, and any residual cement was removed through the fracture site. The loose acetabular prosthesis was removed and replaced by a noncemented prosthesis with two screws for added rotational stability. The intact distal femoral shaft was then reamed to the diameter required for the definitive prosthesis. A trial prosthesis 4 mm smaller in diameter was inserted into the shaft, and the fracture was reduced around the temporary trial prosthesis in situ (👁 **10.12-2**). The cable plate and allograft were applied at 90° to each other, and the cables were tensioned to the maximum. This trial construct was then reduced with a trial head in situ.

After removal of the trial prosthesis, the proximal canal was broached and the definitive prosthesis inserted. Retensioning of the cables can be performed, if necessary.

Rehabilitation and follow-up

IV.3-B2

Toe-touch weight bearing was allowed for the first 8 weeks postoperatively. Partial to full weight bearing was then introduced over the next 4 weeks. Prophylaxis for deep vein thrombosis continued with use of compression stockings and oral aspirin for 6 weeks postoperatively. Follow-up x-rays obtained 1 year postoperatively showed fracture union and incorporation of the allograft (👁 **10.12-3a–b**). The patient could ambulate independently around her home but used a walking frame when outdoors.

Points to remember

- The sciatic nerve may be damaged during the approach. Therefore, staying on the bone during dissection of the external rotators and capsule is necessary to protect it. Another option is to find healthy tissue either above or below the previous surgical dissection and then trace the nerve along its course, but this option also puts the nerve at risk.
- Soft-tissue stripping of bone fragments can occur with an extended lateral approach; thus, soft-tissue dissection must be kept to a minimum.
- The cable plate needs to be contoured while maintaining reduction, and fixation is done with the temporary prosthesis in situ.
- A burr is used to smooth the edges of the allograft, which will ensure cortical contact of the allograft to the side of the femoral shaft.
- The cable plate has to be secured first, followed by the allograft to ensure equal tension and fixation of both constructs.
- Retensioning of the cables once the definitive prosthesis is inserted allows adjustments to be made to tensioning the overall construct, preventing both premature loosening of the construct and subsequent subsidence of prosthesis, which is an advantage.

IV.3-B2

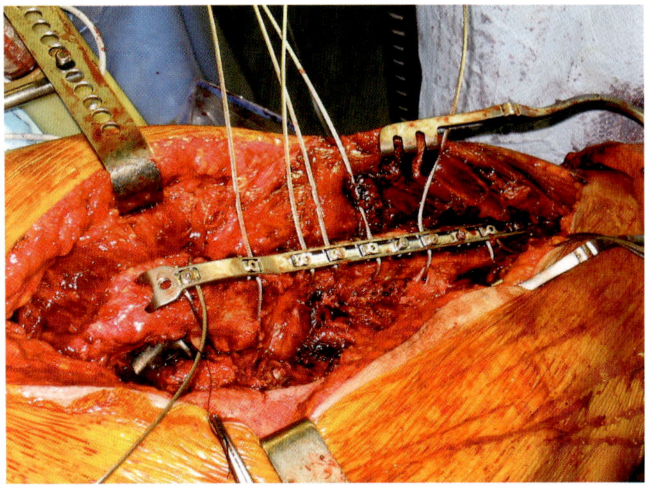

10.12-2 Reduction of a periprosthetic fracture of the femur over a temporary prosthesis. The cable plate and strut graft were then applied and preliminarily tensioned.

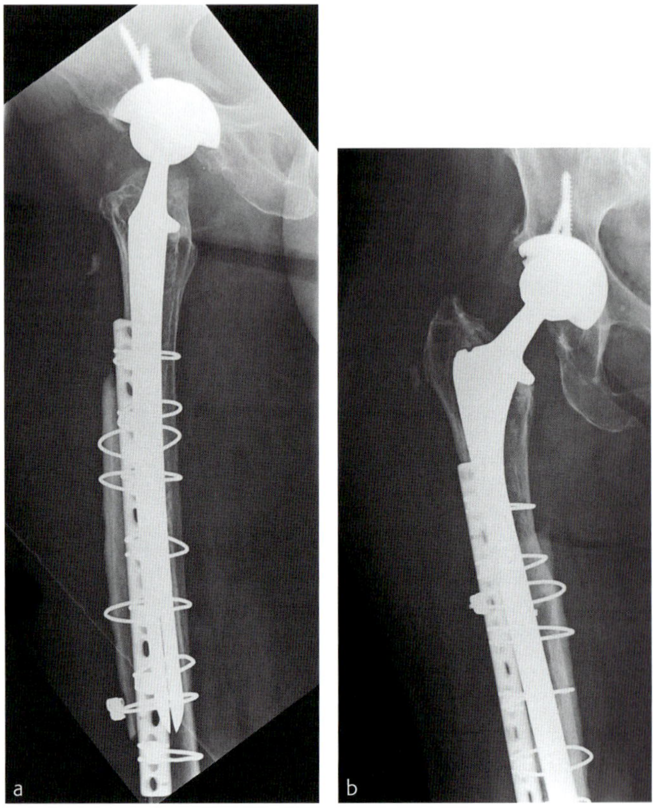

10.12-3a–b X-rays obtained 1 year postoperatively.
a AP view.
b Lateral view.

10.13 Subtrochanteric fracture, loose prosthesis

Revision: arthroplasty with cerclage wires and corticocancellous autograft

Author **Takeshi Sawaguchi**

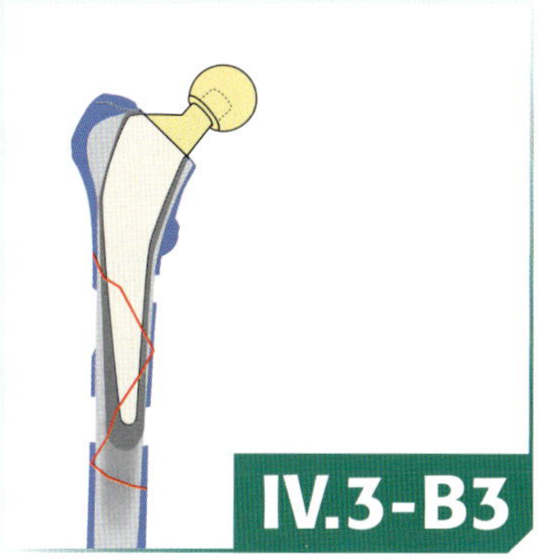

Case description

A 77-year-old woman, who presented with pain in the right thigh and no history of trauma, underwent cemented total hip arthroplasty 4.5 years ago for osteoarthritis at another hospital. She now had severe osteolysis of the proximal femur with a cement fracture and stem loosening. Current x-rays showed that the stem also had subsided significantly compared with the postoperative x-ray of the index procedure (**10.13-1a–c**).

Classification: Type IV.3-B3

Diagnosis: Periprosthetic fracture of the proximal femur, with a loose prosthetic stem

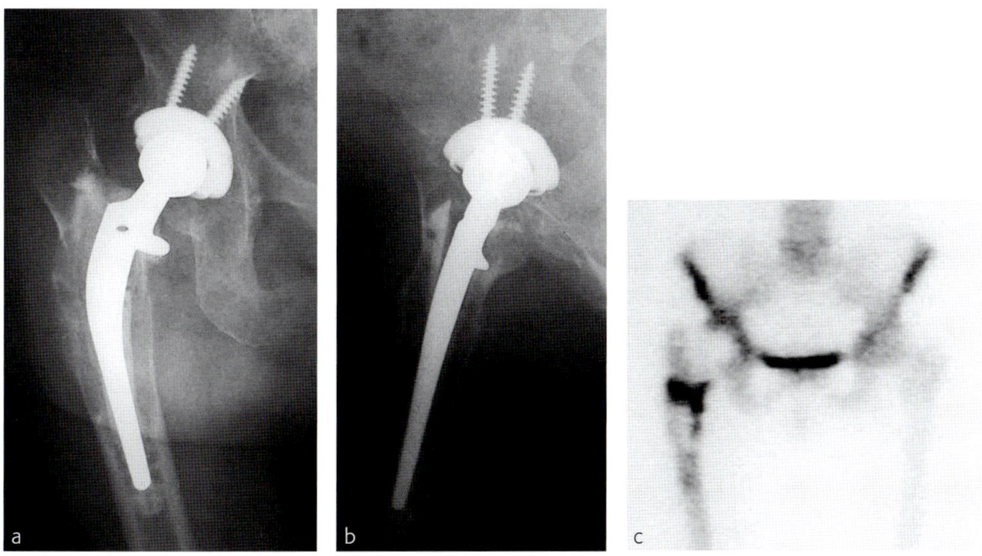

10.13-1a–c Severe osteolysis of the proximal femur with a cement fracture and stem loosening. Note the significant subsidence compared with that in the postoperative x-ray of the index procedure.
a AP view.
b Lateral view.
c Bone scan.

Decision making

IV.3-B3

The patient had severe osteolysis of the proximal femur with significant stem subsidence, loosening, and cement fracture, as well as a simple transverse fracture in the subtrochanteric area. The patient required revision of the prosthesis together with reconstruction of the bone stock of the proximal femur (chapter 5.5).

Treatment options included impaction allograft with a long-stem cemented prosthesis, a structural allograft with a long-stem cemented prosthesis, autograft for the proximal femur with a long-stem cemented prosthesis, and tumor prosthesis. Since allograft was not available at that time in the hospital, then autograft for the proximal femur with a cemented long-stem prosthesis was chosen.

Preoperative planning

Equipment

- Long-stem cemented prosthesis
- Cerclage wires
- Greater trochanter grip device

Patient preparation and positioning

- First- or second-generation cephalosporin for antibiotic prophylaxis
- Low-molecular-weight heparin for thrombosis prophylaxis
- Lateral decubitus position

Reduction and fixation

A large full-thickness corticocancellous bone graft was first harvested from the contralateral iliac crest. The defect in the ilium was restored with hydroxyapatite bone substitute.

With the patient in a lateral decubitus position, a transfemoral approach was used, extending from the greater trochanter to the distal end of the prosthetic stem. Careful attention was required to preserve the soft-tissue attachment to the thin eggshell-like cortex of the proximal femur.

The loose femoral prosthesis and cement were easily removed. The cup insert was also removed, and cup stability was tested after removal of the screws. The cup was considered stable and well fixed even without screws, so only the cup insert was exchanged. The soft tissue inside the proximal femur was completely removed with curettage. A long-stem revision prosthesis was fixed distally with cement after adjusting to the correct length of the lower extremity. The corticocancellous autograft was packed around the proximal part of the prosthesis and around the osteotomy site. To secure the closed cortical shell, three cerclage wires were applied. The greater trochanter was fixed with a cable grip system. Careful attention was paid to preserve the soft-tissue attachment to the thin cortex. The postoperative result was verified radiologically (**10.13-2**).

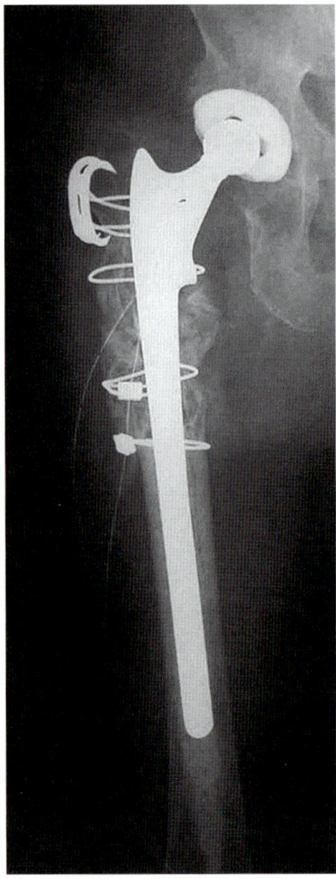

10.13-2 The AP x-ray obtained postoperatively shows the stem well fixed with cement distally. The proximal femoral canal was filled with autogenous corticocancellous bone. The thin cortex was fixed with three cerclage wires, and the greater trochanter attached with a cable grip system.

The histology of the tissue around the stem showed lacunae with numerous polymethylmethacrylate particles. These particles were produced by the matte-finished surface of the stem (👁 **10.13-3**), abrading the cement around the stem. The particles were a likely cause of early loosening of the femoral component and severe osteolysis, which finally resulted in subsidence of the prosthesis and the fatigue fracture of the subtrochanteric femur.

Rehabilitation and follow-up

Partial weight bearing was allowed after 4 weeks, increasing after 10 weeks to full weight bearing at 6 months. At the 1-year follow-up, the patient could walk with a cane and perform the activities of daily living independently. An x-ray obtained at this time showed union of the fracture and the osteotomy (👁 **10.13-4a**). Partial restoration of the bone stock of the proximal femur also was observed. Two years postoperatively, x-rays showed good restoration of the bone stock of the proximal femur and the internal bone structure, except for slight proximal migration of the greater trochanter, although it was united (👁 **10.13-4b**). Even 13 years later, there were no signs of implant loosening (👁 **10.13-4c**). IV.3-B3

Points to remember

- Spontaneous fractures or fatigue fractures can occur in the subtrochanteric area in which patients usually are asymptomatic prior to the fracture.
- Subsequent radiological follow-up and early detection of severe osteolysis before the fracture event are essential.
- Early revision in progressive osteolysis is recommended.
- Extensive soft-tissue dissection around the bone may cause nonunion and implant failure. Preservation of the soft-tissue attachment to the bone is critical to preserve the blood supply.
- Gradual weight bearing helps restore internal bone structure.
- In selected cases, autogenous corticocancellous bone may be used instead of an allograft, if the latter is not available.

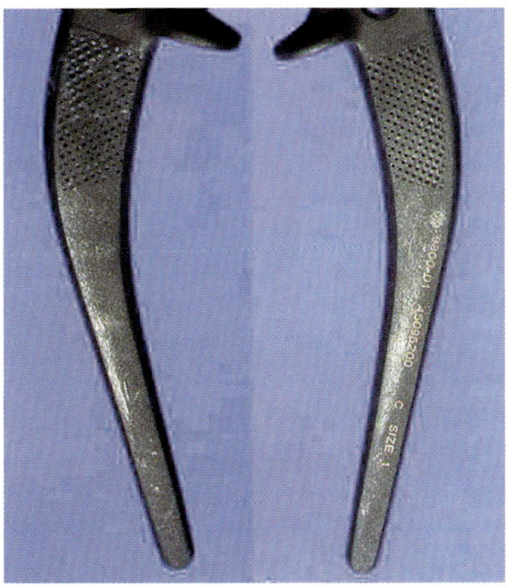

👁 **10.13-3** Retrieved implant with a matte-finished surface that abraded bone cement, creating a large volume of polymethylmethacrylate particles that eventually led to severe osteolysis and early loosening.

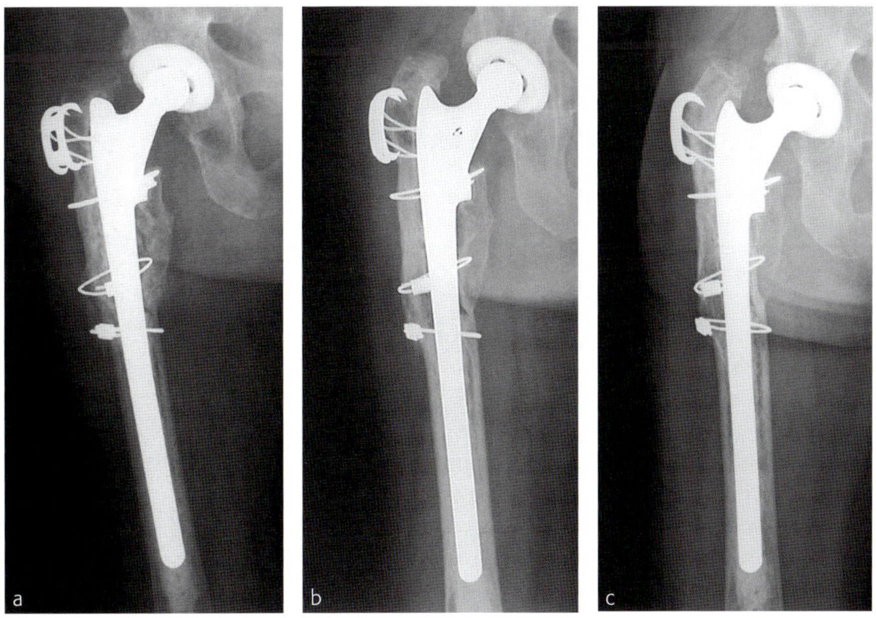

👁 **10.13-4a–c** Follow-up x-rays.

a AP view at 1 year shows fracture union of the osteotomy, and partial restoration of the bone stock.

b AP view at 2 years shows good restoration of bone stock of the proximal femur, as well as restoration of the internal bone structure except for slight proximal migration of the greater trochanter.

c AP view at 13 years shows continued good restoration of bone stock of the proximal femur and no sign of implant loosening.

IV.3-B3

10.14 Multifragmentary proximal femoral fracture, loose prosthesis

Revision: new femoral component, impaction grafting, steel mesh, bridging plate

Author **Emilio Fantin**

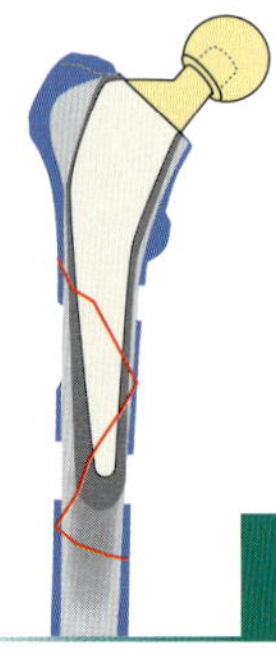

IV.3-B3

Case description

A 64-year-old man with dementia who presented with pain in the right hip after falling from a step at home had undergone total hip arthroplasty 14 years ago. X-rays showed a complex fracture of the proximal femur with apparent loosening of the cemented stem (👁 **10.14-1**).

Classification: Type IV.3-B3

Diagnosis: Compex periprosthetic fracture of the proximal femur, with a loose prosthesis

Decision making

Due to the loose prosthetic stem and bone deficiency at the proximal femur, the only treatment option was a revision procedure combining a long-stem prosthesis with fixation of the complex fracture (chapter 5.5). The goal was to achieve a construct that would allow immediate full weight bearing.

The femoral component had to be exchanged for a device with a longer stem, which has to be compatible with the acetabular cup. A long bridging locking compression plate (LCP) was selected to fix the fracture. To improve the bone stock impaction grafting with fresh frozen allograft was planned, to be held in place with a steel mesh.

Preoperative planning

Equipment

- Instruments to remove the prosthesis and cement
- Instruments for revision of the femoral component to a long-stem device
- Instruments and implants for locking compression plating
- Fresh-frozen allograft bone
- Steel mesh and wires
- Two doses of polymethylmethacrylate bone cement
- Image intensifier intraoperatively

Patient preparation and positioning

- Lateral position on a conventional table
- General anesthesia

Reduction and fixation

After removal of the loose femoral component and cement in the proximal femur, the fracture fragments were reduced and held in place with the steel mesh and cerclage wires. The femoral canal was filled with allogenic bone chips using an impaction technique. After testing the correct position of the 22 cm long prosthesis, a resorbable cement stopper was placed into the medullary canal. The bone cement was then introduced, followed by insertion of the prosthesis. To stabilize the construct, a long bridging LCP was added after reduction of the prosthesis and then fixed with locking-head screws proximally and distally of the prosthesis (👁 **10.14-2a–b**).

Rehabilitation and follow-up

The patient was confined to bed for the first 7 days postoperatively because of his mental state. He was then allowed to start walking with full weight bearing. He did not report any pain, and his ability to walk gradually improved. At the 6-month follow-up, he was doing well and living in an institution for geriatric patients (**10.14-3**).

Points to remember

- Use of cemented implants is an option in older, low-demand patients only. When a cemented stem is used, additional bone grafting increases the stability of the bone-cement interface.
- In patients with type B3 fractures with a loose femoral component, the only possibility for salvage is revision with a long-stem prosthesis.
- With inadequate stability of the prosthesis or fragments, additional osteosynthesis (eg, bridge plating) is mandatory.
- A metal mesh can be applied before the cement and prosthesis are inserted to hold the reduced fragments and bone graft in place.
- The prosthetic stem must reach across the fracture, and the bridging plate should be much longer than the stem.

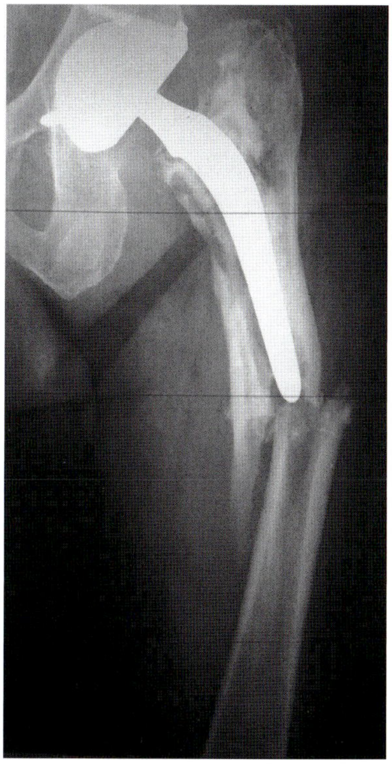

10.14-1 AP view shows a complex fracture of the proximal femur with evident loosening of the femoral component of the total hip arthroplasty and possible bone deficiencies.

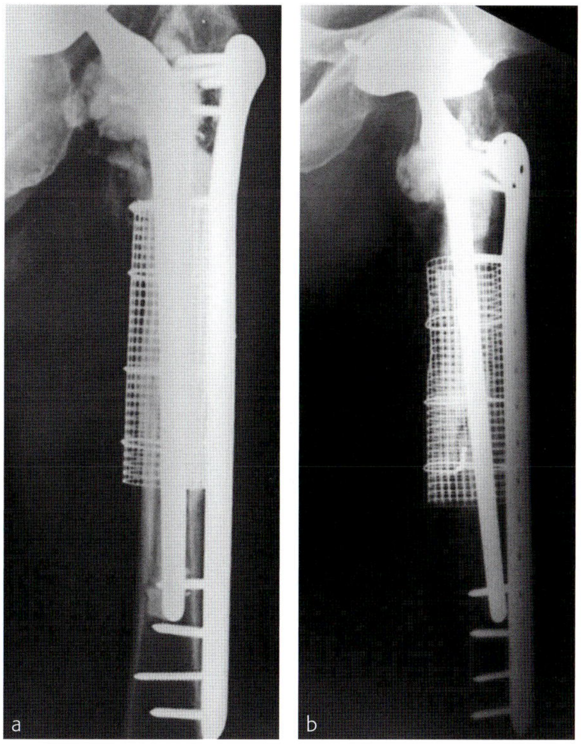

10.14-2a–b Postoperative x-rays show a long locking compression plate protecting the fixation of the newly placed femoral prosthesis. The steel mesh serves to hold the fragments and grafts in place.

a AP view.
b Lateral view.

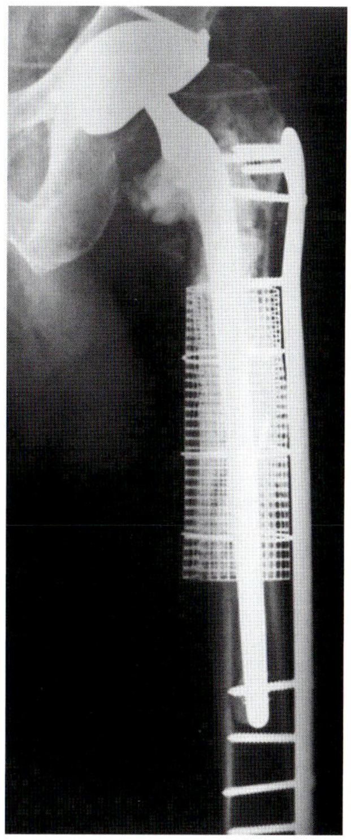

10.14-3 X-ray obtained 6 months postoperatively shows signs of fracture consolidation.

IV.3-C

10.15 Femoral butterfly fracture distal to stable prosthesis

MIPO: lag screws and LCP 4.5/5.0 distal femur

Author **Rodrigo Pesantez**

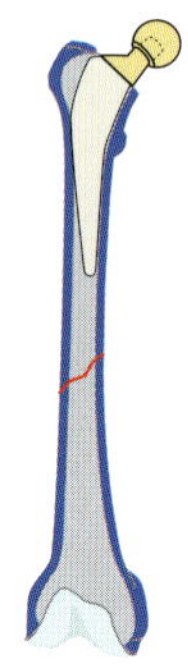

IV.3-C

Case description

An 80-year-old woman with severe osteoporosis sustained an intertrochanteric fracture after a fall from standing height. She was initially treated with closed reduction and an intramedullary nail (trochanteric femoral nail). A few weeks postoperatively, the spiral blade cut out and the intramedullary nail was replaced with a cemented bipolar arthroplasty. Almost 2 years later, the patient fell again from standing height, sustaining a spiral fracture with a large butterfly fragment distal to the cemented and well-fixed arthroplasty (👁 **10.15-1a–b**).

Classification: Type IV.3-C

Diagnosis: Periprosthetic butterfly fracture of the femur distal to the stable implant

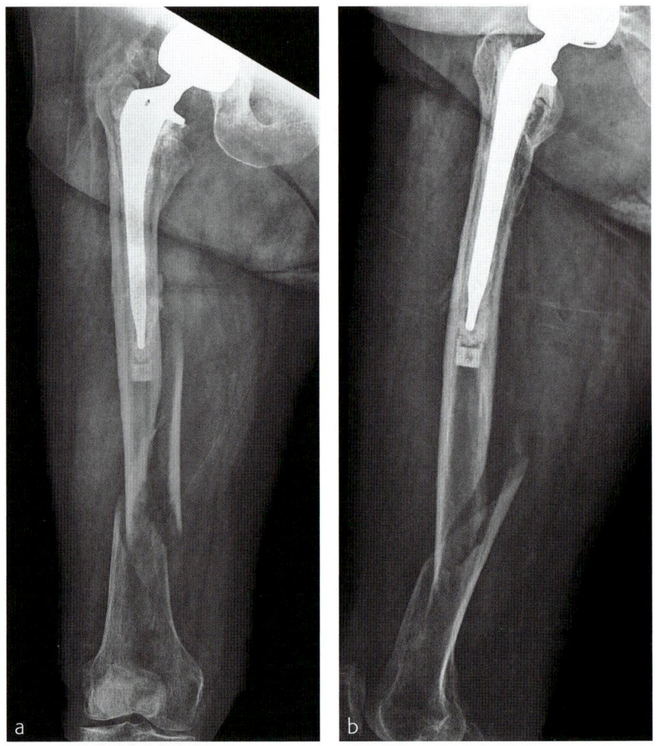

👁 **10.15-1a–b** X-rays show a periprosthetic type C spiral fracture with a large butterfly fragment distal to the cemented stem.

a AP view.
b Lateral view.

Decision making

In view of the patient's considerable history, specifically three previous interventions, severe osteoporosis, and the current injury, the best treatment option appeared to be fixation that spans the fracture zone and overlaps the prosthesis, thereby avoiding additional fracture. A long bridging locking compression plate (LCP) (chapter 5.4.1) extending from the femoral condyles to the tip of the trochanter seemed appropriate.

Preoperative planning

Equipment

- Distal femoral LCP or less invasive stabilization system (LISS)
- 7.3/5.0 mm locking-head screw
- 4.5 mm cortex screws
- 3.5 mm cortex screws

Patient preparation and positioning

- Supine position on a radiolucent table with a bolster under the ipsilateral buttock
- First- or second-generation cephalosporin for antibiotic prophylaxis
- Low-molecular-weight heparin for thrombosis prophylaxis

Reduction and fixation

Three separate lateral incisions (trochanter, fracture focus, and femoral condyles) were made in line with the femur. Open reduction was performed with manual traction and placement of bone forceps under image intensification. Several independent lag screws were then inserted to hold the fracture reduction, which due to the poor bone stock was neither easy nor perfect. After a submuscular tunnel was prepared from distal to proximal, the 16-hole distal femur LCP was inserted, bridging the fracture zone. The plate was centered through the proximal incision to the greater trochanter. Distal fixation was secured with locking-head screws, whereas proximally fixation was secured with well-spaced, 4.5 mm cortex screws at different angles to avoid the prosthesis. Postoperative x-rays were obtained (👁 **10.15-2a–b**).

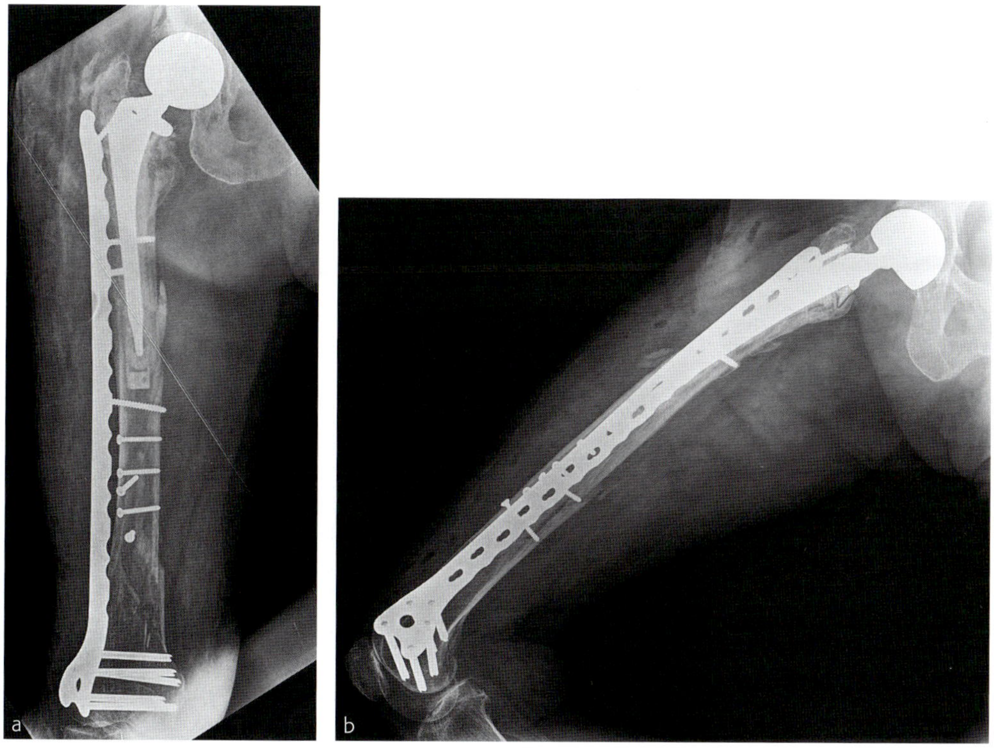

👁 **10.15-2a–b** X-rays obtained immediately postoperatively show lag screw fixation of the fracture and the long 16-hole plate spanning the femur from the condyles to the greater trochanter.
a AP view.
b Lateral view.

IV.3-C Rehabilitation and follow-up

Immediate physiotherapy was initiated to restore hip and knee motion. Partial weight bearing for 6 weeks was advised with progression to full weight bearing at 12 weeks. Prophylaxis for deep vein thrombosis included low-molecular-weight heparin for 35 days and compression stockings. Follow-up occurred at 3, 6, and 12 weeks, 6 months, and 1 year (**10.15-3a–e**). Two years postoperatively, the patient could perform all activities of daily living independently (**10.15-4a–b**).

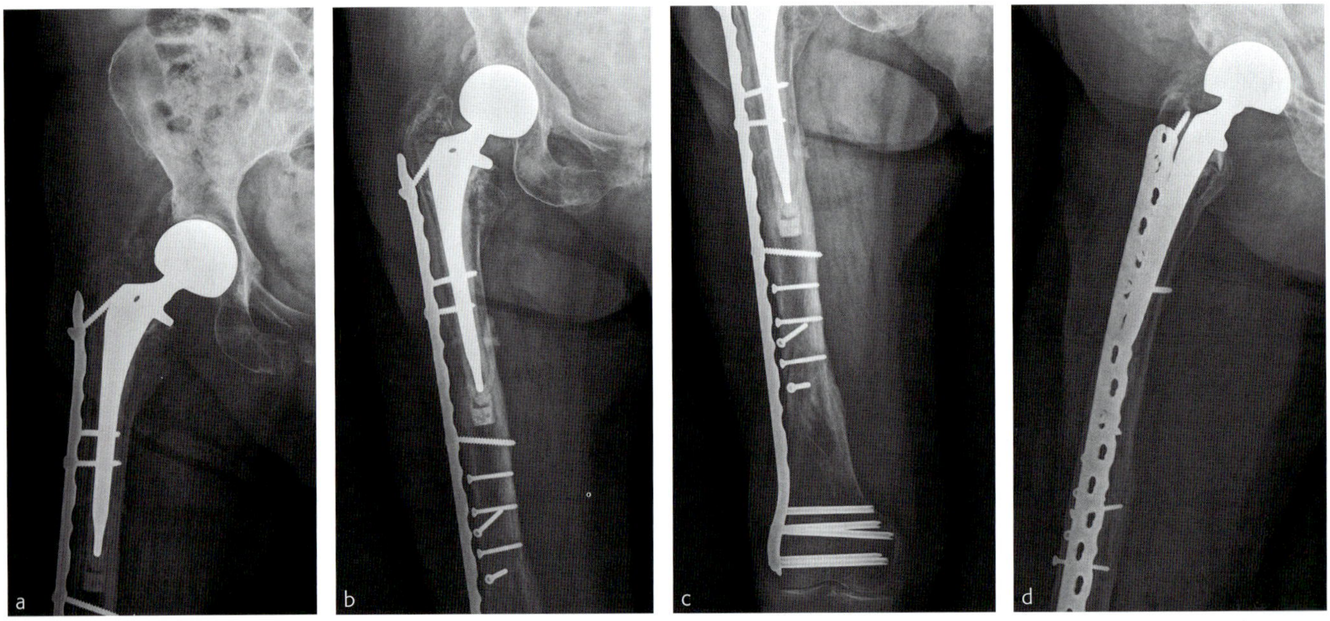

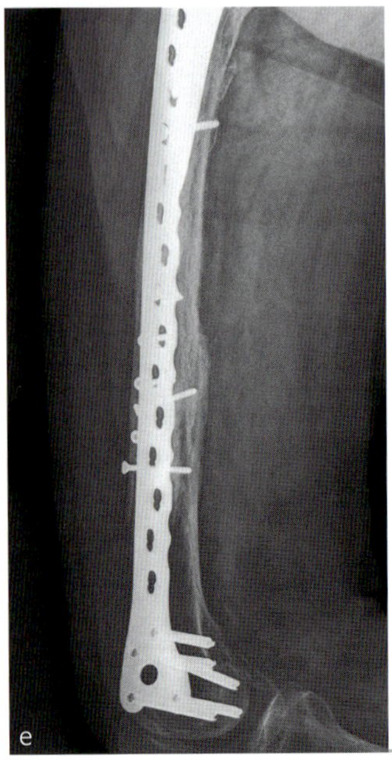

10.15-3a–e X-rays obtained 1 year postoperatively show a well-consolidated fracture.
- **a** AP view of the pelvis.
- **b** AP view of the proximal femur shows some signs of loosening of the cemented prosthesis.
- **c** AP view of the distal two thirds of the femur.
- **d** Lateral view of the proximal femur.
- **e** Lateral view of the distal femur.

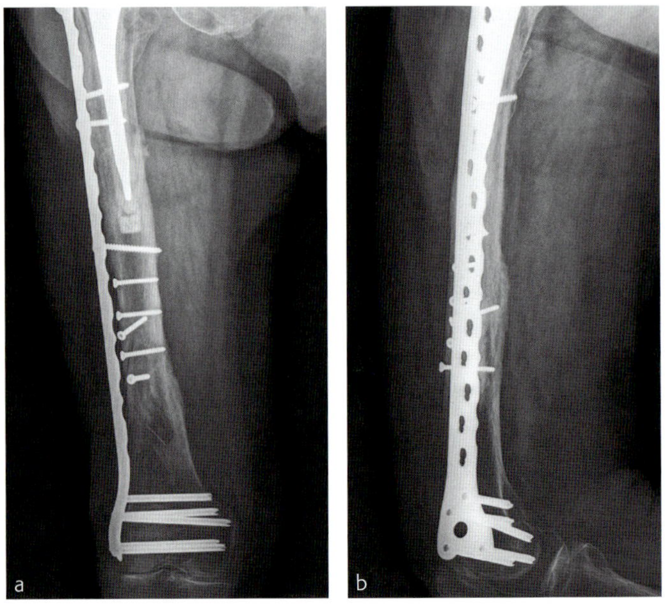

10.15-4a–b Follow-up x-rays obtained 2 years postoperatively.
- **a** AP view.
- **b** Lateral view.

Points to remember

- The combination of lag screws and bridging plate technique used in this patient has a limited indication only.
- Use a radiolucent table. Place a bolster under the ipsilateral buttock to obtain AP and lateral views of the femur.
- Position the C-arm on the opposite side of the fracture with the screens distally (at the patient's feet).
- Use the image intensifier to identify the skin incisions for plate and forceps placement. IV.3-C
- Ensure that cables and attachments for cables are available.
- Another option is the locking attachment plate 3.5.
- If locking-head screws are not available, conventional 4.5 mm cortex screws may be used. If cortex screws are inserted at different angles, they have a higher resistance to pull-out.

IV.3-C

10.16 Femoral shaft butterfly fracture distal to stable prosthesis

MIPO: distal femur LCP 4.5/5.0 and LAP

Author **Michael Wagner**

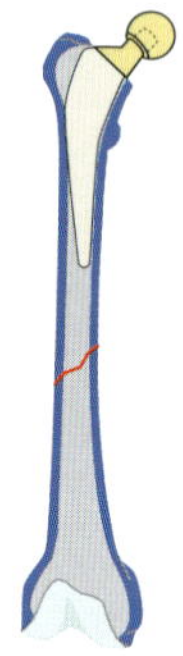

IV.3-C

Case description

A 76-year-old woman sustained a displaced butterfly fracture distal to a clinically stable noncemented hip arthroplasty as a result of a fall at home. Before the incident, the patient could walk without crutches and was asymptomatic. While the patient was being prepared and waiting for surgery, the leg was placed in traction to reduce pain (👁 **10.16-1a–b**).

Classification: Type IV.3-C

Diagnosis: Displaced butterfly femoral shaft fracture distal to a stable total hip arthroplasty

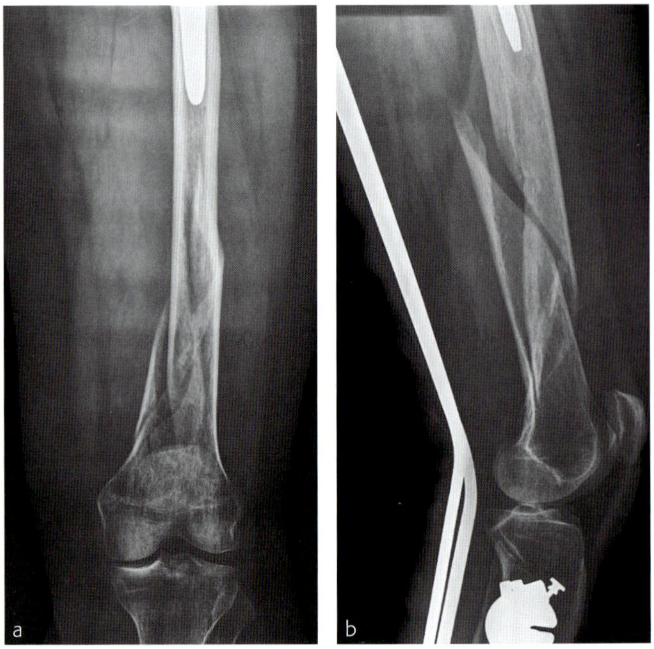

👁 **10.16-1a–b** Low-energy butterfly fracture of the distal femur in osteoporotic bone in traction.
a AP view.
b Lateral view.

Decision making

Internal fixation was the best solution for this patient because she was asymptomatic before the fall and had no clinical signs of prosthetic loosening. Nonoperative treatment with traction is associated with prolonged bed rest and typically is not an option for elderly patients. Of the two possibilities for internal fixation, retrograde intramedullary nailing or application of a bridging locking compression plate (LCP) with an additional locking attachment plate (LAP) (chapter 5.4.1) for plate fixation in the proximal fragment, the latter was preferred as the tip of the prosthesis was not suitable for coupling with a nail.

This displaced butterfly fracture distal to a noncemented hip arthroplasty should be treated according to the AO principles of splinting with a long LCP in a minimally invasive plate osteosynthesis (MIPO) technique and closed indirect reduction.

The use of anatomically preshaped plates and locking-head screws is technically helpful in this minimally invasive technique. Additional fixation of the main plate with a LAP is helpful in the operative treatment of periprosthetic fractures, as it provides secure fixation to the main fragment with the prosthetic stem in the medullar channel. In osteoporotic bone the LAP provides more rotational stability and avoids lateral pull-out of the plate compared to short monocortical periprosthetic locking-head screws. The goal of treatment is uneventful fracture healing with indirect bone healing and early full weight bearing.

Preoperative planning

Equipment

- 13-hole distal femur LCP 4.5/5.0
- Locking-head screws
- Periprosthetic locking-head screws
- 8-hole LAP
- Connecting screw
- 3.5 mm cortex screws
- Distal femoral LCP aiming device/insertion guide
- Collinear reduction forceps

Patient preparation and positioning

- Supine position on a radiolucent table
- Fractured leg is positioned with the knee flexed at 20°
- Uninjured leg is elevated to allow a lateral view with the C-arm

Reduction and fixation

Two incisions were made—one over the lateral condyle and the other in the region of the proximal plate end. Two additional stab incisions were made over the distal shaft, which allowed the insertion of the collinear reduction forceps. Indirect reduction of the fracture was done with manual traction. Direct percutaneous reduction was performed with the collinear reduction forceps after insertion of the distal femur LCP into a submuscular tunnel from distal to proximal. Intraoperative x-ray control was used to confirm axial and rotational alignment. Distal fixation of the plate continued with self-drilling, self-tapping locking-head screws. In the proximal fragment, two short monocortical periprosthetic locking-head screws and two bicortical locking-head screws were used. For additional rotational stability and to avoid lateral screw pull-out, a LAP was placed over and fixed to LCP with the two components of the connecting screw. This construct allows insertion of either 3.5 mm locking-head screws or 3.5 mm cortex screws, which do not interfere with the prosthetic stem. Immediate postoperative x-rays showed good fracture reduction and plate position (**10.16-2a–b**).

IV.3-C

Rehabilitation and follow-up

Continuous passive motion was initiated on the first postoperative day. Mobilization with partial weight bearing for 8–10 weeks is indicated, depending on postoperative x-rays obtained after 6 weeks. Uneventful fracture healing and full weight bearing was achieved. X-rays obtained at the 1-year follow-up showed indirect bone healing with callus formation as a result of the indirect closed reduction and splinting method in this butterfly fracture pattern (**10.16-3a–b**).

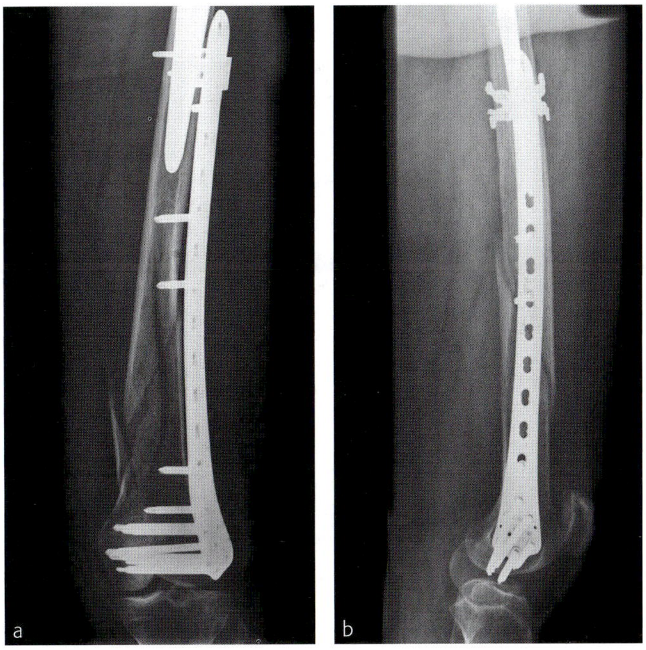

10.16-2a–b Postoperative x-rays show good fracture reduction and correct positioning of the plate with a locking attachment plate securing the fixation around the stem.
a AP view.
b Lateral view.

IV.3-C

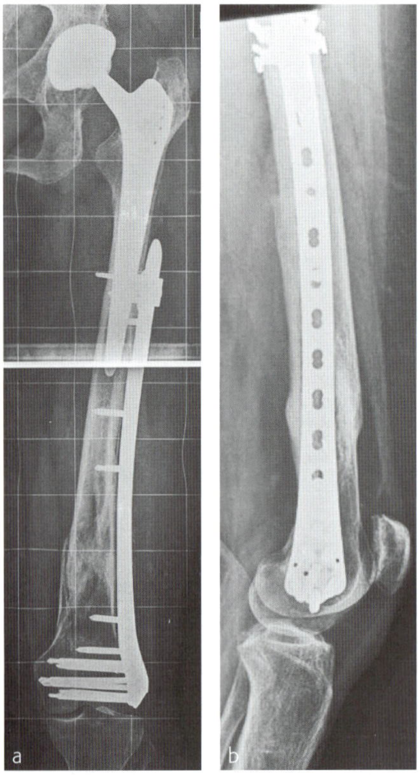

10.16-3a–b X-rays obtained 1 year postoperatively show indirect bone healing with callus formation due to the indirect reduction and bridge plating with relative stability of the fracture.
a AP view.
b Lateral view.

Points to remember

- Closed indirect reduction of shaft fractures and MIPO using the bridging method is technically demanding but results in good indirect bone healing.
- The use of anatomically preshaped plates and locked screws (internal fixators) is technically helpful in the minimally invasive technique and provides the best fixation in osteoporotic bone.
- The LAP is helpful for insertion of screws around the stem without interfering with it or the bone cement. This plate also provides more rotational stability and avoids lateral pull-out of the plate in osteoporotic bone.

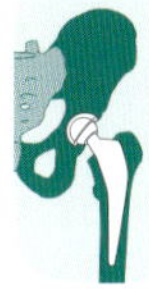

10.17 Interprosthetic femoral fracture, stable hip and knee prosthesis

ORIF: bridging LCP 4.5/5.0

Author Tak-wing Lau

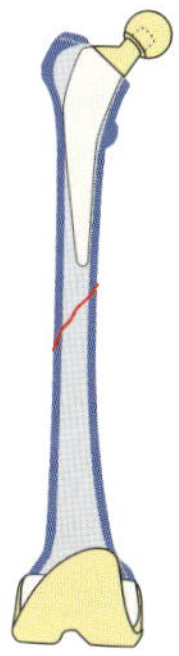

IV.3-D

Case description

A 53-year-old woman with rheumatoid arthritis, a previous total hip arthroplasty, and ipsilateral total knee arthroplasty sustained a simple diaphyseal fracture after a fall on level ground (**10.17-1a–b**).

Classification: Type IV.3-D

Diagnosis: Interprosthetic fracture of the femur between a total hip arthroplasty and a total knee arthroplasty

Decision making

This patient has very poor bone quality as a result of rheumatoid arthritis. Intramedullary nailing was not possible due to the presence of both hip and knee arthroplasties. Because both prosthetic components appeared to be well fixed in bone, this simple diaphyseal fracture is best stabilized with a long locking compression plate (LCP) bridging the fracture and extending as far proximally and distally as possible (chapter 5.4.1). An open approach was planned because minimally invasive plate osteosynthesis (MIPO) may not achieve adequate reduction. As monocortical locking-head screws of the proximal end of the osteoporotic femur may not provide enough purchase, augmentation with cerclage wires was used to improve the proximal fixation.

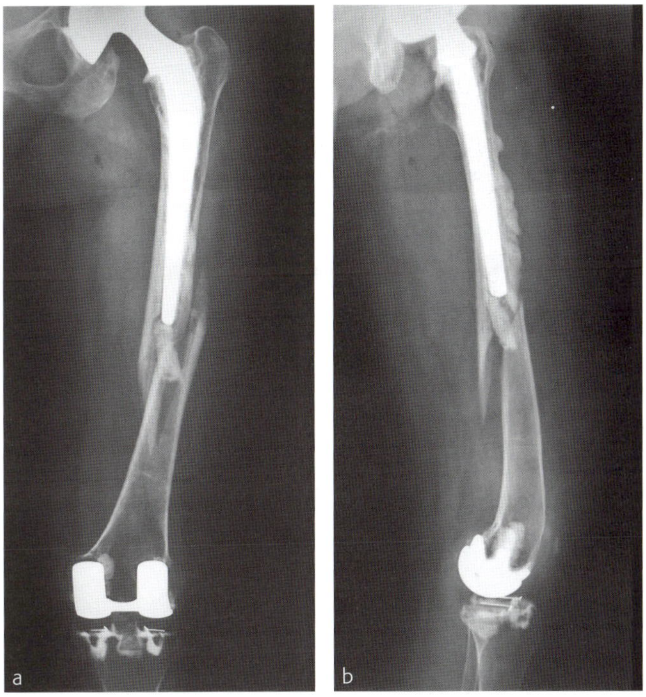

10.17-1a–b Preoperative x-rays show an intercalary fracture of the left femur situated close to the tip of the femoral component.
a AP view.
b Lateral view.

IV.3-D

Preoperative planning

Equipment
- Broad straight LCP 4.5/5.0
- 4.5 mm cortex screw
- 5 mm locking-head screws
- 1.8 mm cerclage wires
- Wire-mounting nuts for LCP

Patient preparation and positioning
- First-generation cephalosporin as antibiotic prophylaxis
- Low-molecular-weight heparin as thrombosis prophylaxis
- Supine or lateral position on a radiolucent table

Reduction and fixation

Lateral incisions were made over the proximal femur, the fracture site, and the distal femur. The vastus lateralis muscle was mobilized anteriorly in order to expose the fracture site. The fracture was reduced with a femoral distractor and reduction forceps, with care to minimize any soft-tissue damage (**10.17-2**). Reduction was maintained temporarily with cerclage wires and a 3.5 mm lag screw. A precontoured, 14-hole, straight broad LCP 4.5/5.0 was inserted into the submuscular plane from distal to proximal without complete elevation of the muscle. Proximal fixation was achieved with monocortical locking-head screws and cerclage wires through wire-mounting nuts. Distal fixation was performed with multiple locking-head screws (**10.17-3a–b**).

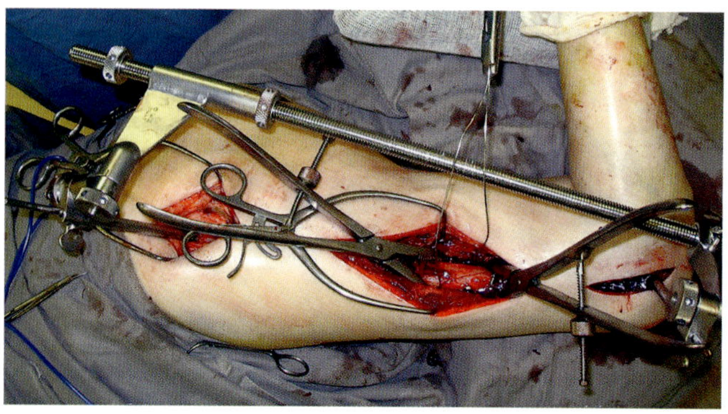

10.17-2 A femoral distractor is used to reduce the fracture and maintain the length and rotation of the femur. Accurate reduction is achieved by bone forceps. Cerclage wires hold the fracture reduction for later definitive fixation with a locking compression plate.

Rehabilitation and follow-up

Protected weight bearing was prescribed for 6–8 weeks with full active knee and hip mobilization exercise allowed. The patient was pain free and could walk without assistance 3 months postoperatively. With additional physiotherapy, the patient had full extension and flexion up to 90° of the knee, which was the preinjury range of movement (**10.17-4a–b**).

Upon regular follow-up, the patient reports satisfaction with the operative result. She continues to have mild hip and knee discomfort due to previous arthroplasties. Two years postoperatively, the patient is pain free at the fracture site, and range of motion of the hips and knee are unchanged. X-rays obtained 2 years later showed complete fracture remodeling and no evidence of loosening of the screws (**10.17-5a–b**).

Points to remember

- Reduction in simple diaphyseal fractures should be accurate enough to allow compression plating, whereas in comminuted fractures bridge plating is preferred. The fracture may need to be exposed if reduction cannot be achieved by closed means.
- The broad LCP 4.5/5.0 provides good stability and strength for early weight bearing. If a curved plate that fits the natural form of the femur had been available, an even longer plate could have been applied.
- The use of bicortical locking-head screws in the distal femur improves fixation in osteoporotic bone.
- Monocortical locking-head screws inserted proximally around the stem may not provide enough purchase in osteoporotic bone. Augmentation with cerclage wires or cables may be required.
- In addition to the monocortical locking-head screws, wire-mounting nuts in the LCP secure the position of the cerclage wires for proximal fixation.

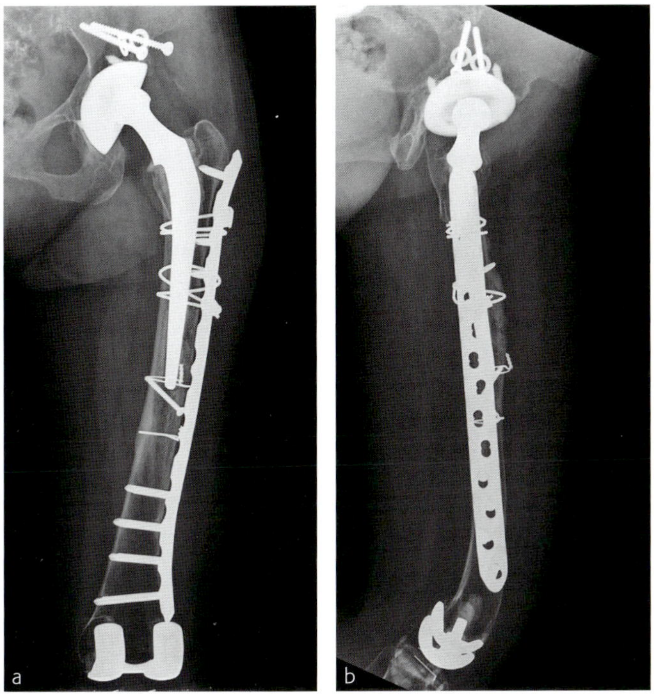

10.17-3a–b Postoperative x-rays show a reduced and well-fixed fracture. A slightly curved and distally longer plate would have been preferable.
a AP view.
b Lateral view.

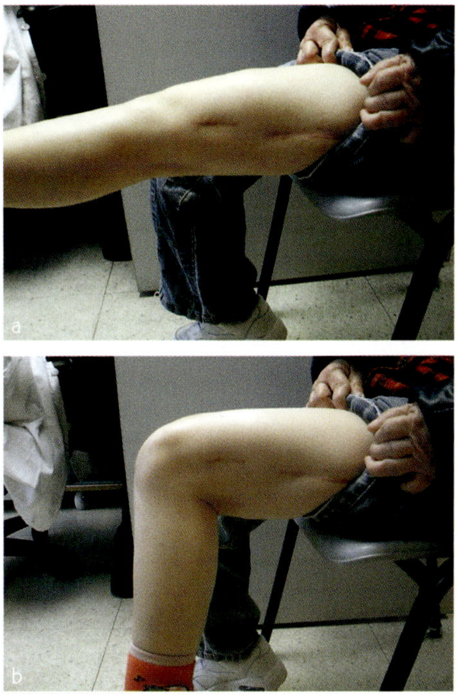

10.17-4a–b The patient has good knee function and uneventful wound healing 6 months postoperatively.
a Full extension.
b Flexion to 90°.

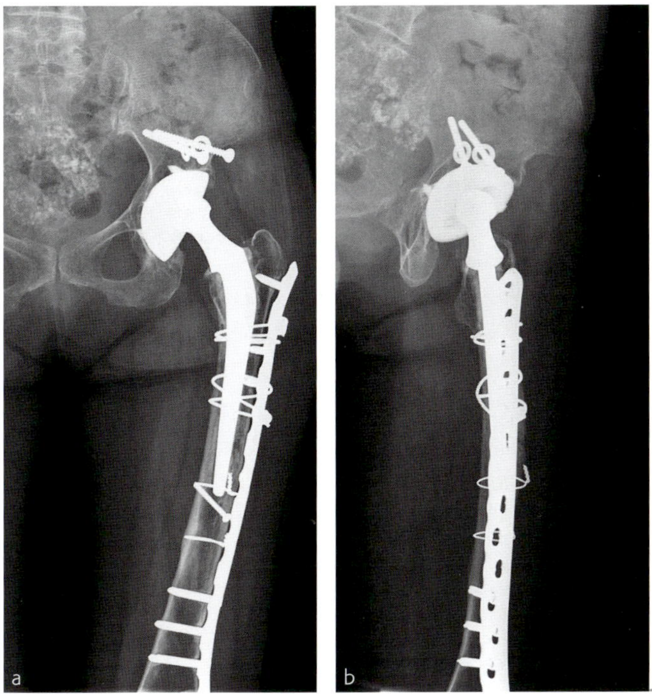

10.17-5a–b X-rays obtained 2 years postoperatively show good fracture union with complete remodeling. Note mild polyethylene wear at the total hip arthroplasty. The loose screws in the acetabulum are unrelated to the actual problem.
a AP view.
b Lateral view.

IV.3-D

10.18 Interprosthetic femoral refracture, plate breakage, stable prosthesis

ORIF: locked antegrade intramedullary nail

Authors **Christof Meyer, Gabor Szalay**

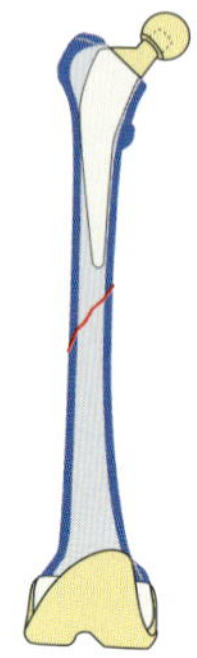

IV.3-D

Case description

An 84-year-old woman sustained an intercalary periprosthetic femoral shaft fracture as a result of a fall. The fracture was initially stabilized with a straight locking compression plate (LCP). She also had a history of total knee arthroplasty 7 years ago and a healed peritrochanteric fracture after gamma nailing 4 years ago. Five months after the current stabilization, the LCP broke due to fatigue without any new trauma (**10.18-1a–b**).

Classification: Type IV.3-D

Diagnosis: Intercalary periprosthetic delayed union of the femur with fatigue fracture of the LCP

Decision making

Salvage options ranged from a second plate fixation bridging the entire femur, revision knee arthroplasty with a longer intramedullary stem or antegrade intramedullary nailing to total femur replacement. Osteosynthesis was initially selected because of the absence of arthrosis of the hip joint and the stable, well-functioning knee prosthesis.

Bony consolidation of the former proximal femoral fracture was confirmed by CT, and the diameter of the medullary canal and size of the prosthesis were measured.

Because of the disadvantages and risks associated with a second plate osteosynthesis and according to the principles of treating a delayed union of the femoral shaft by intramedullary nailing, an in situ extension of the knee prosthesis with an antegrade intramedullary nail was considered to be the least invasive and safest procedure (chapter 5.4.2).

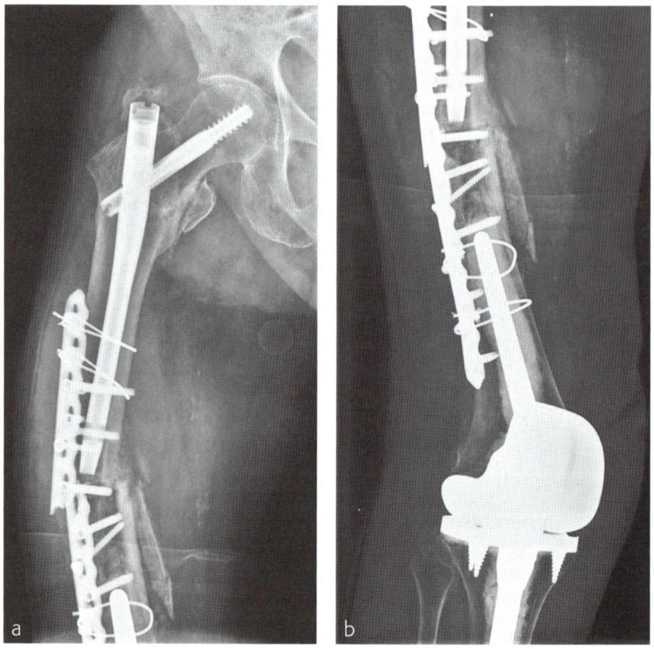

10.18-1a–b X-rays show an intercalary periprosthetic delayed union with a fatigue fracture of a locking compression plate that was applied 5 months ago.

- **a** AP view of the proximal femur, including the hip joint. The former peritrochanteric fracture fixed with a gamma nail looks consolidated.
- **b** AP view of the distal femur with the knee joint shows that the femoral component appears well fixed.

Preoperative planning

Equipment

- Custom-made antegrade intramedullary nail (Grosse-Kempf)
- Grosse-Kempf locking nail system

Patient preparation and positioning

- Supine position on a normal surgical table

Reduction and fixation

The gamma nail was first removed, allowing access to the intramedullary canal. The broken plate and cerclage wires were then removed through the original lateral incision. Reaming of the proximal fragment up to 13 mm diameter followed. The reaming debris was collected and later used as an autogenous bone graft. The tip of the stem of the total knee arthroplasty was prepared by removing adherent cement. After antegrade insertion, the intramedullary nail and the prosthesis were coupled under direct visualization and impacted with radiological control (👁 **10.18-2**). The last step consisted of proximal locking once the correct length was verified.

Rehabilitation and follow-up

IV.3-D

Postoperative x-rays showed a stable fixation as a result of in situ extension of the prosthesis by coupling with an intramedullary nail. The patient was allowed weight bearing as tolerated. After 1 week, she could walk independently with crutches, and after 4 weeks she could walk for short distances without a walking aid. X-rays obtained after 3 months showed progressive bony consolidation (👁 **10.18-3a–c**). Six months after the last surgery, the patient was hospitalized with severe pneumonia and died several weeks later of the consequences of this illness.

Points to remember

- In situ extension of a prosthetic stem with a custom-made slotted hollow intramedullary nail has several advantages, including stable docking between the prosthesis and the intramedullary nail with an implant-overlapping distance of 3–4 cm.
- Early mobilization under full weight bearing is possible.
- Bony consolidation of the fracture occurs despite previous plate fixation with subsequent impairment of the periosteal blood flow.
- Reaming debris seems to have a positive influence on fracture healing.

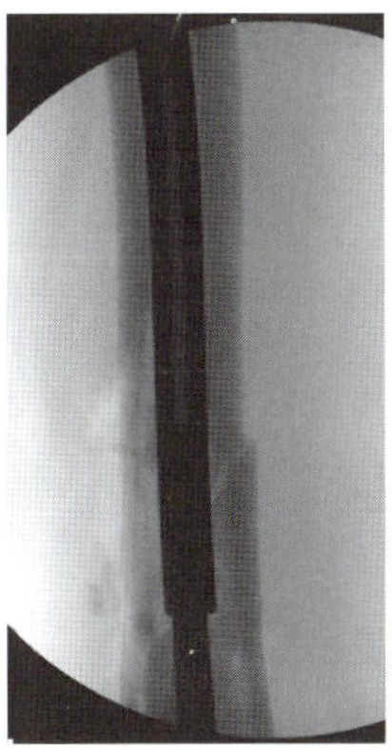

👁 **10.18-2** Intraoperative image after the docking maneuver shows the slotted nail safely inserted over the stem of the total knee arthroplasty overlapping it by about 4 cm.

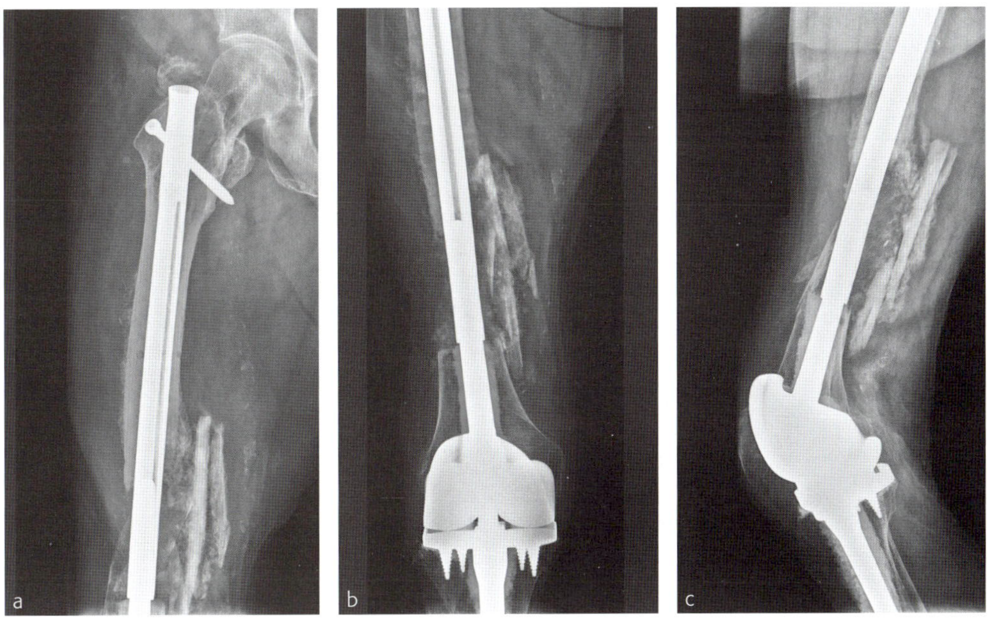

👁 **10.18-3a–c** X-rays obtained 3 months postoperatively show clear signs of progressive fracture consolidation with callus formation.

a Lateral view of the proximal femur.
b AP view of the distal femur.
c Lateral view of the distal femur.

11

Knee cases

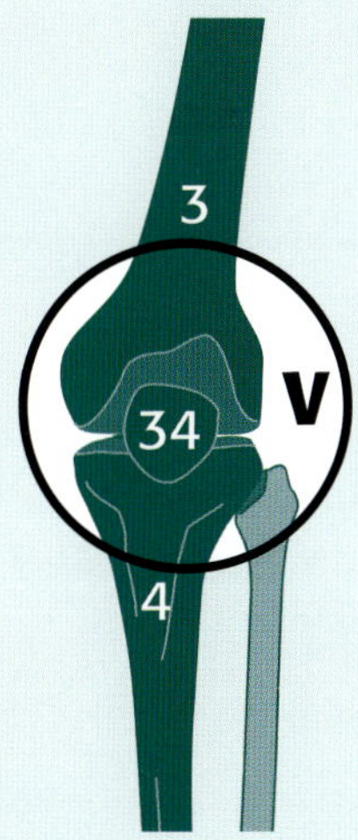

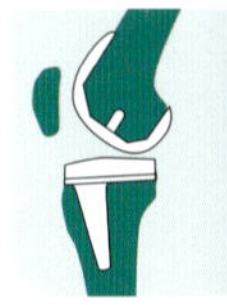

11.1 Open patellar fracture dislocation, stable prosthesis

ORIF: tension-band fixation

Authors **Marschall B Berkes, Dean G Lorich**

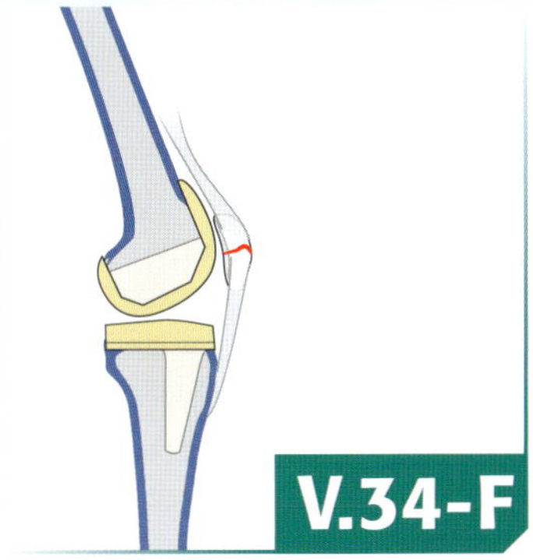

Case description

A 53-year-old woman, who previously underwent total knee arthroplasty of the right knee, sustained a grade IIIA open posterior dislocation of the prosthesis and a displaced patellar fracture as a result of a low-energy fall (**11.1-1a–b**). She was unable to raise a straightened leg or extend her right knee. The right knee was reduced in an emergency procedure and the wound irrigated and debrided before definitive treatment of the patellar fracture (**11.1-2a–b**).

Classification: Type V.34-F

Diagnosis: Open transverse midpole patellar fracture

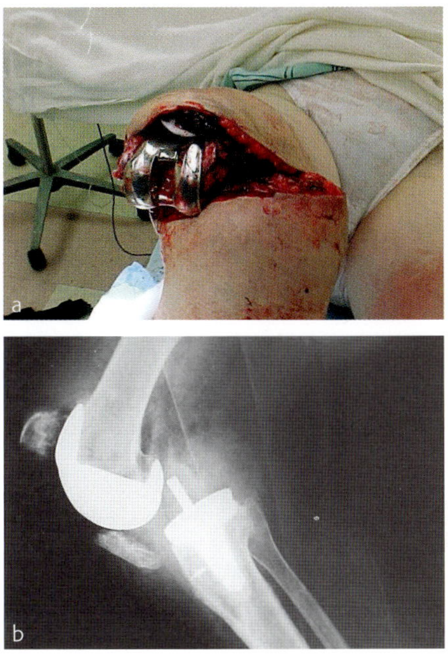

11.1-1a–b Situation on admission.
a Open knee dislocation with a large anterior transverse traumatic wound.
b Lateral view obtained before reduction. Note the widely displaced patellar fracture.

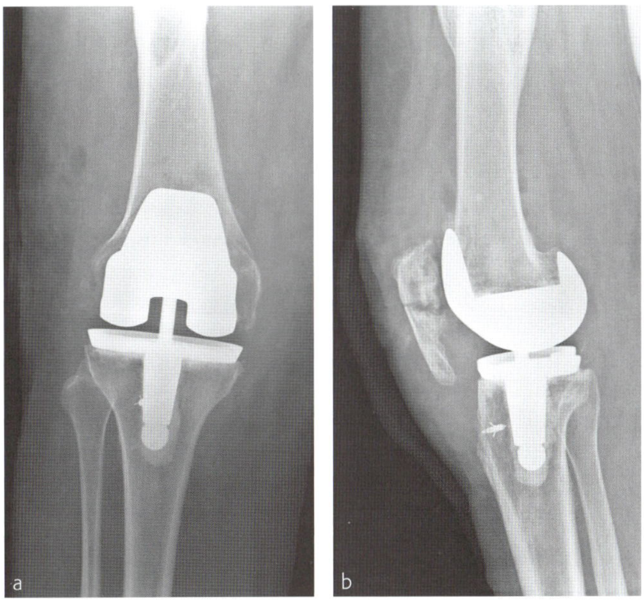

11.1-2a–b X-rays obtained immedately after reduction.
a AP view.
b Lateral view shows residual displacement at the patellar fracture site.

V.34-F
Decision making

The prosthesis was a posteriorly stabilized design with a cam and post mechanism. The dislocation very likely occurred because the cam jumped the post with hyperflexion, which is a known mechanism for dislocation of a total knee arthroplasty. This situation was unique in that although the energy that caused the dislocation was low, it was high enough to result in an open dislocation with disruption of the extensor mechanism by virtue of the patellar fracture. After reduction of the dislocation, all aspects of joint stability must be assessed. In this case, medial and lateral ligamentous stability was sufficient, and anterior posterior stability was restored after the correct relationship between the cam and post was reestablished.

Two treatment strategies are available for open fracture dislocations of a knee arthroplasty. One strategy involves an aggressive algorithm consisting of arthroplasty explantation, placement of an antibiotic spacer, debridement, and osteosynthesis of the patella, followed by a staged revision arthroplasty after fracture union. This strategy assumes that the joint is by definition infected as a result of the open fracture. The other strategy follows a more limited approach, consisting of only open fracture debridement and irrigation, followed by patellar fracture osteosynthesis.

The latter strategy was selected for this patient and was favored over a more radical surgical approach, including explantation, for several reasons. First, the femur and tibial components were well fixed. Second, there was no gross contamination of the joint despite the open fracture. Finally, after reduction of the knee joint, the collateral ligaments were found to be competent, with good stability to varus and valgus stress. This stability was undoubtedly aided by the constrained design of the prosthesis. These factors led to the decision to pursue a less aggressive strategy.

Following irrigation and debridement, osteosynthesis of the patella is best achieved with a tension-band construct.

Preoperative planning

Equipment

- K-wires
- 18-gauge wire
- Pliers
- C-arm
- Nonresorbable suture

Patient preparation and positioning

- Cefazolin and gentamicin for antibiotic prophylaxis (given as soon as possible in the emergency department)
- Subcutaneous heparin for thrombosis prophylaxis
- Supine position on a radiolucent table with a bolster under the ipsilateral hip to prevent external rotation of the limb
- A nonsterile tourniquet (applied but not necessarily inflated)

Reduction and fixation

An anterior approach to the knee was chosen because it offered direct access to the patella through the traumatic transverse wound. Any devitalized skin, subcutanous tissue, bone, or muscle was debrided. All components were tested for stability.

The fracture was reduced with pointed Weber forceps. Two K-wires were inserted from proximal to distal just superficial to the articular surface to purchase subchondral bone. An 18-gauge wire was used to create a figure-of-eight tension band. The wire was passed deep to the patellar and quadriceps tendons, beneath the exposed ends of the K-wires and tightened on the anterior surface with pliers. X-rays with the fixation in place were obtained immediately postoperatively (👁 **11.1-3a–b**). The retinaculum was repaired with a nonresorbable suture; the traumatic wound was repaired with deep absorbable suture and nylon.

Rehabilitation and follow-up

The extremity was placed in a hinged knee brace, locked in extension with no knee range of motion for the first 2 weeks postoperatively. Weight bearing was allowed as tolerated immediately after surgery.

At 2 weeks postoperatively, knee range of motion was progressed to active and active-assisted exercises from 0–30° until 6 weeks postoperatively. After this time, active and passive range-of-motion exercises with no limits were initiated.

No major complications were encountered during the patient's postoperative course, and healing occurred without any secondary surgeries. X-rays obtained 8 months postoperatively demonstrated bony union (👁 **11.1-4a–b**). The patient reported hardware prominence, which led to removal of the tension band and K-wires 8 months postoperatively. Follow-up at 12 months demonstrated a healed patella (👁 **11.1-5a–b**).

More than 9 years after the date of injury the patient required no additional surgery on the right knee. Despite having limited knee flexion, she remained active on a daily basis. She can ambulate more than 1 mile, with the occasional use of a cane. She also continues to participate in recreational activities, such as yoga and kayaking.

Points to remember

- A deep infection as the result of the open fracture must be considered. Daily wound control and routine control of C-reactive protein and erythrocyte sedimentation rate are mandatory.
- The tension-band wire must pass beneath the exposed ends of the longitudinal K-wires.
- The twisted ends of the 18-gauge wire must be buried laterally to decrease subcutaneous irritation over the anterior aspect of the knee.
- Fixation can be enhanced by passing nonresorbable sutures through bone tunnels in the patella and incorporating the patellar tendon with a running locking stitch.
- The stability of the construct should be tested prior to leaving the operating room with gentle range of motion of the knee.

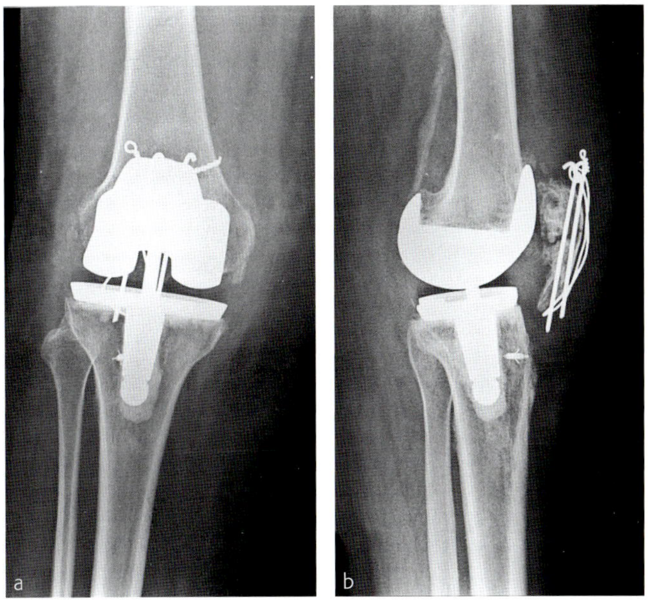

11.1-3a–b X-rays of the right knee obtained immediately after open reduction and internal fixation with tension-band wiring.
a AP view.
b Lateral view.

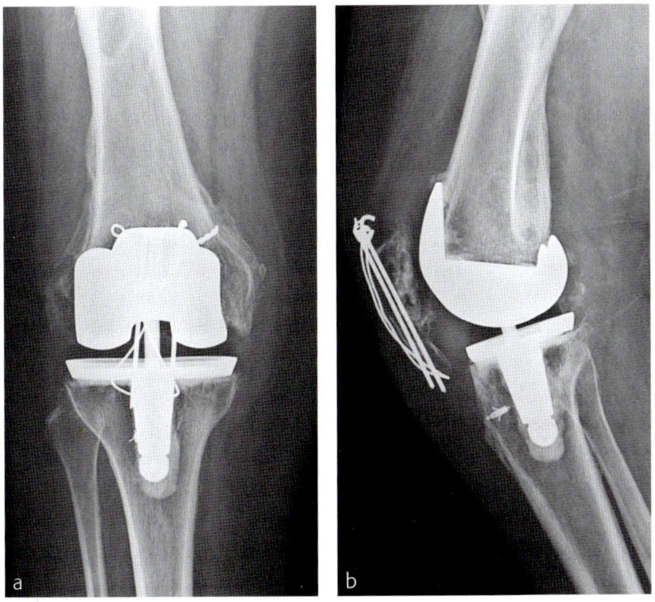

11.1-4a–b X-rays of the right knee obtained 8 months postoperatively show fracture union with the hardware in place.
a AP view.
b Lateral view.

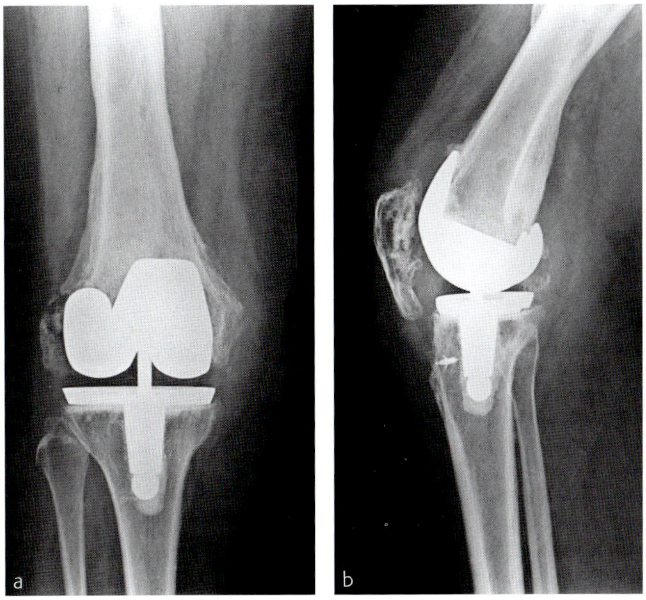

11.1-5a–b Final x-rays of the right knee obtained 12 months after interval removal of hardware. Note bony union at the fracture site.
a AP view.
b Lateral view.

V.3-B2

11.2 Pediatric femoral fracture, stable tumor prosthesis

ORIF: reverse LISS proximal tibia

Author Peter Kloen

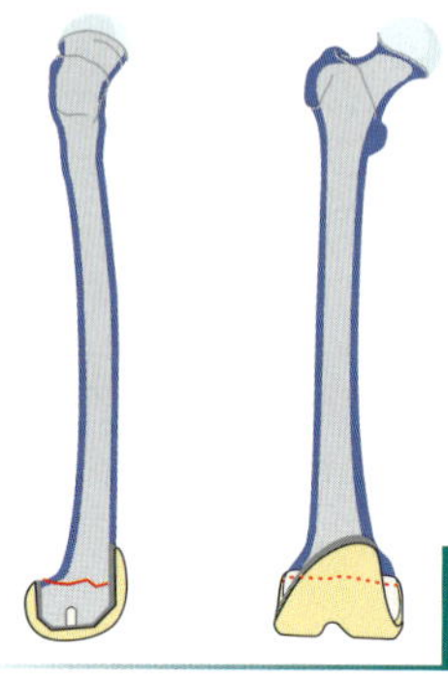

V.3-B2

Case description

An 11-year-old boy presented with a periprosthetic spiral fracture of the femoral shaft above a tumor prosthesis after a low-energy fall (👁 **11.2-1a–c**). He had a history of telangiectatic osteosarcoma in the proximal tibia for which he initially received chemotherapy, followed by resection of the distal femur and proximal tibia, and knee reconstruction. The immediate postoperative course was complicated by a deep infection for which multiple debridements and ultimately a two-stage exchange were required. The newly placed silver-coated prosthesis was noncemented. The soft tissues were reconstructed with a vascularized free flap using the rectus abdominis muscle. He had done well for a few months prior to falling. There was no evidence of infection and he was mobilizing, albeit with a fairly stiff knee and a pes equinus deformity. He had not taken antibiotics for a few weeks.

Classification: Type V.3-B2

Diagnosis: Periprosthetic fracture of the proximal femur to a stable tumor prosthesis

Decision making

Given the patient's complicated history before the fall, a revision to a long-stem prosthesis bypassing the fracture was believed to be too risky. Similarly, an imperfect reduction in a long-leg cast would compromise the healing potential of the fracture and also further harm his already limited knee function. An above-knee amputation had been discussed prior during his protracted and complicated reconstruction but was not yet an option for the family, partly for religious and cultural reasons. Of note is that there was no evidence of metastatic disease at this time. Hence, osteosynthesis was felt to be the only feasible treatment. The space for plate osteosynthesis obviously was limited given the large prosthesis and the relatively small bone size in this 11-year-old boy. Various plating options were considered. It was felt that a less invasive stabilization system (LISS) proximal tibia plating system might be a relatively good fit and would allow monocortical locking (chapter 5.4.1).

Preoperative planning

Equipment

- Carbon table
- LISS proximal tibia plating system
- 5.0 mm locking-head screws
- 4.5 mm conventional screws
- Periprosthetic screws

Patient preparation and positioning

- Cephalosporin for antibiotic prophylaxis
- Low-molecular-weight heparin for thrombosis prophylaxis

V.3-B2

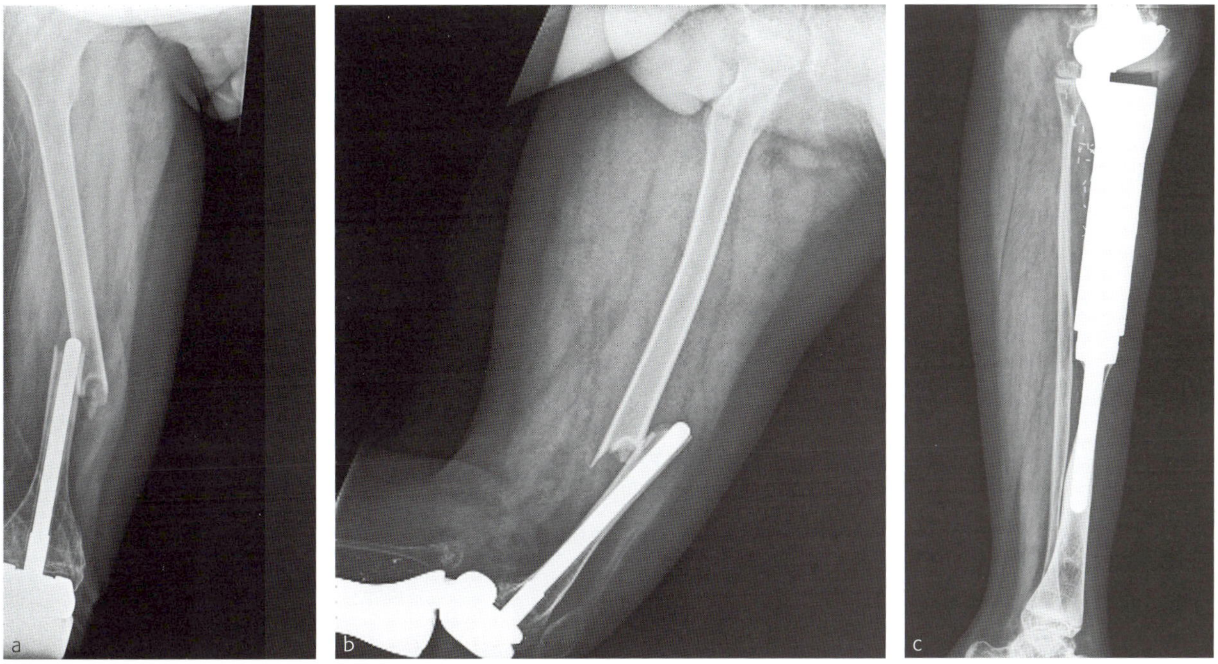

11.2-1a–c X-rays of the spiral fracture of the femoral shaft starting at the tip of the femoral stem. Some notching and resorption of the cortex was already present.

- **a** AP view.
- **b** Lateral view shows possible signs of osteolysis around the tip of the long stem.
- **c** AP view shows the large tibial tumor component.

Reduction and fixation

Although a minimally invasive plate osteosynthesis (MIPO) technique could have been used, a formal lateral approach was selected to make anatomical reduction possible. The soft-tissue reconstruction was on the anteromedial side, and the plastic surgeon saw no problems with the lateral approach.

Open reduction with manual traction allowed exact repositioning of the fracture. The tip of the stem was reduced in the proximal fracture fragment. A right 15-hole tibia LISS was placed laterally and upside down onto the femur and had an almost-perfect fit. Distally, the plate was fixed with locking-head screws. The femoral component precluded placement of more than one long bicortical screw. To prevent contact of the locking-head screws with the prosthesis, specific periprosthetic screws were used around the stem. These screws have a blunt tip as not to damage the prosthesis. Proximal from the stem, bicortical conventional screws were used.

Rehabilitation and follow-up

The patient was allowed toe-touch weight bearing for the first 6 weeks postoperatively. At 6 weeks, x-rays showed early healing with bridging callus. Weight bearing was increased at that time to a level that was tolerated. At 7 months, the patient was able to bear full weight without pain. At 13 months, x-rays showed complete fracture healing and remodeling (**11.2-2a–d**).

V.3-B2

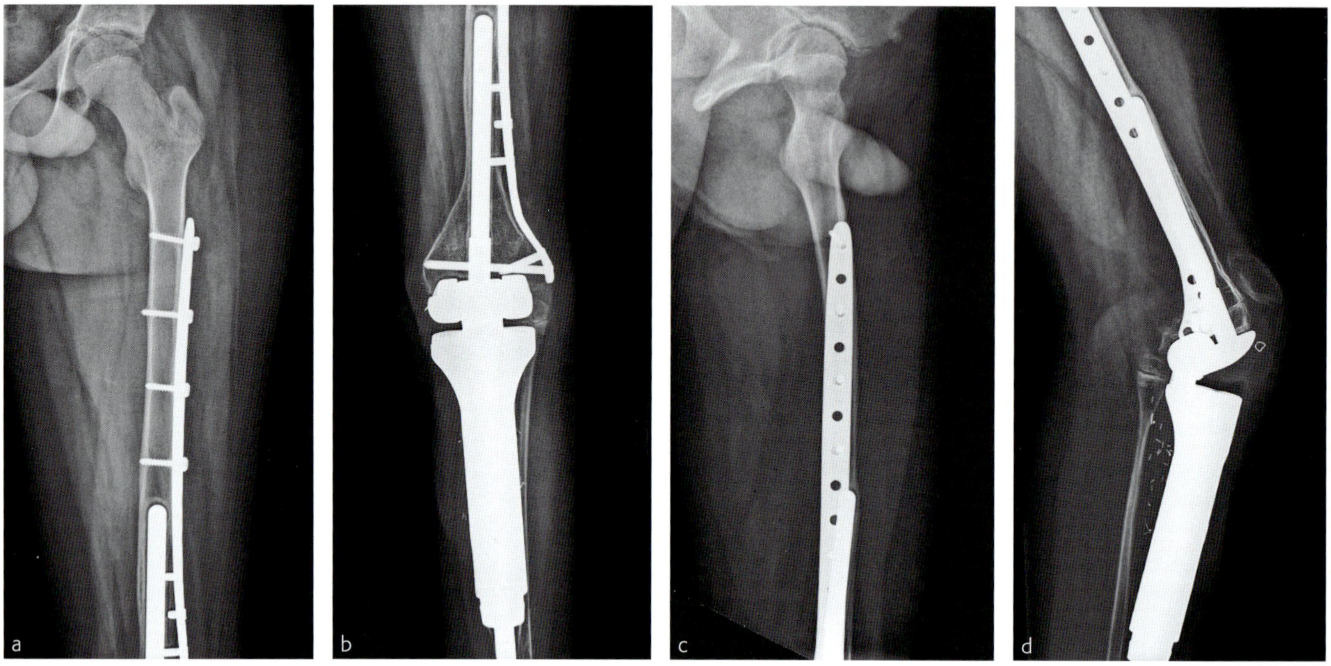

11.2-2a–d X-rays obtained 13 months postoperatively show a healed fracture and a stable prosthesis.
a–b AP views. The prosthesis shows no evidence of loosening.
c–d Lateral views. There is no further progression of notching around the tip of the prosthetic stem.

Points to remember

- Notching and resorption around the tip of the femoral stem is of concern and should be monitored closely.
- Use of a short plate will compromise stability of fixation; therefore, the longest plate possible should be used.
- Varus deformity of the femur can develop if stability is suboptimal.
- Unusual circumstances call for unusual solutions. Being comfortable with various plating systems will help decide between possible alternatives.
- A second smaller plate or allograft strut on the anteromedial side augments stability and prevents varus deformity.
- Special periprosthetic screws will prevent abutment of the screw tip with the prosthesis while still providing monocortical fixation.
- Healing capacity in the femur of a child is much better than in the femur of an elderly person.

11.3 Refracture of a nonunited distal femoral fracture, stable prosthesis

ORIF: locked retrograde intramedullary nail

Authors **Stephen L Kates, Natasha O'Malley**

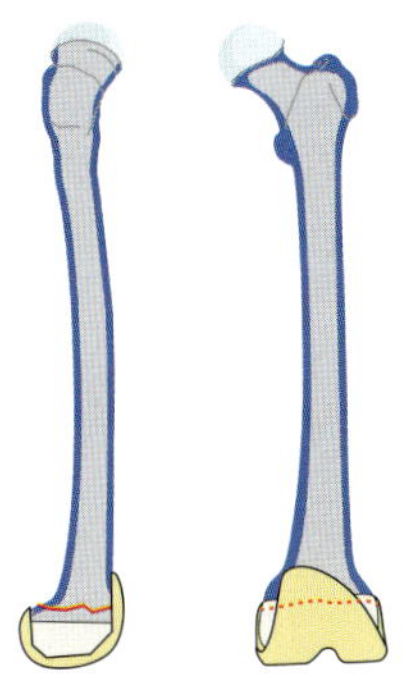

V.3-B1

Case description

An 83-year-old woman sustained a periprosthetic fracture of the distal femur that was originally fixed with a minimally invasive locking compression plate (LCP). Sixteen months later, x-rays showed fracture nonunion and fatigue failure of the hardware (**11.3-1a–b**).

Classification: Type V.3-B1

Diagnosis: Plate breakage after ORIF of a distal femoral periprosthetic nonunion, with stable prosthesis

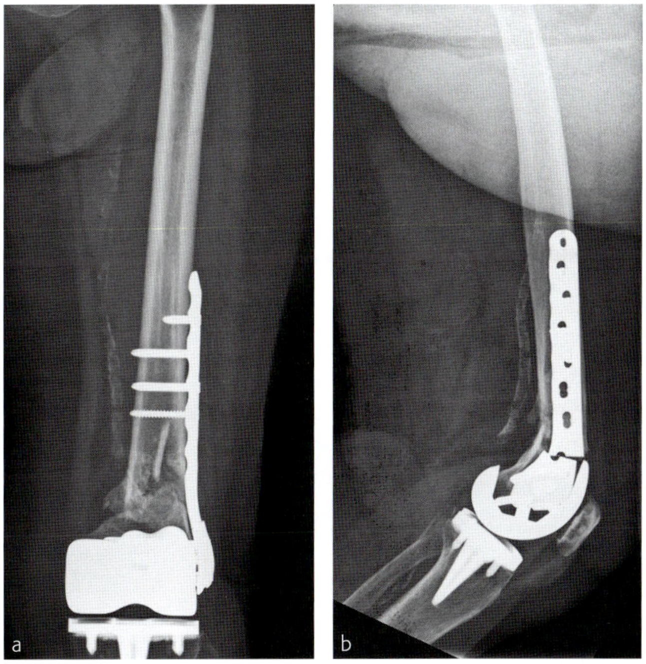

11.3-1a–b X-rays of the broken distal femoral plate, with nonunion of a periprosthetic fracture above the in situ total knee arthroplasty.
a AP view.
b Lateral view.

Decision making

Revision plating and bone grafting were discussed, but this approach would have required a prolonged period of no weight bearing and was therefore rejected. Other options included revision with insertion of a long-stem femoral component or use of a retrograde intramedullary nail (chapter 5.4.2). The latter was considered a good option as it allowed earlier weight bearing in this fragile elderly patient.

Preoperative planning

Infection was excluded. The total knee arthroplasty implant brand and size was confirmed to ensure the intercondylar notch of the femoral component will permit entry of the available retrograde femoral intramedullary nail, and that the appropriate-sized femoral nail is available.

V.3-B1 **Equipment**

- LCP extraction set
- Broken-screw removal set
- Intraoperative imaging
- Retrograde femoral nailing set and reamers
- Appropriately sized retrograde femoral nail
- Sterile radiolucent knee rest
- Revision total arthroplasty equipment as secondary option in case of failure

Patient preparation and positioning

- Spinal or general anesthesia
- Supine position on radiolucent table

Reduction and fixation

The broken plate was removed through minimal incisions (👁 **11.3-2**). A midline incision with medial parapatellar arthrotomy was then made to prepare for guide wire access and eventual insertion of the supracondylar nail. After correct guide wire placement was confirmed with imaging and sequential reaming was completed, the retrograde intramedullary nail was inserted and then locked in the short distal fragment. Local bone graft (reaming debris) was then distributed at the fracture site.

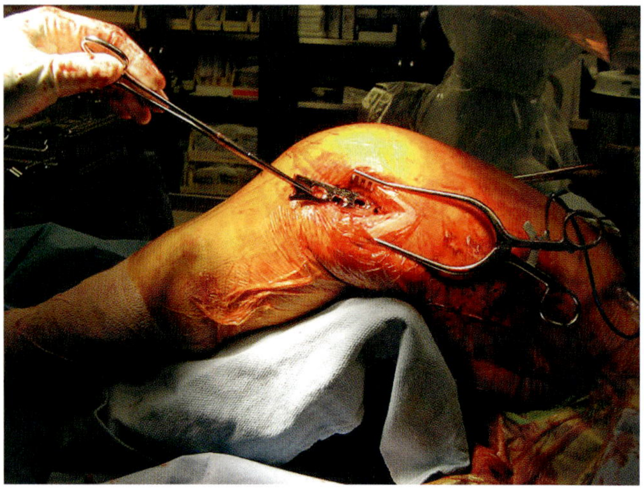

👁 **11.3-2** Intraoperative photograph shows extraction of the broken proximal plate.

Rehabilitation and follow-up

A supervised rehabilitation program was initiated on the first postoperative day, specifically weight bearing as tolerated in an unlocked hinged knee brace. X-rays obtained 6 months postoperatively confirmed healing with clinical range of motion of 0–100° (👁 **11.3-3a–b**).

Points to remember

- Undiagnosed medical reasons for nonunion have to be identified, including metabolic deficiencies, infection, or other causes.
- Correct planning is mandatory to ensure the intramedullary nail passes through the prosthesis.
- A secondary plan, such as revision prosthesis, is also required.
- In case of polyethylene wear, there must be the possibility to replace the spacer during surgery.
- Intramedullary reaming debris can be used as bone graft.

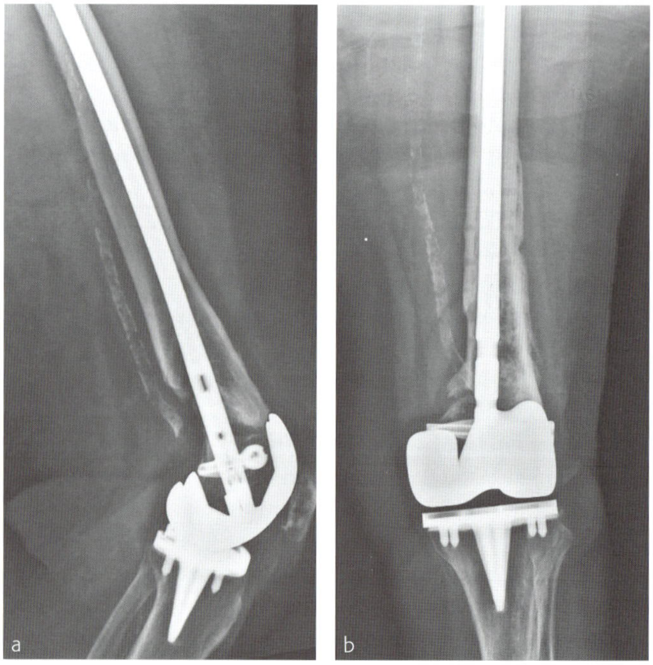

👁 **11.3-3a–b** X-rays obtained 6 months after conversion to intramedullary nail. Patient had range of motion of 0–100°.
a AP view.
b Lateral view.

11.4 Distal femoral fracture, loose prosthesis

Revision: tumor prosthesis

Authors **Richard J Jenkinson, Hans J Kreder**

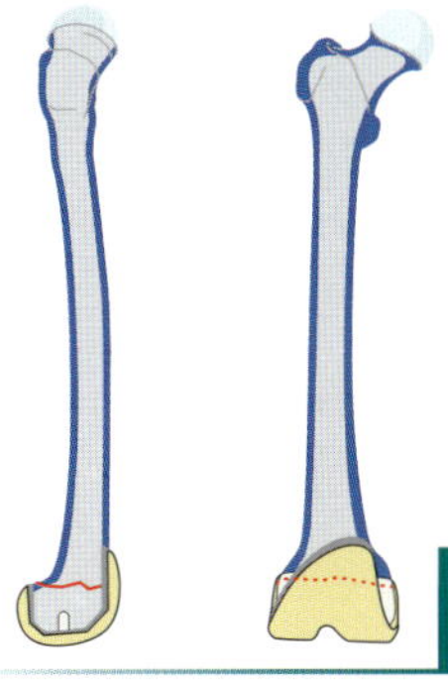

V.3-B2

Case description

A 75-year-old woman presented with an inability to bear weight and instability above the knee after a fall from standing height in her home. Before the fall, she ambulated independently and lived in her own home. Twelve years ago she underwent successful right total knee arthroplasty for osteoarthritis. She has a history of coronary artery disease and had a myocardial infarction 8 years ago. Physical examination showed a well-healed midline scar over her right knee. Pulses and results of neurological exam were normal. Imaging studies obtained on presentation showed a distal femoral periprosthetic fracture, with poor-quality osteoporotic bone and only a small amount of bone fixed to the prosthesis (**11.4-1a–c**). Preinjury x-rays were unavailable.

Classification: Type V.3-B2

Diagnosis: Periprosthetic fracture of the distal femur, with a loose prosthesis

Decision making

The patient had an extremely distal fracture above her primary total knee arthroplasty, with acute flexion at the fracture site. The goal of treatment was to restore independent functioning, if possible. General options for treatment included nonoperative care with casting/bracing, fracture fixation with retention of the prosthesis, revision total knee arthroplasty, restoring bone stock with bulk allograft, and replacement of the distal femur with a tumor prosthesis.

The risks associated with surgery in this patient were deemed acceptable, but a regional technique and a relatively short surgery were suggested. Nonoperative care avoided the risks of surgery and anesthesia but had an unacceptably high complication rate.

Fracture fixation with prosthesis retention was considered challenging in this patient given the extremely distal extent of the fracture coupled with osteoporotic bone. An intramedullary nail would have no distal anchorage and is a poor implant choice. A distal femoral locking compression plate could possibly achieve a small amount of fixation in the distal segment. However, this option was not selected given the poor bone quality and minimal amount of bone available.

Revision arthroplasty (chapter 5.5) was selected because it allowed for early ambulation and restored stability in the joint and limb after the reconstructive procedure. Revision arthroplasty with a distal femoral allograft (chapter 5.6) would also be a viable reconstruction option, as it would potentially restore bone stock if future reconstruction was required. However, this procedure is technically demanding, often requiring significant amounts of operative time to both fashion a graft and revise the knee components. Postoperatively, partial weight bearing usually is required. A distal femoral replacement prosthesis must be implanted with attention to detail but should require less operative time than a distal allograft procedure and allows for immediate full weight bearing.

V.3-B2

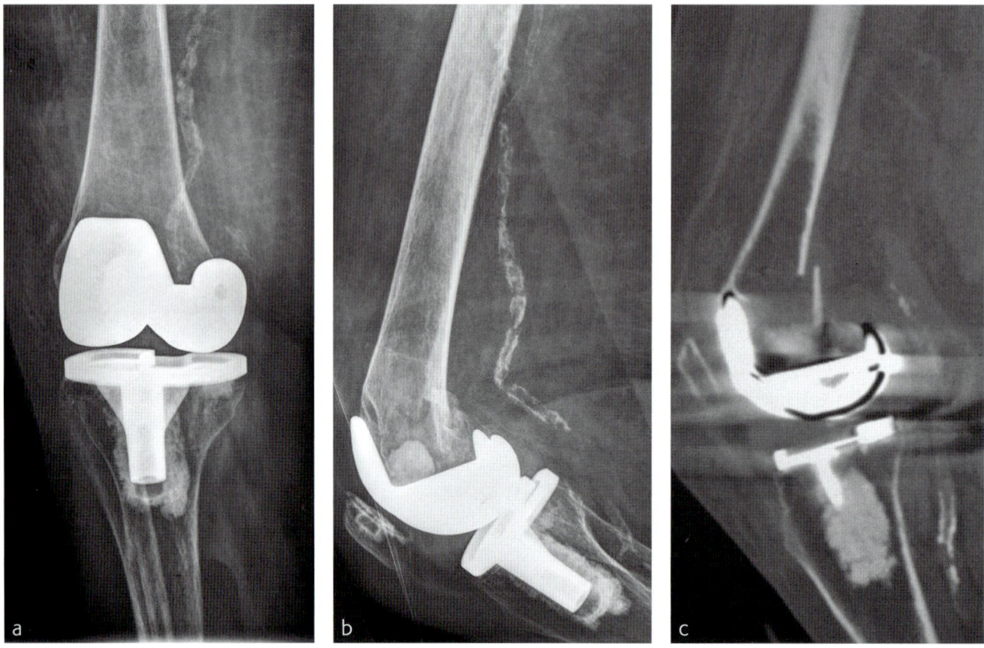

11.4-1a–c Preoperative imaging studies of the distal femur show a very low distal femoral periprosthetic fracture in poor-quality bone. The stability of the prosthesis is questionable.
- **a** AP view.
- **b** Lateral view.
- **c** CT scan showing minimal bone available for internal fixation.

Preoperative planning

Equipment

- Chisels, osteotomes for component removal
- Distal femoral replacement constrained prosthesis system
- Experienced arthroplasty nursing support
- Prosthesis company service representative

Patient preparation and positioning

- Supine position with a bolster under the ipsilateral hip to neutralize natural hip external rotation
- Tourniquet on thigh
- Preoperative antibiotics
- Foot plate to support leg at 90° of knee flexion

Reduction and fixation

The previous midline incision with slight proximal and distal extension was used. Full-thickness soft-tissue flaps were elevated, followed by a medial parapatellar arthrotomy with eversion of the patella (**11.4-2**). After removal of the distal femur, extensive slack was seen in the soft tissues; therefore, extensile arthroplasty exposures were not necessary.

The distal femur was exposed, and both the distal femoral component and the attached bone were removed while working through the fracture. During this step the origins of the medial and lateral collateral ligaments were also removed. In this patient, a very thin shell of bone was adhered to the component laterally, but the medial bone was actually loose from the prosthesis. This finding would have made nonoperative treatment or open reduction and internal fixation unlikely to be successful.

With the distal femur removed, the tibial component was easily exposed. The polyethylene and tibial tray and metaphyseal cement were removed with osteotomes. After the distal femur and arthroplasty components were removed, a large defect was seen between the residual distal femur and the proximal tibia (**11.4-3**).

The tibial component was first prepared to restore a stable platform upon which to establish the joint line. Femoral landmarks are not available to guide this level. However, the distal pole of the patella is useful to guide restoration of the joint line. The tibial component must be implanted with appropriate external rotation. Because femoral rotation landmarks are not available, tibial rotation is the only guidance.

Fixation is possible with either noncemented or cemented stems. In this case, a cemented stem was chosen due to the desire for immediate weight bearing and the poor bone quality.

Internal rotation must be avoided. Once the trial components are in place, assessment of patellar tracking is of paramount importance. Flexion and extension balancing should be optimized but is of less importance than in a nonhinged arthroplasty. A hinged prosthesis does not constrain the patellofemoral joint so prosthesis rotation must be accurate (**11.4-4a–b**). Postoperative x-rays showed the joint reconstruction with the distal femoral replacement (**11.4-5a–b**). V.3-B2

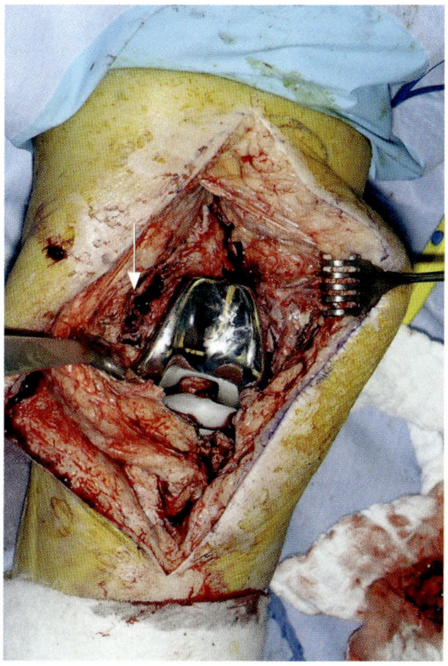

11.4-2 Surgical exposure through a midline incision with medial parapatellar arthrotomy. The fracture line can be seen just proximal to the femoral component (white arrow).

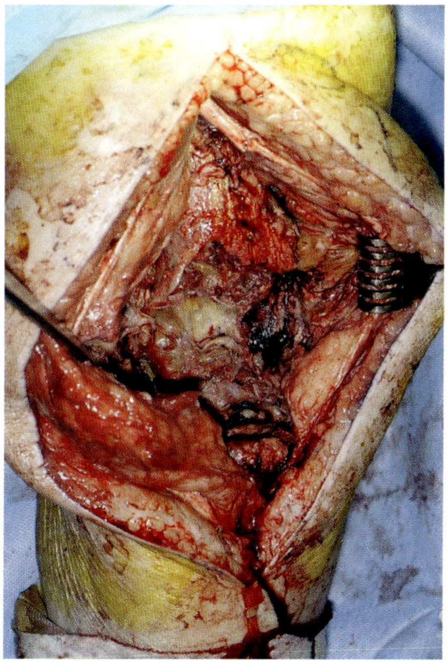

11.4-3 Bone defect after the removal of previous knee arthroplasty components.

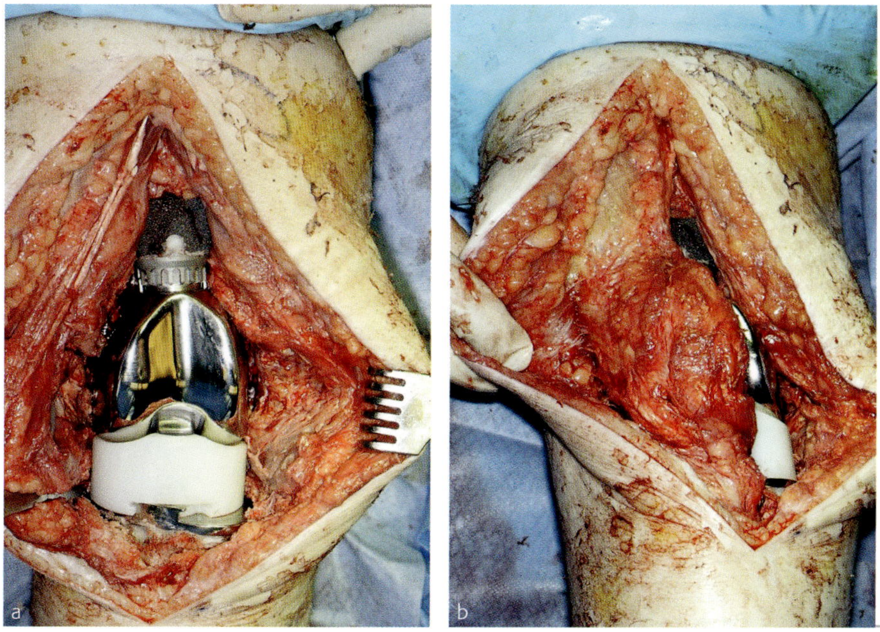

11.4-4a–b Prosthetic reconstruction.
- **a** Reconstruction using a rotating hinge distal femoral arthroplasty prosthesis.
- **b** Reconstruction with reduced extensor mechanism shows good restoration of the joint line. Patellofemoral tracking must be performed to ensure accurate component rotation.

V.3-B2

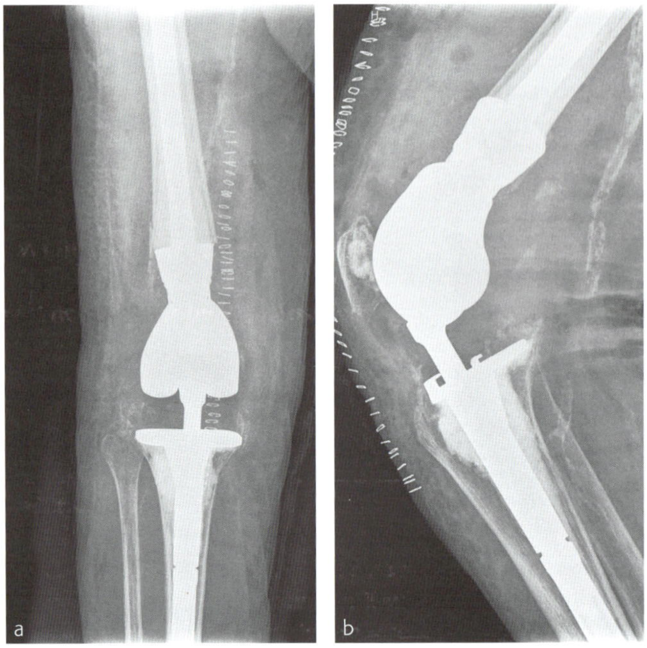

11.4-5a–b X-rays obtained immediately postoperatively show prosthetic reconstruction.
a AP view.
b Lateral view.

Rehabilitation and follow-up

The initial bulky dressing and extension splint were left in place for 48 hours. After dressing reduction, gentle range-of-motion exercises were initiated, and the patient was mobilized with full weight bearing. Perioperative antibiotic prophylaxis was used for 24 hours. Prophylaxis for deep vein thrombosis was administered until the patient was discharged to a rehabilitation facility.

No important early medical or surgical complications developed in this patient. Her wound healed without incident, and she was discharged to rehabilitation after 2 weeks where she was able to walk with a walker and assistance. Nine months postoperatively the patient's knee was functioning without any complaints. She was not willing to come for a comprehensive follow-up due to general frailty.

Points to remember

- Treatment of distal femoral periprosthetic fractures with revision knee arthroplasty is best performed by experienced providers.
- Strict adherence to antibiotic prophylaxis and sterile technique is required as deep infection is a catastrophic complication.
- The surgical approach rarely requires extensile arthroplasty exposure; however, if a tibial tubercle osteotomy is considered, fixation will be difficult given the osteoporosis seen in these patients.
- The tibial component also must be revised to allow for a compatible stemmed tibial component.
- The joint line is established first by restoring the tibial platform.
- The inferior patellar pole guides the level of the joint line. If a tibial tubercle osteotomy or quadriceps turndown has been used, this needs to be taken into account when landmarking the joint line.
- Correct rotation of the femoral component is difficult to achieve given the lack of landmarks, but it is vital to a good outcome.
- Careful attention to patellofemoral tracking is required before definitive component implantation.
- A constrained prosthesis using a rotating hinge is required for stability in these cases due to incompetent collateral ligaments.
- A modern hinged prosthesis with some rotational freedom should decrease transmitted stress to the bone prosthesis interphase and improve component longevity.

11.5 Bilateral distal femoral interprosthetic fractures, stable prosthesis

MIPO: bilateral LCP 4.5/5.0 distal femur, LAP, secondary medial buttress plate

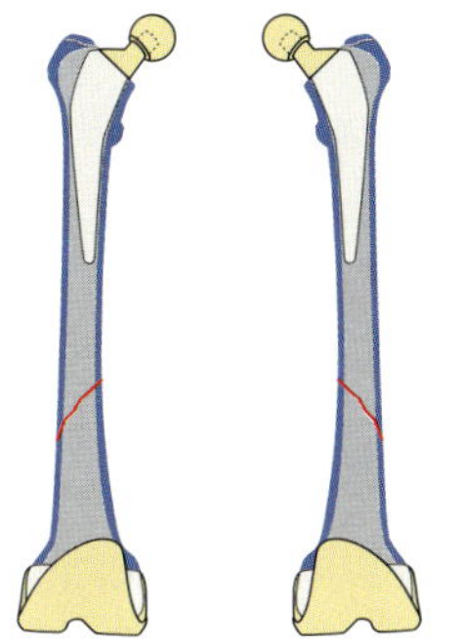

V.3-D
V.3-D

Author **Christoph Sommer**

Case description

A 64-year-old woman sustained bilateral distal metaphyseal femoral fractures (closed on the left side, open grade 1 on the anterior right side) after falling down a flight of stairs (👁 **11.5-1a–d**). She has a 35-year history of chronic rheumatoid arthritis and has taken steroids for more than 20 years. More recently, she started taking immunosuppressive medication. She has diabetes mellitus and a body mass index of 31. Fifteen years ago she underwent bilateral total hip arthroplasties, and more than 11 years ago had bilateral total knee arthroplasties. She also had osteoporosis for which she has taken calcium and vitamin D3 for many years. Although there were no objective parameters to specify the degree of osteoporosis, marked thinning of the cortical bone at the distal metaphysis and shaft of both femora suggested poor local bone quality in that region.

Classification: Types V.3-D

Diagnosis: Bilateral interprosthetic multifragmentary metaphyseal distal femoral fractures with osteoporosis and a stable prosthesis

Decision making

Operative intervention was mandatory to get the patient mobilized. CT was ordered to confirm the stability of the femoral components of the total knee arthroplasties. Despite the metallic artifacts, stable fixation of both prostheses was verified. Although the type of femoral component permitted use of a retrograde intramedullary nail, fixation with a long locking plate seemed more appropriate. Compared to retrograde nailing that comprises a few locking bolts, a long locking plate allows insertion of multiple locking-head screws, resulting in a larger bone-implant interface. Long plates overlapping the stem of the total hip arthroplasty (at least 6 cm) also avoid the critical junction and stress concentration between a retrograde nail and the distal end of the stem. Similarly, a revision prosthesis with a long stem increases the risk of a stress fracture between the two stems. Finally, by planning a minimally invasive plate osteosynthesis, periosteal and muscular attachments to the fracture fragments would be preserved best (chapter 5.4.1).

In patients with a very short distal periarticular main fragment, a second medial plate combined with polymethylmethacrylate might be an option to better anchor the locking-head screws in this region. However, this decision must be made intraoperatively, depending on the quality of fixation achieved.

Long plates generally are recommended in such circumstances, overlapping the distal end of the proximal prosthetic stem by at least 6 cm. The number of screws must be adjusted to the length of the plate and the quality of the bone. In the distal main fragment of this patient, insertion of as many screws as possible was planned due to the poor bone quality and the short periarticular fragment. The proximal end of the plate would be fixed with one periprosthetic screw (monocortical with flat tip) and a locking attachment plate (LAP) to prevent drilling into the cement mantle. Together with two bicortical locking, head screws below the tip of the stem (one close to the fracture), eight cortices, which is the minimal number recommended, would be grabbed proximally.

V.3-D
V.3-D

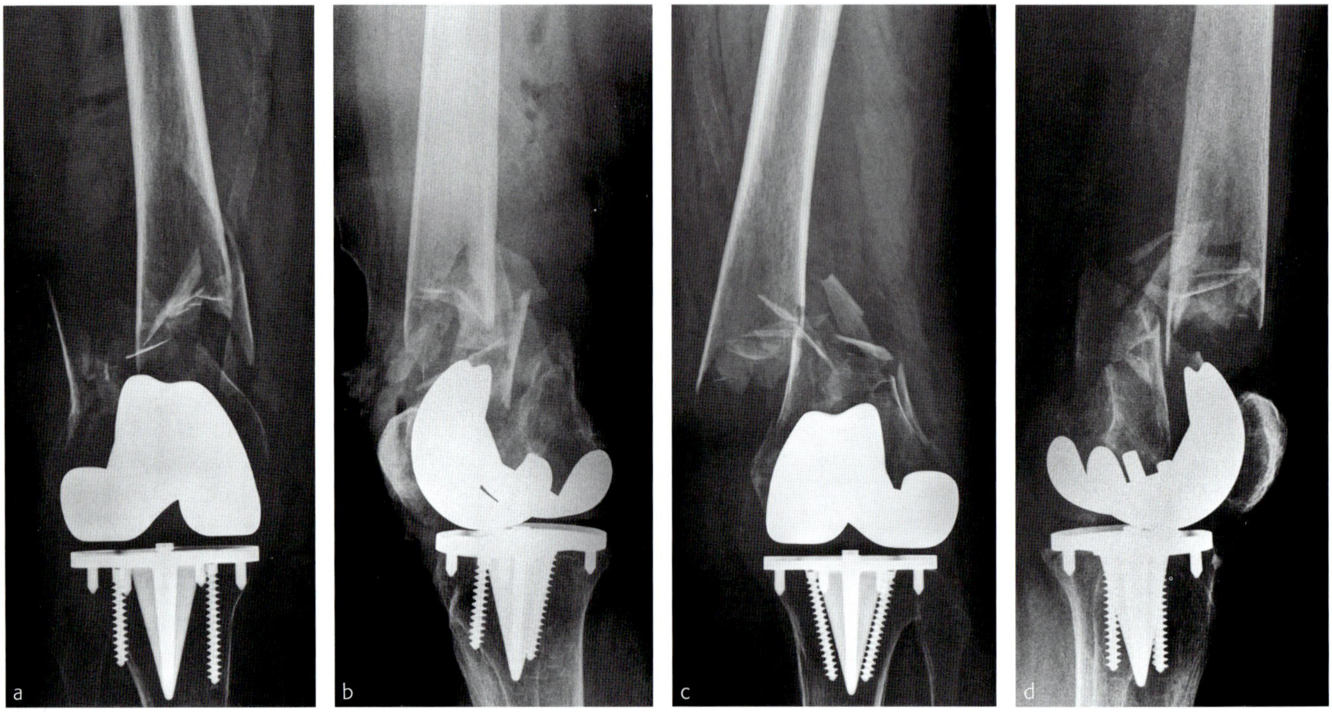

11.5-1a–d X-rays obtained immediately after injury.
a AP view of the right knee shows a highly comminuted distal fracture in osteoporotic bone.
b Lateral view of the right knee.
c AP view of the left knee shows considerable medial displacement of the femoral shaft.
d Lateral view of the left knee.

Preoperative planning

Equipment

- 13-hole distal femur locking compression plate (LCP), left and right (with or without aiming device) (longer plates with 15 holes would have been preferred but were not available)
- Instruments and locking-head screws for a LCP 4.5/5.0
- Conventional 4.5 mm cortex screws
- LAP
- Instruments and locking-head screws for a LCP 3.5 (for the LAP)
- 2.0 mm K-wires

Patient preparation and positioning

- Antibiotic prophylaxis
- Supine position with both legs prepared up to the hip
- Knees flexed 20–30° (hinged leg holder or pad, towel roll under the knees)

Reduction and fixation

A short lateral extraarticular approach was used. The incision began just above the lateral joint space and continued proximally for about 6 cm. It was placed at the border between the anterior and middle third of the lateral femoral condyle at the level of the planned plate position. The bone was exposed only distal to the fracture area, leaving the fracture hematoma untouched.

The distal femur LCP was first inserted through a submuscular tunnel running distal to proximal. For this purpose, a threaded drill sleeve that was firmly screwed to the most distal plate hole was used as a handle. Correct plate positioning in relation to the distal femur was confirmed using an image intensifier in both planes. Axial alignment in the frontal plane was adjusted by manipulating the lower leg (varus/valgus position) until the joint space was absolutely parallel to the drill sleeve (**11.5-2a**). By inserting two

K-wires through the corresponding anterior and posterior K-wire holes of the plate, the plate was held in position distally. Then, a 5.0 mm locking-head screw was inserted into the most distal plate hole parallel to the joint space. Proximally, the plate was centered over the femur, and once correct rotation and length of the leg was established and confirmed, a conventional 4.5 mm cortex screw was inserted through a stab incision (**11.5-2b**). This step approximates the femoral shaft to the plate. In this case with bilateral comminuted fractures and severe osteoporosis, a moderate, symmetrical shortening by longitudinal impaction of the fracture was part of the plan.

Axial alignment in the sagittal plane (lateral view) was then checked. A genu recurvatum malalignment often is present but can be corrected by placing a towel roll or a bump under the fracture site and applying manual force, or by flexing the knee, as was done for this patient (**11.5-2c–d**). This V.3-D
step correctly centered the femoral shaft onto the full length V.3-D
of the plate after which time additional screws were inserted. Distally, all threaded holes were used to optimize the critical purchase of the locking-head screws in the patient's poor-quality bone.

Proximally, two bicortical locking-head screws were used, one just proximal to the fracture, the other just distal to the stem of the proximal prosthesis. The screws were placed wide apart to allow a flexible fixation of the long plate. Proximally, overlapping the stem by 3–4 cm, a short monocortical periprosthetic screw was placed in the uppermost hole. The LAP was positioned over the second most proximal hole and optimized plate fixation at that level of the stem with four 3.5 mm locking-head screws, which did not interfere with the stem or bone cement.

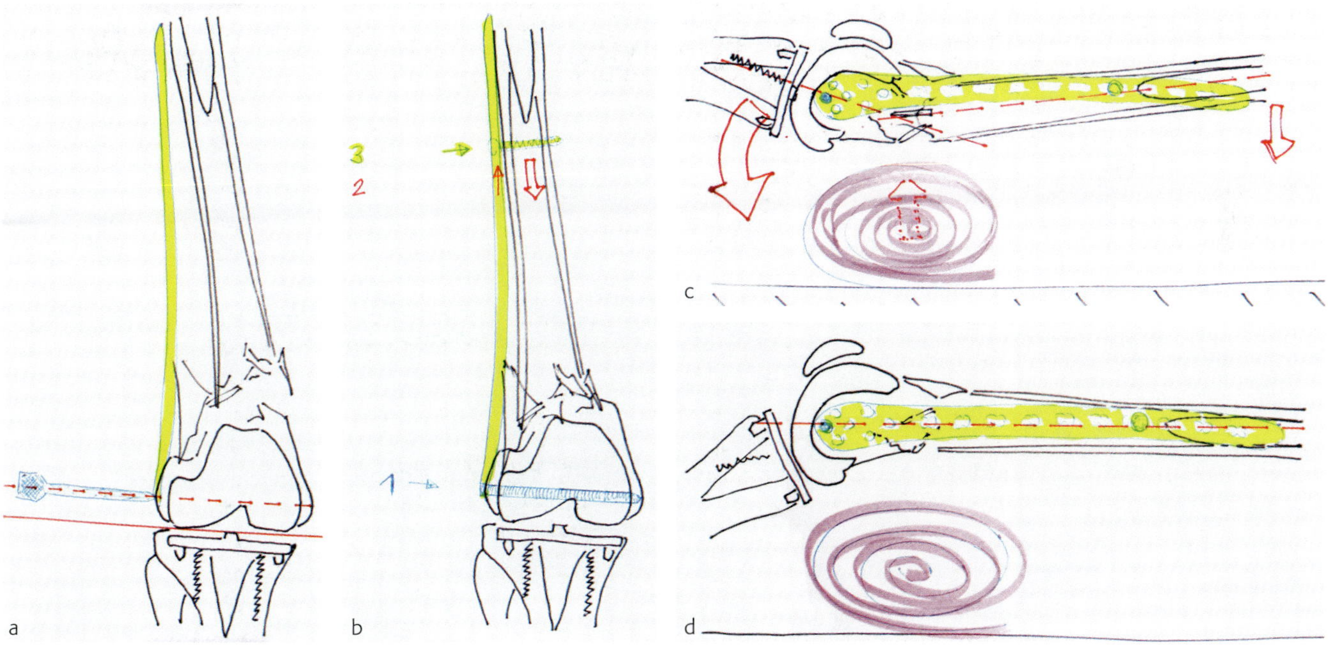

11.5-2a–d Steps of reduction and fixation.

- **a** Correct alignment after valgus displacement of the distal main fragment (joint block) by manipulating the lower leg. The drill sleeve is now oriented parallel to the joint space.
- **b** Preliminary fixation distally with a locking-head screw and proximally with a 4.5 mm cortex screw to approximate the femur to the plate. This allows correction of any malalignment in the frontal plane.
- **c** Typical genu recurvatum malalignment with the knee in extension.
- **d** Correction of a genu recurvatum by placing a towel roll or bolster under the leg at the level of the fracture or by flexing the knee.

V.3-D At the end of the procedure, the stability of the fracture
V.3-D fixation, the prosthesis, and the knee joint was tested under image intensification by varus-valgus and flexion-extension maneuvers. Slight instability of the knee joint was noted, which was most likely preexisting before trauma.

Postoperative x-rays confirmed correct alignment of both reconstructed femurs in both planes. On the left side, there was a slight medial offset, probably due to the forced shortening of the fracture. Stress concentration was avoided by overlapping the plates over the stem of the total hip arthroplasty by 3–4 cm, although this was considered critically short (at least 6 cm are preferred) (**11.5-3a–d**).

Rehabilitation and follow-up

Immediate active and continuous passive knee and hip motion was initiated. The patient was mobilized on postoperative day 2 in a wheelchair. At 10 days, walking exercises in water were encouraged. After 2 months, the patient started to walk on firm ground with partial weight bearing of 30–40 kg on each side with two crutches (4-point walking). At 6 months postoperatively, the patient was pain free, well mobilized on crutches, and ready to go home from the rehabilitation clinic. On the right side, x-rays confirmed slow but ongoing healing. However, the left side showed a secondary loss of reduction without bone healing (**11.5-4a–d**), necessitating another procedure despite the absence of pain and instability.

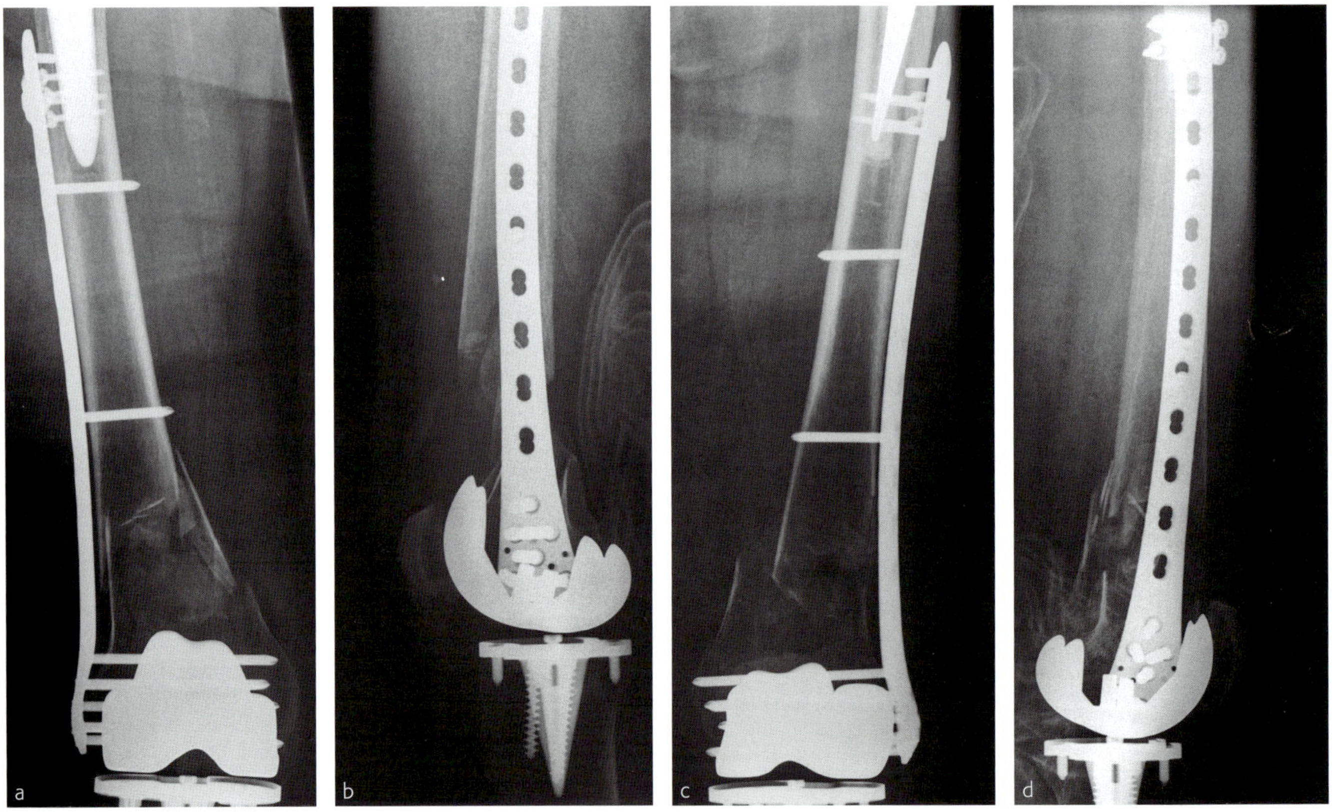

11.5-3a–d X-rays obtained immediately postoperatively.

- **a** AP view of the right knee shows correct axial alignment. The long plate is acting as a bridge across the comminuted fracture zone. At the proximal end, the plate overlaps the stem of the hip prosthesis by about 3–4 cm (as a minimum). It is fixed to the femur with a short locking-head screw and a locking attachment plate, which allows insertion of four 3.5 mm locking-head screws without interfering with the stem or bone cement. The locking attachment plate is an alternative to cerclage wires.
- **b** Lateral view of the right knee shows good correction of recurvation. Note the ventral bone defect.
- **c** AP view of the left knee shows considerable medial off-set of the joint block, either due to shortening of the fracture zone or by a posterior position of the plate in relation to the lateral condyle, or both.
- **d** Lateral view of the left knee shows good alignment of the axis.

Reoperation was performed in two stages. First, atrophic scar tissue from the delayed union site was excised for microbiological culture, resulting in a large bone defect. All distal locking-head screws were removed with no change proximally. The second step allowed a reduction of the distal joint block to the plate. A second plate (reversed anterolateral proximal tibia LCP 3.5) was inserted with a minimally invasive technique on the medial side from distal to proximal. After preliminary supracondylar fixation with a 3.5 mm locking-head screw, a large reduction forceps was placed onto both plates (acting as large washers) for the final reduction (👁 **11.5-5**). All distal screws were augmented by polymethylmethacrylate to optimize the distal anchoring in the patient's severely osteoporotic bone.

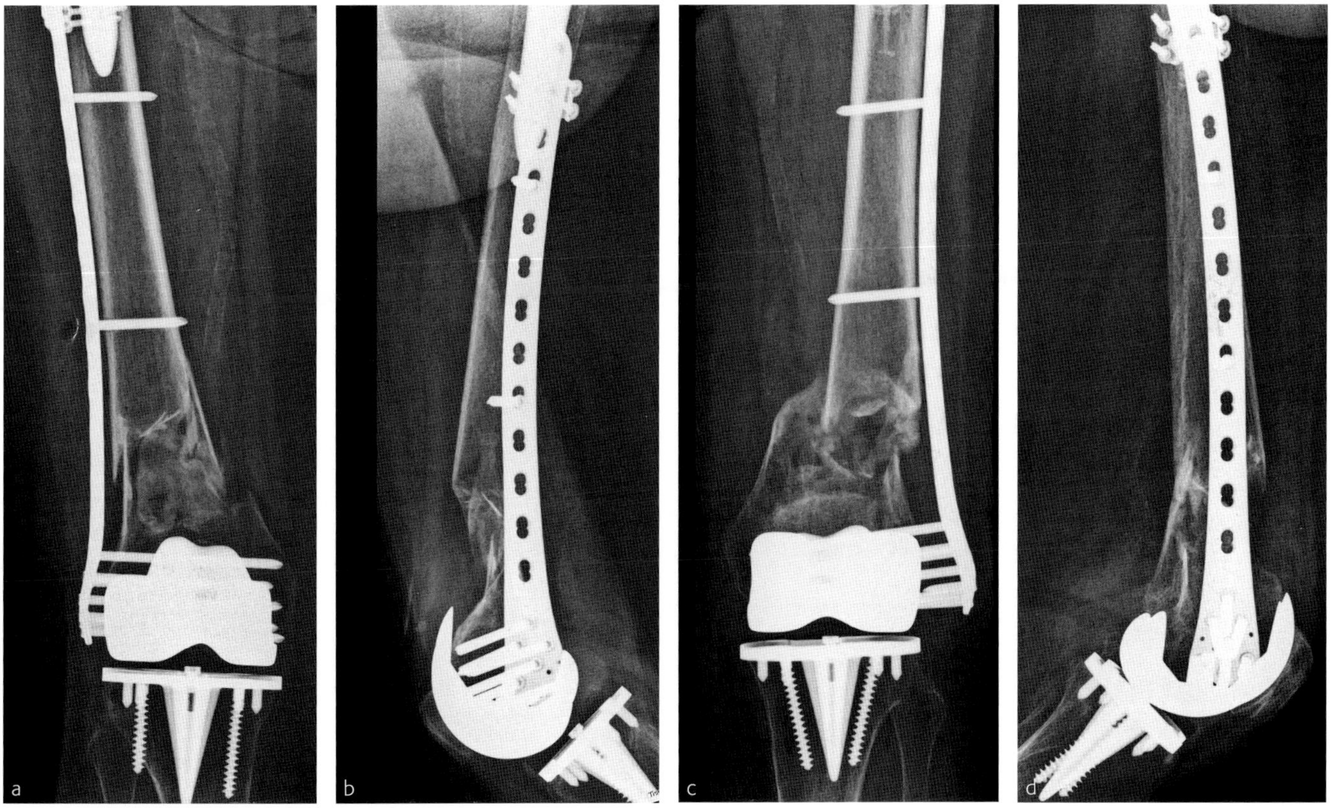

👁 **11.5-4a–d** X-rays obtained 6 months postoperatively.
a AP view of the right knee shows visible but slow healing with little callus formation.
b Lateral view of the right knee shows good axial alignment. The ventral defect persists but healing is progressing.
c AP view of the left knee shows secondary loss of reduction with medialization of the distal femur and delayed union at the fracture site due to partial en bloc pull-out of the distal fixation, whereas proximally there is no change.
d Lateral view of the left knee shows maintenance of axial alignment.

V.3-D Results of tissue cultures were negative. The second surgery
V.3-D was performed 6 days later by filling the bone defect with a mixture of autogenous bone graft from the posterior iliac crest and artificial bone (👁 **11.5-6a–b**).

Further rehabilitation and healing were uneventful. Sixteen months after the injury (and 10 months after reoperation on the left side), the patient mobilized on two elbow crutches, as before injury. Both fractures were completely healed and alignment was good, with the prostheses and implants apparently stable. Implant removal was not advised (👁 **11.5-7a–d**).

Points to remember

- An LCP provides good stability, even in patients with very distal fractures and osteoporotic bone.
- Long overlap between the plate and prosthesis (at least 6 cm) in interprosthetic fractures is advised.
- As an alternative to cerclage wires, the LAP provides good, rigid fixation between the plate and bone at the level of the stem without interfering with the prosthesis or bone cement.
- At the end of the operation, stability of the fracture fixation, the prosthesis, and the knee joint must be tested.

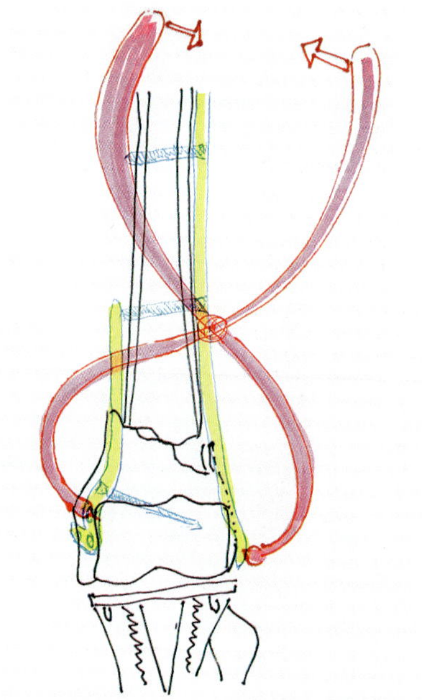

👁 **11.5-5** Plan shows how to perform the reduction maneuver by applying a second plate medially and a large reduction forceps across the knee. Insertion of a bone graft is done as a second step.

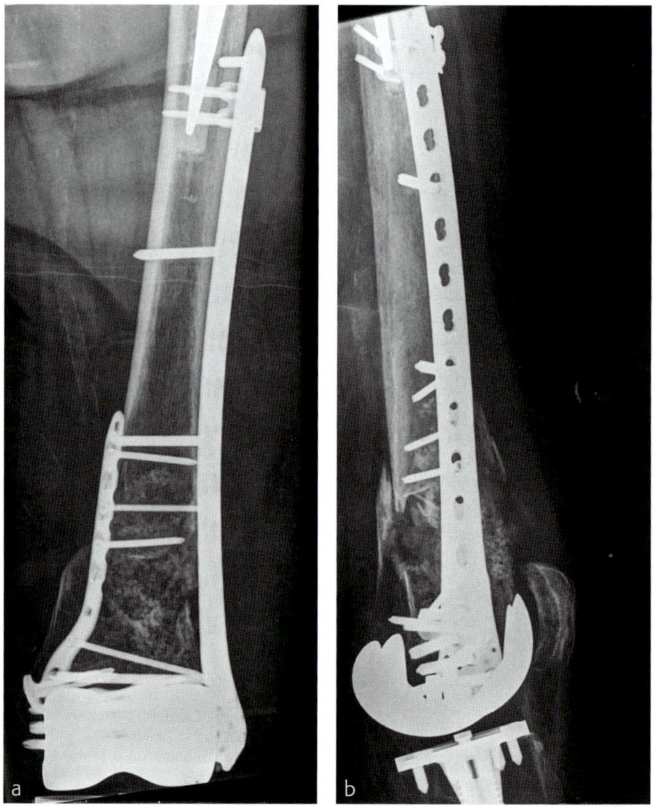

👁 **11.5-6a–b** X-rays obtained after the second surgery and bone grafting of the left knee.

a AP view shows correct alignment and good fixation. All distal screws were augmented with polymethylmethacrylate for better purchase.

b Lateral view.

However, sometimes a slight or moderate instability may already exist before trauma. Only significant instability needs revision arthroplasty.

- Bilateral cases are challenging. Undesired overloading is possible.
- In case of loss of reduction due to poor-quality bone and overloading, a second plate or, if preferred, a strut graft medially can increase stability. This step also could be done primarily. V.3-D
- Screw augmentation with polymethylmethacrylate in the condylar part can optimize the bone-implant interface and might be a good technique even in primary surgery in situations of critical fixation quality (extremely poor-quality bone or distal fracture). V.3-D

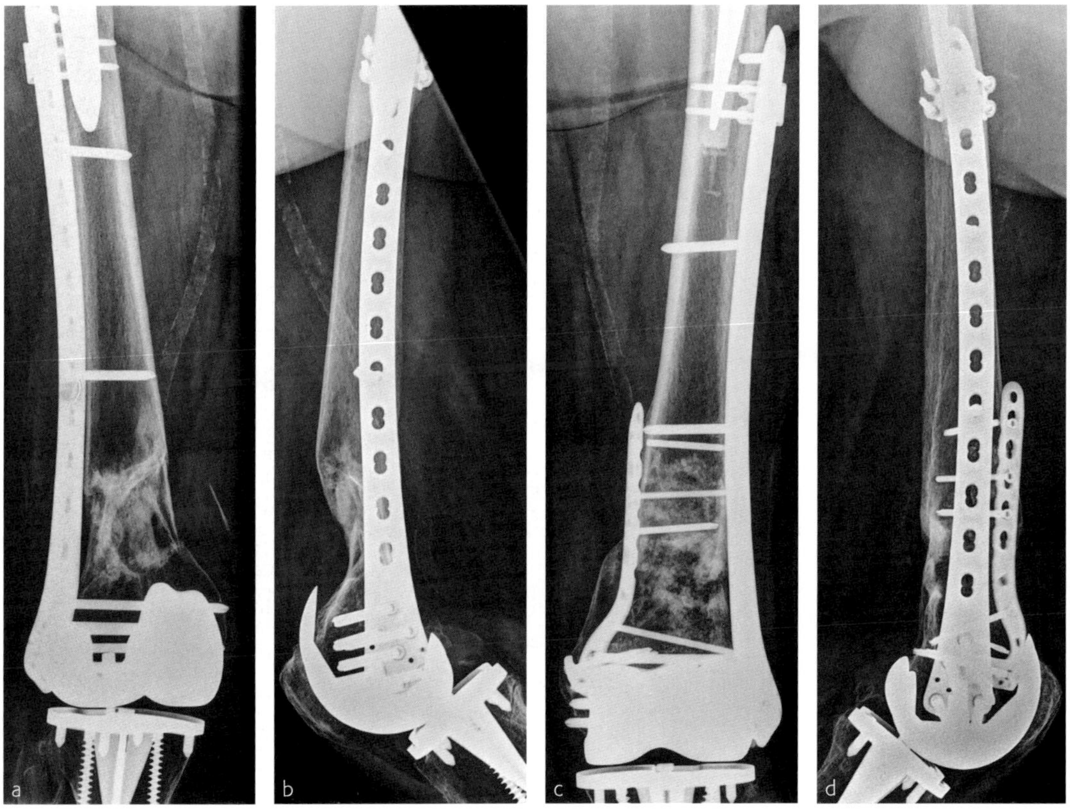

11.5-7a–d X-rays obtained 16 months after injury and 10 months after reoperation on the left side.

a AP view of the right knee shows good alignment.
b Lateral view of the right knee shows alignment is unchanged and the healed aspect of the fracture zone, which looks thin. Implant removal is not recommended.
c AP view of the left knee shows consolidation of the comminuted fracture with integration of the bone graft. The alignment is unchanged compared with the aspect after the reoperation. Medially, the most proximal screw is broken.
d Lateral view of the left knee.

V.3-D

11.6 Interprosthetic distal femoral fracture, stable prosthesis and hip screw

MIPO: polyaxial noncontact plate and secondary addition of a strut graft

Author **Peter Kloen**

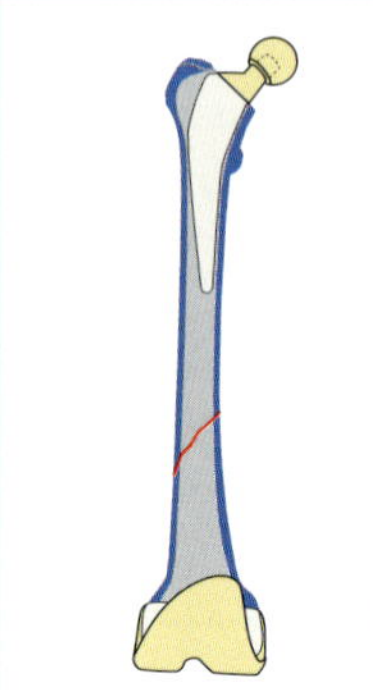

V.3-D

Case description

An otherwise healthy, active 88-year-old woman presented with pain in the right leg after a low-energy fall. In the distant past, she sustained a hip fracture on the same side (treated with a gamma nail) and underwent total knee arthroplasty (TKA). The TKA functioned well, with no evidence of loosening on x-rays (**11.6-1a–c**). A previous attempt at fracture fixation was discontinued when the fracture site was opened because the surgeon did not feel capable to continue nor had the correct plating system available to fix her fairly distal comminuted interprosthetic fracture. The wound was closed, and the patient referred the next day for definitive treatment.

Classification: Type V.3-D

Diagnosis: Interprosthetic femoral fracture between TKA and gamma nail

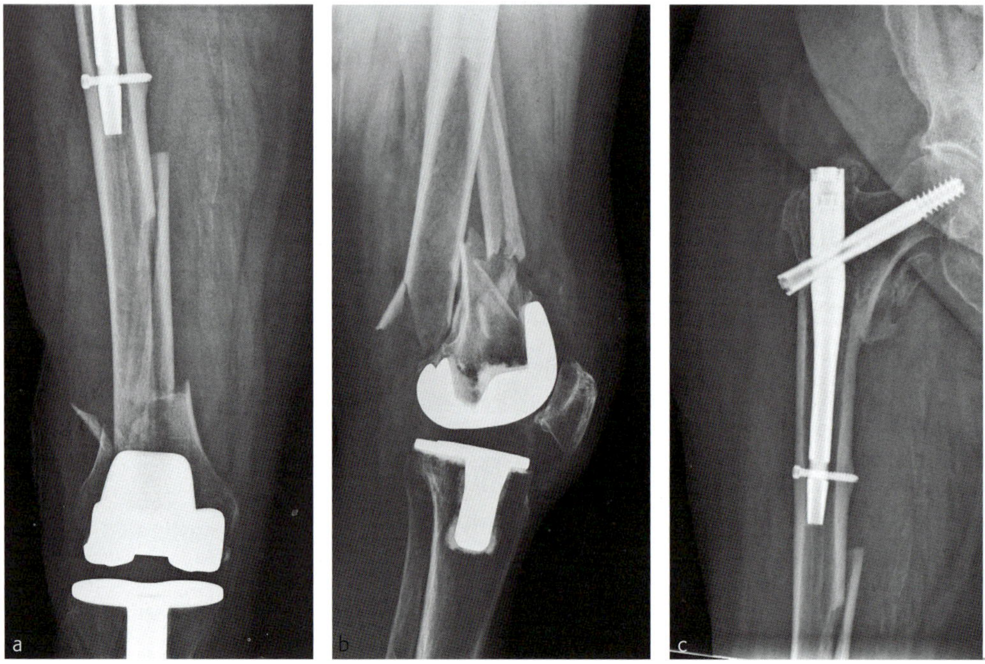

11.6-1a–c X-rays of the distal femoral fracture. Both the total knee arthroplasty and gamma nail appear well fixed.

- **a** AP view.
- **b** Lateral view.
- **c** Gamma nail in situ.

Decision making

The femoral component of the TKA was well fixed; thus, osteosynthesis was the first option to fix the fracture. Retrograde intramedullary nailing was not considered an option because of the closed-box design of the knee prosthesis. A third option was application of a long locking compression plate (LCP) because there appeared to be adequate bone quality (chapter 5.4.1). Revision with a long-stem femoral component or tumor prosthesis would be the last option but would require removal of the gamma nail.

Preoperative planning

Equipment

- LCP system for the distal femur
- Plates of various lengths
- Locking-head screws (ideally bicortical)
- Removal set for the gamma nail
- Bone-graft harvesting tools and/or some type of artificial bone graft (eg, demineralized bone graft)

Patient preparation and positioning

- First- or second-generation cephalosporin for antibiotic prophylaxis
- Low-molecular-weight heparin for thrombosis prophylaxis

Reduction and fixation

The midline incision used for the TKA, which had been reopened by the referring surgeon 2 days before, was used instead of making a new lateral one. Ideally, a lateral incision would have been used; however, a midline approach was used, turning the previous incision more lateral proximally. To apply a long lateral plate, the gamma nail was removed through the old incision. The femoral component of the TKA was well fixed without evidence of loosening. As expected, based on preoperative CT, there was limited bone stock distally.

By placing the leg on a few strategically placed towel rolls, the fracture was reduced anatomically, based on perfect alignment of the metaphyseal lateral cortex. Temporary fixation was obtained by placing two 3.0 mm K-wires from distal to proximal. The large medial butterfly fragment was pulled gently laterally but could not be reduced anatomically. This fragment was not in continuity with any soft-tissue attachment. Although the fragment may have been used as a "strut" graft, it could not be reduced anatomically without further stripping and devascularization of the medial side of the femur. Therefore, the butterfly fragment, which measured about 12 × 1 cm proximally and widened to about 2.5 cm distally, was removed entirely. V.3-D

To optimize screw fixation in the condylar fragment, the femoral less invasive stabilization system (LISS) was considered suboptimal, given its fixed-angle screw option. Instead, a polyaxial noncontact plate was selected because it allows variation in screw direction of up to 30° (chapter 5.4.1). This increased variation in screw direction would allow the screw to be directed toward the bone that is best available. The 13-hole plate was inserted with the targeting device using a minimally invasive surgical technique.

With the assistance of the targeting device, the plate was inserted between the vastus lateralis muscle and the periosteum. Selecting periprosthetic femur plate system, anatomically contoured with a good distal fit. The image intensifier showed that proximally the plate overlapped with the gamma nail; therefore, the nail was removed. Some of the distal screws were placed into the cement, and the proximal locking-head screws were inserted percutaneously. Note that currently no strict guidelines specify how many screws are needed proximally and distally. In this situation, four locking-head screws were planned on either side (ideally locking and bicortical). In the proximal aspect bicortical screws were used, whereas in the area opposite the removed medial butterfly fragment short monocortical screws were used as there was no opposite cortex. The defect was filled with 20 mL of demineralized bone matrix (👁 **11.6-2a–d**).

Rehabilitation and follow-up

Toe-touch weight bearing was allowed for 6 weeks. At regular follow-up visits a delay in bone healing was noted. At 6 months postoperatively, CT showed no medial bridging where the large cortical butterfly cortical fragment had been removed in the initial surgery (👁 **11.6-3a–c**).

Although the patient reported no pain and the plate fixation seemed to be stable, full weight bearing was a concern because the large medial defect could lead to plate fatigue and failure. A second surgery was performed in which a fibular allograft was placed anteromedially as a strut graft in an effort to increase stability and optimize biology. The graft was impacted distally in the condylar block and proximally press-fitted under the medial cortex. The strut graft was fixed with two 3.5 mm screws from medial to lateral and with a 4.5 mm screw from lateral to medial through the

V.3-D

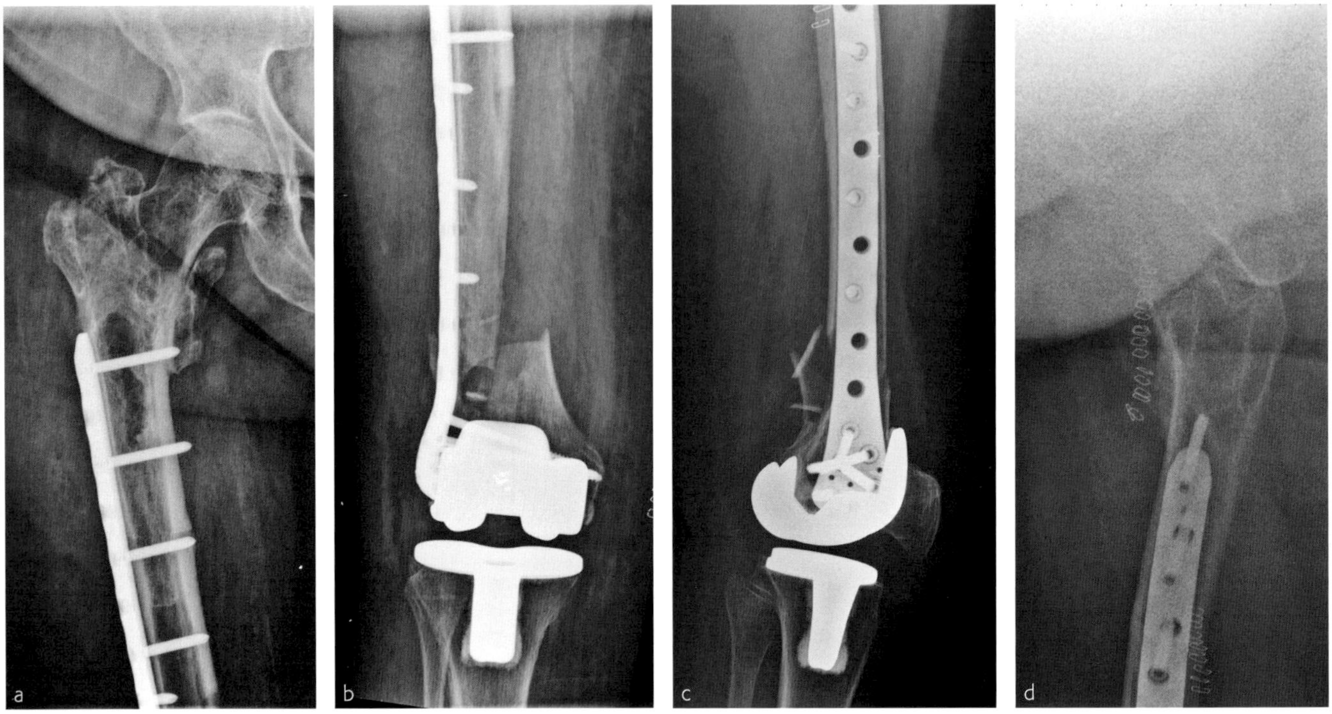

11.6-2a–d X-rays obtained immediately postoperatively.
a–b AP views.
c–d Lateral views.

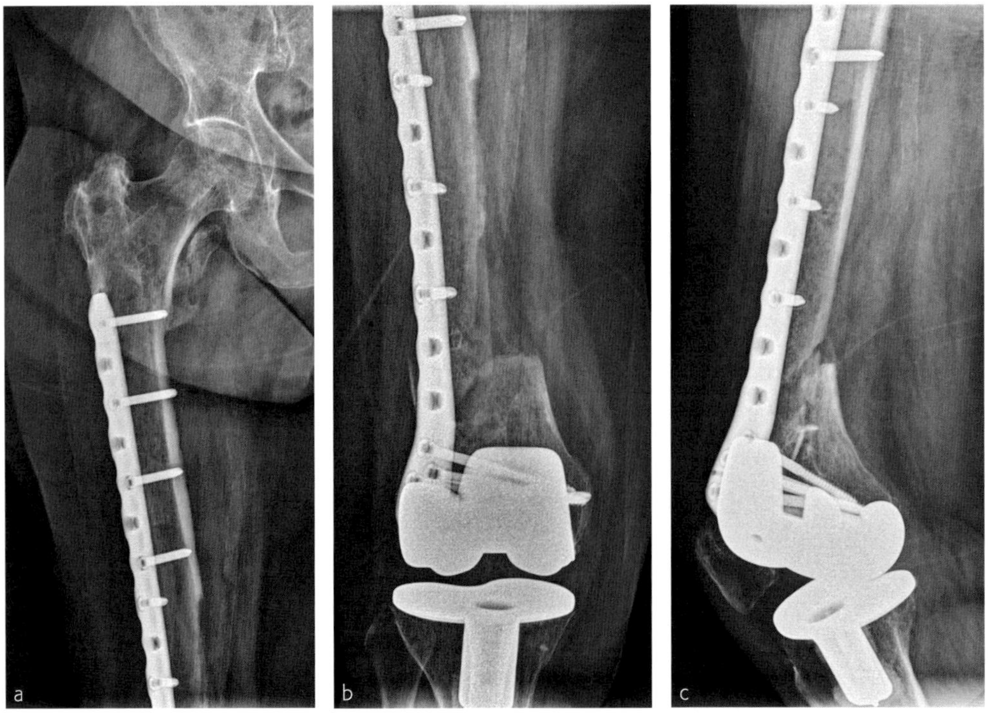

11.6-3a–c X-rays show delayed healing at 6 months postoperatively.
a–b AP views.
c Lateral view.

plate and the strut graft. A large volume of iliac crest graft mixed with 10 mL of demineralized bone matrix also was added. The iliac crest graft was harvested from the posterior iliac crests when the patient was in a prone position before repositioning her into a supine position.

Partial weight bearing was now allowed. At 2 months postoperatively, the patient was doing well and progressed to full weight bearing. Range of motion was similar to preinjury levels. At 9 months postoperatively, there was incomplete incorporation of the fibular allograft but good range of motion (👁 **11.6-4a–c**). Despite screw failure and incomplete incorporation of the fibular allograft distally, the patient was pain free and tolerated full weight bearing in good alignment.

Fifteen months after the strut grafting procedure, full weight bearing was tolerated. X-rays showed further incorporation of the allograft (👁 **11.6-5a–c**). The patient had good range of motion, which was now similar to prefracture levels (👁 **11.6-6a–b**). She could walk for longer than an hour and had no pain.

Points to remember

- Careful preoperative planning is needed with these critical fracture situations.
- Inability to fix the fracture might require conversion to a revision TKA. If a long-stem revision TKA is not immediately available, surgery should be delayed to assemble to all available options.
- The large butterfly fragment could have been used as a medial strut graft, similar to what was done in the second surgery with the fibular graft. The fibular allograft is incorporated by creeping substitution.
- Polyaxial screws allow more freedom, as they can be directed into the area of best available bone stock.
- The plate must overlap with potential stress risers. When in doubt, a longer plate is preferred over a shorter plate.
- Despite presence of a TKA, valuable information can be obtained with preoperative CT.
- Good alignment of the plate proximally should be confirmed. A small incision can help with manual realignment of the plate proximally before fixation distally.

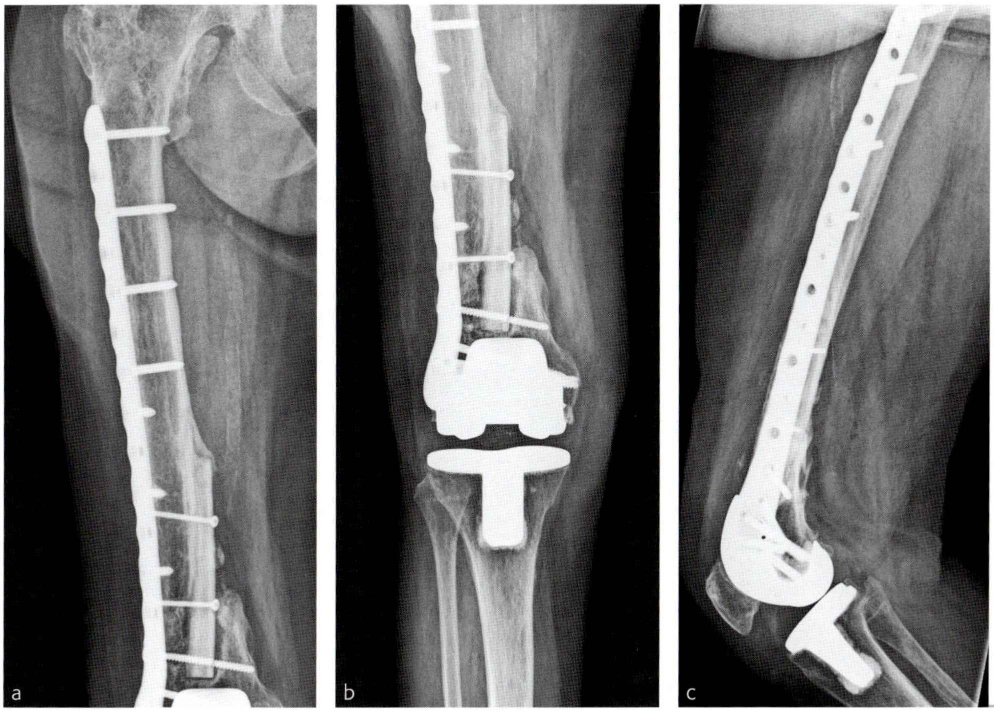

👁 **11.6-4a–c** X-rays obtained 9 months after the last surgery show incorporation of the fibular allograft proximally. Distally, the conventional screw through the plate, lateral femoral cortex, fibular allograft (two cortices), and medial femoral cortex has failed. Compared with x-rays obtained earlier, there is increased bridging distally, although an area of lysis can be seen around the distal aspect of the allograft.
a–b AP views.
c Lateral view.

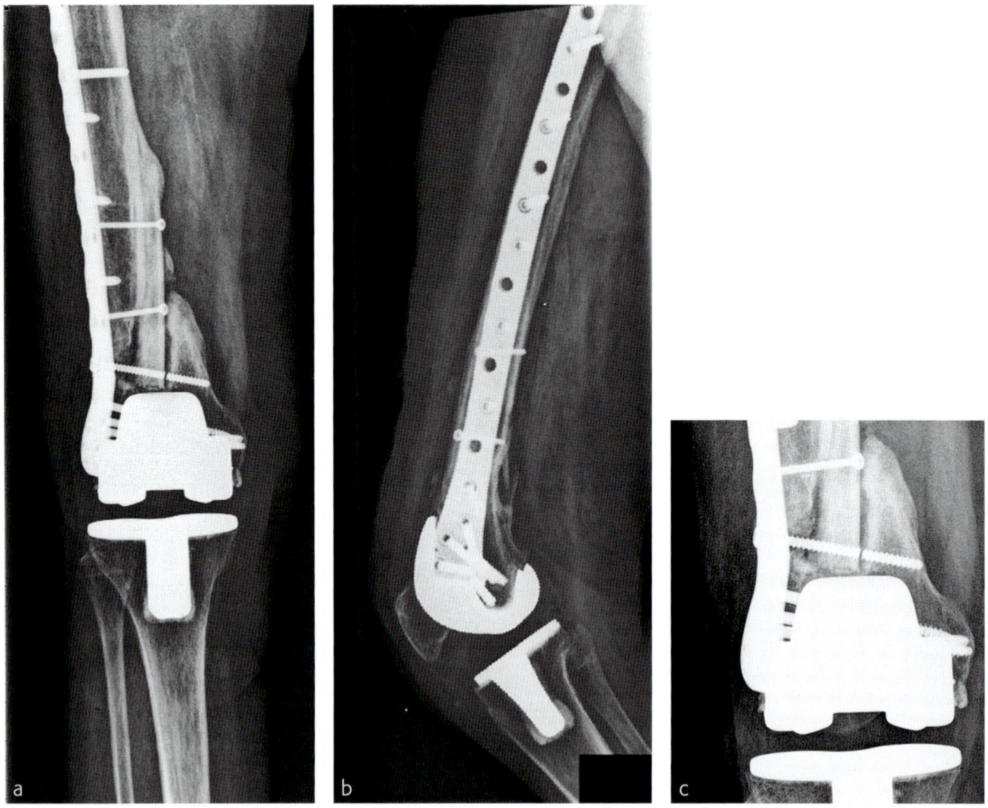

11.6-5a–c X-rays obtained 15 months after the last surgery show incorporation of the fibular allograft proximally. Distally, there is still incomplete incorporation of the allograft. However, there is good consolidation on the lateral side.

a AP view.
b Lateral view.
c Detailed view of the distal part of the allograft.

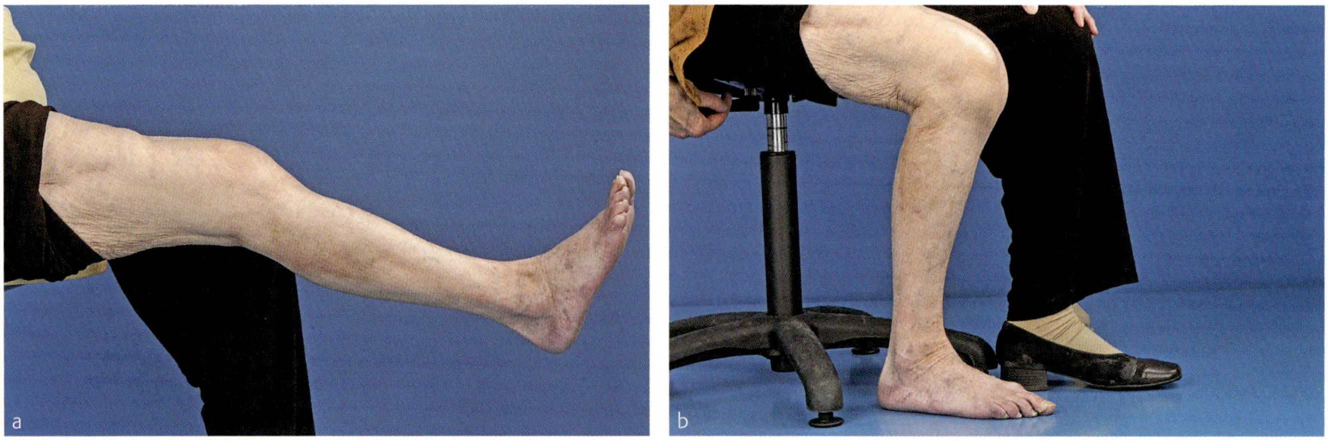

11.6-6a–b The patient has good range of motion at her last follow-up, similar to her status before the fracture.

11.7 Distal femoral fracture complicated by contralateral intercalary fracture, stable prostheses

ORIF: bilateral retrograde intramedullary nails

Author **Emilio Fantin**

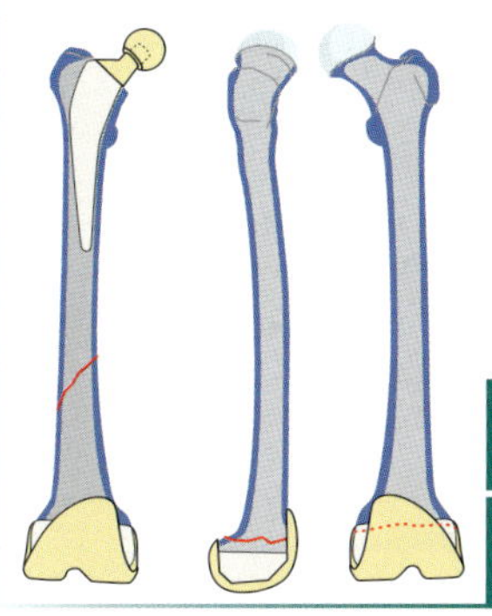

V.3-D

V.3-B1

Case description

A 68-year-old woman who presented with a painful left knee as a result of a fall at home (**11.7-1a–b**) has had rheumatoid arthritis since age 16 treated with corticosteroids and multiple medications for many years. Comorbidities included diabetes mellitus and hypertension, and she had a history of multiple surgeries on the hands and feet, a total hip arthroplasty on the right side, and bilateral total knee arthroplasties at age 52.

Classification: left: Type V.3-D
right: Type V.3-B1

Diagnosis: Supracondylar periprosthetic fracture of the left femur with a well-fixed femoral prosthesis, followed by interprosthetic fracture of the right femur

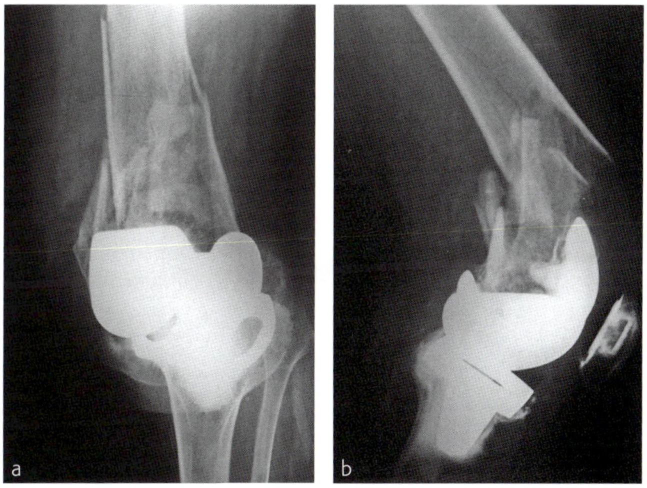

11.7-1a–b X-rays obtained shortly after the injury show a total knee arthroplasty with supracondylar femoral fracture on the left side.
- **a** AP view.
- **b** Lateral view.

Decision making

Because the patient had multiple comorbidities, several different treatment options were considered, ranging from revision of the total knee arthroplasty to osteosynthesis with plates or nails. Retrograde intramedullary nailing was chosen because it is a minimally invasive technique, with the possibility to offer a certain amount of stability to the fracture.

V.3-D
V.3-B1

Preoperative planning

Equipment

- Retrograde femoral nail
- Radiolucent operating table
- Image intensifier
- Bone cement (PMMC)

Patient preparation and positioning

- Supine position on fracture table with a support placed under the knee (👁 **11.7-2**)

Reduction and fixation

A minimally invasive surgical approach was used for a medial patellar tendon arthrotomy. Indirect reduction was performed, and a retrograde intramedullary nail was used. Due to insufficient fixation between the nail and the distal fracture fragment, an augmentation technique with polymethylmethacrylate bone cement was necessary (👁 **11.7-3**).

Rehabilitation and follow-up

Four weeks postoperatively, the patient returned to her home in a wheelchair. She started walking with a cane at 20 weeks postoperatively. X-rays showed fracture union (👁 **11.7-4a–b**).

Contralateral fracture

Eight months after the first fracture on the left side, the patient sustained an interprosthetic supracondylar fracture of the right femur, with stable total knee arthroplasty and total hip arthroplasty, as a result of another fall at home (👁 **11.7-5a–b**). Plate fixation was the first choice of treatment for this fracture, retrograde intramedullary nailing being the second choice. Because of the patient's general condition, intramedullary nailing via minimally invasive surgery was selected on the right side as well. X-rays obtained 4 months after the second operation showed good consolidation (👁 **11.7-6a–c**).

Points to remember

- Careful preoperative planning is critical to confirm that the knee prosthesis can tolerate retrograde nailing.
- In case of an additional hip prosthesis, a potential disadvantage of the technique is having an extremely short zone of stress rising between the stem of the prosthesis and the nail, as present in the right side of this case.
- In patients with multiple comorbidities, many treatment options must be evaluated, including staged procedures.

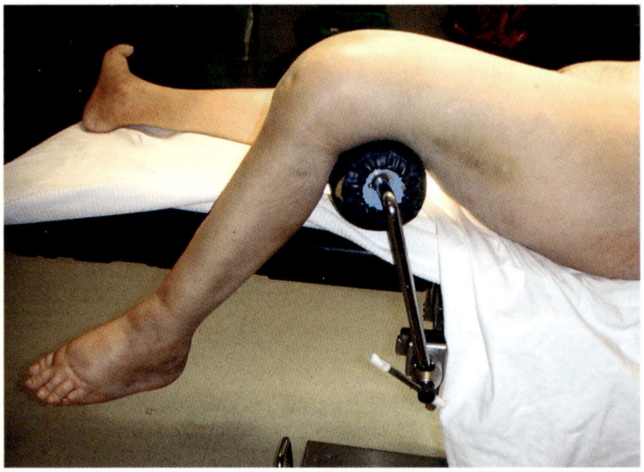

👁 **11.7-2** Patient placed in a supine position with a support under the knee.

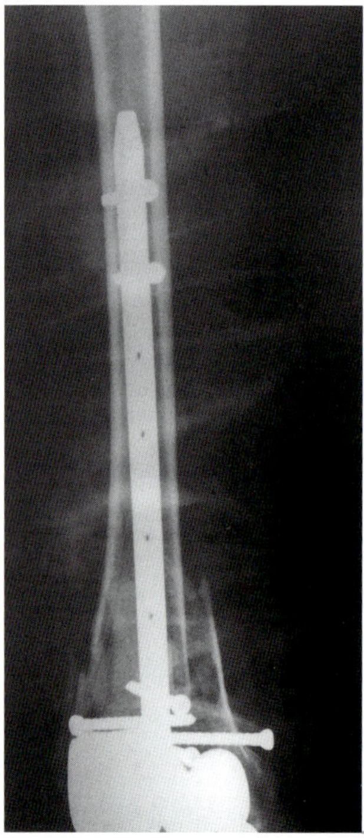

👁 **11.7-3** X-ray of the left distal femur obtained immediately postoperatively.

11.7 **Distal femoral fracture complicated by contralateral intercalary fracture, stable prostheses**

ORIF: bilateral retrograde intramedullary nails

V.3-D
V.3-B1

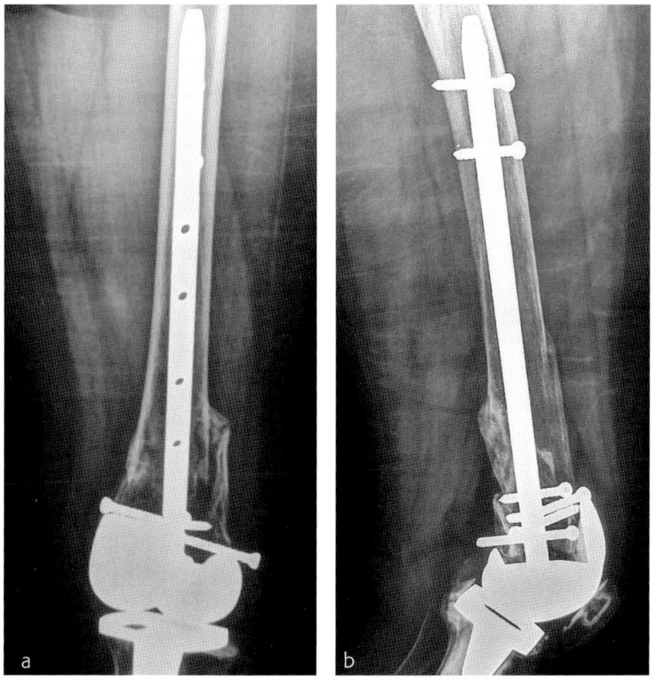

11.7-4a–b X-rays of the left femur obtained 5 months postoperatively show fracture union. Treatment with a retrograde intramedullary nail and augmentation with polymethylmethacrylate bone cement were successful.
- **a** AP view.
- **b** Lateral view.

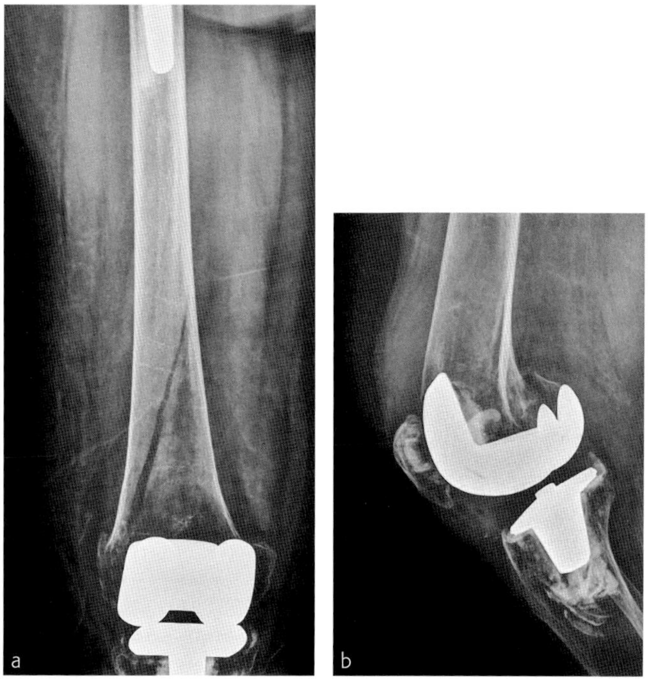

11.7-5a–b X-rays of the right side with a new periprosthetic fracture, which occurred 8 months after the first periprosthetic fracture on the left side.
- **a** AP view.
- **b** Lateral view.

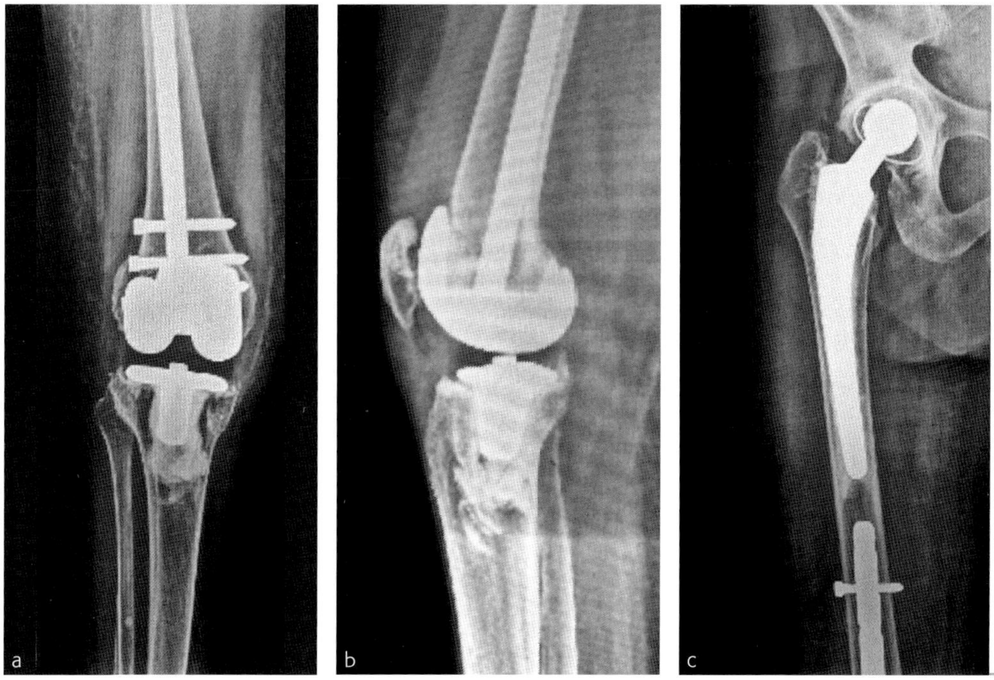

11.7-6a–c X-rays of the right side obtained 4 months after minimally invasive intramedullary nailing.
- **a** AP view.
- **b** Lateral view.
- **c** AP view of proximal femur with the critical zone as stress riser between the two implants.

V.4-B1

11.8 Proximal tibial fracture, stable unicondylar prosthesis

MIPO: LISS proximal tibia and LCP

Author **Peter Kloen**

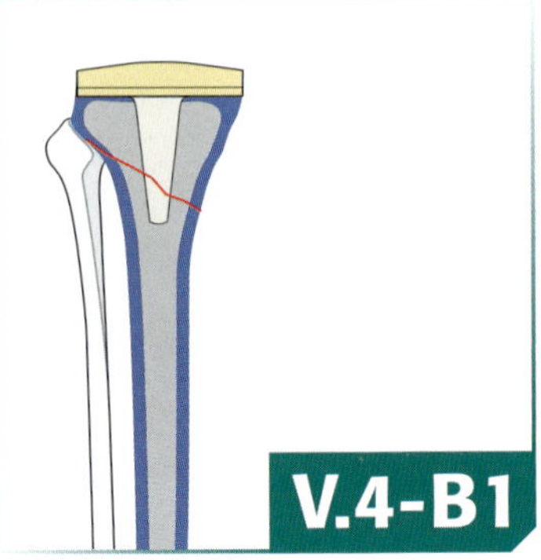

Case description

A 60-year-old man, who had a medial hemiarthroplasty of the right nee several years ago, was unable to bear weight on the right leg after a low-energy fall. Examination revealed moderate soft-tissue swelling with a large area of ecchymosis and bruising (**11.8-1a–b**). Results of a neurovascular examination were within normal limits. There was no evidence of loosening of the well-functioning prosthesis before the patient fell. The patient also had a long history of alcohol abuse.

Classification: Type V.4-B1

Diagnosis: Periprosthetic fracture of the proximal tibia, with a stable hemiarthroplasty

Decision making

Cast bracing of the patient's unstable fracture was inappropriate because of the necessity for long-term immobilization and the anticipated poor patient compliance. Osteosynthesis possibly would be compromised by noticeable osteopenia and the poor condition of the soft tissues. If the tibial component had been obviously loose, revision total knee arthroplasty would have been considered with a long-stem tibial component. However, the knee had been well functioning prior to the fall, with no radiological or clinical evidence of loosening. Due to the soft-tissue swelling, knee-spanning external fixation was selected as an initial step to provide pain control, alignment, and soft-tissue healing. Ten days later, the soft tissues had healed completely, and definitive open reduction and internal fixation with plates was planned (chapter 5.4.1).

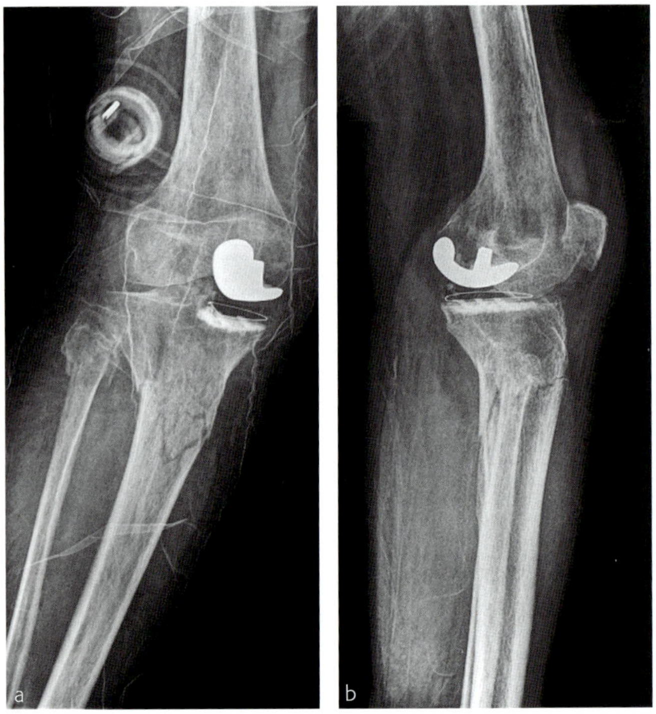

11.8-1a–b X-rays obtained shortly after the injury. Due to considerable swelling, a joint-spanning external fixator was applied as a first step.
a AP view.
b Lateral view.

Preoperative planning

Equipment

- Less invasive stabilization system proximal tibia (LISS PTL)
- Locking compression plate (LCP) 3.5
- 5.0 and 3.5 mm locking-head and conventional 4.5 mm cortex screws
- 2 mm K-wires

Patient preparation and positioning

- First- or second-generation cephalosporin for antibiotic prophylaxis
- Low-molecular-weight heparin for thrombosis prophylaxis

Reduction and fixation

The external fixator was removed before surgical preparation and draping. Use of a femoral distractor was not anticipated; otherwise, one of the Schanz screws would have been left in place in the distal tibia. The external fixator pin sites in the proximal femur were maintained outside the surgical field.

A hockey-stick incision of approximately 5 cm was made, starting from Gerdy's tubercle, with dissection down to the periosteum. V.4-B1

After the anterior lateral compartment was opened and the anterior tibial muscle released from the proximal aspect of the tibia, the fracture was reduced under direct vision. Gentle varus stress was applied to the lower leg until the lateral cortex was aligned anatomically (**11.8-2a**). A collapsed joint surface should be gently elevated, if necessary. A tunnel was then made for epiperiosteal insertion of a 9-hole LISS PTL with a MIPO technique. The presence of an associated longitudinal split in the plateau was inconclusive on CT scan. A large pointed Weber forceps was placed to compress the plateau in the event of an intraarticular fracture. The LISS PTL was temporarily fixed with 2 mm K-wires inserted at either end through the drill sleeve. Correct alignment in the lateral plane was verified radiologically (**11.8-2b**). The LISS PTL was then fixed to the tibia with locking-head screws. The unicondylar medial plateau knee arthroplasty prevented use of all proximal screws holes; therefore, application of a second small medial plate as a buttress was believed to be beneficial to augment the lateral fixation. The plate was applied via two small incisions that allowed placement of a reconstruction LCP 3.5 with four locking-head screws. Postoperative x-rays showed good joint congruency (**11.8-3a–b**).

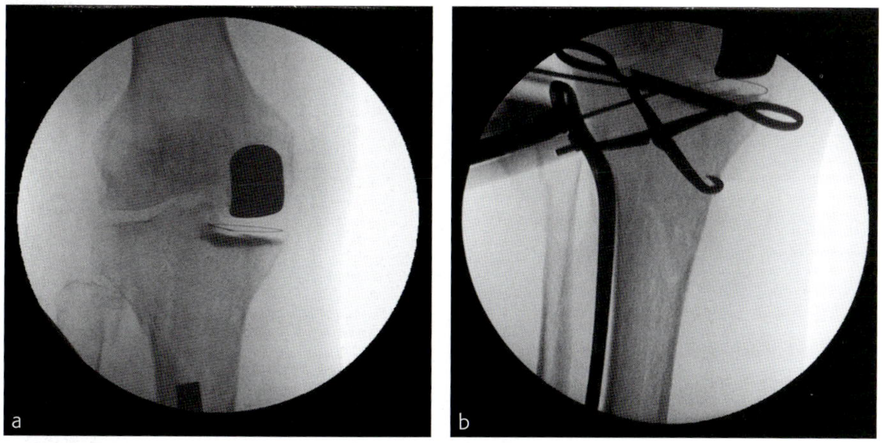

11.8-2a–b Intraoperative images.
a Reduction is verified under traction.
b Situation after insertion of the LISS PTL with the Weber forceps still in place.

V.4-B1

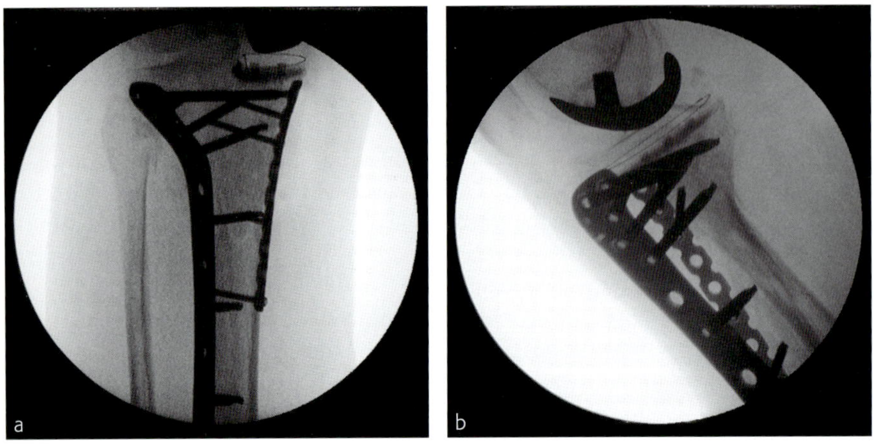

11.8-3a–b Final postoperative x-rays after fixation with the LISS-PTL and the medial reconstruction plate.
a AP view.
b Lateral view.

Rehabilitation and follow-up

Immediate toe-touch weight bearing was allowed and gradually increased to full weight bearing from 6 weeks to 3 months. X-rays were obtained at 6 and 12 weeks postoperatively. At the 12-week follow-up, the fracture appeared consolidated (**11.8-4a–b**). The patient was ambulating without pain and had an excellent range of motion. One year postoperatively, the patient could walk an unlimited distance without pain, and had excellent range of motion and stability in the knee, despite a mild effusion. The patient succumbed 2 months later to pancreatic cancer.

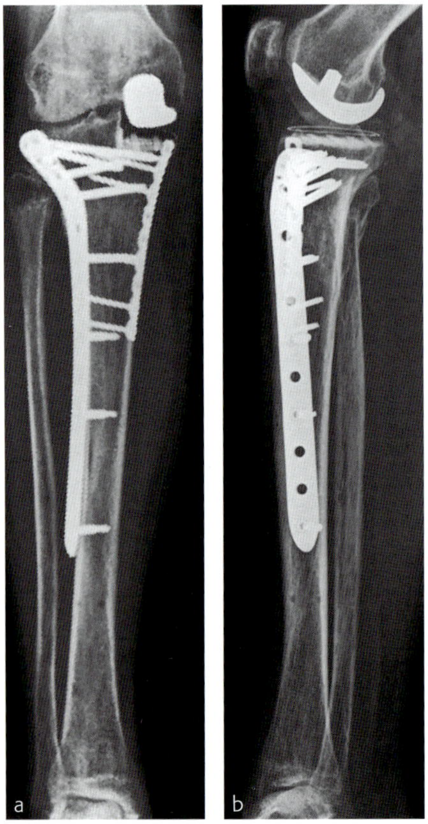

Fig 11.8-4a–b Follow-up x-rays obtained 12 weeks postoperatively, show good functional result.
a AP view.
b Lateral view.

Points to remember

- If the patient has a recent midline incision (eg, for a total knee arthroplasty), a second separate incision made more laterally might compromise wound healing. A plastic surgeon should be consulted in case of doubt.
- Correct positioning of the plate at the tibial head is crucial and must be anticipated for the approach and preparation.
- Longer plates are always preferred to plates that are too short, especially in patients with osteoporotic bone in which case bicortical locking-head screws are mandatory.
- Use of a minimally invasive approach preserves the blood supply to the soft tissues and bone.
- Intraoperative x-rays are necessary to ensure that the plate is properly aligned to the lateral side of the tibia in two planes.

11.9 Proximal tibial fracture, stable prosthesis

ORIF: buttress plate 4.5 and tension band

Author Emilio Fantin

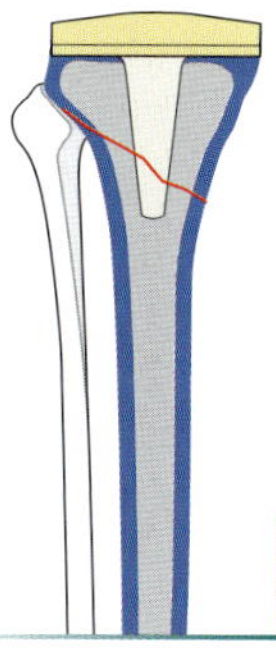

V.4-B1

Case description

A 72-year-old man presented with pain and inability to fully extend his left knee after a fall. He underwent total knee arthroplasty 5 years ago and previous fixation with an angled blade plate for a supracondylar fracture of the distal femur. X-rays showed a nondisplaced periprosthetic fracture of the proximal tibia (**11.9-1a–b**).

Classification: Type V.4-B1

Diagnosis: Transverse periprosthetic fracture of the proximal tibia with slight displacement of the anterior tibial tuberosity, with a stable prosthesis

Decision making

Three options were available to treat this minimally displaced proximal tibial fracture: knee bracing, revision of the tibial prosthetic component with a stem version, and internal fixation with a plate. Bracing would be cumbersome and the outcome questionable. Revision of the prosthesis would be invasive and associated with a high morbidity rate. Plate fixation combined with a tension band for the tuberosity appeared to be the most rational solution (chapter 5.4.1).

Preoperative planning

Equipment

- Proximal tibia locking compression plate (LCP) and corresponding locking-head screws
- 4.5 mm conventional screw set
- Image intensifier
- Radiolucent table
- Instruments and wire for tension-band fixation

Patient preparation and positioning

- Supine position, with a support below the knee
- Prophylactic antibiotics

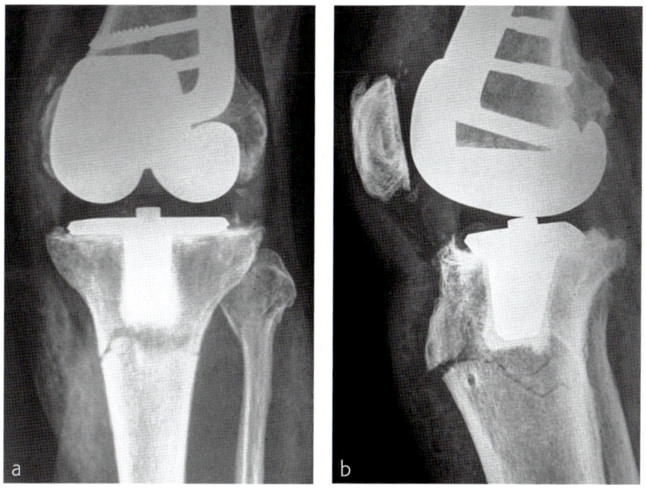

11.9-1a–b X-rays of a transverse periprosthetic fracture around the tibial component of a total knee arthroplasty with avulsion of the tibial tuberosity. Both lesions are minimally displaced.
a AP view.
b Lateral view.

V.4-B1
Reduction and fixation

Two approaches were selected. The anterior longitudinal scar was used for tension-band wiring of the tibial tuberosity, and a more direct posteromedial incision was used for the posteromedial buttress plate.

Fixation of the tibial tuberosity was initiated with the knee in extension. A 2 mm wire was run through the insertion of the patellar tendon at the apex of the tuberosity, forming a figure of eight around a 4.5 mm cortex screw, which was placed more distally in an anteroposterior direction into the tibia. The posteromedial incision was used to approach and reduce the transverse tibia fracture. The proximal tibia LCP was positioned posteriorly so that all three screws were inserted dorsal to the tibial prosthesis. Distal to the fracture, three additional bicortical screws were well spaced apart. This construct resulted in stable fixation, allowing for immediate active movement of the knee (👁 **11.9-2a–b**).

Rehabilitation and follow-up

Immediate active mobilization with partial weight bearing was allowed during the first 3 weeks postoperatively. Callus formation was observed at the lateral side of the fracture 8 weeks postoperatively (👁 **11.9-3a–b**). The patient resumed his normal activities of daily living, with full function and no pain. Follow-up x-rays were obtained after 24 months (👁 **11.9-4a–b**).

Points to remember

- Preserving a well-functioning prosthesis after a periprosthetic fracture has priority if the components of the prosthesis are still well fixed.
- Stable fixation allows early mobilization of the joint, preventing posttraumatic stiffness.
- An avulsed tibial tuberosity is best fixed with tension-band wiring. However, extended healing time may be a consequence.

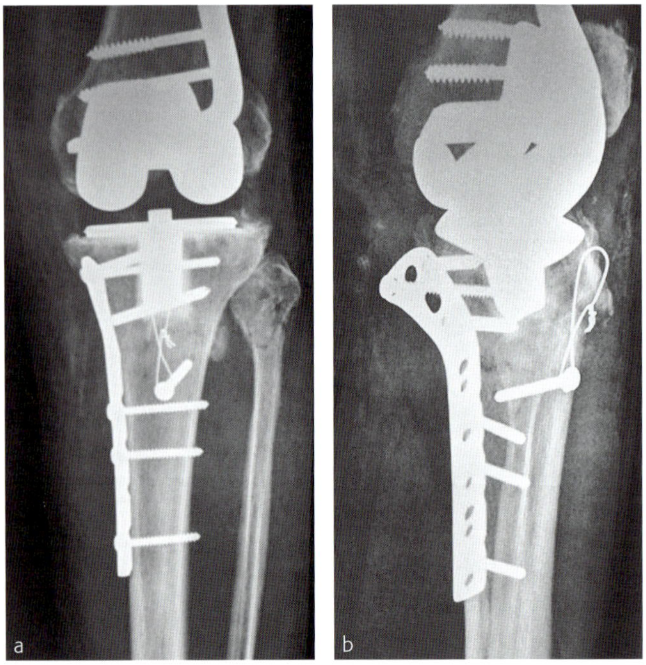

👁 **11.9-2a–b** Immediate postoperative x-rays.
a AP view.
b Lateral view.

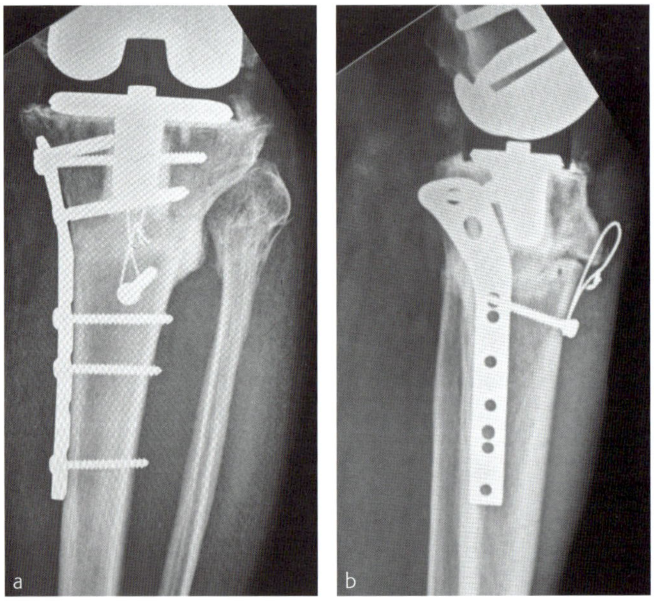

👁 **11.9-3a–b** X-rays obtained 8 weeks postoperatively show progressive callus formation.
a AP view.
b Lateral view.

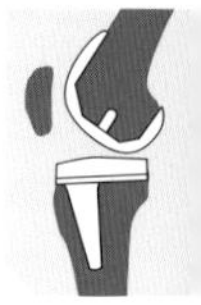

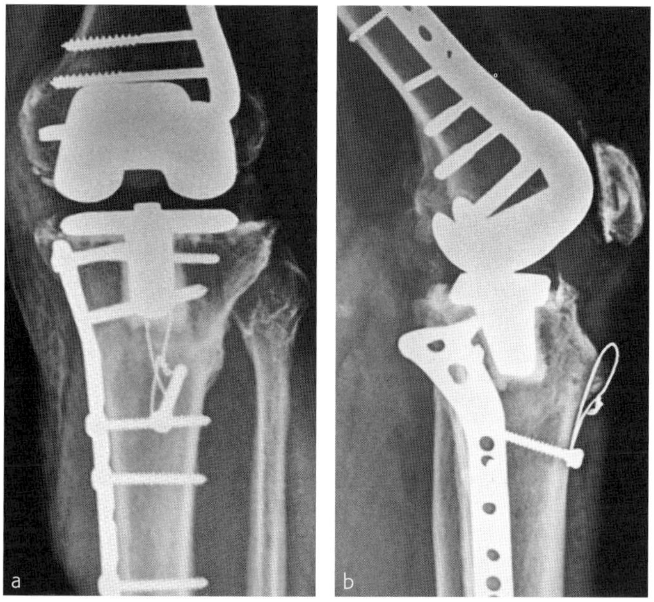

11.9-4a–b X-rays obtained 24 months postoperatively show the fracture consolidation. The patient has excellent functional outcome without pain.

a AP view.

b Lateral view.

V.4-B1

11.10 Proximal tibial fracture, stable prosthesis

ORIF: LCP 3.5 proximal tibia and LCP 2.0

Authors **Andrew D Carrothers, Richard J Jenkinson**

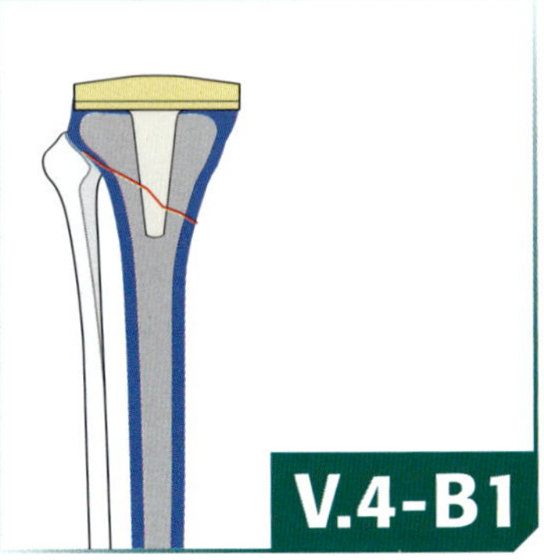

Case description

A 74-year-old woman sustained a low-energy accident in a pedestrian versus motor vehicle collision in a parking garage. She was living independently at home and had a successful total knee arthroplasty for osteoarthritis of the right knee 4 years ago. Her medical history included hypercholesterolemia, hypertension, and a 3-year history of type 1 diabetes mellitus with no end-organ sequelae. Examination revealed a well-healed scar over the knee with good peripheral pulses. X-rays showed a periprosthetic fracture of the proximal tibia in which the implant appeared to be stable (**11.10-1a–b**).

Classification: Type V.4-B1

Diagnosis: Periprosthetic fracture of the proximal tibia, with a stable total knee arthroplasty

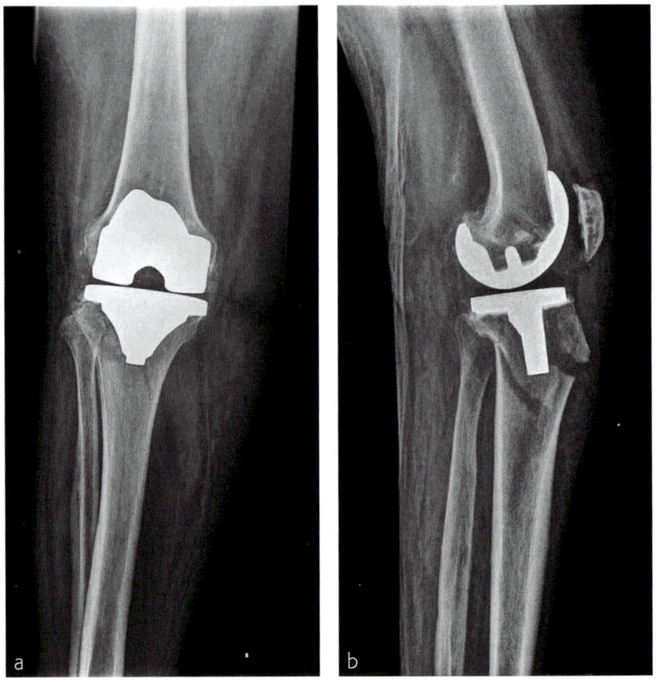

11.10-1a–b Preoperative x-rays of the periprosthetic fracture of the proximal tibia show displacement via the distracting force of the extensor mechanism.
a AP view.
b Lateral view.

Decision making

The patient's proximal tibial fracture was located just below the native well-fixed total knee arthroplasty tibial base plate, with anterior distraction caused by pull of the intact extensor mechanism on the tibial tuberosity. The goal of treatment was to restore an independent level of function. A number of treatment options were considered. Nonoperative care with casting and/or bracing was not promising. The surgical options were internal fixation with retention of the prosthesis and revision total knee arthroplasty.

Fracture fixation and revision to a long-stem tibial component could help maintain bone stock. However, because the primary tibial component was well fixed, the process of removal would compromise the proximal tibial bone stock and likely require allograft or prosthetic replacement. The addition of a constrained component provides initial stability and the possibility of early weight bearing. It also requires changing the femoral component to a compatible long-stem component.

Open reduction and internal fixation was selected because it helps maintain host bone stock, allows retention of the stable total knee arthroplasty prosthesis, and offers early ambulation after a short period of protected weight bearing. The procedure would be challenging, given the extremely proximal extent of the fracture coupled with osteoporotic bone. Locking compression plate (LCP) fixation can optimize hardware anchorage in the small proximal fracture segment (chapter 5.4.1).

Preoperative planning

Equipment

- Radiolucent operating table
- Intraoperative image intensification
- Various sized pointed reduction forceps
- K-wires for temporary fixation
- Small-fragment locking instruments and implants
- Precontoured medial proximal tibia LCPs
- Minifragment LCPs and instruments

Patient preparation and positioning

- Supine position
- Bolster under the ipsilateral hip to neutralize natural hip external rotation
- Tourniquet on thigh
- Preoperative antibiotics
- Sterile triangles or bolsters to adjust knee flexion

Reduction and fixation

With the patient under general anesthesia and tourniquet control, the distal aspect of the previous midline incision with distal extension was used. Full-thickness soft-tissue flaps were elevated and the patellar tendon and deep knee capsule identified. The approach remained extraarticular to avoid further compromise to the knee or extensor mechanism. The tibial base plate was assessed intraoperatively using direct examination and image intensification and determined to be stable.

The proximal tibia was exposed and the fracture configuration identified. The knee was extended to relax the extensor mechanism, which allowed the fracture to be anatomically reduced and held provisionally with reduction forceps and K-wires. Satisfactory fracture reduction was confirmed with two-plane image intensification. A medial proximal tibial locking plate was applied in a buttress mode, placed over the medial fracture axilla component. After the position of the locking plate was verified with image intensification, the plate was secured distally with conventional 3.5 mm cortex screws (securing the plate to the tibial diaphysis and buttressing the proximal medial fracture) and 3.5 mm locking-head screws proximally. As the deforming moment of the extensor mechanism was poorly neutralized by the medial plate, an additional tension-band method was used. A minifragment locking Y-plate 2.0 was contoured and applied over the tibial tuberosity to function as a tension band. Conventional cortex screws were used distally to secure the plate to the tibial diaphysis and locking-head screws were used proximally (**11.10-2a–b**). Once the fracture was fixed, the in situ total knee arthroplasty was carefully assessed for stability, patellar tracking, and satisfactory soft-tissue balancing both in flexion and extension.

Rehabilitation and follow-up

After 48 hours, the leg was placed in extension in a locked hinged knee brace, and the patient did not bear weight for the first 2 weeks postoperatively.

Perioperative antibiotic prophylaxis was administered for 24 hours. Prophylaxis for deep vein thrombosis with low-molecular-weight heparin was administered for 4 days (national guidelines should be considered). No early medical or surgical complications developed.

Wound healing was uneventful. After the 2-week follow-up, range-of-motion exercises were initiated in a hinged

V.4-B1 brace. Partial weight bearing was allowed after 6 weeks. At 3 months postoperatively, x-rays showed fracture healing (👁 **11.10-3a–b**), and full unprotected weight bearing was allowed. At 6 months, the patient had a range of motion of 0–120° and no extensor lag.

Points to remember

- Treatment of proximal tibial periprosthetic fractures should be performed by surgeons with experience in both trauma surgery and revision knee arthroplasty.
- Intraoperative assessment of implant position is mandatory. In case of abnormal implant position, revision knee arthroplasty is required.
- If prosthetic components are found to be loose intraoperatively, early failure can be expected and conversion to revision total knee arthroplasty should be considered.
- Proximal fixation is limited by the tibial component of the arthroplasty.
- Plates that accept locking-head screws are ideally suited to maximize holding anchorage in short osteoporotic proximal segments.
- The tibial component limits screw length and placement. Thought must be given to the distracting force of the extensor mechanism. Conventional placement of the plate, medially or laterally, may not sufficiently resist such sagittal displacement. Thus, an additional tension-band method may be necessary.
- Strict adherence to antibiotic prophylaxis and sterile technique is required because deep infection is a devastating complication.

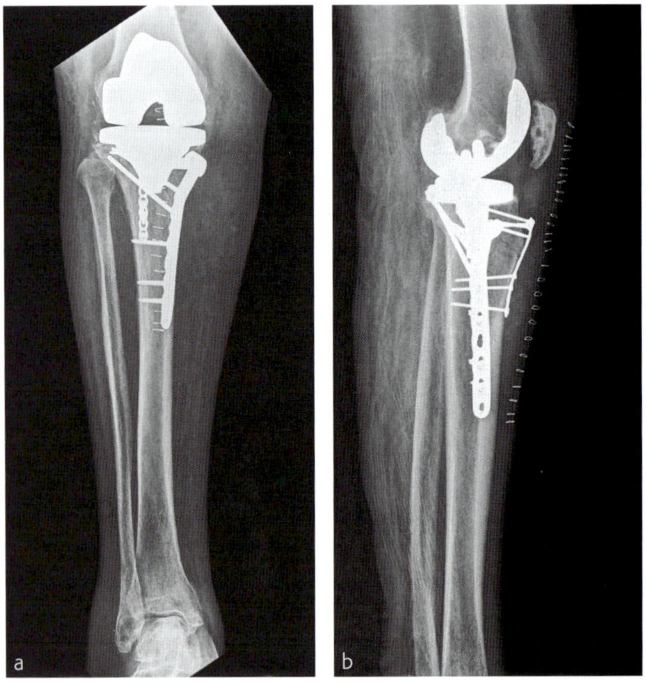

👁 **11.10-2a–b** X-rays obtained after open reduction and internal fixation with a medially applied proximal tibia locking compression plate and an anteriorly placed locking compression plate 2.0 with tension-band function.
a AP view.
b Lateral view.

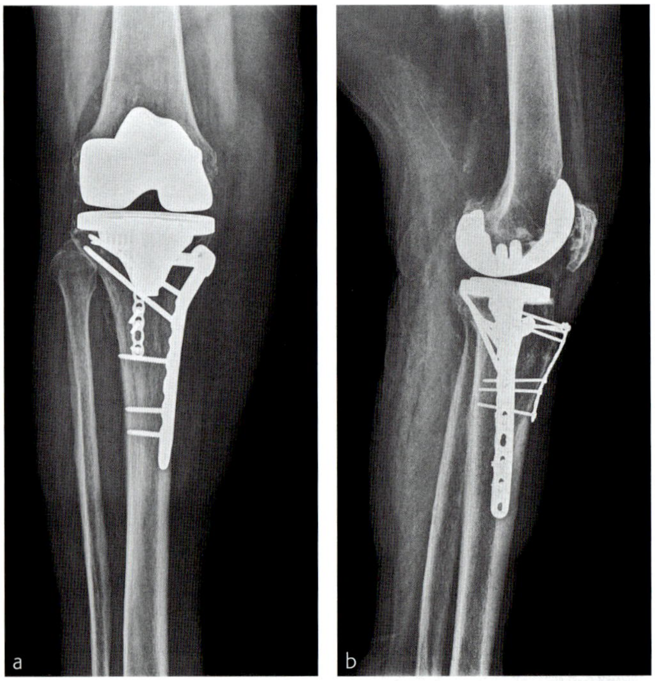

👁 **11.10-3a–b** X-rays obtained 6 months postoperatively show a well-healed periprosthetic fracture. Full functional recovery was achieved.
a AP view.
b Lateral view.

11.11 Segmental tibial shaft fracture, stable prosthesis

MIPO: lateral LISS proximal tibia and medial distal tibia LCP

Author **Philipp Schwabe**

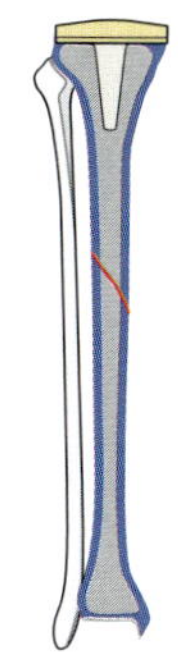

V.4-C

Case description

A 72-year old man was hit on the right side by a motor vehicle 5 months after undergoing total knee arthroplasty. Preoperative x-rays revealed a periprosthetic segmental tibial shaft fracture (**11.11-1a–d**).

Classification: Type V.4-C

Diagnosis: Periprosthetic segmental tibial fracture and fibular fracture, with a stable prosthesis

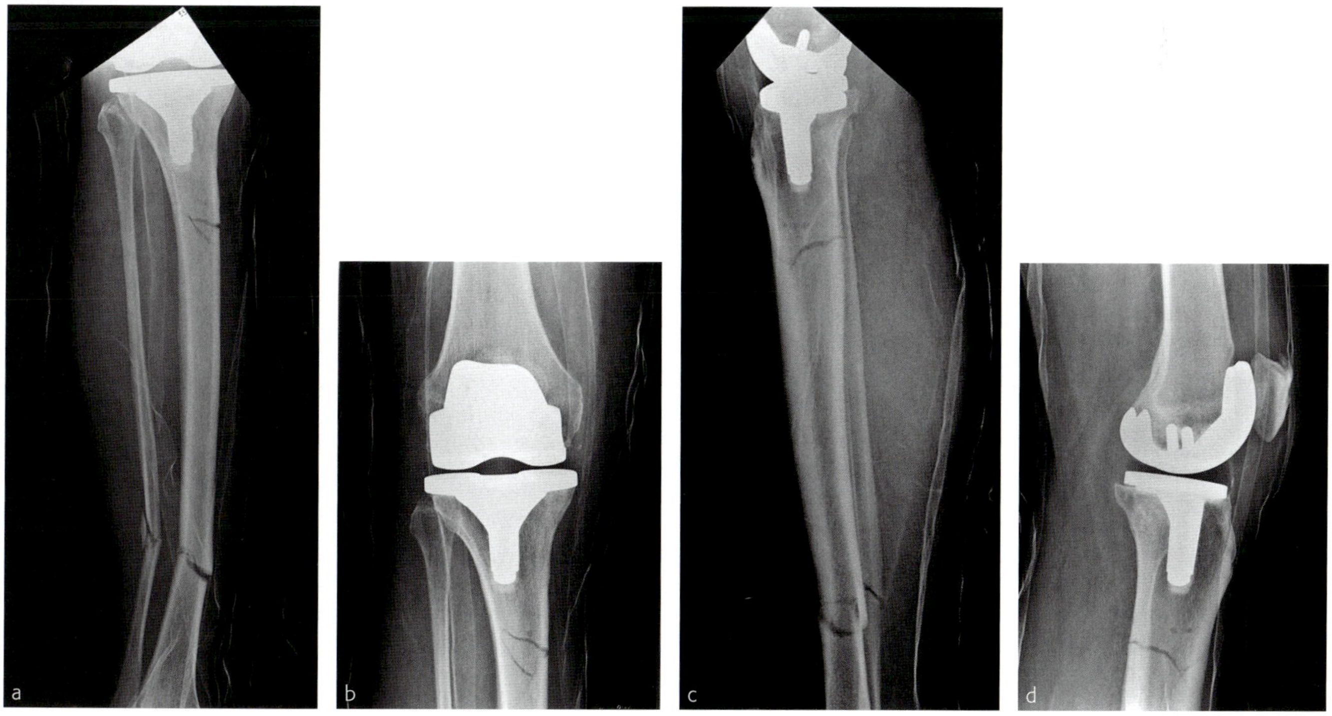

11.11-1a–d X-rays of the knee and lower leg with segmental fracture after injury.
a–b AP views.
c–d Lateral views.

V.4-C
Decision making

The cemented knee prosthesis appeared clinically and radiologically well fixed; therefore, osteosynthesis was an option for fixation of the segmental fracture distal to the prosthesis. Intramedullary nailing, however, was not an option because of the knee prosthesis; thus, plating appeared to be the only choice. The patient's severe soft-tissue injury and swelling required initial treatment with external fixation for emergency fracture reduction and stabilization. The fractures should be bridged with two anatomically preshaped locking plates using minimally invasive plate osteosynthesis technique. Because this was a segmental fracture, each fracture component had to be treated separately using a different approach. The proximal fracture was stabilized with a less invasive stabilization system proximal lateral tibia (LISS PLT) and the distal fracture with a distal tibia locking compression plate (LCP) (chapter 5.4.1).

Preoperative planning

Equipment

- LISS PLT
- 5.0 mm locking-head screws
- Low-bend distal tibia LCP 3.5
- 3.5 mm locking-head screws
- 2.0 mm K-wires

Patient preparation and positioning

- Supine position with the contralateral leg lowered to allow improved access to the lateral view on image intensification
- Gel wedge under the ipsilateral buttock to allow improved access for AP positioning of the leg
- Single-shot intravenous antibiotics
- Low-molecular-weight heparin for thrombosis prophylaxis

Reduction and fixation

For the proximal fracture, a 5 cm incision was made at the lateral proximal tibia, beginning at Gerdy's tubercle and ending distally close to the tibial tubercle. Sharp dissection to the periosteum was required for percutaneous insertion of the lateral LISS PLT; the distal locking-head screws were inserted via stab incisions.

The plate bed was prepared epiperiostally along the anterior tibial muscle with a bone raspatory. The proximal fracture was reduced manually with the fixator pins used as joysticks. The LISS PLT was inserted with an aiming device, and its position confirmed with image intensification in both AP and lateral planes. The plate was fixed temporarily, both proximally and distally, with 2.0 mm K-wires inserted through the drill sleeves. The pulling device can be used for reduction, if necessary. Locking-head screws were alternatingly inserted distally and proximally. At the level of prosthetic stem, monocortical screws were used, distally bicortical ones.

For the distal fracture, a 3 cm incision was made over the medial malleolus. Sharp dissection to the periosteum was required, with care to preserve the great saphenous vein and saphenous nerve. The distal tibia LCP was inserted medially in a percutaneous manner and the screws were inserted via stab incisions.

The distal fracture was reduced manually with the fixator pins used as joysticks. If necessary, the fracture can temporarily be fixed with two crossed K-wires, which are removed after plate fixation. The plate bed was prepared epiperiosteally with a bone raspatory, and the plate was inserted from distal to proximal. A drill sleeve firmly attached to a distal plate hole can act as a handle. The tips of the two plates should overlap by at least four plate holes to avoid development of stress risers. Stab incisions were made over a proximal plate hole and a K-wire was inserted through a drill sleeve to temporarily hold the plate. Plate position and reduction were confirmed with image intensification in both planes. Open placement of the locking-head screws occurred distally and proximally through stab incisions.

Rehabilitation and follow-up

X-rays obtained 2 days postoperatively confirmed the stable construct (**11.11-2a–b**).

Physiotherapy starting at day 2 postoperatively consisted of continuous active and passive motion of the knee and the ankle joint. Partial weight bearing (half body weight) was prescribed for 6 weeks, progressing to full weight bearing. X-rays obtained 6 months postoperatively showed good consolidation of both fractures (**11.11-3a–b**). Clinical follow-up 6 months later showed no limitation in range of motion, similar to the contralateral leg, and uneventful soft-tissue healing (**11.11-4**). The patient continued to do well.

11.11 **Segmental tibial shaft fracture, stable prosthesis**

MIPO: lateral LISS proximal tibia and medial distal tibia LCP

Points to remember

- A minimally invasive procedure is recommended in patients with extensive fracture configuration.
- No bending of implants is required with use of anatomically precontoured plates.
- Double locking plate osteosynthesis provides good stability in selected fracture situations.
- The superficial peroneal nerve can be injured during insertion of the distal screws of the lateral plate.
- Exact positioning of the precontoured plate to the tibia facilitates accurate indirect fracture reduction.
- The saphenous vein and nerve must be protected to prevent injury during preparation of medial distal approach.
- Patient discomfort can occur as a result of limited soft-tissue coverage of the distal plate.

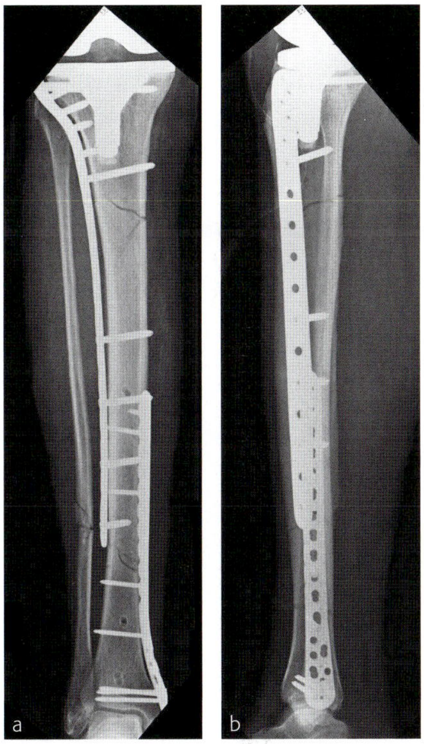

11.11-2a–b X-rays obtained 2 days postoperatively show a stable construct.
a AP view.
b Lateral view.

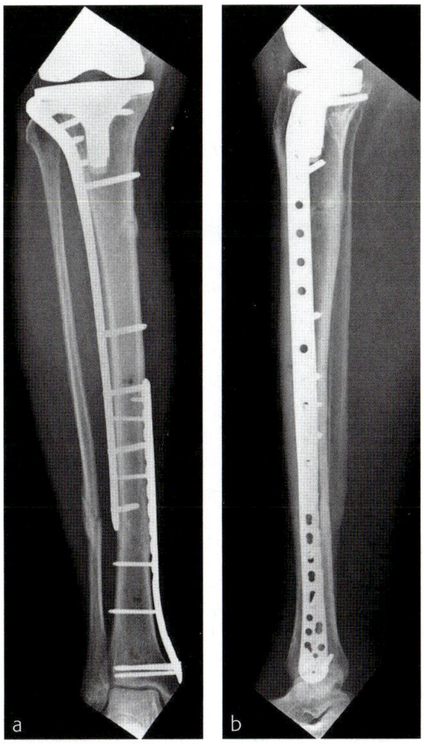

11.11-3a–b X-rays obtained 6 months postoperatively show consolidation of both fractures.
a AP view.
b Lateral view.

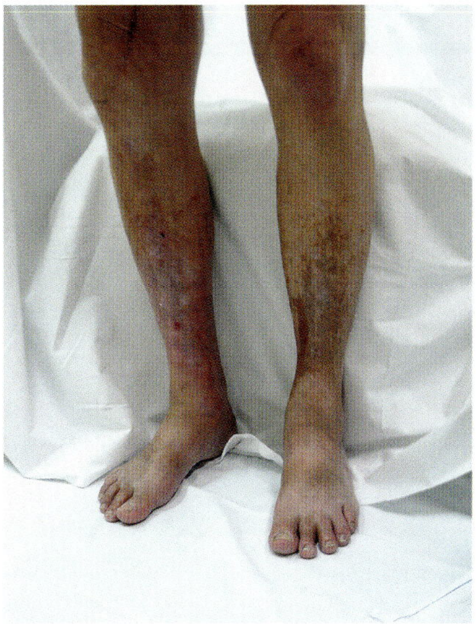

11.11-4 Clinical follow-up after 6 months.

12

Ankle cases

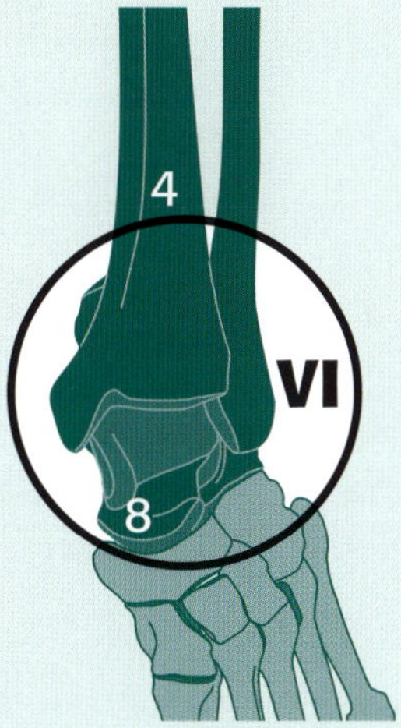

12.1 Medial malleolar fracture, stable prosthesis

Nonoperative treatment: cast

Author **Sebastian Manegold**

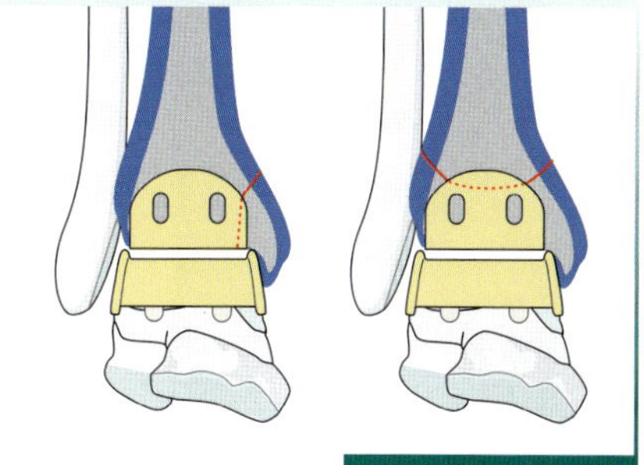

VI.4-B1

Case description

A 72-year-old man has had posttraumatic arthritis following a fracture of the right ankle that occurred more than 20 years ago. The weight-bearing x-ray showed lateralization of the talus with an increased medial clear space, and the tibia tarsal joint space almost obliterated compared with the uninjured side (👁 **12.1-1**). The tibial joint line was parallel to the ground, so a total ankle arthroplasty was performed (👁 **12.1-2**). The patient was noncompliant with postoperative instructions and started with full weight bearing against medical recommendations.

The patient then presented with a stress fracture of the medial malleolus with no clear evidence of trauma. An x-ray showed that the source of the fracture was the varus malposition of the prosthesis together with a hindfoot valgus deformity in the frontal plane (👁 **12.1-3**). Impingement of the talar component at the medial malleolus resulted in overload and ultimately a stress fracture.

Classification: Type VI.4-B1

Diagnosis: Periprosthetic fracture of the medial malleolus, with a stable prosthetic component

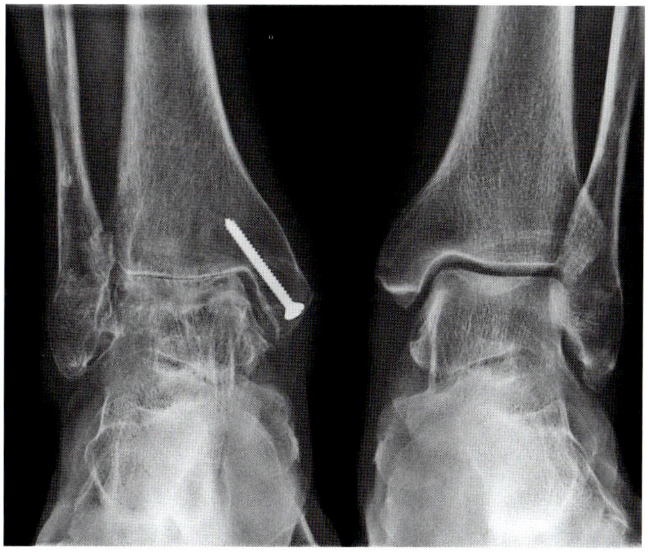

👁 **12.1-1** AP x-ray of both ankles under weight-bearing. The right ankle shows posttraumatic arthritis that developed over a period of 20 years after a fracture caused by valgus malalignment of the fibula. The joint space is almost obliterated.

VI.4-B1

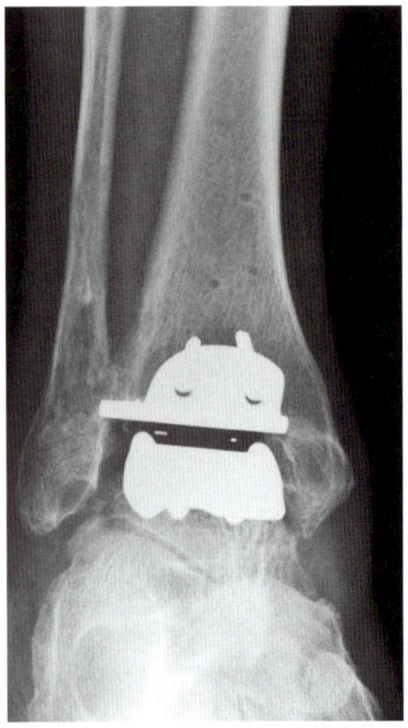

12.1-2 AP x-ray obtained after implantation of a total ankle arthroplasty.

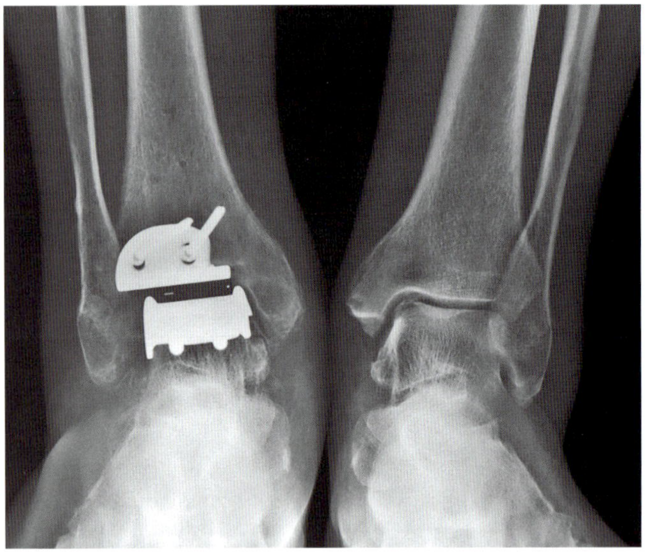

12.1-3 AP x-ray under weight-bearing which shows a non-displaced fracture caused by overload of the medial malleolus.

Decision making

Varus or valgus malposition of the prosthesis, especially with concomitant hindfoot deformity in the coronal plane, represents a deterioration of the mechanical axis that can trigger a fatigue fracture. In this case, the varus malposition of the prosthesis caused a nondisplaced fracture of the medial malleolus. Surgical correction of the malpositioned but stable prosthesis with supramalleolar osteotomy is indicated to restore the mechanical axis of the leg and to reposition the prosthesis so that it is parallel to the ground with weight bearing. The additional hindfoot deformity can be addressed simultaneously with medial translational osteotomy of the calcaneus. However, because of the patient's poor compliance issues, nonoperative treatment with cast immobilization and partial weight bearing was initiated (chapter 5.3).

Rehabilitation and follow-up

Weight-bearing x-rays obtained at 4, 8, 12, and 25 months following total ankle arthroplasty (**12.1-4a–b**) showed callus formation at the medial cortex of the distal tibia.

Points to remember

- Prosthetic loosening must be excluded.
- The mechanical axis of the leg must be carefully analyzed with weight-bearing x-rays.
- The mechanical axis of the leg can be restored with a corrective osteotomy of the tibia and hindfoot (if necessary) to achieve a balanced prosthesis.
- The patient's personality and reliability must be considered when planning treatment.
- Nonoperative treatment with immobilization of the ankle and a strict program of progressive weight bearing can be successful.

12.1 **Medial malleolar fracture, stable prosthesis**

Nonoperative treatment: cast

VI.4-B1

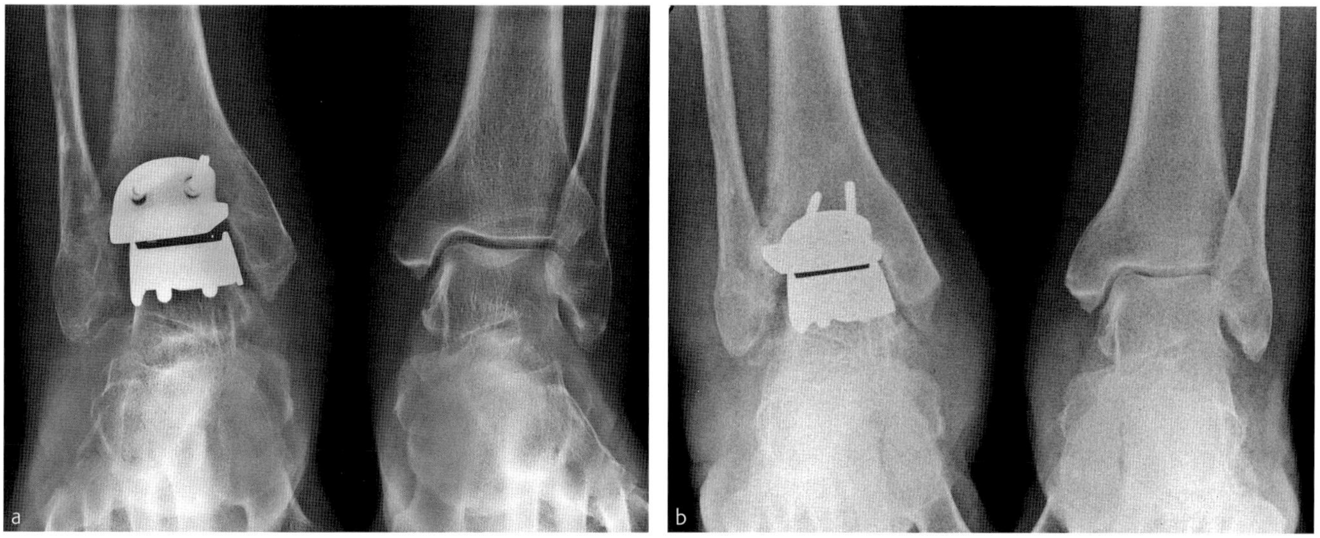

12.1-4a–b X-rays obtained after total ankle arthroplasty. Nonoperative treatment consisted of cast immobilization and partial weight bearing. Note callus formation at the medial cortex of the distal tibia.

a AP view obtained 4 months postoperatively.

b AP view obtained 25 months postoperatively.

VI.4-B1

12.2 Distal tibial and fibular stress fracture, stable prosthesis

ORIF: LCP 3.5

Authors **Alexej Barg, Beat Hintermann**

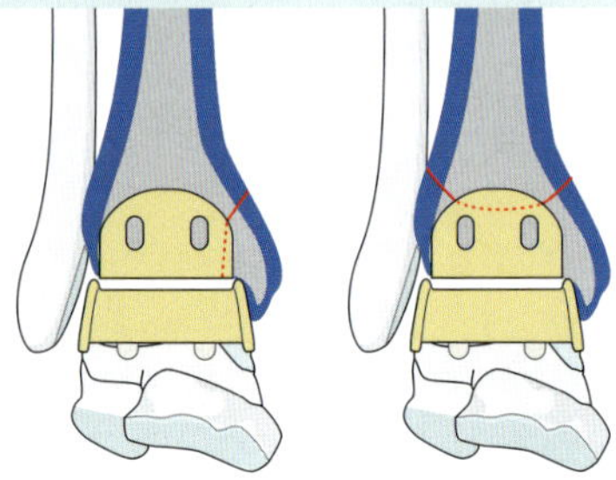

VI.4-B1

Case description

A 56-year-old woman underwent total ankle arthroplasty with a total ankle prosthesis 6 months ago for painful rheumatoid ankle osteoarthritis. The patient had significant hindfoot and midfoot deformities for which double arthrodesis and medial sliding osteotomy were performed in the same procedure.

The initial postoperative course consisted of 8 weeks of full weight bearing in a walking boot and was uneventful. However, with unprotected ambulation, the patient experienced increasing lower leg pain under loading. No traumatic event was recorded. At the 4-month follow-up, examination revealed minimal swelling of the ankle, but no redness or local hyperthermia. Range of motion of the "replaced" ankle was 5°/12° (dorsiflexion/plantar flexion), but all movements were painful. Weight-bearing x-rays of the ankle obtained at that time showed stress fractures of the distal tibia and fibula with signs of osseous consolidation (👁 **12.2-1a–c**). However, the distal tibia showed significant valgus and recurvatum deformity with dislocation of the tibial component. The hindfoot alignment view (Saltzman view) also showed a significant valgus hindfoot deformity.

Classification: Type VI.4-B1

Diagnosis: Stress fracture of the distal tibia and fibula (under osseous consolidation), valgus recurvatum deformity of the hindfoot, dislocation of the tibial component

Decision making

Although there were signs of osseous consolidation, nonoperative treatment was not considered an option because of the significant hindfoot deformity and dislocation of prosthetic component as a result of the stress fractures. Surgical realignment of the tibia and fibula was selected to address the valgus recurvatum deformity with different plates (chapter 5.4.1), with revision of the tibial component to address the ventral dislocation of the ankle prosthesis (chapter 5.5).

Preoperative planning

Equipment

- 7-hole locking compression plate (LCP) 3.5
- T-shaped LCP 3.5
- 2.0 mm K-wires

Patient preparation and positioning

- First- or second-generation cephalosporin for antibiotic prophylaxis
- Low-molecular-weight heparin for thrombosis prophylaxis
- Supine position
- X-ray assessment in the lateral and frontal planes with the image intensifier

Reduction and fixation

Incisions from the initial surgery were used to expose the ankle joint and extended proximally to approach the distal tibial fracture. After exposure of the fracture, the existing callus was removed. The fracture and physiological axis of the lower leg was restored under traction. After the reduction was verified with the image intensifier, the fracture was fixed anteriorly with a T-shaped LCP 3.5 and laterally with a LCP 3.5. The fibula had already healed, although it was now significantly shorter and malrotated, which required a corrective osteotomy and fixation with another plate. Finally, the tibial component of the prosthesis was replaced to address the anterior dislocation.

Rehabilitation and follow-up

Partial weight bearing in a stable walker was allowed for 6 weeks postoperatively. X-rays obtained at that first follow-up showed good consolidation of the fractures and osteotomy (**12.2-2a–b**). Follow-up after 6 weeks found the patient to be pain free.

Points to remember

- The extent of the fracture should be carefully assessed and any loosening of the prosthesis must be excluded (eg, using CT or SPECT-CT) preoperatively.
- Fracture reduction should result in a well-aligned hindfoot.
- In patients with poor bone quality (eg, osteoporosis, Charcot arthropathy, rheumatoid diseases) stable fixation is important (eg, using two or more plates).
- Any malalignment of a prosthetic component associated with the fracture should be addressed, if necessary by revision of components. Malalignment can adversely affect the clinical outcome or even cause the failure of the prosthesis.

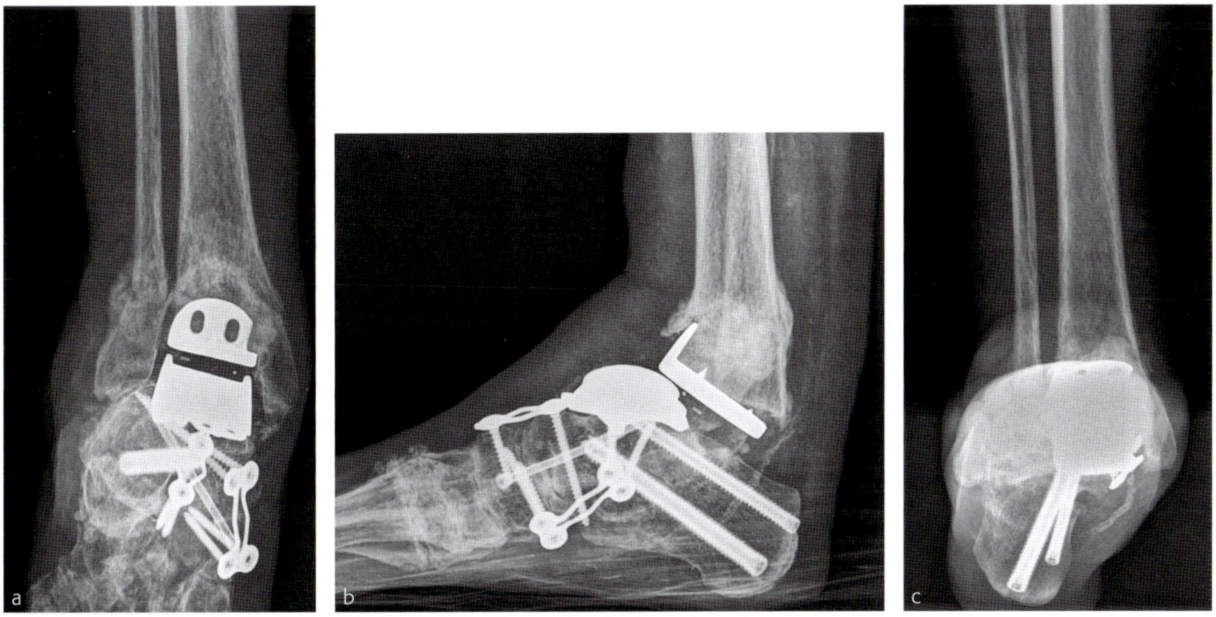

12.2-1a–c X-rays of the stress-induced periprosthetic fracture of the distal tibia and fibula obtained 4 months after an ankle arthroplasty and hindfoot corrective osteotomy.
a AP view shows that the fibular and tibial fractures display considerable callus formation.
b Lateral view shows obvious subluxation of the ankle joint.
c Hindfoot alignment view (Saltzman view).

VI.4-B1

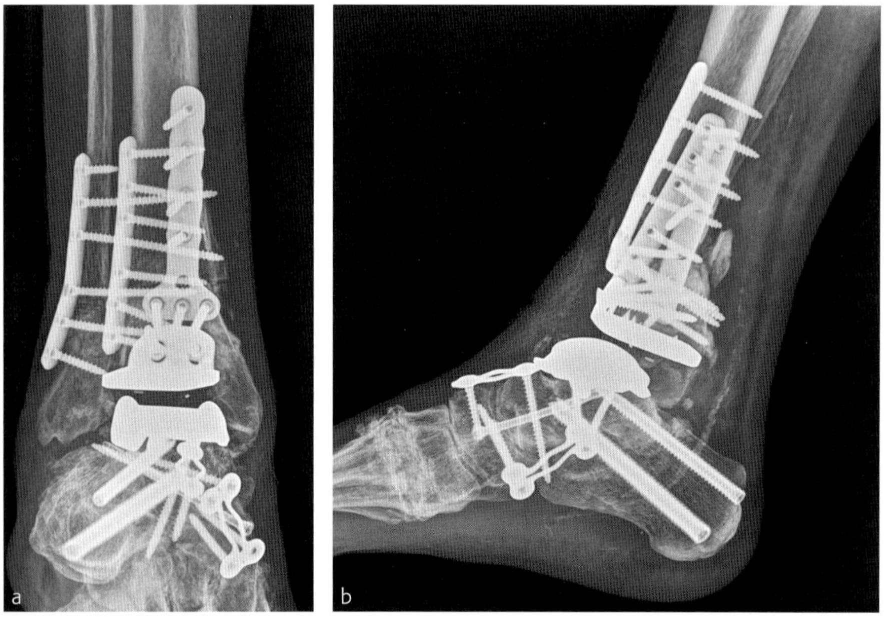

12.2-2a–b Postoperative x-rays obtained 6 weeks after revision surgery. The fractures and osteotomy already appear consolidated, and the prosthesis appears well fixed and in correct alignment.
a AP view.
b Lateral view.

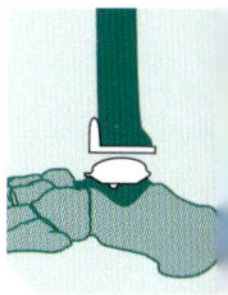

12.3 Medial malleolar stress fracture, stable prosthesis

ORIF: LCP 3.5 and T-LCP 3.5

Authors **Alexej Barg, Beat Hintermann**

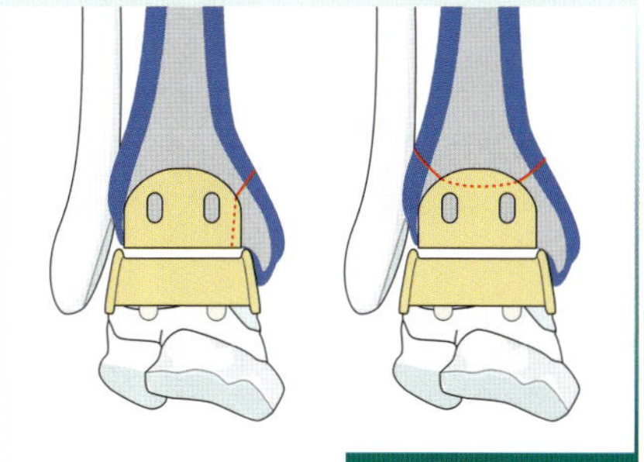

VI.4-B1

Case description

A 52-year-old man with posttraumatic arthritis of the left ankle underwent total ankle arthroplasty 8 months ago. A z-shaped calcaneal osteotomy and lengthening osteotomy of the fibula were done simultaneously to correct a significant varus deformity of the hindfoot. The initial postoperative course was uneventful.

Two years later, the patient felt a sharp pain on the medial aspect of the ankle during a 30-minute session on a home cycle trainer. Nonoperative treatment initiated by the family physician failed. He presented with minimal swelling with no signs of inflammation. Range of motion in the left ankle was 19°/32° (dorsiflexion/plantar flexion), and there was no pain with movement. Examination revealed a varus deformity of the hindfoot with significant lateral ligamentous instability (**12.3-1a–c**). Weight-bearing x-rays showed a fatigue fracture of the medial malleolus with no evidence of prosthetic component loosening (**12.3-2a–b**). However, the polyethylene inlay was displaced. The z-shaped calcaneal osteotomy had completely healed with appropriate screw position.

Classification: Type VI.4-B1

Diagnosis: Stress fracture of medial malleolus after ankle prosthesis with subsequent varus deformity of the hindfoot, subluxation of the polyethylene inlay, and lateral ligamentous instability

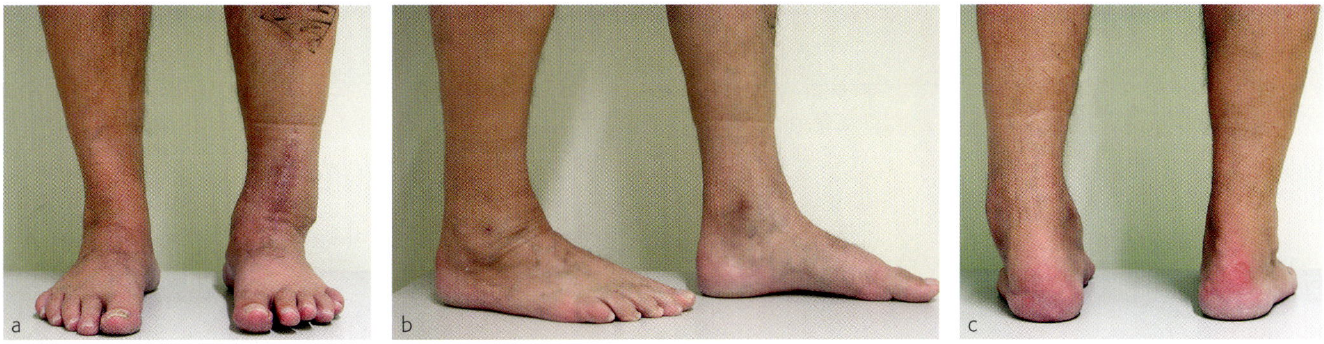

12.3-1a–c A 52-year-old man with a fatigue fracture of the medial malleolus and significant varus deformity of the hindfoot.
a Front view.
b Lateral view.
c Back view.

VI.4-B1

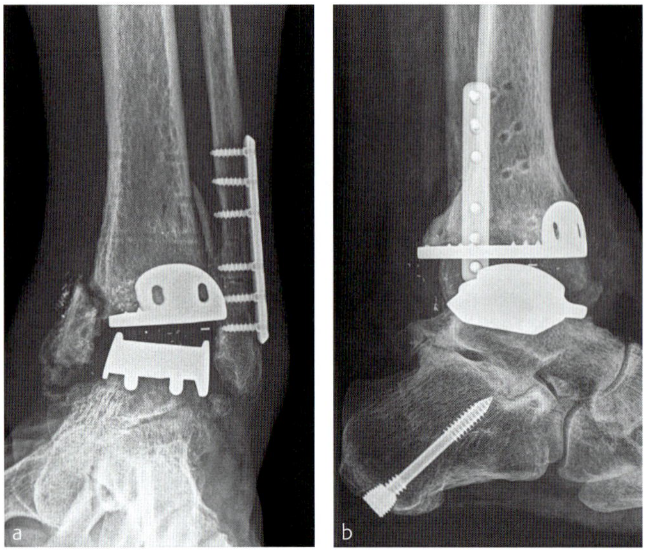

12.3-2a–b X-rays of the distal tibia and foot obtained 8 months after total ankle arthroplasty and subsequent fatigue fracture of the medial malleolus.
a AP view.
b Lateral view.

Decision making

Nonoperative treatmen t was not an option because of significant hindfoot deformity and dislocation of the polyethylene inlay. The stress fracture of medial malleolus had to be anatomically reduced and stabilized. The dislocated polyethylene inlay needed to be exchanged because a damaged surface may result in increased wear. Depending on the intraoperative situation, realignment of fibula would be necessary to restore the anatomical relationship of the mortise. Finally, the lateral ligamentous instability should be addressed to avoid recurrent varus deformity.

Preoperative planning

Equipment

- 7-hole locking compression plate (LCP) 3.5
- Tibial buttress plate
- Custom-made 2-hole LCP
- 2.0 mm K-wires
- Exchange inlay
- Image intensifier

Patient preparation and positioning

- First- or second-generation cephalosporin for antibiotic prophylaxis
- Low-molecular-weight heparin for thrombosis prophylaxis
- Supine position

Reduction and fixation

A standard incision over the medial malleolus was used to expose the stress fracture. On the lateral side, the original incision was used to expose the fibula, exchange the inlay, and address the lateral ligamentous instability.

After exposure of the medial malleolus, the fracture was reduced and the reduction verified with the image intensifier. A tibial buttress plate (tibial axis plate) was used for the fixation (chapter 5.4.1). To improve initial stability, two additional 2-hole plates (anteriorly and posteriorly) were applied. The polyethylene inlay was exchanged using the lateral approach. A lengthening osteotomy of the fibula was done to restore proper alignment of the ankle mortise.

Rehabilitation and follow-up

The patient was allowed partial weight bearing in a stable walker for the first 8 weeks postoperatively. Follow-up x-rays obtained after 8 weeks showed bony consolidation of the medial malleolus and appropriate position of prosthetic components (**12.3-3a–b**). One year after revision surgery, the patient was pain free. Clinically, the hindfoot was well aligned (**12.3-4a–b**) and the medial malleolus had healed (**12.3-5a–b**).

Points to remember

- The extent of the fracture should be carefully assessed and prosthetic loosening must be excluded (eg, using CT or SPECT-CT).
- Fracture reduction should include correct alignment of the hindfoot.
- Patients with a fatigue fracture of the medial malleolus often present with a subluxation of the polyethylene inlay. Therefore, the inlay should be exchanged to avoid the increased wear, which may damage the surface of the inlay.

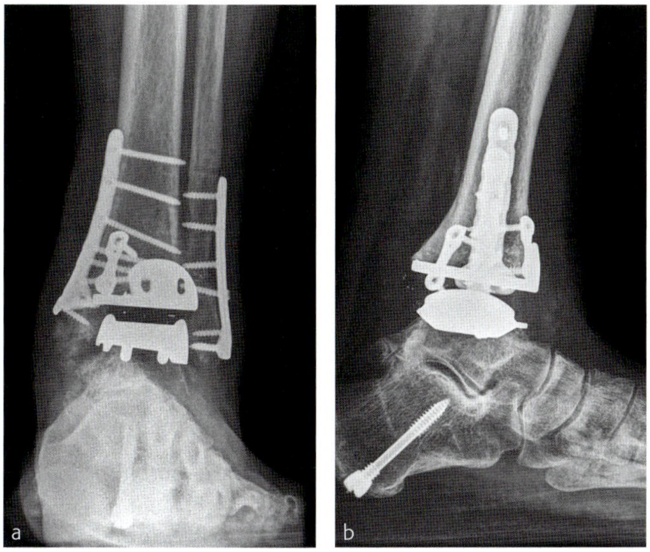

12.3-3a–b X-rays obtained 8 weeks after revision surgery with buttressing of the medial malleolus, corrective osteotomy of the fibula, and exchange of the inlay.
a AP view.
b Lateral view.

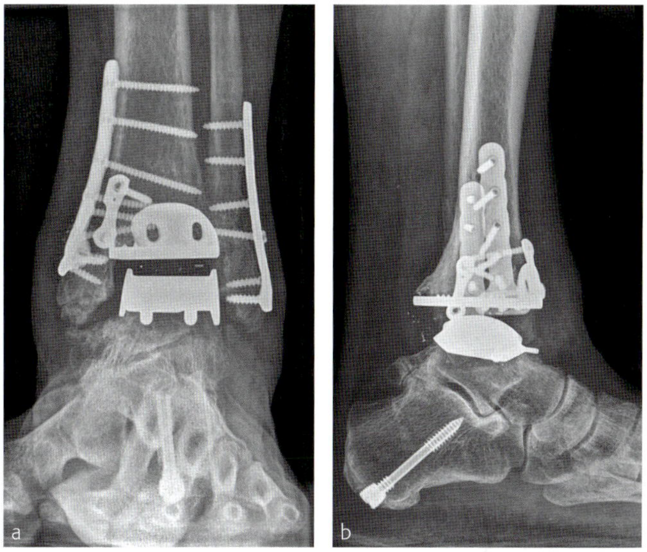

12.3-4a–b Follow-up x-rays obtained one year after revision surgery.
a AP view.
b Lateral view.

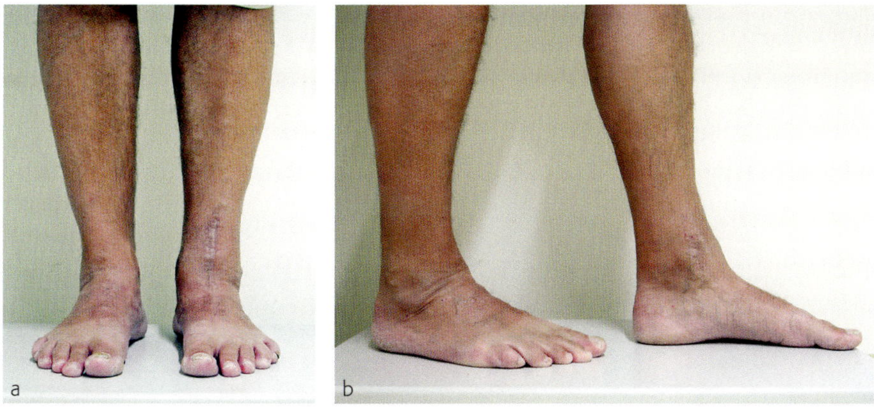

12.3-5a–b Clinical photograph taken one year after revision surgery. The patient is asymptomatic.
a AP view.
b Lateral view.

VI.4-C

12.4 Lower-leg fracture, stable ankle prosthesis

MIPO: LCP 3.5, metaphyseal LCP 4.5

Author **Sebastian Manegold**

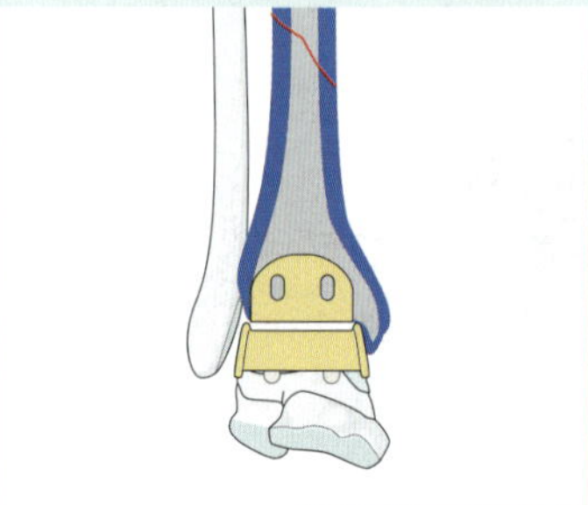

VI.4-C

Case description

A 47-year-old woman presented with a severe flatfoot deformity and posttraumatic ankle arthritis after a pilon fracture (**12.4-1a–b**). She reported pain while walking and standing. A triple arthrodesis of the flatfoot deformity was performed initially, followed by total ankle arthroplasty (TAA) 9 months later (**12.4-2a–b**). The initial two surgeries were successful with no reported complications. Seven months after undergoing the TAA, the patient fractured her lower leg proximal to the TAA as a result of a fall (**12.4-3a–b**). Radiologically, the TAA appeared to be well fixed.

Classification: Type VI.4-C

Diagnosis: Periprosthetic fracture of the lower leg proximal to total ankle arthrodesis

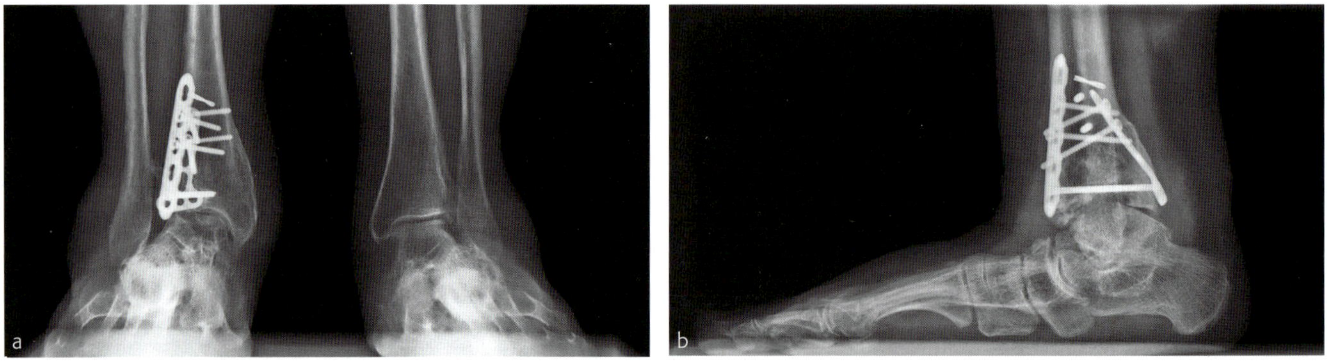

12.4-1a–b Weight-bearing x-rays show severe flatfoot deformity and posttraumatic ankle arthritis after pilon fracture.
a AP view.
b Lateral view.

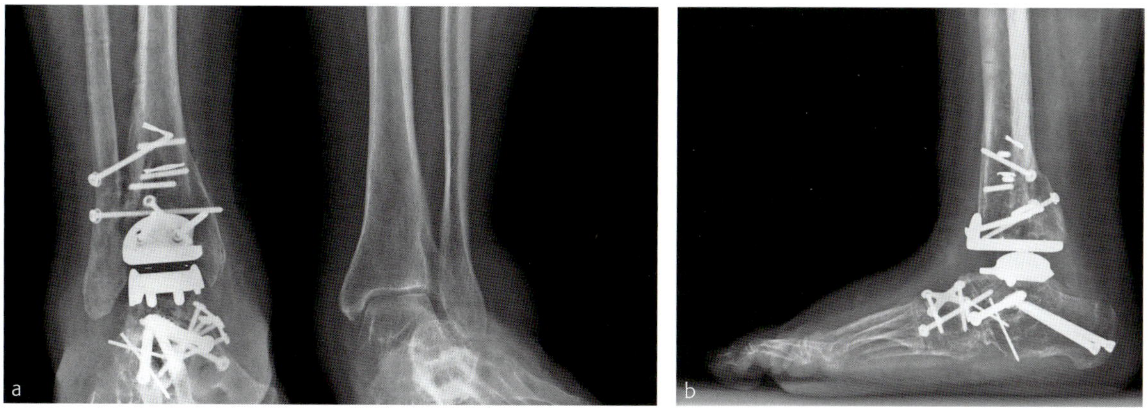

12.4-2a–b Postoperative x-rays show triple arthrodesis of the foot and implantation of a total ankle arthroplasty (TAA).
a AP view.
b Lateral view.

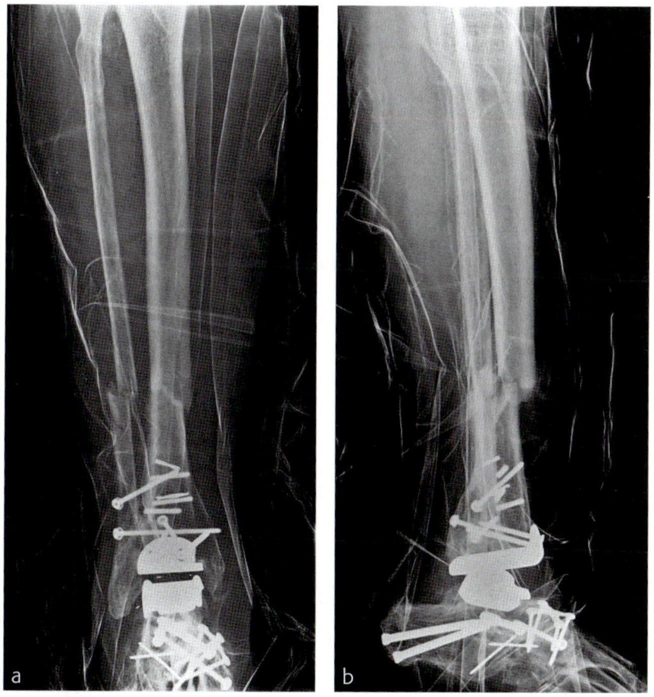

12.4-3a–b X-rays obtained 7 months after TAA implantation. The patient fractured the distal third of the tibia and fibula as a result of a fall.
a AP view.
b Lateral view.

Decision making

Due to the unstable fracture pattern, nonoperative treatment was not an option. Preoperatively, two basic questions needed to be answered:

- Is the fracture related to loosening of the prosthesis? If the cause is in doubt (preexisting cysts or a fracture line involving the prosthesis), CT could help analyze the fracture pattern.
- Is the fracture independent of loosening of the prosthesis? If infection is suspected, a history of pain, clinical, and radiological signs, as well as results of laboratory tests (C-reactive protein) and analysis of a bacteriological sample obtained by joint aspiration may help exclude infection.

Finally, the mechanical axis and position of the prosthesis needed careful evaluation. In case of malposition of the prosthesis, a corrective osteotomy or a revision arthroplasty should be considered.

Although intramedullary nailing is considered state-of-the-art treatment for tibial shaft fractures, it was not appropriate in this case because insertion of the nail by hammering could harm both the TAA and the triple fusion. Moreover, any remaining hardware (broken screws and drill bits) from previous surgeries prevent correct nail insertion and impede distal locking.

To reduce soft-tissue damage and achieve maximum stability, the use of a bridging plate as an internal fixator inserted with a minimally invasive plate osteosynthesis technique was considered the preferred type of osteosynthesis.

VI.4-C Preoperative planning

Equipment

- Metaphyseal locking compression plate (LCP) (3.5/4.5/5.0 of variable lengths)
- LCP 3.5
- 3.5 and 4.5 mm locking-head screws
- 3.5 and 4.5 mm cortex lag screw (optional)
- Reduction forceps
- K-wires and guiding sleeve
- Set for revision arthroplasty (in the event of TAA loosening)

Patient preparation and positioning

- Supine position on a radiolucent operating table
- Injured foot elevated at the end of the table and the contralateral leg lowered for easier x-ray assessment
- Tourniquet (optional)
- Use of perioperative antibiotics and thrombosis prophylaxis

Reduction and fixation

A short incision was made over the medial malleolus. Epiperiostal dissection of the medial malleolus was performed with care to avoid injuring the greater saphenous vein and the saphenous nerve. Blunt preparation of the subcutaneous tunnel was then carried out with a bone raspatory to insert a metaphyseal plate. The fibula was approached with a longitudinal incision with blunt surgical dissection, preserving the peroneal muscles and the superficial peroneal nerve.

Closed reduction can be attempted by manual traction under image intensification. Final fine tuning of the reduction to restore axis, length, and rotation is best done with a percutaneously applied reduction forceps. In patients with comminuted fractures, a medially placed external fixator can be helpful. A precontoured metaphyseal LCP was inserted on the anteromedial aspect of the tibia by sliding it proximally, where it was met through a short incision. The plate was centered on the tibial diaphysis and the position checked with the image intensifier. Temporary fixation was achieved with K-wires inserted through the guiding sleeves. Locking-head screws were inserted in the distal and proximal tibia to bridge the fracture zone, which remained untouched. Finally, open reduction and internal fixation of the fibula was performed.

Rehabilitation and follow-up

Postoperatively, the patient was immobilized in a walking caliper, allowing partial weight bearing for up to 12 weeks until fracture healing was complete. Follow-up after 3 years showed a well-consolidated fracture and a nondisplaced TAA (**12.4-4a–b**).

Points to remember

- Prior to surgery the possibility of prosthesis loosening and/or low-grade infection should be excluded.
- The greater saphenous vein and the saphenous nerve must be preserved during the medial approach.
- The mechanical axis must be restored to achieve balanced load bearing of the prosthesis. Lack of reduction can lead to a malpositioned TAA.
- In case of TAA loosening, an anterior approach is necessary for revision arthroplasty. Therefore, it is advantageous to reduce soft-tissue damage by using a minimally invasive approach for osteosynthesis of periprosthetic ankle fractures, especially in the distal tibia.

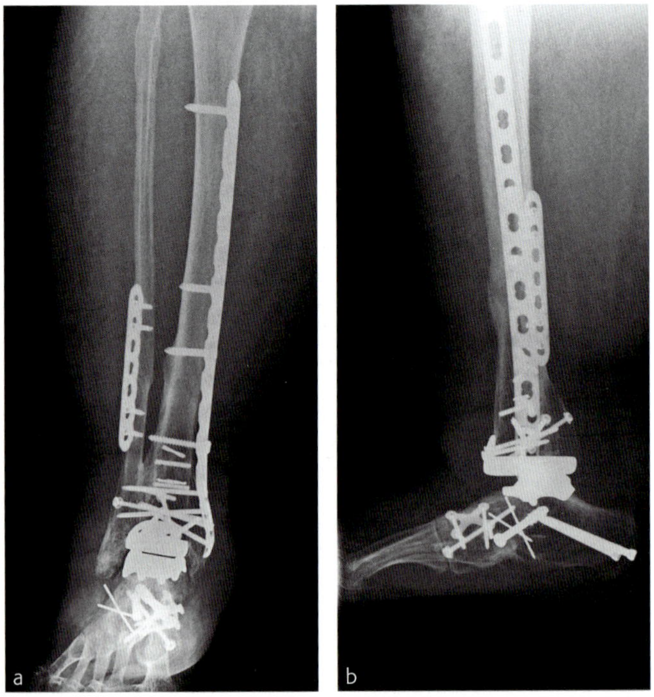

12.4-4a–b X-rays obtained at the 3-year follow-up show undisturbed fracture healing without TAA loosening.
a AP view.
b Lateral view.